FLOW CYTOMETRY – RECENT PERSPECTIVES

Edited by **Ingrid Schmid**

Flow Cytometry – Recent Perspectives
Edited by Ingrid Schmid

Published by InTech

Janeza Trdine 9, 51000 Rijeka, Croatia

Publishing Process Manager Martina Blecic

Technical Editor Teodora Smiljanic

Cover Designer InTech Design Team

Additional hard copies can be obtained from orders@intechopen.com

Flow Cytometry – Recent Perspectives, Edited by Ingrid Schmid
p. cm.
ISBN 978-953-51-0626-5

For EU product safety concerns:
IN TECH d.o.o., Prolaz Marije Krucifikse Kozulić 3, 51000 Rijeka, Croatia,
info@intechopen.com or visit our website at intechopen.com.

Meet the editor

Mag. Schmid is an Academic Research Specialist in the Department of Medicine, Division of Hematology-Oncology, at the University of California at Los Angeles and the technical director of the UCLA Flow Cytometry Shared Resource. Mag. Schmid received her degree in the Pharmaceutical Sciences from the University of Vienna, Austria. She immigrated to the United States of America in 1981 and joined the UCLA laboratory of Dr. John Fahey, a noted immunologist, in 1983. She started working in flow cytometry at that time, and in 1989, working with Dr. Janis Giorgi, a well-known HIV researcher, she established the UCLA Flow Cytometry Core Facility. Mag. Schmid published twenty-seven peer-reviewed, first author papers, reviews, and book chapters and has co-authored an additional twenty-eight papers and two chapters. Her present interests include the development of accurate methods for the flow cytometric assessment of circulating epithelial progenitor cells as biomarkers of cardiovascular disease as well as the formulation of documents that provide guidance to the flow cytometry community at large for creating Standard Operating Procedures for cell sorting that contain appropriate safeguards.

Contents

Preface

Advances in cell biology have always been closely linked to the development of critical quantitative analysis methods. Flow cytometry is such a pivotal methodology. It can be applied to individual cells or organelles allowing investigators interested in obtaining information about the functional properties of cells to assess the differences among cells in a heterogeneous cell preparation or between cells from separate samples. It is characterized by the use of a select wavelength of light (or multiple ones) to interrogate cells or other particles one at a time providing statistically relevant, rapid correlated measurements of multiple parameters with excellent temporal resolution. These intrinsic attributes, as well as advances in instrumentation and fluorescent probes and reagents, have contributed to the tremendous growth of applications in flow cytometry and to the world-wide expansion of laboratories which use this technology since its inception in the late 1960s.

This publication reflects these facts as indicated by the global author panel and the wide range of sample types, assays, and methodologies described. The compendium will give readers a historical perspective as well as the current state of important topics in flow cytometry. Openly accessible, the book is intended to introduce novices to this powerful technology and also provide experienced professionals with valuable insights and an opportunity to refresh or up-date their knowledge in various subject areas of flow cytometry.

Ingrid Schmid, Mag. pharm.
Department of Medicine
Division of Hematology-Oncology
University of California, Los Angeles
USA

1

What Flow Cytometry Can Tell Us About Marine Micro-Organisms – Current Status and Future Applications

A. Manti, S. Papa and P. Boi
Department of Earth, Life and Environmental Sciences, University of Urbino "Carlo Bo", Italy

1. Introduction

Born in the field of medicine for the analysis of mammalian cell DNA, flow cytometry (FCM) was first used in microbiology studies in the late 1970s thanks to optical improvements and the development of new fluorochromes (Steen & Lindmo, 1979; Steen, 1986). Its initial applications in clinical microbiology are dated to the 1980s (Steen & Boyne, 1981; Ingram et al., 1982; Martinez et al., 1982; Steen 1982; Mansour et al., 1985), and, by the end of that decade, FCM had also become popular in environmental microbiology (Burkill, 1987; Burkill et al., 1990; Yentsch et al., 1983; Yentsch & Pomponi, 1986; Yentsch & Horan, 1989; Phinney & Cucci, 1989). Today, it is a poweful and commonly used tool for the study of aquatic micro-organisms. FCM has thus become a precise alternative to microscopic counts, increasing the number of both the micro-organisms detected and the samples that can be analyzed. The advantages of FCM include single-cell detection, rapid analysis (5000 cells per second or more), the generation of multiple parameters, a high degree of accuracy and statistically relevant data sets.

The significance of flow cytometry can be summarized as the measure (-metry) of the optical properties of cells (cyto-) transported by a liquid sheath (flow) to a light source excitation (most often a laser) (Shapiro, 2003).

FCM facilitates single cell analyses of both cell suspension, such as eukariotic and prokariotic cells, and "non cellular" suspension, such as microbeads, nuclei, mitochondria and chromosomes.

A typical flow cytometer is formed by different units: the light source, the flow cell, the hydraulic fluidic system, several optical filters, a group of photodiodes or photomultiplier tubes and, finally, a data processing unit (Veal et al., 2000; Longobardi, 2001; Shapiro, 2003; Robinson, 2004; Diaz et al., 2010).

In a flow cytometer, individual cells pass in a single file within a hydrodynamically focused fluid stream. Single cells are centered in the stream so that they intercept an excitation source, meaning that scatter and/or fluorescence signals can be collected and optically separated by dichroic filters and detectors. The data collected are then converted into digital information. Finally, software displays data as events along with their relative statistics.

The light scattering properties are detected as FALS (forward angle light scatter) and RALS (right angle light scatter). FALS, collected in the same direction as the incident light (0-13° conic angle with respect to the incident point of the laser), is measured in the plane of the laser beam and provides information on cell size, while RALS is usually measured at 90° (70-110° conic angle) to the beam and provides data on cell granularity or the internal structure of the cell (Hewitt & Nebe-Von-Caron, 2004) (Fig. 1).

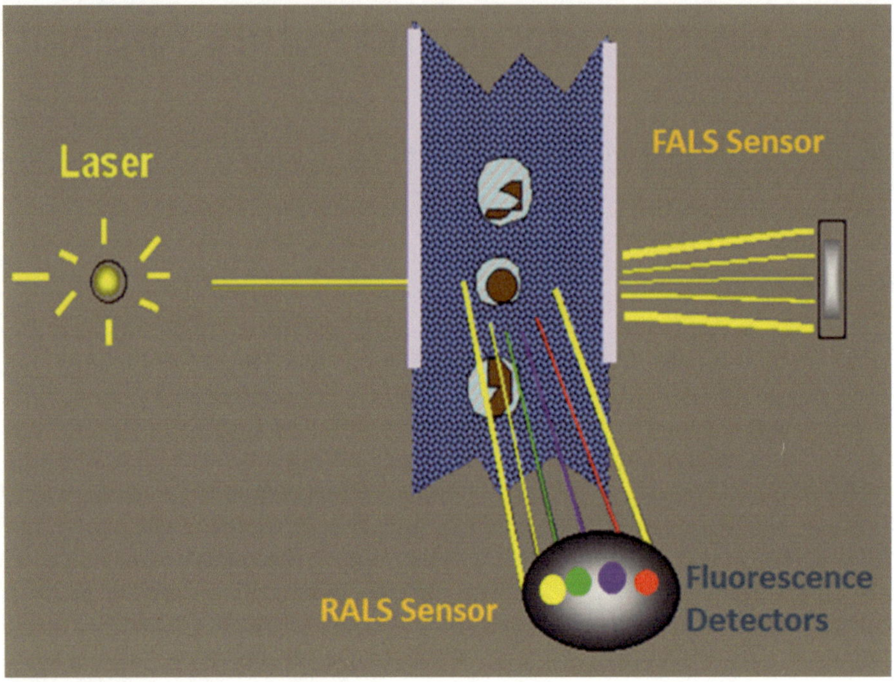

Fig. 1. Light fractions scattered and fluorescence by an excited single cell

Together with the FALS and RALS data, fluorescent information can also be collected, which includes signals from autofluorescence or induced fluorescence.

Each single value can be amplified, and stored events are commonly represented in a monoparametric histogram or biparametric dot plot. One-parameter histograms represent the number of cells or particles per channel (y-axis) versus the scattering or fluorescence intensity (x-axis). Dot plots are the most common graphic representations of the relative distribution of different cell populations.

Regions and gates can be made to better separate and analyze populations of interest. Furthermore, on the basis that the dyes used to stain cells have overlapping emission spectra, the compensation is normally made to reduce interference.

While basic instruments may only permit the simultaneous collection of two or three fluorescence signals, the more complex and expensive research instruments mean that it is possible to obtain more than 14 parameters (Winson & Davey, 2000; Chattopadhyay et al., 2008) depending on the laser equipment utilized. Selection of the lasers will depend on the range of wavelengths needed for the excitation of the selected fluorochromes.

Some flow cytometers have the ability to physically separate different sub-populations of interest (cell sorting) depending on their cytometric characteristics (stream-in-air), thus permitting the recovery and purification of cell subsets from a mixed population for further applications (Bergquist et al., 2009; Davey, 2010).

In natural samples in particular, a very important advantage of FCM is the opportunity to analyze micro-organisms with minimal pre-treatment and without the need for cultivation steps, also taking into account that the most of natural bacteria are resistant to cultivation (Fig. 2). Furthermore, FCM is particularly well-suited for the investigation of natural picoplankton. This is because of their small size (<2 µm; Sierbuth, 1978), which renders the analysis thereof difficult by more traditional methods. Particularly due to the rapidity with which data can be obtained, flow cytometry has been routinely used over the last few decades for the analysis of different types of micro-organisms in marine samples (Porter et al., 1997; Yentsch & Yentsch, 2008; Vives-Rego et al., 2000; Wang et al., 2010). It is now commonly accepted as a reference technique in oceanography.

Knowledge of seawater microbial diversity is important for understanding community structure and patterns of distribution. In the ocean water column, organisms <200 µm include a variety of taxa, such as free viruses, autotrophic bacteria (cyanobacteria, which include the group known formerly as prochlorophytes), heterotrophic bacteria, protozoa (flagellates and ciliates) and small metazoans (Legendre et al., 2001), all of which have different morphological, ecological and physiological characteristics.

Heterotrophic and autotrophic bacteria, viruses and authotrophic picoeukaryotes represent marine picoplankton (2- 0,2 µm), while the larger fraction of micro-organisms is divided into nano-plankton (20-2 µm) and micro-plankton (200-20 µm).

Among these taxa, bacteria are very important because they play a crucial role in most biogeochemical cycles in marine ecosystems (Fenchel, 1988), taking part in the decomposition of organic matter and the cycling of nutrients. Bacteria are also an important source of food for a variety of marine organisms (Das et al., 2006), and their activity has a major impact on ecosystem metabolism and function. Both autotroph and heterotroph micro-organisms constitute two fundamental functional units in ecosystems, where the former generally dominate eutrophic systems and the latter generally dominate oligotrophic systems (Dortch & Postel, 1989; Gasol et al., 1997). An extensive body of literature has documented the great importance of the activity of algae in terms of the size of picoplankton in the global primary production of aquatic ecosystems (Craig, 1985; Stockner & Antia, 1986; Stockner, 1988; Callieri & Stockner, 2002). Picocyanobacteria are a diverse and widespread group of photosynthetic prokaryotes and belong to the main group of primary producers (Castenholz & Waterbury. 1989; Rippka, 1988). Picoeukaryotes, meanwhile, are a diverse group that is widely distributed in the marine environment, and they have a fundamental role in aquatic ecosystems because of their high productivity. Like bacteria, marine viruses are thought to play important roles in global and small-scale biogeochemical cycling. They are also believed to influence community structure and affect bloom termination, gene transfer, and the evolution of aquatic organisms. Viruses are the most numerous 'lifeforms' in aquatic systems, being about 15 times more abundant than total of bacteria and archaea. Data from literaure seem to indicate that the abundance of marine viruses is linked to the abundance of their hosts, so that changes in the prokaryotic host populations will affect viral abundance (Danovaro et al., 2011).

Given that the vast majority of the biomass [organic carbon (OC)] in oceans consists of micro-organisms, it is expected that viruses and other prokaryotic and eukaryotic micro-organisms will play important roles as agents and recipients of global climate change (Danovaro et al., 2011).

Accordingly, the accurate determination of micro-organism abundance, biomass and activity is essential for understanding the aquatic ecosystem. Consequently, the aim of this review is to provide a general overview of the applications of flow cytometric tecniques to studies in marine microbiology.

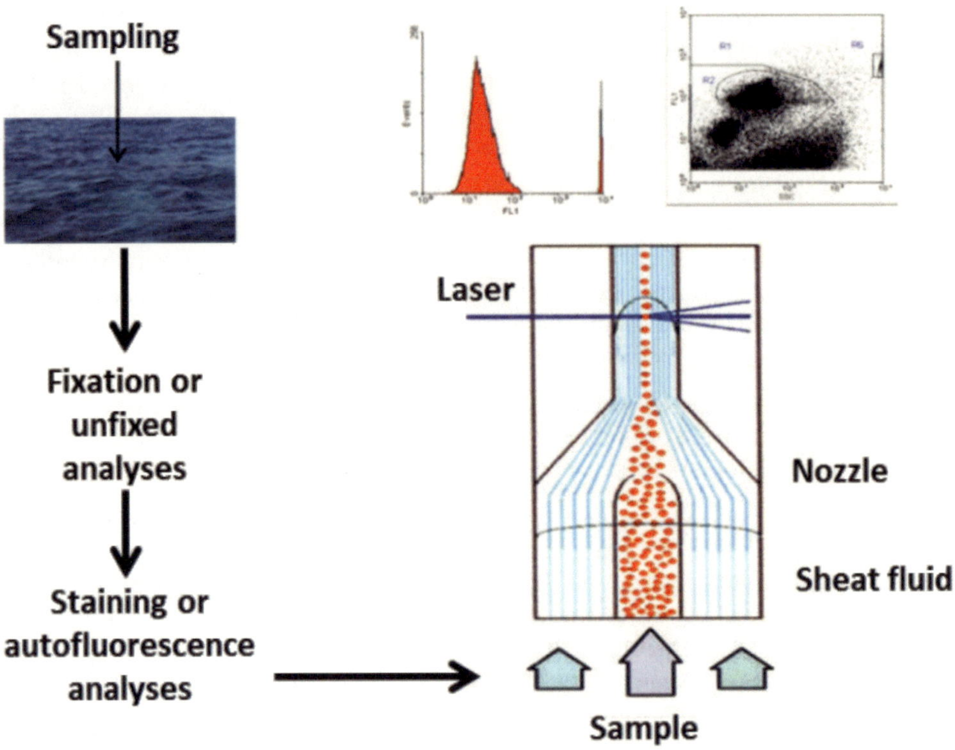

Fig. 2. Scheme of the main step: from sampling to the flow cytometric data

2. Autofluorescence analyses

The opportunity to measure fluorescence by flow cytometry is a key aspect in microbial ecology, since light-scattering characteristics alone are not usually enough to uncover much detail about either the taxonomic affinities or the physiological status of micro-organisms (Davey & Kell, 1996). Phytoplanktonic micro-organisms are an ideal subject for flow cytometric analysis because they are naturally autofluorescent by virtue of their complement of photosynthetic pigments. Most of these pigments can absorb the blue light of the 488 nm line of an Argon laser, meaning that they can be distinguished because of their unique fluorescence emission spectra. Standard filter arrangements in a dual laser system (488 and 633 nm lasers) can distinguish and quantify chlorophyll fluorescence (red ex, em > 630 nm), phycoerythrin (PE) fluorescence (blue ex, em 570 nm) and phycocyanine (PC) fluorescence (red ex, em >630 nm) (Callieri, 1996; Callieri & Stockner, 2002). Accordingly, flow cytometric data collected from natural phytoplankton assemblages can be used to identify and classify phytoplankton based on scattering characteristics (size) and fluorescence (pigmentation) (for an example, see Figure 3).

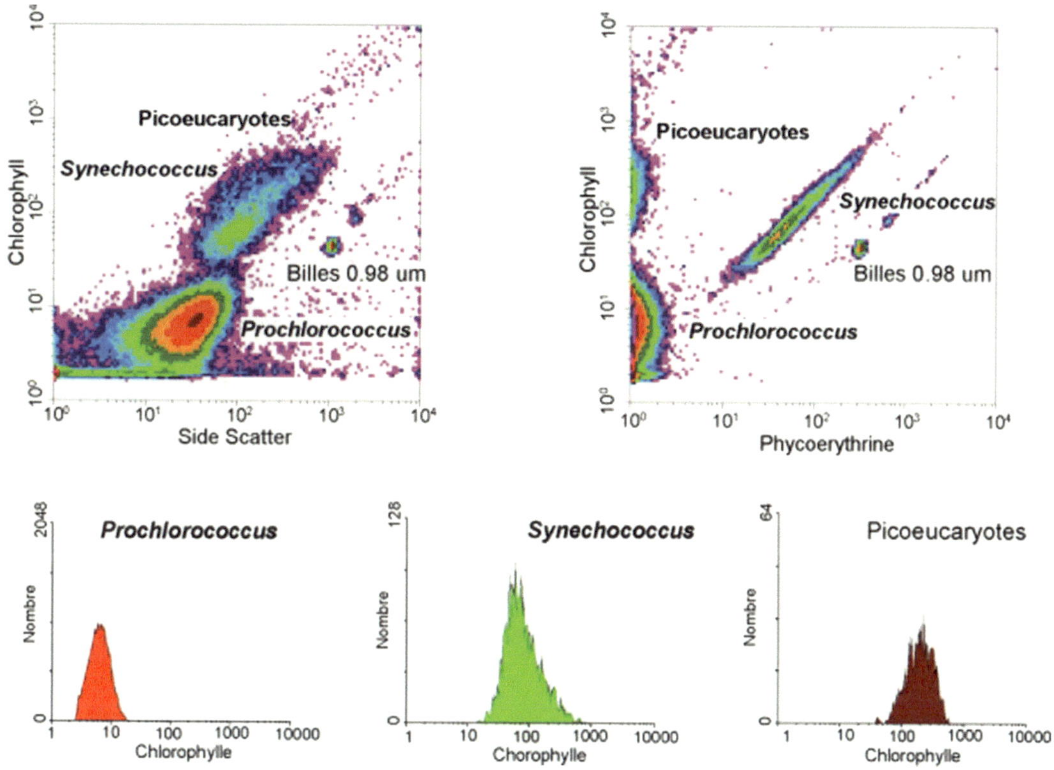

Fig. 3. Autotrophic picoplankton by flow cytometry. Image provided by Daniel Vaulot, CNRS, Station Biologique de Roscoff, France

The use of flow cytometry in aquatic microbial ecology increased our knowledge of the structure of phytoplankton assemblages (Olson et al., 1993). Based on flow cytometric analyses, phytoplankton are typically divided into Cyanobacteria (*Synechococcus*, *Prochlorococcus*) and small (pico-) and large eukaryotes. They are also able to define the distributions and dynamics of each group (e.g. Olson et al., 1990; Campbell et al., 1994; Li, 1995; Lindell & Post, 1995; Partensky et al., 1996; Campbell et al., 1997). The phycoerythrin (PE)-containing *Synechococcus* can be distinguished from *Prochlorococcus,* which are similar in size, but do not produce the 'orange' fluorescence that is typical of phycoerythrin. Eukaryotic phytoplankton, meanwhile, are distinguished based on their larger scatter and chlorophyll fluorescence signals.

The application of flow cytometry to marine samples led to the discovery of a primitive, prokaryotic picocyanobacteria of the Prochlorophyta group (Chisholm et al., 1988), with divinyl chlorophyll-*a* (chl-*a*) as the principal light-harvesting pigment and divinyl chlorophyll b (chl-*b*), zeaxanthin, alfa-carotene and a chl-*c*-like pigment as the main accessory pigments (Goericke & Repeta, 1993).

In some cases, the larger cells may be further distinguished based on their scattering characteristics (coccolithophorids) or the presence of both PE and chlorophyll (cryptophytes) (Olson et al., 1989; Collier & Campell, 1999).

Many authors have reported the distributions and dynamics of each photosynthetic group in the water column in different marine environments (Li, 1995; Campbell & Vaulot, 1993; Vaulot & Marie, 1999). As both cyanobacteria and picoeukaryotes are widely distributed in the marine environment, they play a fundamental role in aquatic ecosystems because of their high productivity.

Cyanobacteria are a diverse group of unicellular and multicellular photosynthetic prokaryotes (Castenholz & Waterbury, 1989; Rippka, 1988); they are often referred to as blue-green algae, even though it is now known that they are not related to any of the other algal groups.

Seasonal patterns of picoplankton abundance have been observed in many studies, revealing a strong relation with water temperature. A study on picophytoplankton populations conducted by Alonso and colleagues (2007) in north-west Mediterranean coastal waters showed a peak during the winter for picoeukaryotes, and peaks in spring and summer for *Synechococcus*. Meanwhile, *Prochlorococcus* was more abundant from September to January.

Zubkov et al. (2000) found that *Prochlorococcus spp.* were the dominant cyanobacteria in the northern and southern Atlantic gyres and the equatorial region, giving way to *Synechococcus* spp. in cooler waters. *Synechococcus* cells also become more numerous and even reach blooming densities near the tropical region affected by the Mauritanian upwelling. Finally, the concentrations of Picoeukaryotes tend to be at their height in temperate waters.

The small coccoid prochlorophyte species, *Prochlorococcus marinus*, were found to be abundant in the North Atlantic (Veldhuis & Kraay, 1990), the tropical and subtropical Pacific Ocean (Campbell et al., 1994), the Mediterranean (Vaulot et al., 1990) and in the Red Sea (Veldhuis & Kraay, 1993).

A monitoring study conducted in the Central Adriatic Sea (authors' unpublished results) revealed the presence of cyanobacteria, pico-eukariotes and nano-plankton (Fig. 4), while prochlorococcus were absent throughout the entire year.

Other authors (Marie et al., 2006) have underlined the similarity of the distribution of picoeukariotes to that of total chlorophyll-*a* in the Mediterranean Sea, with maximum concentrations reaching around $2x10^2$ cell/ml.

Shi and co-authors (2009) have characterized photosynthetic picoeukaryote populations by flow cytometry in samples collected in the south-east Pacific Ocean, registering abundances from $6x10^2$ to $3,7x10^4$ cell/ml. Meanwhile, 18S rRNA gene clone libraries were constructed after flow sorting.

3. Total cell counting

Total cell counting is one of the most important functions of flow cytometry. The rapidity and accuracy of the data obtained overcome the limitations (e.g. time-consuming, subjectiveness linked to the operator) of other techniques such as epifluorescence microscopy.

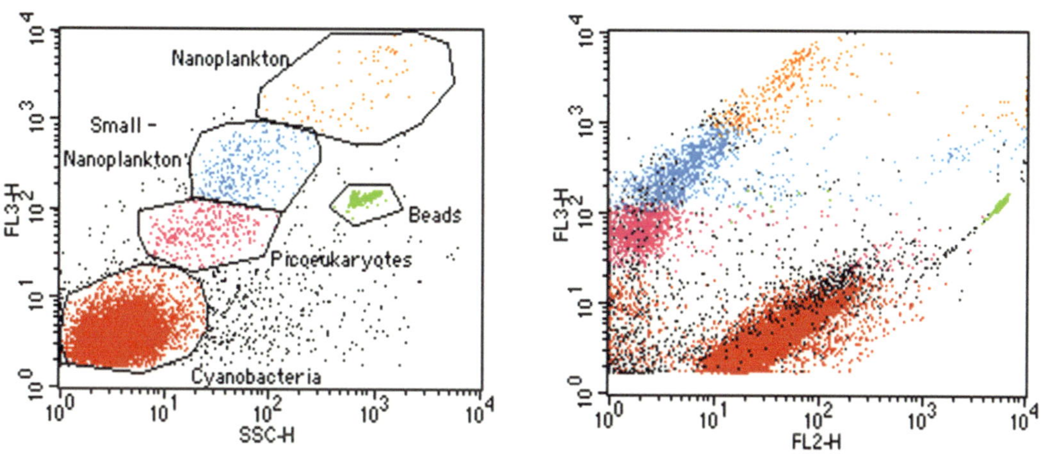

Fig. 4. Example of dot plot showing autothrophic micro-organisms in the Central Adriatic Sea

Flow cytometric countings can be determined with high statistical confidence. Some flow cytometers are equipped with volumetric counting hardware that enables the absolute cell count to be made through a predefined volume. Yet most cytometers do not have this equipment, and, in such circumstances, cell counting is perfomed by: 1) the addition of synthethic counting beads; 2) the calibration of the flow rate; and 3) weighing the sample before and after conducting any analyses. The addition of precounted beads is now also possible with commercially available beads for "absolute counting" (e.g. Coulter Flowcount beads, Cytocount counting beads, DakoCytomation, and Trucount tubes by Becton Dickinson). Accompanying datasheets provide the exact number per μl of beads to use (Cantineaux et al., 1993; Brando et al., 2000, Manti et al., 2008). The number of cells per microlitre is obtained by the following formula:

$$\text{Number of cells} = (\text{cell events}/\text{beads events})^* \\ (\text{bead number}/\mu\text{l})^* \text{ Dilution Factor}$$

Other methods have proposed the use of standard beads (Polysciences latex beads), as well described by Gasol and del Giorgio in 2000. Briefly, the beads have to be counted every day and must be sonicated to avoid aggregation.

Flow rate calibration can be performed by weighing a tube containing water, processing various volumes, estimating the time needed for each volume to go through and then reweighing the tube. This makes it possible to calculate the mean of the flow rate per minute (Paul, 2001).

The third method is comprised of estimating volume differences: the volume of the sample is measured by a micro-pipette before and after the run through the flow cytometer. However, these measurements are not as precise as those obtained using weight differences.

The flow cytometric counting of non-fluorescent cells is possible through the staining of nucleic acids (or other cellular components) with fluorescent dyes. There are commercially available probes that allow the direct counting of marine bacteria, such as, for example, the nucleic acid dyes Syto-9, Syto-13 (Lebaron et al., 1998; Vives-Rego et al., 1999), SYBR Green I and II (Lebaron et al., 1998; Marie et al., 1997), Pico Green (Sieracki et al., 1999; Marie et al., 1996), TO-PRO 1, and TOTO-1 (Li et al., 1995). Their use permits the separation of cells from abiotic particles and background signals in a water sample. An initial selection step is represented by the threshold, usually in the typical channel fluorescence (e.g. green fluorescence when SYBR Green I is used). In order to better visualize cells, a dot plot containing the scatter signal (FCS or SSC) against fluorescence signals (green or red fluorescence) is recommended.

Figure 5 shows a marine sample stained with SYBR Green I and analyzed by a FACScalibur flow cytometer (Becton Dickinson).

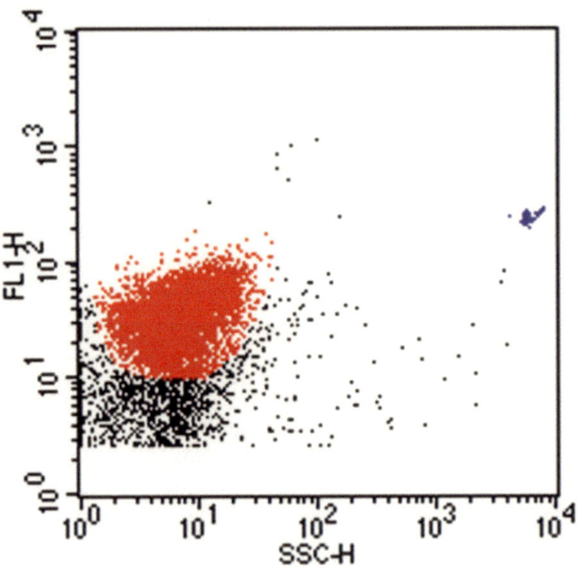

Fig. 5. Dot plot SSC *vs.* FL1 showing bacteria population stained with SYBR Green I

The affinity of the cyanine dyes, TOTO- 1 and YOYO- 1, and their monomeric equivalents, YO-PRO- 1 and TO-PRO-l, decreases significantly with increasing ionic strength, meaning that their use is inappropriate for the analysis of seawater samples (Marie et al., 1996). Other dyes, such as the SYBR Greens I and II, SYTOX Green and the SYTO family, are less dependent on medium composition and can therefore be used to count marine bacteria (Marie et al., 1999b; Lebaron et al., 1998). As SYBR Green I (SYBR-I) has a very high fluorescence yield, its use is recommended for enumerating bacteria from marine samples (Table 1).

Zubkov and collegues (2000) determined the total number of picoplankton in marine samples using the fluorochromes TOTO-1 iodide and SYBR Green I. These dyes bind strongly to nucleic acids, but SYBR Green 1 penetrates cell membranes, whereas it is necessary to use detergent to aid the penetration of TOTO-1 into cells (Li et al., 1995; Marie, et al., 1996; Marie, et al., 1997). The number of bacteria found in subsamples stained by SYBR Green I were the same as the TOTO-1 counts for the same samples. The results obtained were evidence that the intensity of fluorescence with SYBR Green 1 was greater than with TOTO-1; at the same time, SYBR Green I improved the recognition of cells with low staining, helping the separation of their signal from the background noise level. This confirms that SYBR Green is more adaptable for the analysis of marine bacteria.

In a study reported by Gregori and colleagues (2001), SYBR Green II expresses a higher selectivity for RNA, with a quantum yield of 0.54, while also maintaining a strong affinity for double-stranded DNA, with a quantum yield of 0.36, about half that of SYBR Green I.

In 1999, Gasol and co-workers published a study on a comparison of different nucleic acid dyes and techniques, such as flow cytometric and epifluorescence microscopy. They found that Syto13 counts correlate well with DAPI and SYBR Green I counts, generating slightly lower fluorescence yields than those of the other fluorochromes. This was particularly true in seawater, meaning that, without dismissing the potential of other stains, this fluorochrome is a viable alternative to the total counting of marine planktonic bacteria.

Alonso and co-authors published (Alonso et al., 2007) a monthly study in Blanes Bay, which revealed that the abundance of heterotrophic prokaryotes (ranging from 0,5 $x10^6$ to $1,5x10^6$ cell/ml) roughly followed the pattern of Chl-a.

In general, heterotrophic bacterial abundances followed the distribution of total picophytoplankton, revealing seasonal changes in their distribution, as reported for the subtropical northern Pacific Ocean (Campbell & Vaulot, 1993; Zubkov et al., 2000).

Lasternas and colleagues (2010) produced results from a cruise on the Mediterranean Sea during the summer of 2006. The composition and viability of pelagic communities were studied in relation to nutrient regimes and hydrological conditions. It was found that the picoplankton fraction dominated the pelagic community across the study region, with bacterioplankton being the most abundant (mean ± SE 7,73 ± $0,39x10^5$ cells/ml) component.

4. Detection of viruses

Viruses control microbial and phytoplankton community succession dynamics (Fuhrman & Suttle, 1993; Suttle, 2000; Castberg et al., 2001; Weinbauer, 2004; Weinbauer & Rassoulzadegan, 2004; Sawstrom et al., 2007; Rohwer & Thurber, 2009). They also play an important role in nutrient (Wilhelm & Suttle, 1999) and biogeochemical cycling (Fuhrman, 1999; Mathias et al., 2003; Wang, et al., 2010).

Initial studies of viruses in aquatic environments were performed using either transmission electron microscopy (TEM) (Bergh et al., 1989; Borsheim et al., 1990; Sime-Ngando et al., 1996; Field, 1982) or epifluorescence microscopy (EFM) (Hennes & Suttle, 1995; Chen et al., 2001; Danovaro et al., 2008). The use of EFM combined with the development of a variety of highly fluorescent nucleic acid specific dyes soon became the accepted study method, because it involved faster and less expensive technology. Nowadays, viruses (especially bacteriophages) are still typically counted by EFM using fluorochromes such as SYBR Green I, SYBR Green II, SYBR Gold or Yo- Pro I (Xenopoulos & Bird, 1997; Marie et al., 1999a,b; Shopov et al., 2000; Hewson et al., 2001a,b,c; Chen et al., 2001; Middelboe et al., 2003; Wen et al., 2004; Duhamel & Jacquet, 2006). These techniques are selective for viruses that are infectious to a specific host, but they are very time-consuming.

In 1999, however, Marie and colleagues (Marie et al., 1999a,b) successfully proposed the use of flow cytometry for the analysis of viruses in the water column. Other authors then applied FCM to virus studies (Marie et al., 1999a,b; Brussaard et al., 2000; Chen et al., 2001; Jacquet et al., 2002a,b).

The protocol proposed by Marie and collagues in 1999 included the use of SYBR Green I to stain virus nucleic acids. This protocol was revised and optimized by Broussard in 2004.

Viruses are too small in particle size (less than 0.5 micron) to be discriminated solely on the basis of their light scatter properties using the standard, commercially available, benchtop flow cytometers. As most flow cytometers are not designed for the analysis of these small and abundant particles, attention to detail must be paid to obtain high quality data. It is, therefore, crucial to determine the level of background noise with the use of an adequate negative control such as a 0. 2μm pore-size filtered liquid of a comparable composition.

Brussaard (2004) has shown that a variety of viruses of different morphologies and genome sizes could be detected by flow cytometry. Indeed, flow cytometry (FCM) data suggested that two virus groups (V-I and V-II) were present in natural water samples (Marie et al., 1999; Wang et al., 2010).

In their research, Wang et al. (2010) revealed a viral abundance ranging from 7,06x10^6 VLP ml^{-1} to 5,16x10^7 VLP ml^{-1}, with the average being 2,47 x10^7 VLP ml^{-1}. The V-II group was the dominant virioplankton, and had lower DNA compositions than the V-I group.

5. DNA content

The use of nucleic acid dyes for the detection of bacterioplankton cells revealed a tendency to cluster into distinct fractions based on differences in individual cell fluorescence (related to the nucleic acid content) and side and forward light scatter signals. There were at least two major fractions: cells with a high nucleic acid content (HNA cells) and cells with a low nucleic acid content (LNA cells) (Robertson & Button, 1989; Li et al., 1995; Marie et al., 1997; Gasol et al., 1999; Troussellier et al., 1999; Zubkov et al.,2001; Lebaron et al., 2001; Sherr et al., 2006) (Fig. 6). In a recent study, Bouvier and co-authors (2007) underlined that despite the large presence of these clusters in aquatic ecosystems (fresh to salt water, eutrophic to oligotrophic environments), there is still no consensus among scientists about their ecological significance.

The results obtained by Bouvier and others (Bouvier et al., 2007) support the notion that it is more likely that the existence of these two fractions in almost all of the bacterioplankton assemblages is the result of complex processes involving both the passage of cells from one fraction to another as well as bacterial groups that are characteristic of either HNA or LNA fractions.

The findings by Zubkov et al., (2007), which were based on the results of fluorescence *in situ* hybridization, revealed that 60% of heterotrophic sorted bacteria, with low nucleic acid content, were comprised of SAR11 clade cells.

The SAR11 clade has the smallest genome size among free-living bacteria (Giovannoni et al., 2005), and they are also the most abundant class of the bacterial ribosomal RNA genes detected in seawater DNA by gene cloning.

Many authors have presented data about the presence of HNA and LNA, not only in marine environments, but also in freshwater (Boi et al., in prep.) and in lakes (Stenuite et al., 2009).

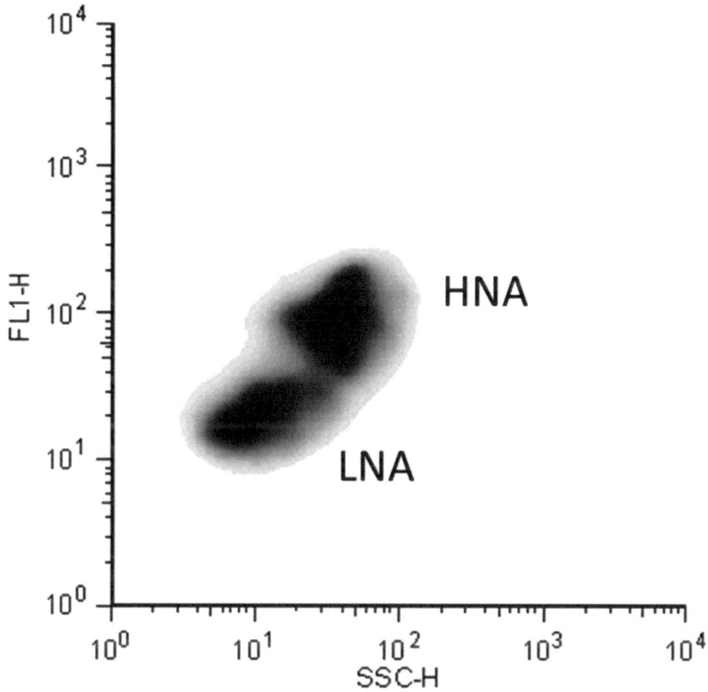

Fig. 6. Dot plot SSC *vs.* FL1 showing HNA and LNA cells stained with SYBR Green I

6. Physiological states

There is a wide and extensive variety of stains used in combination with FCM, with different degrees of specificity (Collier & Campell, 1999). Numerous classifications are available according to several criteria (Davey & Kell, 1996; Vives -Rego et al., 2000; Shapiro, 2000).

The most valuable source lists on fluorescent probes for flow cytometry are the *Handbook of Fluorescent Probes and Research Chemicals* (Haugland, 1996) and the catalogue of Molecular Probes, Inc. (Eugene, OR, USA; www.invitrogen.com). The current edition, which is the 11th, lists a range of dyes with different spectral characteristics and high specificities for nucleic acids.

Some fluorochromes bind specifically to cell molecules (nucleic acids, proteins and lipids) while increasing their fluorescence. Others accumulate selectively in cell compartments, or modify their properties through specific biochemical reactions in response to changes in the environment, such as pH, membrane polarization (cyanines, oxonols) or enzymatic activity (fluorogenic substrates) (Fig. 7).

A number of commercial kits are available which allow microbiologists to enumerate and determine physiological states and Gram status (Davey et al., 1999; Haugland et al., 1996; Winson & Davey, 2000).

Knowledge of the living/non-living and active/inactive states of cell populations is fundamental to understanding the role and importance of micro-organisms in natural ecosystems. Several probes, or a combination thereof, have been used to assess bacteria physiological states (Lebaron et al., 1998; Joux & Lebaron, 2000; Gregori et al., 2001). Among others, an interesting application of FCM in microbiology is the determination of viability, even if this is one of the most fundamental properties of a cell that is difficult to define and measure.

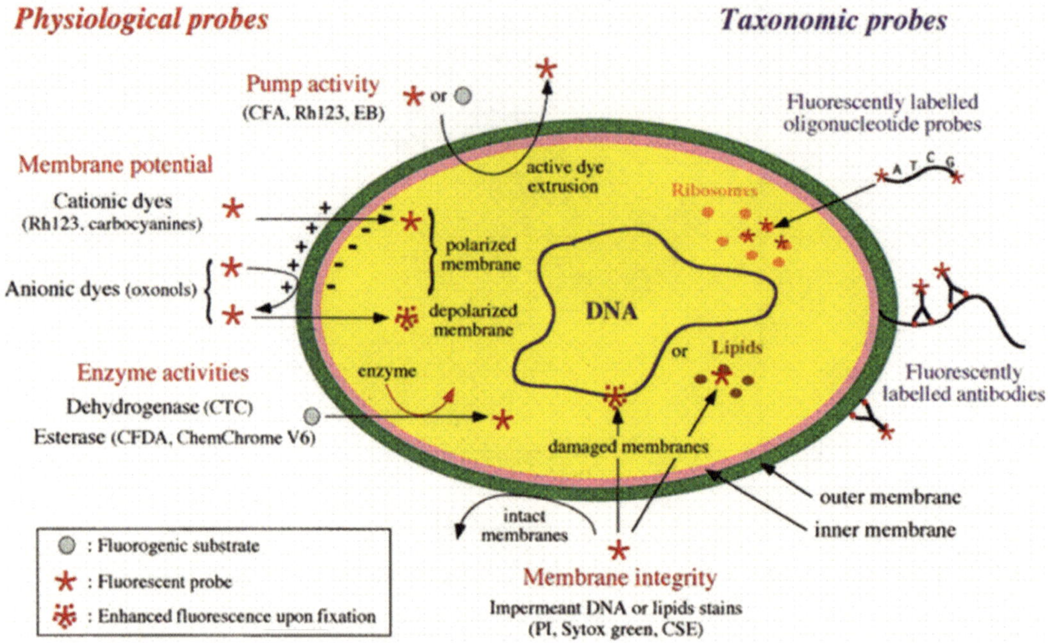

Fig. 7. Different cellular target sites for physiological and taxonomic fluorescent dyes from Joux & Lebaron, 2000

Many approaches are based on membrane integrity, such as the Life/Dead kits (e.g. the LIVE/DEAD BacLight bacterial viability kit from Molecular Probes) that are based on the rely of the propidium iodide based assessment of dead cells. Usually, a combination of SYBR Green dyes or Sytox 9 and PI is used to analyze dead cell numbers.

Barbesti and co-authors (2000) proposed a protocol for the assessment of viable cells based on nucleic acid double staining (NADS). The NADS protocol uses, simultaneously, a permeant dye, such as SYBR Green (Lebaron et al., 1998), and an impermeant one, as propidium iodide (Jones & Senft. 1985; Lopez-Amoros, 1997; Sgorbati et al., 1996; Williams et al., 1998). The efficiency of the combined staining is magnified by the energy transfer from SYBR Green to PI when both are bound to the nucleic acids, as described by Barbesti and colleagues (2000). Both dyes can be readily excited with the blue light from the laser or arc lamp of relatively simple and portable flow cytometers; the green nucleic acid probes lead to energy transfer from SYBR Green to the red PI fluorescence in the case of double staining (Barbesti et al., 2000; Falcioni et al., 2008; Manti et al., 2008). In order to better distinguish dead from viable cells, a dot plot containing fluorescence signals (green *vs* red fluorescence) is recommended (Fig. 8). Membrane intact cells that are considered to be viable emit a green fluorescence that is only due to the incorporation of SYBR Green. Cells with a damaged membrane will enable PI to enter and to bind some nucleic acids, with a corresponding increase in red and a decrease in green fluorescence.

In 2001, Gregori and co-authors optimized the double staining protocol, comparing two dyes belonging to the SYBR Green family. SYBR Green II expresses greater selectivity for RNA, while keeping a strong affinity for double-stranded DNA of about half that of SYBR Green I. The authors thus concluded that using SYBR Green II on marine samples was better.

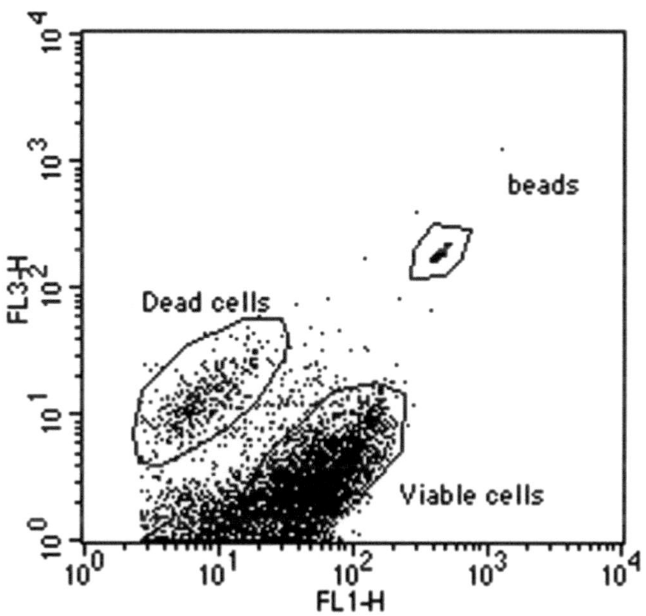

Fig. 8. Dot plot FL1 *vs.* FL3 of a marine sample stained with SYBR Green I and PI

Cell viability can be tested by assessing esterase activity or bacterial respiration. 5-cyano-2,3-ditolyl tetrazolium chloride (CTC) in flow cytometry has been used to assess "active bacteria" in seawater (del Giorgio et al., 1997), and is referred to cells that have an active electron transport system and are capable of reducing the tetrazolium salt (CTC) (Table 1). Because CTC is reduced to a brightly fluorescent formazan, it is possible to enumerate respiring cells with great sensitivity, precision and speed.

While the use of this method has increased over the last few years (e.g. Sherr et al. 1999; Jugnia et al., 2000; Haglund et al., 2002), there have also been a number of studies that are highly critical of CTC as a means of distinguishing metabolically active cells (e.g. Ullrich et al., 1996, 1999; Karner & Fuhrman, 1997; Servais et al., 2001). Some authors have stated that CTC could be toxic for some bacteria, while in some cases the results obtained would underestimate the real activity of bacteria, especially in natural seawater (Gasol & del Giorgio, 2000). Although abundances of CTC+ cells in natural samples tend to be well correlated to measures of either bacterial production (e.g. del Giorgio et al., 1997; Sherr et al., 1999) or respiration (Smith, 1998), the proportion of total cells scored as CTC+ tends to be too low, generally less than 20%, and sometimes less than just a few percent (Smith & del Giorgio, 2003).

5 (and 6)-carboxyfluorescein diacetate (CFDA) was employed to detect esterase activity in living cells in seawater samples. CFDA is a non-fluorescent molecule, but upon intracellular

enzymatic cleavage produces a green fluorescent compound that can be detected by FCM (Gasol & del Giorgio, 2000) (Table 1). Some authors (Yamaguchi et al., 1994; Schupp & Erlandsen, 1987; Yamaguchi & Nasu, 1997) coupled 6CFDA with proidium iodide to distinguish active from inactive cell membranes. Accordingly, after 6CFDA-PI double staining, bacterial cells with esterase activity display only green CFDA fluorescence, while damaged cells show only red PI fluorescence.

	DYE	EX/EM	REFERENCE
NUCLEIC ACID PROBES	SYTO- 13	485-508/ 498-527	Andrade et al., 2003 Gasol et al., 1999 Gasol & del Giorgio, 2000 Alonso et al., 2007
	SYBR Green I/II	497-520	Lebaron et al., 1998, Gregori et al., 2001, Marie et al., 1997
	Propidium Iodide (PI)	536-623	Barbesti et al., 2000 Gregori et al., 2001
	TOTO-1	509-533	Guindulain et al., 1997; Zubkov et al., 2000
DEHYDROGENASE ACTIVITY	CTC	480/580-660	Gasol et al., 1995, Sherr et al. 1999, Servais et al., 2001; Pearce et al., 2007
ENZIMATIC ACTIVITY	CFDA	492/517	Gregori et al., 2001; Pearce et al., 2007

Table 1. Shows some available dyes used for the analysis of marine micro-organisms, their excitation and emission maximal wavelengths, along with some selected references

Another interesting application of FCM to microbiology requires the use of fluorochromes conjugated to antibodies or oligonucleotides for the detection of microbial antigens or DNA and RNA sequences to directly (Vives-Rego et al., 2000; Amann et al., 1990a; Marx et al., 2003; Temmerman et al., 2004) identify micro-organisms in natural ecosystems (Amann et al., 1990b; Amann et al., 2001; Wallner et al., 1997; Biegala et al., 2003).

7. Bacteria identification with antibodies and nucleic acid probes (FISH)

Immunodetection techniques utilize the specificity of the antibody/antigen association as a probe for recognizing and distinguishing between micro-organisms. Parallel, immunological detection methods can provide quantitative data, including in relation to the sensitivity of the method used. The application of immunology in phytoplankton research started when Bernhard and co-authors (1969) developed antibodies against two species of diatoms, but it was in the 1980s that immunological techniques for species identification were actually applied in marine research. The first species investigated were prokaryotes (Dahl & Laake, 1982; Campbell et al., 1983); later Hiroish et al. (1988) and Shapiro et al. (1989) conducted studies on eukaryotic organisms.

The use of antibodies in combination with FCM is a powerful tool for the specific detection and enumeration of micro-organisms in medical, veterinary and environmental microbiology

(Cucci & Robbins, 1988; Porter et al., 1993; Vrieling *et al.*, 1993a; McClelland & Pinder, 1994; Vrieling & Anderson, 1996; Kusunoki et al., 1998; Chitarra et al., 2002). Antibodies also have a role to play in determinations of the physiological characteristics of cells; Steen and colleagues used fluorescently labelled antibodies as part of a flow cytometric method of antigenicity determination (Steen et al., 1982) that may vary according to growth conditions (Davey & Winson, 2003).

The availability of antibodies against bacteria is limited mostly to the research and identification of pathogens (e.g. Kusunoki et al., 1996; Kusunoki et al., 1998; McClelland & Pinder, 1994; Tanaka et al., 2000).

Barbesti and colleagues (Barbesti et al., 2000) performed bacterial viability measurement and identification tests using a Cy5-labelled monoclonal antibody combined with SYBR Green I and propidium iodide.

A recent study (Manti et al., 2010) conducted in natural seawater samples reports the immunodetection of *Vibrio parahaemolyticus* and an examination of the specificity and sensitivity of the polyclonal antibody used.

As described above for antibodies, oligonucleotides allow the detection and recognition of micro-organisms in a mixed population. The phylogenetic heterogeneity of micro-organisms can be studied with analyses of ribosomal RNA sequences. Fluorescence *in situ* hybridization (FISH) is based on the omology of an oligonucletide probe with a target region in an individual microbial cell.

In natural samples, however, the signal derived from the use of labelled oligonucleotide probes is often undetectable because of the low rRNA content. Among other methods, FISH with horseradish peroxidase (HRP)-labelled oligonucleotide probes and tyramide signal amplification, also known as catalyzed reporter deposition (CARD), is especially suitable for aquatic habitats with small, slow growing, or starving bacteria (Diaz et al., 2007).

Oligonucleotide probes labelled (directly or indirectly) with fluorescent markers can be detected by epifluorescence and confocal microscopy, or by flow cytometry (Giovannoni et al, 1988; De Long et al, 1989; Amann et al., 1990a; 1990b; 2001; Pernthaler et al., 2001). Several publications have reported the combination of rapidity and the multi-parametric accuracy of flow cytometry, with the phylogenetic specificity of oligonucleotide FISH probes as a powerful emerging tool in aquatic microbiology (Yentsch & Yentsch, 2008; Hammes & Egli, 2010; Muller & Vebe-Von-Caron, 2010; Wang et al., 2010).

The combination of FCM and FISH has been successfully applied to describe microbial populations dispersed in a liquid suspension derived from different media (Lim et al., 1993; Joachimsthal et al., 2004; Rigottier-Gois et al., 2003; Barc et al., 2004; Lange et al., 1997; Wallner et al., 1993 and 1995; Miyauchi et al., 2007).

Only a few studies (Lebaron et al., 1997; Gerdts & Luedk, 2006; Kalyuzhnaya et al., 2006; Yilmaz et al., 2010) have combined FISH and FCM for the analysis of acquatic microbial communities. The main limitation of combining CARD-FISH and FCM is that the former is commonly performed and optimized on a solid support (i.e. polycarbonate membrane filters; Pernthaler et al., 2002), while the latter requires liquid samples with a well dispersed suspension of single cells (Shapiro, 2000). Schonhuber and co-authors (1997) have bridged the two methodologies while working with liquid suspensions, although the proposed permeabilization procedure was not ideal for the detection of large bacterial groups with different cell walls. Meanwhile, Biegala and colleagues (2003) successfully performed a CARD-FISH-FCM protocol for the detection of marine picoeukaryotes, while Sekar and co-authors (2004) proposed the enumeration of bacteria by flow cytometry identified by *in situ* hybridization.

A recent study (Manti et al., 2011) proposed an improved protocol for the flow cytometric detection of CARD-FISH stained bacterial cells, remarking on the importance of improving the identification and quantification of phylogenetic populations within heterogeneous, natural microbial communities.

8. Conclusions

Flow cytometry is a powerful technique with a wide variety of potential applications in marine microbiology. Due to its characteristics, FCM has contributed to the knowledge of free living planktonic microbial community structures and their distribution.

The employment of new techniques and probes normally used in other ecosystems or in clinical microbiology could enhance the field of application of flow cytometry and so the studies of marine assemblages.

Furthermore, modern flow cytometers also provide quantitative data and image analyses for the detection of microbial subgroups, thereby extending the field of flow cytometry applications (Andreatta et al., 2004; Olson & Sosik, 2007).

Last but not least, the development of a portable and cheap flow cytometer, and/or imaging system with a reliable interpretation may render the monitoring of microbial communities in marine ecosystems faster and efficient.

9. References

Alonso-Saez, L., Balaguè, V., Sa, E.L., Sanchez, O., Gonzalez, J.M., Pinhassi, J., Massana, R., Pernthaler, J., Pedros-Aliò, C. & Gasol, J.M. (2007). Seasonality in bacterial diversity in north-west Mediterranean coastal waters: assessment through clone libraries, fingerprinting and FISH. *FEMS Microbiology and Ecology*, 60, pp. 98–112

Amann R., Krumholz L. & Stahl, D.A. (1990b). Fluorescent-oligonucleotide probing of whole cells for determinative, phylogenetic, and environmental studies in microbiology. *Journal of Bacteriology*, 172, pp. 762-770

Amann, R.I., Binder, B.J., Olson, R.J., Chisholm, S.W., Devereux, R. & Stahl, D.A. (1990a). Combination of 16S rRNA-targeted oligonucleotide probes with flow cytometry for analyzing mixed microbial populations. *Applied Environmental Microbiology*, 56, pp. 1919–1925

Amann, R.I., Fuchs, B.M. & Behrens, S. (2001). The identification of micro-organisms by fluorescence in situ hybridization. *Current Opinion in Microbiology*, 12, pp. 231–236

Andrade, L., Gonzalez, A.M., Araujo, F.V. & Paranhos, R. (2003). Flow cytometry assessment of bacterioplankton in tropical marine environments. *Journal of Microbiological Methods*, 55, pp. 841-850

Andreatta, S., Wallinger, M.M., Piera, J., Catalan, J., Psenner, R., Hofer, J.S. & Sommaruga, R. (2004). Tools for discrimination and analysis of lake bacterioplankton subgroups measured by flow cytometry in a high-resolution depth profile. *Aquatic Microbial Ecology*, 36, pp. 107-115

Barbesti S., Citterio S., Labra M., Baroni M.D., Neri M.G. & Sgorbati, S. (2000). Two and three-color fluorescence flow cytometric analysis of immunoidentified viable bacteria. *Cytometry*, 40, pp. 214-218

Barc, M.C., Bourlioux, F., Rigottier-Gois, L., Charrin-sarnel, C., Janoir, C., Boureau, H., Doré, J. & Collignon, A. (2004). Effect of amoxicillin-Clavulanic acid on human fecal flora in a gnotobiotic mouse assessed with fluorescence hybridization using group-specific 16S rRNA probes in combination with flow cytometry. *Antimicrobial Agents Chemotherapy*, 48, pp. 1365–1368

Bergh, O., Borsheim, K.Y., Bratbak, G. & Heldal, M. (1989). High abundances of viruses found in aquatic environments. *Nature*, 340, pp. 467–468

Bergquist, P.L., Hardiman, E.H., Ferrari, B.C. & Winsley, T. (2009). Applications of flow cytometry in environmental microbiology and biotechnology. *Extremophiles*, 13, pp. 389-401

Bernhard, M.B., Lomi, G., Riparbelli, G., Saletti, M. & Zattera, A. (1969). Un metodo immunologico per la caratterizzazione del fitoplancton. *Estratto dalle Pubblicazioni Stazione Zoologica Napoli*, 37, pp. 64-72

Biegala, I.C., Not, F., Vaulot, D. & Simon, N. (2003). Quantitative assessment of picoeucaryotes in natural environment by using taxon-specific oligonucleotide probes in association with tyramide signal amplification-fluorescence in situ hybridization and flow cytometry. *Applied Environmental Microbiology*, 69, pp. 5519–5529

Borsheim, K.Y., Bratbak, G. & Heldal, M. (1990). Enumeration and biomass estimation of planktonic bacteria and viruses by transmission electron microscopy. *Applied Environmental Microbiology*, 56, pp. 352- 356

Bouvier, T., del Giorgio P. A. & Gasol, J.M. (2007). A comparative study of the cytometric characteristics of High and Low nucleic-acid bacterioplankton cells from different aquatic ecosystems. *Environmental Microbiology*, 9(8), pp. 2050–2066

Brando B., Barnett D., Janossy G., Mandy F., Autran B., Rothe G., Scarpati B., D'Avanzo G., D'Hautcourt J.L., Lenkei R., Schmitz G., Kunkl A., Chianese R., Papa S. & Gratama, J.W. (2000). Cytofluorimetric methods for assessing absolute numbers of cell subsets in blood. *Cytometry*. 42, pp. 327-346

Brussaard, C.P.D. (2004). Optimization of Procedures for Counting Viruses by Flow Cytometry. *Applied Environmental Microbiology*, 70, pp. 1506- 1513

Brussaard, C.P.D., Marie, D. & Bratbak, G. (2000). Flow cytometric detection of viruses. *Journal of Virology Methods*, 85, pp. 175–182

Burkill P.H., Mantoura, R.F.C. & Cresser, M. (1990). The rapid analysis of single marine cells by flow cytometry. *Philosophical Transactions of the Royal Society*, 333, pp. 99-112

Burkill, P.H. (1987). Analytical flow cytometry and its application to marine microbial ecology, In: *Microbes in the sea*, Sleigh, M.A., pp. 139-166, Wiley, New York, Chichester

Callieri, C. (1996). Extinction coefficient of red, green and blue light and its influence on picocyanobacterial types in lakes at different trophic levels. *The journal Memorie dell'Istituto Italiano di Idrobiologia*, 54, pp. 135-142

Callieri, C. & Stockner, J.G. (2002). Freshwater autotrophic picoplankton: a review. *Journal of Limnology* 61, 1-14

Campbell, L. & Vaulot, D. (1993). Photosynthetic picoplankton community structure in the subtropical North Pacific Ocean near Hawaii (station ALOHA). *Deep Sea Research Part I: Oceanographic Research Papers*, 40, pp. 2043-2060

Campbell, L., Carpenter, E.J. & Iacono, V.I. (1983). Identification and enumeration of marine chroococcoid cyanobacteria by immunofluorescence. *Applied Environmental Microbiology*, 46, pp. 553-559

Campbell, L., Nolla, H. A. & Vaulot, D. (1994). The importance of Prochlorococcus to community structure in the central North Pacific Ocean. *Limnololy and Oceanography*, 39, pp. 954–961

Campbell, L., Liu, H., Nolla, H. A. & Vaulot, D. (1997). Annual variability of phytoplankton and bacteria in the subtropical North Pacific Ocean and Station ALOHA during the 1991–1994 ENSO event. *Deep Sea Research*. 44, pp.167–192

Cantineaux, B., Courtoy, P. & Fondu, P. (1993). Accurate flow cytometric measurement of bacteria concentrations. *Pathobiology*, 61, pp. 95-97

Castberg, T., Larsen, A., Sandaa, R.A., Brussaard, C.P.D., Egge, J.K., Heldal, M., Thyrhaug, R., van Hannen, E.J. & Bratbak, G. (2001). Microbial population dynamics and diversity during a bloom of the marine coccolithophorid *Emiliania huxleyi* (Haptophyta). *Marine Ecology Progress Series*, 221, pp. 39–46

Castenholz, R. W. & Waterbury, J. B. (1989). Group I. Cyanobacteria, In: *Bergey's Manual of Systematic Bacteriology*, Staley, J.T., Bryant, M.P., Pfennig, N. & Holt, J.G., pp. 1710-1728, Williams &Wilkins, Baltimore

Chattopadhyay, P.K., Hogerkorp C.M. & Roederer, M. (2008). A chromatic explosion: the development and future of multiparameter flow cytometry. *Immunology*, 125, pp. 441–449

Chen, F., Lu, J.-R., Binder, B.J., Liu, Y.C. & Hodson, R.E., (2001). Application of digital image analysis and flow cytometry to enumerate marine viruses stained with SYBR Gold. *Applied Environmental Microbiology*, 67, pp. 539–545

Chisholm, S.W., Olson, R.J. Zettler, R., Goericke, R., Waterbury, J.B. & Welschmeyer, N.A. (1988). A novel free-living prochlorophyte abundant in the oceanic euphotic zone. *Nature*, 334, pp. 340-343

Chitarra, L.G., Langerak, C.J., Bergervoet, J.H.W. & Bulk, R.W. (2002). Detection of the plant pathogenic bacterium Xanthomonas campestris pv. campestris in seed extracts of Brassica sp. applying fluorescent antibodies and flow cytometry. *Cytometry*, 47, pp. 118–126

Collier, J.L. & Campbell, L. (1999). Flow cytometry in molecular aquatic ecology. *Hydrobiologia*, 401, pp. 33-53

Craig, S.R. (1985). Distribution of algal picoplankton in some European freshwaters, *Proceedings of 2nd International Phycology Congress*, Copenhagen, August 1985

Cucci, T.L. & Robins, D. (1988). Flow cytometry and immunofluorescence in aquatic sciences, In: *Immunochemical approaches to coastal, estuarine and oceanographic questions*, Yentsch, C.M., Mague F.C., & Horan P.K., pp. 184-193, Springer- Verlag, Berlin

Dahl, A.B. & Laake, M. (1982). Diversity dynamics of marine bacteria studied by immunofluorescent staining on membrane filters. *Applied Environmental Microbiology*, 43, pp. 169-176

Danovaro, R., Dell'Anno, A., Corinaldesi, C., Magagnini, M., Noble, R., Tamburini, C. & Weinbauer, M. (2008). Major viral impact on the functioning of benthic deep-sea ecosystems. *Nature*, 454, pp. 1084-1087

Danovaro, R., Corinaldesi, C., Dell'Anno, A., Fuhrman J.A., Middelburg, J.J., Noble, R.T. & Suttle, C.A. (2011). Marine viruses and global climate change. *FEMS Microbiology Reviews*, 35, pp. 993–1034

Das, S., Lyla P.S. & Khan, S.A. (2006). Marine microbial diversity and ecology: importance and future perspectives. *Current Science*, 90, pp. 1325-1335

Davey, H.M. (2010). Prospects for the automation of analysis and interpretation of flow cytometric data. *Cytometry Part A*, 77, pp. 3-5

Davey, H.M. & Kell, D.B. (1996). Flow cytometry and cell sorting of heterogeneous microbial populations: the importance of single-cell analyses. *Microbiology and Molecular Biology Reviews*, 60, pp. 641-696

Davey, H.M. & Winson, M.K. (2003). Using Flow Cytometry to Quantify Microbial Heterogeneity. *Current Issues in Molecular Biology*, 5, pp. 9-15

Davey, H.M., Kaprelyants, A.S., Weichart, D.H. & Kell, D.B. (1999). Microbial Cytometry, In: *Current protocols in cytometry*, J. P. E. A. Robinson, John Wiley & Sons, Inc., New York. N.Y

del Giorgio, P.A., Prairie, Y.T. & Bird, D.F. (1997). Coupling Between Rates of Bacterial Production and the Abundance of Metabolically Active Bacteria in Lakes, Enumerated Using CTC Reduction and Flow Cytometry. *Microbial Ecology*, 34, pp. 144–154

DeLong, E.F., Wickham, G.S. & Pace, N.R. (1989). Phylogenetic stains: ribosomal RNA-based probes for the identification of single cells. *Science*, 243, pp. 1360-1363

Diaz, E. González, T., Joulian, C. & Amils, R. (2007). The Use of CARD-FISH to Evaluate the Quantitative Microbial Ecology Involved in the Continuous Bioleaching of a Cobaltiferrous Pyrite. *Advanced Materials Research*, 21, pp. 565-568

Diaz, M., Herrero, M., Garcia, L.A. & Quiros, C. (2010). Application of flow cytometry to industrial microbial bioprocesses. *Biochemical Engineering Journal*, 48, pp. 385–407

Dortch, Q. & Postel, J.R. (1989). Biochemical indicators of N utilization by phytoplankton during upwellings off the Washington coast. *Limnology and Oceanography*, 34, pp. 758-773

Duhamel, S. & Jacquet, S. (2006). Flow cytometric analysis of bacteria- and virus-like particles in lake sediments. *Journal of microbiological methods*, 64, pp. 316-332

Falcioni, T., Papa, S. & Gasol, J.M. (2008). Evaluating the Flow-Cytometric Nucleic Acid Double-Staining Protocol in Realistic Situations of Planktonic Bacterial Death. *Applied Environmental Microbiology*, 74, pp. 1767-1779

Fenchel, T. (1988). Marine plankton food chains. *Annual Review of Ecology, Evolution, and Systematics*, 19, pp. 19-38

Field, A.M. (1982). Diagnostic virology using electron microscopy. *Advances in virus research*, 27, pp. 1 -69

Fuhrman, J.A. (1999). Marine viruses and their biogeochemical and ecological effects. *Nature*, 399, pp. 541–548

Fuhrman, J.A. & Suttle, C.A. (1993). Viruses in marine planktonic systems. *Oceanography*, 6, pp. 51–63

Gasol J.M., del Giorgio P.A. & Duarte, C.M. (1997). Biomass distribution in marine planktonic communities. *Limnology and Oceanography*, 45, pp. 789-800

Gasol J.M., del Giorgio P.A., Massana R. & Duarte, C.M. (1995). Active versus inactive bacteria: size-dependence in a coastal marine plankton community. *Marine Ecology Progress Series*, 128, pp. 91-97

Gasol, J.M., Zweifel U.L., Peters, F., Fuhrman, J.A. & Hagstro, A. (1999). Significance of Size and Nucleic Acid Content Heterogeneity as Measured by Flow Cytometry in Natural Planktonic Bacteria. *Applied Environmental Microbiology*, 65, pp. 4475–4483

Gasol, J.P. & Del Giorgio, P.A. (2000). Using flow cytometry for counting natural planktonic bacteria and understanding the structure of planktonic bacterial communities. *Scientia Marina*, 64, pp. 197-224

Gerdts, G. & Luedk, G. (2006). FISH and chips: Marine bacterial communities analyzed by flow cytometry based on microfluidics. *Journal of Microbiolial Methods*, 64, pp. 232–240

Giovannoni, S.J., Tripp, H.J., Givan, S., Podar, M., Vergin, K.L., Baptista, D., Bibbs, L., Eads, J., Richardson, T.H., Moordewier, M., Rappè, M.S., Short, J.M., Carrington, J.C. & Mathur, E.J. (2005). Genome streamlining in a cosmopolitan oceanic bacterium. *Science*, 309, pp. 1242–1245

Giovannoni, S.J.,Delong, E.F., Olsen, G.J. & Pace, N.R. (1988). Phylogenetic Group-Specific Oligodeoxynucleotide Probes for Identification of Single Microbial Cells. *Journal of Bacteriology*, 170, pp. 720-726

Goericke, R. & Repeta, D.J. (1993). Chlorophylls a and b and divinyl-chlorophylls a and b in the open subtropical North Atlantic Ocean. *Marine Ecology Progress Series*, 101, pp. 307-313

Gregori, G., Citterio, S., Ghiani, A., Labra, M., Sgorbati, S., Brown, S. & Denis, M. (2001). Resolution of viable and membrane-compromised bacteria in freshwater and marine waters based on analytical flow cytometry and nucleic acid double staining. *Applied and Environmental Microbiology*, 67, pp. 4662-4670

Guindulain T., Comas, J. & Vives-Rego, J. (1997). Use of Nucleic Acid Dyes SYTO-13, TOTO-1, and YOYO-1 in the Study of Escherichia coli and Marine Prokaryotic Populations by Flow Cytometry. *Applied and Environmental Microbiology*, 63, pp. 4608-4611

Haglund, A.L., Tornblom, E., Bostrom, B. & Tranvik, L. (2002). Large differences in the fraction of active bacteria in plankton, sediments, and biofilm. *Microbial Ecology*, 43, pp. 232–241

Hammes, F. & Egli, T. (2010). Cytometric methods for measuring bacteria in water: advantages, pitfalls and applications. *Analytical and bioanalytical chemistry*, 397, pp. 1083–1095

Haugland, R. P. (1996). In: *Molecular Probes Handbook of Fluorescent Probes and Research Chemicals*, 6th ed., Spence, M.T.Z., Molecular Probes, Eugene, OR

Hennes, K.P. & Suttle, C.A. (1995). Direct counts of viruses in natural waters and laboratory cultures by epifluorescence microscopy. *Limnololgy and Oceanography*, 40, pp.1050–1055.

Hewitt, C. J. & Nebe-Von-Caron, G. (2004). The application of multi-parameter flow cytometry to monitor individual microbial cell physiological states. *Advances in Biochemical Engineering/Biotechnology*, 89, pp. 197-223

Hewson, I., O'Neil, J.M. & Dennison, W.C. (2001a). Virus-like particles associated with Lyngbya majuscula (Cyanophyta; Oscillatoria) bloom decline in Moreton Bay, Australia. *Aquatic Microbial Ecology*, 25, pp. 207- 213

Hewson, I., O'Neil, J.M., Furhman, J.A. & Dennison, W.C. (2001c). Virus-like particle distribution and abundance in sediments and overlying waters along eutrophication gradients in two subtropical estuaries. *Limnology and Oceanography*, 47, pp. 1734- 1746

Hewson, I., O'Neil, J.M., Heil, C.A., Bratbak, G. & Demison, W.C. (2001b). Effects of concentrated viral communities on photosynthesis and community composition of co-occurring benthic microalgae and phytoplankton. *Aquatic Microbial Ecology*, 25, pp. 1-10

Hiroishi, S., Uchida, A., Nagasaki, K. & Ishida, Y. (1988). A new method for identification of inter- and intra-species of the red tide algae Chattonella antiqua and Chatonella marina (Raphidophyceae) by means of monoclonal antibodies. *Journal of Phycology*, 24, pp. 442-444

Ingram, M., Cleary, T. J, Price, B. J. & Castro, A. (1982). Rapid detection of Legionella pneumophila by flow cytometry. *Cytometry*, 3, pp. 134–147

Jacquet, S., Havskum, H., Thingstad, F.T. & Vaulot, D. (2002a). Effect of inorganic and organic nutrient addition on a coastal microbial community (Isefjord, Denmark). *Marine Ecology Progress Series*, 228, pp. 3–14

Jacquet, S., Heldal, M., Iglesias-Rodriguez, D., Larsen, A., Wilson, W. & Bratbak, G., (2002b). Flow cytometric analysis of an Emiliana huxleyi bloom terminated by viral infection. *Aquatic Microbial Ecology*, 27, pp. 11-124

Joachimsthal, E.L., Ivanov, V., Tay, S.T.-L. & Tay, J.-H. (2004). Bacteriological examination of ballast water in Singapore harbor by flow cytometry with FISH. *Marine Pollution Bulletin*, 423, pp. 334–343

Jones, K.H. & Senft, J.A. (1985). An improved method to determine cell viability by simultaneous staining with fluorescein diacetate-propidium iodide. *Journal of Histochemistry and Cytochemistry*, 33, pp. 77–79

Joux, F. & Lebaron, P. (2000). Use of fluorescent probes to assess physiological functions of bacteria at single-cell level. *Microbes and Infection*, 2, pp. 1523−1535

Jugnia, L.B., Richardot, M., Debroas, D., Sime-Ngando, T.S. & Devaux, J. (2000). Variations in the number of active bacteria in the euphotic zone of a recently flooded reservoir. *Aquatic Microbial Ecology*, 22, pp. 251–259

Kalyuzhnaya, M.G., Zabinsky, R., Bowerman, S., Baker, D.R., Lidstrom, M.E. & Chistoserdova, L. (2006). Fluorescence in situ hybridization-flowcytometry-cell sorting-based method for separation and enrichment of type I and 335 type II methanotroph populations. *Applied and Environmental Microbiology*, 72, pp. 4293-4301

Karner, M. & Fuhrman, J.A. (1997). Determination of active marine bacterioplankton: a comparison of universal 16S rRNA probes, autoradiography, and nucleoid staining. *Applied and Environmental Microbiology*, 63, pp. 1208–1213

Kusunoki, H., Kobayashi, K., Kita, T., Tajima, T., Sugii, S. & Uemura, T. (1998). Analysis of enterohemorrhagic Escherichia coli serotype 0157: H7 by flow cytometry using monoclonal antibodies. *Journal of Veterinary Medical Science*, 60, pp. 1315–1319

Kusunoki, H., Tzukamoto, T., Gibas, C.F.C., Dalmacio, I.F. & Uemura, T. (1996). Application of flow cytometry for the detection of Escherichia coli O157. *Journal of Food Hygiene Japanese Society*, 37, pp. 390-394

Lange, J.L., Thorne, P.S. & Lynch, N. (1997). Application of flow cytometry and fluorescent in situ hybridization for assessment of exposures to airborne bacteria. *Applied and Environmental Microbiology*, 63, pp. 1557–1563

Lasternas, S., Agustí, S. & Duarte, C.M. (2010). Phyto- and bacterioplankton abundance and viability and their relationship with phosphorus across the Mediterranean Sea. *Aquatic Microbial Ecology*, 60, pp. 175-191

Lebaron, P., Català, P., Fajon, C., Joux, F., Baudart, J. & Bernard, L. (1997). A new sensitive, whole-cell hybridization technique for the detection of bacteria involving a biotinylated oligonucleotide probe targeting rRNA and tyramide signal amplification. *Applied and Environmental Microbiology*, 63, pp. 3274-3278

Lebaron, P., Parthuisot, N. & Catala, P. (1998). Comparison of Blue Nucleic Acid Dyes for Flow Cytometric Enumeration of Bacteria in Aquatic Systems. *Applied and Environmental Microbiology*, 64, pp. 1725–1730

Lebaron, P., Servais, P., Agogue, H., Courties, C. & Joux, F. (2001a). Does the high nucleic acid content of individual bacterial cells allow us to discriminate between active cells and inactive cells in aquatic systems? *Applied Environmental Microbiology*, 67, pp. 1775–1782

Legendre, L., Courties, C. & Troussellier, M. (2001). Flow cytometry in oceanography 1989-1999: environmental challenges and research trends. *Cytometry*, 44, pp. 164-172

Li, W. K. W., Jellett, J. F. & Dickie, P. M. (1995). DNA distribution in planktonic bacteria stained with TOTO or TO-PRO. *Limnology and Oceanography*, 40, pp. 1485–1495

Li, W.K.W. (1995). Composition of ultraphytoplankton in the central North Atlantic. *Marine Ecology Progress Series*, 122, pp. 1–8

Lim, E.L., Amaral, L.A., Caron, A. & Delong, F. (1993). Application of rRNA-Based Probes for Observing Marine Nanoplanktonic Protists. *Applied and Environmental Microbiology*, 59, pp. 1647-1655

Lindell, D. & Post, A.F. (1995). Ultraphytoplankton succession is triggered by deep winter mixing in the Gulf of Aqaba (Eilat), Red Sea. *Limnology and Oceanography*, 40, pp. 1130–1141

Longobardi Givan, A. (2001). Flow Cytometry: First Principles. In: *Current protocols in cytometry*, J. P. E. A. Robinson, John Wiley & Sons, Inc., New York. N.Y

Lopez-Amoros, R., Castel, S., Comas-Riu, J. & Vives-Rego, J. (1997). Assessment of Escherichia coli and Salmonella viability and starvation by confocal laser microscopy and flow cytometry using rhodamine 123:DiBAC4(3), propidium iodide, and CTC. *Cytometry*, 29, pp. 298–305

Mansour, J.D., Robson, J.A., Arndt, C.W. & Schulte, T.H. (1985). Detection of Escherichia coli in blood using flow cytometry. *Cytometry*, 6, pp. 186–190

Manti, A., Boi, P., Amalfitano, S., Puddu, A. & Papa, S. (2011). Experimental improvements in combining CARD-FISH and flow cytometry for bacterial cell quantification. *Journal of Microbiological Methods*, 87, pp. 309-315

Manti, A., Boi, P., Falcioni, T., Canonico, B., Ventura, A., Sisti, D., Pianetti, A., Balsamo, M. & Papa, S. (2008). Bacterial Cell Monitoring in Wastewater Treatment Plants by Flow Cytometry. *Water Environmental Research*, 80, pp. 346–354

Manti, A., Falcioni, T., Campana, R., Sisti, D., Rocchi, M. Medina, V., Dominici, S., Papa S. & Baffone, W. (2010). Detection of environmental Vibrio parahaemolyticus using a polyclonal antibody by flow cytometry. *Applied Environmental Reports*, 2, pp. 158-165

Marie, D., Bruussard, C., Bratbak, G. & Vaulot, D., (1999a). Enumeration of marine viruses in culture and natural samples by flow cytometry. *Applied Environmental Microbiology*, 65, pp. 45- 52

Marie, D., Partensky, F., Jacquet, S. & Vaulot, V. (1997). Enumeration and Cell Cycle Analysis of Natural Populations of Marine Picoplankton by Flow Cytometry Using the Nucleic Acid Stain SYBR Green I. *Applied and Environmental Microbiology*, 63, pp. 186–193

Marie, D., Partensky, F., Vaulot, D. & Brussaard, C.P. (1999b). Enumeration of phytoplankton, bacteria, and viruses in marine samples, In: *Current protocols in cytometry*, J. P. E. A. Robinson, John Wiley & Sons, Inc., New York. N.Y

Marie, D., Vaulot, D. & Partensky, F. (1996). Application of the novel nucleic acid dyes YOYO-1, YO-PRO-1, and PicoGreen for flow cytometric analysis of marine prokaryotes. *Applied and Environmental Microbiology*, 62, pp. 1649–1655

Martinez, O.V., Gratzner, H.G, Malinin, T.I. & Ingram, M. (1982). The effect of some beta-lactam antibiotics on *Escherichia coli* studied by flow cytometry. *Cytometry*, 3, pp. 129–133

Marx, A., Hewitt, C.J., Grewal, R., Scheer, S., Vandre, K., Pfefferle, W., Kossmann, B., Ottersbach, P., Beimfohr, C., J. Snaidr, Auge, C. & Reuss, M. (2003). Anwendungen der Zytometrie in der Biotechnologie, *Chemie Ingenieur Technik*, 75, pp. 608–614

Mathias, M., Lasse, R., Grieg, F.S., Vinni, H. & Ole, N. (2003). Virus-induced transfer of organic carbon between marine bacteria in a model community. *Aquatic Microbial Ecology*, 33, pp. 1–10

Mattanovich, D. & Borth, N. (2006). Applications of cell sorting in biotechnology, *Microbial Cell Factories*, 5, pp. 1–11

McClelland, R.G. & Pinder, A.C. (1994). Detection of low levels of specific Salmonella species by fluorescent antibodies and flow cytometry. *Journal of Applied Bacteriology*, 77, pp. 440–447

Middelboe, M., Glud, R.N. & Finster, K. (2003). Distribution of viruses and bacteria in relation to diagenic activity in an estuarine sediment. *Limnology and Oceanography*, 48, pp. 1447-1456

Miyauchi, R., Oki, K., Aoi, Y. & Tsuneda, S. (2007). Diversity of Nitrite Reductase Genes in "Candidatus Accumulibacter phosphatis"-Dominated Cultures Enriched by Flow Cytometric Sorting. *Applied Environmental Microbiology*, 73, pp. 5331–5337

Muller, S. & Nebe-von-Caron, G. (2010). Functional single-cell analyses: flow cytometry and cell sorting of microbial populations and communities. *FEMS Microbial Ecology*, 34, pp. 554–587

Olson, R. J., Zettler, E.R. & Anderson, O.K. (1989). Discrimination of eukaryotic phytoplankton cell types from light scatter and autofluorescence properties measured by flow cytometry. *Cytometry*, 10, pp. 636–643

Olson, R. J., Zettler, E. R. & DuRand M.D. (1993). Phytoplankton analysis using flow cytometry, In: *Handbook of methods in aquatic microbial ecology*, Kemp, P. F., Sherr, B. F., Sherr E. B., & Cole, J. J., Lewis pp. 175-186, Boca Raton, FL

Olson, R.J. & and Sosik, H.M. (2007). A submersible imaging-in-flow instrument to analyze nano and microplankton: Imaging FlowCytobot. Limnology and Oceanograohy: Methods, 5, pp. 195–203

Olson, R.J., Chisholm, S.W., Zettler, E.R. Altabet, M.A. & Dusenberry, J.A. (1990). Spatial and temporal distributions of prochlorophyte picoplankton in the North Atlantic Ocean. *Deep-Sea Research*, 37, pp. 1033- 1051

Packard, T.T. (1985) Measurements of electron transport activity in microplankton. *Advances in Aquatic* Microbiology, 3, pp. 207–261

Partensky, F., Blanchot, J., Lantoine, F., Neveux, J. & Marie, D. (1996). Vertical structure of picophytoplankton at different trophic sites of the tropical northeastern Atlantic Ocean. *Deep Sea Research*, 43, pp. 1191–1213

Paul, J.H. (2001). Marine microbiology, In: *Methods of microbiology*. Whitton, B., & Potts, M., pp. 563–589, The Netherlands: Kluwer Academic Publishers, Elsevier Academic press

Pearce, I., Davidson, A. T., Bell, E. M. & Wright, S. (2007). Seasonal changes in the concentration and metabolic activity of bacteria and viruses at an Antarctic coastal site. *Aquatic Microbial Ecology*, 47, pp. 11–23

Pernthaler, A., Pernthaler, J. & Amann, R. (2002). Fluorescence 359 in situ hybridization and catalysed reporter deposition for the identification of marine bacteria. *Applied Environmental Microbiolology*, 68, pp. 3094–3101

Pernthaler, J., Glöckner, F.O., Schönhuber, W. & R. Amann. (2001). Fluorescence in situ hybridization (FISH) with rRNA-targeted oligonucleotide probes. *Methods in Microbiology*, 30, pp. 208-210

Phinney, D. A. & Cucci, T.L. (1989). Flow cytometry and phytoplankton. *Cytometry*, 10, pp. 511-521

Porter, J., Deere, D., Hardman, M., Clive, E. & Pickup, R. (1997). Go with the flow - use of flow cytometry in environmental microbiology. *Microbiology Ecology*, 24, pp. 93-101

Porter, J., Edwards, C., Morgan, A.W. & Pickup, R.W. (1993). Rapid, automated separation of specific bacteria from lake water and sewage by flow cytometry and cell sorting. *Applied Environmental Microbiology*, 59, pp. 3327–3333

Rigottier-Gois, L., Le Bourhis, A.G., Gramet, G., Rochet, V. & Doré, J. (2003). Fluorescenthybridisation combined with flow cytometry and hybridisation of total RNA to analyse the composition of microbial communities in human faeces using 16S rRNA probes. *FEMS Microbiology and Ecology*, 43, pp. 237–245.

Rippka, R. (1988). Recognition and identification of cyanobacteria. *Methods in enzymology*, 167, pp. 28-67

Robertson, B.R. & Button, D.K. (1989). Characterizing aquatic bacteria according to population, cell-size, and apparent DNA content by flow-cytometry. *Cytometry*, 10, pp. 70–76

Robinson, J.P. (2004). Flow cytometry, In: *Encyclopaedia of Biomaterials and Biomedical Engineering*, Bowlin, G.L., & Wnek, G., pp. 630–640, Marcel Dekker, Inc., New York

Rohwer, F. & Thurber, R.V. (2009). Viruses manipulate the marine environment. *Nature*, 459, pp. 207–212

Sawstrom, C., Graneli, W., Laybourn-Parry, J. & Anesio, A.M. (2007). High viral infection rates in Antarctic and Arctic bacterioplankton. *Environmental Microbiology*, 9, pp. 250–255

Schonhuber, W., Fuchs, B., Juretschko, S. & Amann, R. (1997). Improved Sensitivity of whole-Cell Hybridization by the combination of Horseradish Peroxidase-Labeled Oligonucleotides and Tyramide Signal Amplification. *Applied Environmental Microbiology*, 63, pp. 3268–3273

Schupp, D.G. & Erlandsen, S.L. (1987). A new method to determine Giardia cyst viability: correlation of fluorescein diacetate and propidium iodide staining with animal infectivity. *Applied Antibacterial and Antifungal Agents*, 22, pp. 65–68

Sekar, R., Fuchs, B.M., Amann, R. & Pernthaler, J. (2004). Flow sorting of marine bacterioplankton after fluorescence in situ hybridization. *Applied Environmental Microbiology*, 70, pp. 6210-6219

Servais, P., Agoguè, H., Courties, C., Joux, F. & Lebaron, P. (2001). Are the actively respiring cells (CTC+) those responsible for bacterial production in aquatic environments? *FEMS Microbiology Ecology*, 35, pp. 171-179

Sgorbati, S., Barbesti, S., Citterio, S., Bestetti, G. & De Vecchi, R. (1996). Characterization of number, DNA content, viability and cell size of bacteria from natural environments using DAPI PI dual staining and flow cytometry. *Minerva Biotechnology*, 8, pp. 9–15

Shapiro, H.M. (2000). Microbial analysis at the single-cell level: tasks and techniques. *Journal of Microbiology Methods*, 42, pp. 3–16

Shapiro, H.M. (2003). Practical Flow Cytometry. 4th Edition, Wiley-Liss, New York

Shapiro, L.P., Campbell L. & Haugen, E.M. (1989). Immunochemical recognition of phytoplankton species. *Marine Ecology Progress Series*, 57, pp. 219-224

Sherr, B.F., del Giorgio, P.A. & Sherr, E.B. (1999). Estimating the abundance and single-cell characteristics of respiring bacteria via the redox dye CTC. *Aquatic Microbial Ecology*, 18, pp. 117–131

Sherr, E.B., Sherr, B.F. & Longnecker, K. (2006). Distribution of bacterial abundance and cell-specific nucleic acid content in the Northeast Pacific Ocean. *Deep Sea Res Part I Oceanographic Research Papers*, 53, pp. 713–725

Shopov, A., Williams, S.C. & Verity, P.G. (2000). Improvements in image analysis and fluorescence microscopy to discriminate and enumerate bacteria and viruses in aquatic samples. *Aquatic Microbial Ecology*, 22, pp. 103– 110

Sieburth, J. McN., Smetacek, V. & Lenz, J. (1978). Pelagic ecosystem structure: heterotrophic compartments of the plankton and their relationship to plankton size fractions. *Limnology and Oceanography*, 23, pp. 1256-1263

Sieracki, M. E., Cucci, T.L. & Nicinski, J. (1999). Flow Cytometric Analysis of 5-Cyano-2,3-Ditolyl Tetrazolium Chloride Activity of Marine Bacterioplankton in Dilution Cultures. *Applied and Environmental Microbiology*, 65, pp. 2409-2417

Sime-Ngando, T., Mignot, J.-P., Amblard, C., Bourdier, G., Desvilettes, C. & Quiblier-Lloberas, C. (1996). Characterization of planktonic virus-like particles in a French mountain lake: methodological aspects and preliminary results. *Annual Limnology*, 32, pp. 1–5

Smith, E. M. & del Giorgio, P.A. (2003). Low fractions of active bacteria in natural aquatic communities? *Aquatic Microbial Ecology*, 31, pp. 203–208

Smith, E.M. (1998). Coherence of microbial respiration rate and cell-specific bacterial activity in a coastal planktonic community. *Aquatic Microbial Ecology*, 16, pp. 27–35

Steen, H.B. (1986). Simultaneous separate detection of low angle and large angle light scattering in an arc lamp-based flow cytometer. *Cytometry*, 7, pp. 445–449

Steen, H.B. & Lindmo, T. (1979). Flow cytometry: a high-resolution instrument for everyone. *Science,* 204, pp. 403-404

Steen, H.B., Boye, E., Skarstad, K., Bloom, B., Godal, T. & Mustafa, S. (1982). Applications of flow cytometry on bacteria: cell cycle kinetics, drug effects, and quantitation of antibody binding. *Cytometry,* 2, pp. 249–257

Steen, H. & Boye, E. (1981). Growth of Escherichia coli studied by dual-parameter flow cytometry. *Journal of Bacteriology,* 145, pp. 1091–1094

Stenuite, S., Pirlot, S., Tarbe, A.L., Sarmento, H., Lecomte, M., Thill, S., Leporcq, B., Sinyinza, D., Descy, J.P. & Servais, P. (2009) Abundance and production of bacteria, and relationship to phytoplankton production, in a large tropical lake (Lake Tanganyika). *Freshwater biology,* 54, pp. 1300-1311

Stockner, J.G. & Antia, N.J. (1986). Algal picoplankton from marine and freshwater: a multidisciplinary perspective. *Canadian Journal of Fishers and Aquatic Sciences,* 43, pp. 2472-2503

Stockner, J.G. (1988). Phototrophic picoplankton: an overview from marine and freshwater ecosystems. *Limnology and Oceanography,* 33, pp. 765-775

Suttle, C. (2000). Cyanophages and their role in the ecology of cyanobacteria. In The Ecology of Cyanobacteria. Whitton, B., & Potts, M., pp. 563–589. The Netherlands: Kluwer Academic Publishers

Tanaka, Y., Yamaguchi, N. & Nasu, M. (2000). Viability of *Escherichia coli* O157:H7 in natural river water determined by the use of flow cytometry. *Journal of Applied Microbiology,* 88, pp. 228–236

Temmerman, R., Huys, G. & Swings, J. (2004). Identification of lactic acid bacteria: culture-dependent and culture-independent methods. *Trends in Food Science & Technology,* 15, pp. 348–359

Troussellier, M., Courties, C., Lebaron, P. & Servais, P. (1999). Flow cytometric discrimination of bacterial populations in seawater based on SYTO 13 staining of nucleic acids. *FEMS Microbiology Ecology,* 29, pp. 319–330

Ullrich, S., Karrasch, B. & Hoppe, H.G. (1999). Is the CTC dye technique an adequate approach for estimating active bacterial cells? *Aquatic Microbial Ecology,* 17, pp. 207–209

Ullrich, S., Karrasch, B., Hoppe, H.G., Jeskulke, K. & Mehrens, M. (1996). Toxic effects on bacterial metabolism of the redox dye 5-cyano-2,3-ditolyl tetrazolium chloride. *Applied Environmental Microbiology,* 62, pp. 4587–4593

Vaulot, D. & Marie, D. (1999). Diel variability of photosynthetic picoplankton in the equatorial Pacific. *Journal of geophysical research,* 104, pp. 3297-3310

Vaulot, D., Parternski, F., Neveux,J., Mantoura, R.F.C. & Llewellyn, C.A. (1990). Winter presence of Prochlorophyte in surface waters in the north-western Mediterranean Sea. *Lymnology and Oceanography,* 35, pp, 1156-1164

Veal, D.A., Deere, D., Ferrari, B., Piper, J. & Attfield, P.V. (2000). Fluorescence staining and flow cytometry for monitoring microbial cells. *Journal of Microbiology Methods,* 243, pp. 191–210

Veldhuis, M.J.W. & Kraay, G.W. (2000). Application of flow cytometry in marine phytoplankton research: current applications and future perspectives. *Scientia Marina,* 64, pp. 121-134

Veldhuis, M.J.W. & Kraay, G.W. (1993). Cell abundance and fluorescence of picophytoplankton in relation to growth irradiance and nitrogen availability in the Red Sea. *Netherlands Journal of Sea Research*, 21, pp. 135– 145

Vives-Rego, J., Guindulain, T., Vàzquez-Domínguez, E., Gasol, J.M., Lopez-Amoros, R., Vaquè, D. & Comas, J. (1999). Assessment of the effects of nutrients and pollutants on coastal bacterioplankton by flow cytometry and SYTO-13 staining. *Microbios*, 98, pp. 71–85

Vives-Rego, J., Lebaron P. & Nebe-von-Caron, G. (2000). Current and future applications of flow cytometry in aquatic microbiology. *FEMS Microbiology Ecology*, 24, pp. 429-448

Vrieling, E.G. & Anderson, D.M. (1996). Immunofluorescence in phytoplankton research: applications and potential. *Journal of Phycology*, 32, pp. 1-16

Vrieling, E.G., Gieskes, W.W.C., Colijn, F., Hofstraat, J.W., Peperzak L. & Veenhuis, M. (1993). Immunochemical identification of toxic marine algae: first results with Prorocentrum micans as a model organism, In: *Toxic Phytoplankton Blooms in the Sea*, Smayda, T.J., & Shimizu, Y., pp. 925-931. Elsevier, Amsterdam.

Wallner, G., Amann, R. & Beisker, W. (1993). Optimizing fluorescent in situ hybridization with rRNA-targeted oligonucleotide probes for flow cytometric identification of micro-organisms. *Cytometry*, 14, pp. 136–143

Wallner, G., Erhart, R. & Amann, R. (1995). Flow Cytometric Analysis of Activated Sludge with rRNA-Targeted Probes. *Applied Environmental Microbiology*, 61, pp. 1859–1866

Wallner, G., Steinmetz, I., Bitter-Suermann, I. & Amann, R. (1997). Combination of rRNA-targeted hybridization probes and immuno-probes for the identification of bacteria by flow cytometry. *System of Applied Microbiology*, 19, pp. 569–576

Wang, M., Liang, Y., Bai, X., Jiang, X., Wang, F. & Qiao, Q. (2010). Distribution of microbial populations and their relationship with environmental parameters in the coastal waters of Qingdao, China. *Environmental Microbiology*, 12, pp. 1926–1939

Weinbauer, M.G. (2004). Ecology of prokaryotic viruses. *FEMS Microbiology Reviews*, 28, pp. 127–181

Weinbauer, M.G. & Rassoulzadegan, F. (2004). Are viruses driving microbial diversification and diversity? *Environtal Microbiology*, 6, pp. 1–11

Wen, K., Ortmann, A.C. & Suttle, C.A. (2004). Accurate estimation of viral abundance by epifluorescence microscopy. *Applied Environmental Microbiology*, 70, pp. 3862– 3867

Wilhelm, S.W. & Suttle, C.A. (1999). Viruses and nutrient cycles in the sea. *Bioscience*, 49, pp. 781–788

Williams, S.C., Hong, Y., Danavall, D.C.A., Howard-Jones, M.H., Gibson, D., Frisher, M.E. & Verity, P.G. (1998). Distinguishing between living and non-living bacteria: evolution of the vital stain propidium iodide and its combined use with molecular probes in aquatic samples. *Journal of Microbiology Methods*, 32, pp. 225–236

Winson, M.K. & Davey H.M. (2000). Flow Cytometric Analysis of Micro-organisms. *Methods*, 21, pp. 231-240

Xenopoulos, M.A. & Bird. D. F. (1997). Virus a` la sauce Yo-Pro: microwave-enhanced staining for counting viruses by epifluorescence microscopy. *Limnology and Oceanography*, 42, pp. 1648–1650

Yamaguchi, N. & Nasu, M. (1997). Flow cytometric analysis of bacterial respiratory and enzymatic activity in the natural aquatic environment. *Journal of Applied Microbiology*, 83, pp. 43–52

Yamaguchi, N., Nasu, M., Choi, S.T. & Kondo, M. (1994). Analysis of the life-cycle of Bacillus megaterium by the fluorescein diacetate/propidium iodide double staining method. *Journal of Antibacterial and Antifungal Agents,* 22, pp. 65–68

Yentsch, C. M. & Pomponi, S.A. (1986). Automated Individual Cell Analysis in Aquatic Research. *International Review of Cytology,* 105, pp. 183-243

Yentsch, C. & Yentsch, C.M. (2008). Single cell analysis in biological oceanography and its evolutionary implications. *Journal of Plankton Research,* 30, pp. 107–117

Yentsch, C.M. & Horan, P.H. (1989). Cytometry in the Aquatic Sciences. *Cytometry,* 10, pp. 497-499

Yentsch, C.M., Horan, P.K., Muirhead, K., Dortch, Q., Haugen, E., Legendre, L., Murphy, L.S., Perry, M.J., Phinney, D.A., Pomponi, S.A., Spinrad, R.W., Wood, M., Yentsch C.S. & Zahuranec, B.J. (1983). Flow Cytometry and Cell Sorting: A Technique for the Analysis and Sorting of Aquatic Particles. *Limnology and Oceanography,* 28, pp. 1275-1280

Yilmaz, S., Haroon, M.F., Rabkin, B.A., Tyson, G.W. & Hugenholtz, P. (2010). Fixation-free fluorescence in situ hybridization for targeted enrichment of microbial populations. *ISME Journal,* 4, pp. 1352–1356

Zubkov, M.V, Mary, I. & Woodward E.M.S. (2007). Microbial control of phosphate in the nutrient-depleted North Atlantic subtropical gyre. *Environmental Microbiology,* 9, pp. 2079-2089

Zubkov, M.V., Fuchs, B.M., Burkill, P.H. & Amann, R. (2001). Comparison of cellular and biomass specific activities of dominant bacterioplankton groups in stratified waters of the Celtic Sea. *Applied Environmental Microbiology,* 67, pp. 5210–5218

Zubkov, M.V., Sleigh, M.A., Burkill, P.H. & Leakey, R.J.G. (2000). Picoplankton community structure on the Atlantic Meridional Transect: a comparison between seasons. *Progress In Oceanography,* 45, pp. 369-386

http://www. invitrogen.com

2

Identification and Characterisation of Microbial Populations Using Flow Cytometry in the Adriatic Sea

Danijela Šantić and Nada Krstulović
Institute of Oceanography and Fisheries
Croatia

1. Introduction

Synechococcus, Prochlorococcus and picoeukaryotes have an important role in primary production and also represent significant food resource for protists and small invertebrates (Callieri & Stockner, 2002), thus participating in the role of prey in the energy flow at higher trophic levels. Together with mentioned primary producers, heterotrophic bacteria are important components of marine plankton communities (Azam & Hodson, 1977). On one hand heterotrophic bacteria are consumers of dissolved organic matter (DOM), and as such they are links in the chain of matter and energy flow through an ecosystem (Cole et al., 1988). On the other hand, they decompose organic matter and transform inorganic compounds in forms suitable for primary producers (Ducklow et al., 1986).

Until recently, most determinations of bacterial abundance were usually performed by epifluorescence microscopy of DAPI or Acridine Orange stained samples (Hobbie et al., 1977; Porter & Feig, 1980). During the 1990's flow cytometry was introduced in oceanography (Darzynkiewicz & Crissman, 1990; Allman et al., 1993; Fouchet et al., 1993; Troussellier et al. 1993; Shapiro, 1995; Davey & Kell, 1996; Porter et al., 1997; Collier & Campbell, 1999). Use of flow cytometry in marine microbiology resulted in the discovery of several bacterial groups based on different content of DNA and different amount of fluorescence (Li et al., 1995; Marie et al., 1997): high nucleic acid content group with high amount of fluorescenece (HNA) and group with low nucleic acid and low amount of fluorescence (LNA) content (Gasol & Moràn, 1999; Gasol et al., 1999); and with discovery of cyanobacteria *Prochlorococcus* (Chisholm et al., 1988). So, due to endogenous fluorescence (fluorescing photopigments) and exogenous fluorescence (DNA dyes) it is possible to distinguish the picoplankton cells from other particles in the water column. Detailed, stained heterotrophic bacteria can be detected and discriminated from other non-bacterial particles with a combination of light scatter, green (DNA dyes), orange or red fluorescence (fluorescing photopigments). In addition, the combination of these parameters allows better resolution of the different subpopulation (HNA and LNA) within the heterotrophic bacterial group (Figure 2). Autotrophic picoplankton cells contain plant pigments in a broad of variety, with chlorophyll *a* as the major compound and single source of the red fluorescence. The chlorophyll fluorescence is the principal factor used for discriminating autotrophic cell from other particles, so heterotrophic bacterial cells can easily be distinguished from autotrophic cells in a plot Red vs. Green fluorescence. Further, the orange fluorescence can be used to detect second important fluorescing photopigment respectively phycoeritrin. Phycoeritrin is typical in many *Synechococcus* spp. and some picoeukaryotes, so *Synechococcus*, *Prochlorococcus* and picoeukaryotes can easy be discriminated in a plot Red vs. Orange fluorescence (Figure 3). Flow cytometry also significantly reduce the time employed in each of these determinations (multiparameter analysis of individual cells); increase the level of resolution and provide new insights into the structure and functioning of plankton communities that simply can not be obtained with conventional epifluorescence microscopy (Li et al., 1995; Marie et al., 1996; Marie et al., 1997). Flow cytometry has been routinely used for the analysis of marine samples and now is commonly accepted as a reference technique in oceanography and for the analysis of bacterial community (Monger & Landry, 1993).

Flow cytometry in our studies contributes to better understanding of prokaryotic roles in the Adriatic Sea as a separate ecosystem and as an important part of the Mediterranean Sea. Studies of prokaryotic community by flow cytometry in the eastern part of Adriatic Sea started in year 2003. The first studies were carried out for purposes of comparing two direct counting methods for bacterioplankton (Šantić et al., 2007). The accuracy of epifluorescence microscopy (EM) was assessed against direct counts made by flow cytometry (FCM). Furthermore, flow cytometry is used for investigation and characterization of heterotrophic prokariotic community (Šolić et al., 2008; Šolić et al., 2009; Šolić et al., 2010) and autotrophic prokaryotic community (Vilibić & Šantić, 2008; Šantić et al., 2011). Autotrophic picoplankton community, including *Prochlorococcus* and picoeukarytoes, in the eastern part of Adriatic was described for the first time in the northern Adriatic Sea (Radić et al., 2009).

2. Material and methods

For comparing the two counting methods, epifluorescence microscopy and flow citometry, samples were collected in two geographically different areas: Adriatic Sea, part of the Mediterranean Sea (Figure 1) and English Channel, part of the Atlantic Ocean (50°15′ N, 4° 15′ W, off shore station 6 km off Plymouth, and four shore station from Plymouth Sound UK). From the Adriatic Sea a total of 919 samples comprising both offshore and shore areas were collected on monthly basis from 29 sites during 2005. From the English Channel (N =132) samples were collected at weekly to monthly intervals during winter 2006 from one offshore and four shore sites. In addition, for the purpose of testing repeatability and counting precision, four replicates were made by both direct counting methods, for each sample through vertical profile collected from shore and off shore sites from the Adriatic Sea and the English Channel. For the comparison of the share of biomass within the microbial community samples were collected on monthly basis from the Adriatic Sea (N = 110) from one coastal (ST103) and one open sea (CA009) site during 2010. Seawater samples from the Adriatic Sea sites and offshore site in the English Channel were collected by Niskin bottles through vertical profile. At four shore sites from the English Channel samples were collected manually from the surface. All samples were fixed with formaldehyde (2% final concentration), kept in the dark at 4 °C and analyzed within two weeks. For epifluorescence microscopy (EM) preserved samples were stained with 4'-6-diamidino-2-phenylindole (DAPI) (1 μg mL^{-1} final concentration) for 5 minutes and were filtered through 0.2 μm pore diameter black polycarbonate filters (Millipore, Ireland). Filters were then mounted on microscope slides and stored at 4 °C where they were kept until observation with an Olympus microscope under UV light (Porter & Feig, 1980) at magnification of 1000. From

100 to 400 bacteria were counted per sample, depending on concentration. For flow cytometry analysis (FCM), fixed samples were stained with SYBR GREEN I (add dye at a final concentration of 5 parts in 100 000 and incubated 15 min at room temperature in the dark) (Molecular probes Inc.) (Marie at al., 1997; Lebaron et al., 1998). Samples from the Adriatic Sea were analyzed on a Beckman Coulter EPICS XL-MCL with a high flow rate from 1 to 1.2 μL/sec. Fluorescent beads were added (Level-II Epics DIVISION of Coulter Corporation Hialeah, Florida) for calibration of fluorescence intensity. Samples from the English Channel were analyzed on a flow cytometer FACSort. Beckman Coulter flow set beads at known concentration were used to calibrate the flow rate. Bacterial abundance was determined in scatter plots of particle side scatter versus SYBR GREEN I fluorescence related to cellular nucleic acid content to discriminate bacteria from other particles (Figure 2).

Abundances of *Synechococcus, Prochlorococcus* and picoeukaryotes were determined using flow cytometry (Marie *et al.*, 1997), and different populations were distinguished according to light diffraction, red emission of cellular chlorophyll content and orange emission of phycoerythrin-rich cells (Figure 3). Samples were preserved in 0.5% gluteraldehyde, frozen at -80°C and stored until analysis. Samples were analysed on a Beckman Coulter EPICS XL-MCL with a high flow rate from 1 to 1.2 μL sec^{-1}. Fluorescence beads were added to calibrate the cells' fluorescence intensity (Level-II Epics Division of Coulter Corporation Hialeah, Florida).

Biomasses of *Synechococcus, Prochlorococcus,* picoeukaryotes and heterotrophic bacteria were calculated by using the following volume-to-carbon conversion factors: 250 $fgCcell^{-1}$ for *Synechococcus*, 53 $fgCcell^{-1}$ for *Prochlorococcus,* 2100 $fgCcell^{-1}$ picoeukaryotes and 20 $fgCcell^{-1}$ for heterotrophic bacteria (Zhang et al., 2008).

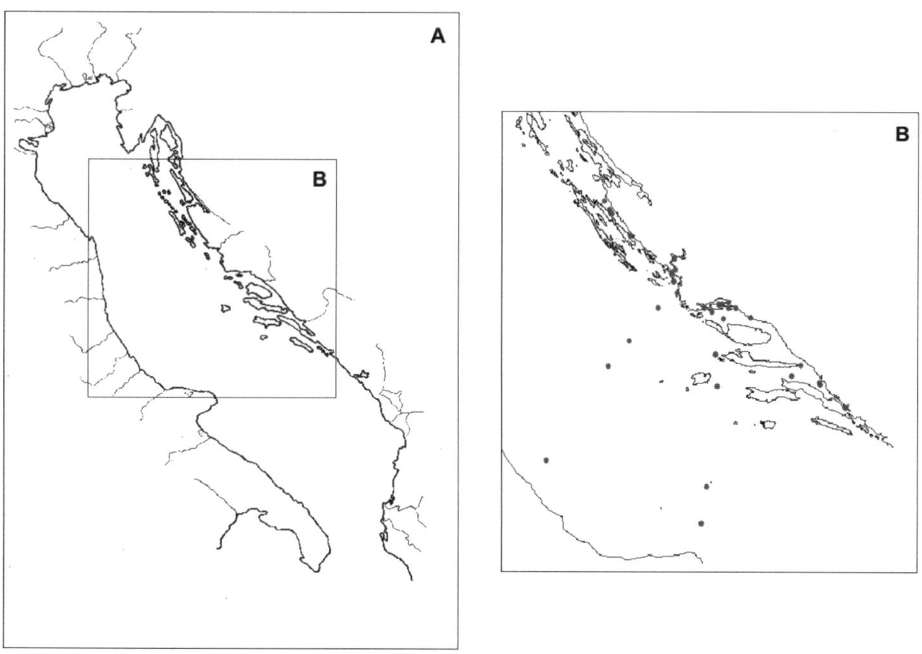

Fig. 1. (A) The Adriatic Sea (B) Locations of the investigated sites

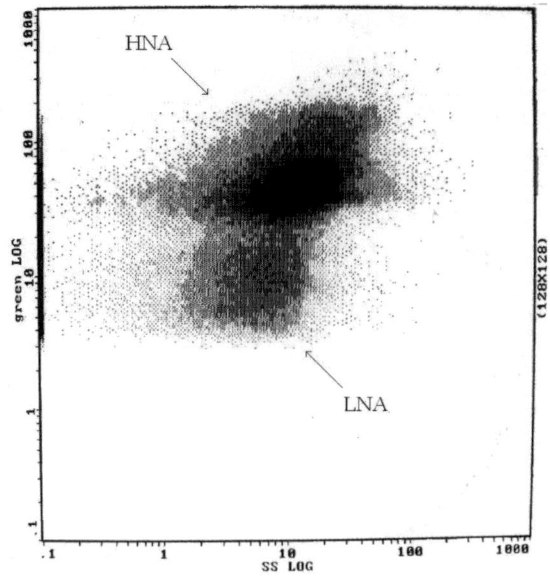

Fig. 2. Two-parametric citogram of heterotrophic prokaryotes

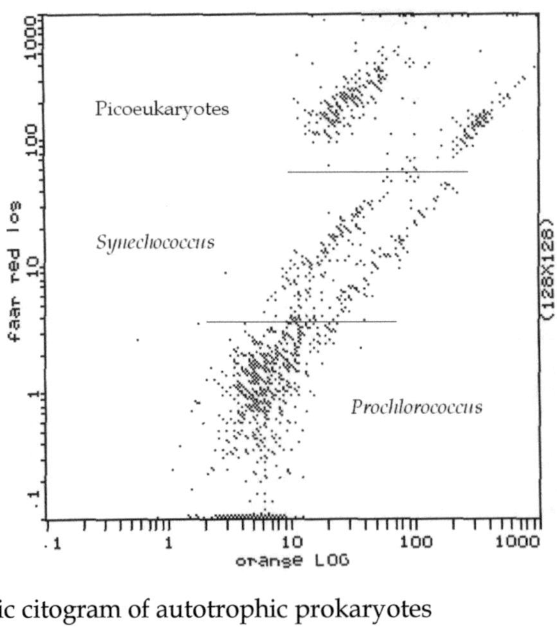

Fig. 3. Two-parametric citogram of autotrophic prokaryotes

3. Results and discussion

Detailed comparison results of two direct counting methods for bacterioplankton in the field samples from different oceanographic regions- the Adriatic Sea and the English Channel showed statistically significant correlation between bacterial counts measured with microscopy and flow cytometry for samples collected in the Adriatic Sea ($r = 0.61$, $n = 919$, $P < 0.001$) and in the English Channel ($r = 0.64$, $n = 33$, $P < 0.001$). Similar significant correlations ($R^2 > 0.8$) were also found in the north-western Mediterranean Sea (Lebaron et al., 1993, 1998; Gasol et al., 1999). Bacterial counts obtained by flow cytometry and microscopy were more similar in the Adriatic Sea than in the English Channel and replicate experiments in both investigated areas showed that coefficients of variation were lower for bacterial counts estimated by FCM than by microscopy (Figure 4).

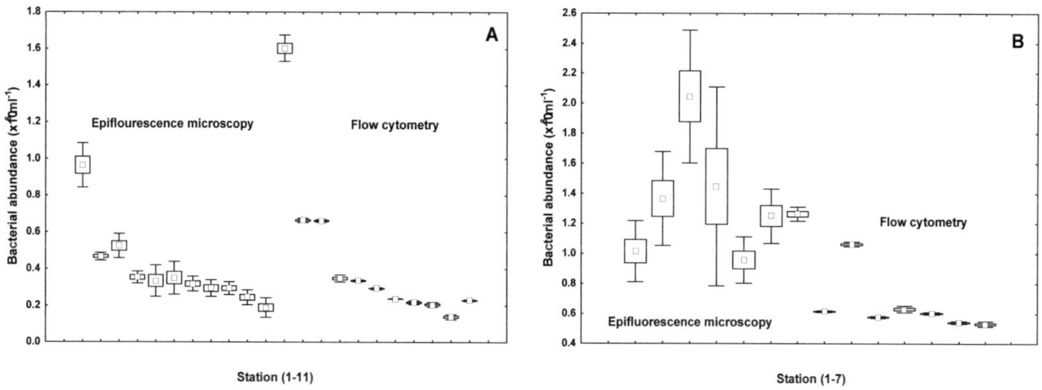

Fig. 4. Box- Whiskers (mean; 50 % conf. int.; std. dev) plot of bacterial abundance obtained by epifluorescence microscopy and flow cytometry from (A) the Adriatic Sea and (B) the English Channel

Noted significant variations in bacterial abundance obtained by microscopy can be explained by the fact that presence of organic and mineral particles and the small sizes of most marine bacteria may result in lower bacterial discrimination (Lebaron et al., 1993; Gasol & Morán, 1999). Use of flow cytometry deals better with that problem because flow cytometer is separating bacteria from other particles on the basis of light scatter (size) and pigment content and has greater precision than microscopy counting (Sieracki et al., 1995; Monger & Landry, 1993; Joachimsthal et al., 2003; Chisholm et al., 1988).

Abundance of heterotrophic bacteria obtained by flow cytometry in the investigated coastal area and in the open Adriatic Sea area ranged from 10^5 to 10^6 cells mL^{-1} and results are similar to previous values obtained by epiflurescence microscopy reported for the eastern coast of Adriatic Sea (Krstulović et al., 1995; Krstulović et al., 1997). Seasonality in the bacterial community in the most investigated coastal areas (Figure 5), with maxima in the spring-summer period and minima during winter was also determined, as in the previous reports on central Adriatic (Krstulović, 1992; Šolić et al., 2001). The average proportion of HNA bacteria in the central and southern coastal area ranged approximately from 20 % to 90 % and LNA bacteria from 10 % to 80 %, while in the open sea HNA and LNA ranged from 30 % to 70 %. In our research the prevalence of the LNA group over HNA was determined, as also established in oligotrophic areas of world's seas and oceans (Zubkov et al., 2001; Jochem et al., 2004; Andrade et al., 2007). In our research of the Adriatic Sea area, the prevalence of the HNA bacterial group in the water column was shown at stations which have a higher trophic level and our finding is consistent with studies that found that the dominance of the HNA over the LNA group in eutrophic areas directly influenced by river inflow (Li et al., 1995; Šolić et al., 2009). The predominance of the LNA group in oligotrophic conditions can be explained by the high surface area to volume ratio of cell and therefore the successful survival in poor conditions (Jochem et al., 2004).

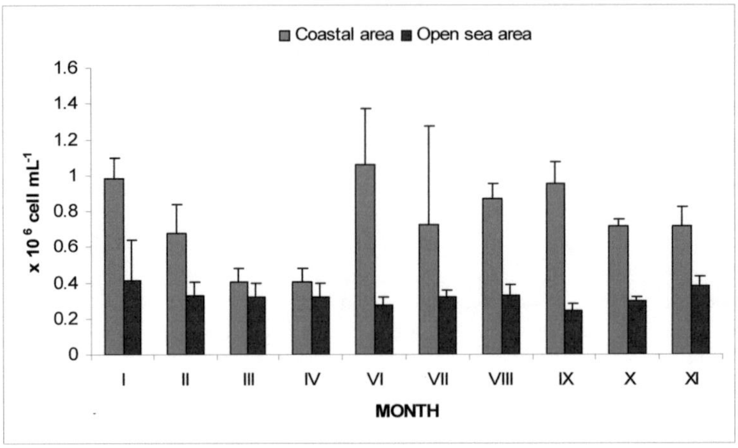

Fig. 5. Seasonal fluctuations of heterotrophic bacteria in the coastal and open sea area. Average values (column) and positive standard deviation (bars) are presented

Average abundance of *Synechococcus* in the central and southern coastal area obtained by flow cytometry ranged from 10^2 to 10^5 cells mL^{-1}, while in the open sea area it ranged from 10^3 to 6.3 x 10^4 cells mL^{-1}. When comparing all investigated areas, the highest individual number of *Synechococcus* was found at the coastal station and was recorded as 4.6 x 10^5 cells mL^{-1} (Figure 6). Abundance of *Synechococcus*, determined in the range of 10^2 to 10^5 cells mL^{-1}, is consistent with previous results obtained by epiflurescence microscopy and reported by Ninčević Gladan *et al.* (2006). According to the literature, similar ranges of *Synechococcus* abundance (10^3 to 10^5 cells mL^{-1}) have also been obtained by flow cytometry in the north-western Mediterranean (Bernardi Aubry *et al.*, 2006), eastern Mediterranean (Uysal & Köksalan, 2006) and the northern Adriatic Sea (Paoli & Del Negro, 2006; Radić *et al.*, 2009).

Our investigations revealed the presence of *Synechococcus* over a wide temperature range in the coastal area, as well as in the open sea. Moreover, increased numbers of *Synechococcus* were found during the warmer seasons, except in the eutrophic coastal area where high values were observed during the colder seasons. Although many authors describe these cyanobacteria as eurythermal organisms (Waterbury et al., 1986; Shapiro & Haugen, 1988; Neuer, 1992), seasonal distribution of *Synechococcus* in the north-western Mediterranean Sea (Agawin *et al.*, 1998) and the northern Adriatic Sea (Fuks *et al.*, 2005) have shown an increased abundance of this genus during the warmer seasons and a lower abundance during the colder seasons. Our research determined abudance of *Synechococcus* over a wide temperature range and showed *Synechococcus* as eurythermal organisms in accordance with the earlier studies (Waterbury *et al.*, 1986; Shapiro & Haugen, 1988; Neuer, 1992).The average cell abundance of *Prochlorococcus* in the central and southern coastal area of eastern Adriatic Sea ranged from 0 to 10^4 cells mL^{-1}, while the average abundance ranged from 10^3 to x 10^4 cells mL^{-1} in the open sea. Similar to *Synechococcus*, variations in the abundances of *Prochlorococcus* were more pronounced in the coastal areas compared to the open sea area (Figure 7). When comparing all investigated areas, the highest individual number of *Prochlorococcus* was found at the station located at the mouth of river Krka and was 7.1 x 10^4 cells mL^{-1} (Figure 7). This is consistent with the high abundance of *Prochlorococcus* recorded in the Mediterranean coastal and open sea waters, where abundance was shown to range, in average order of magnitude, from 10^3 to 10^4 cells mL^{-1} (Sommaruga *et al.*, 2005; Garczarek *et al.*, 2007). For *Prochlorococcus* our research results indicate that cells are detectable within the temperature range of 6.33 °C to 26.93 °C, similar to some reports for the northern Atlantic and north-western Mediterranean Sea (Buck *et al.*, 1996; Agawin *et al.*, 2000; Vaulot *et al.* (1990).

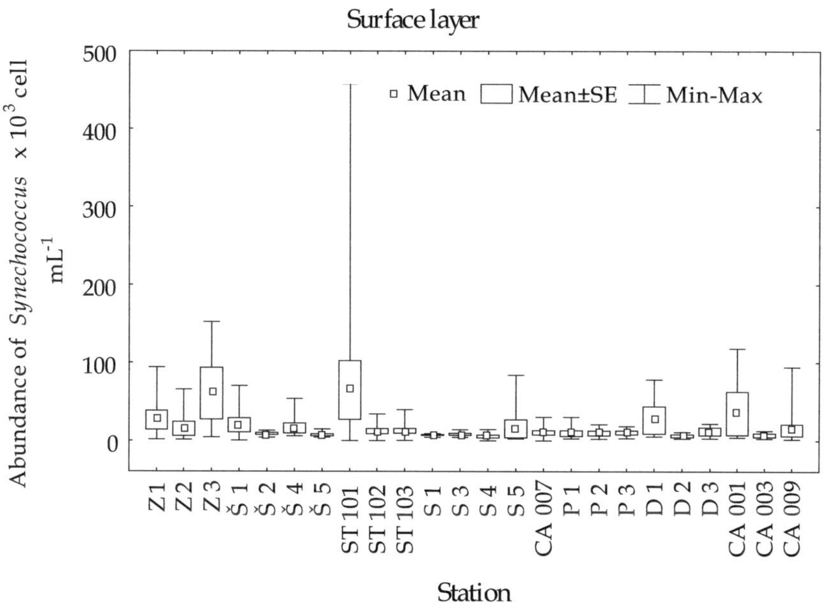

Fig. 6. Abundance of Synechococcus at the surface layer

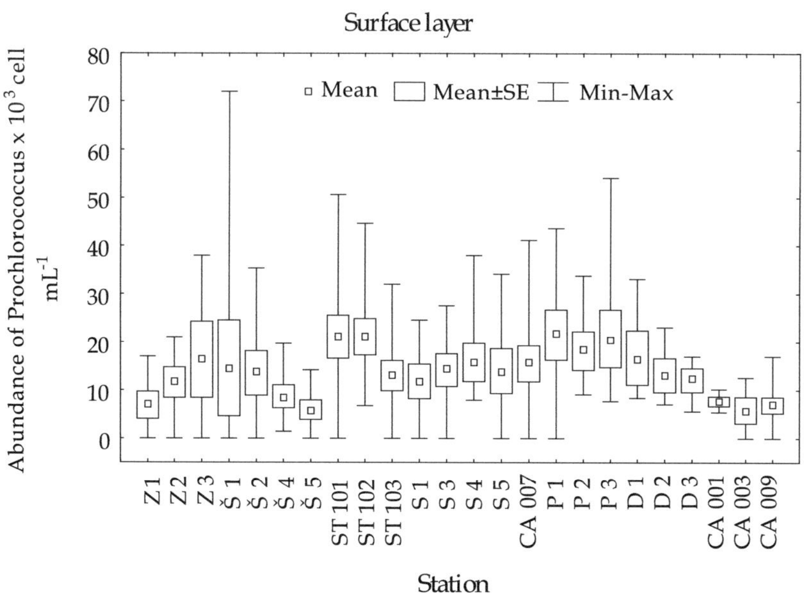

Fig. 7. Abundance of *Prochlorococcus* at the surface layer

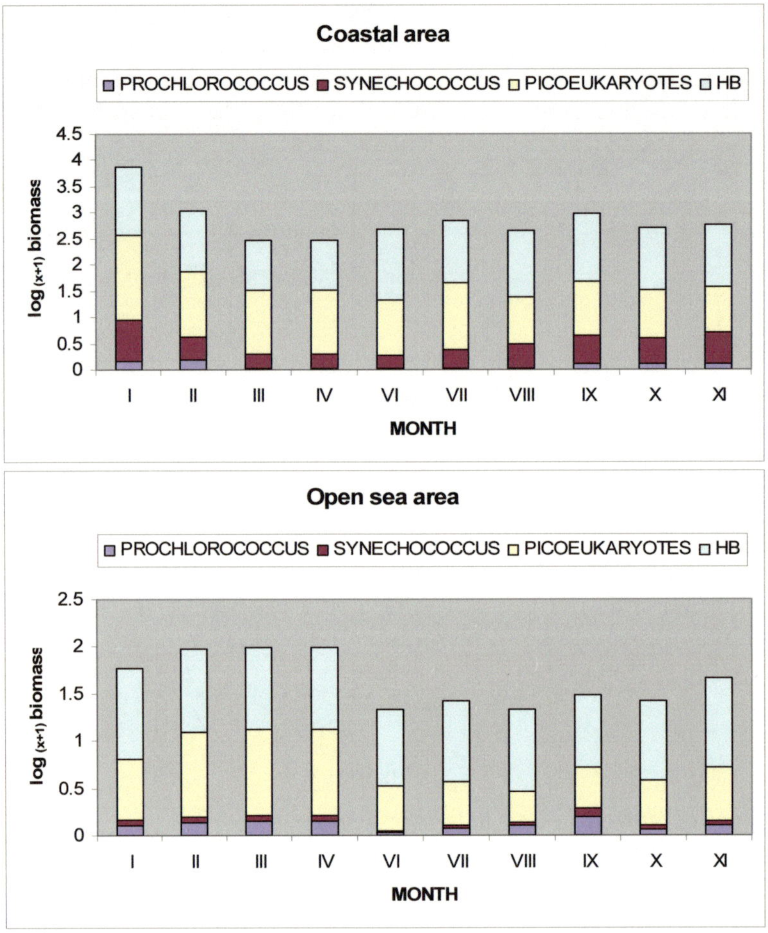

Fig. 8. Seasonal fluctuations of *Synechococcus, Prochlorococcus,* picoeucaryotes and heterotrophic bacterial biomasses in the coastal and open sea area

Use of the flow cytometry, in addition to noted understanding of the abundance and seasonal distribution of *Synechococcus* and *Prochlorococcus,* resulted in the data of vertical distribution of cyanobacteria in the open Adriatic Sea. At deep open sea stations, the high abundance of *Synechococcus* was found in the bottom layers, which agrees with the results of Uysal & Köksalan (2006) for the eastern Mediterranean Sea and of Bernardi Aubry *et al.* (2006) for the northern Adriatic Sea. Therefore, high abundance of *Synechococcus* in the bottom layer is consistent with the finding that *Synechococcus* can successfully live in environments with limited light (Waterbury *et al.,* 1986; Wehr, 1993), due to different pigment ecotypes (Olson *et al.,* 1988). The maximum depth at which *Prochlorococcus* was found in the investigated area of Adriatic Sea was 200 metres at one station located in the Jabuka Pit, with an abundance of 10^3 cells mL^{-1} in February under mixed water column conditions. Previous investigations have revealed high *Prochlorococcus* abundance in deeper layers of the euphotic zone (Wehr, 1993), even at depths of 150 to 200 metres (Partensky *et al.,* 1999a). The most likely reason for their occurrence at this depth is vertical mixing of the water column (Bernardi Aubry *et al.,* 2006) or perhaps the existence of two *Prochloroccocus* ecotypes that inhabit the shallow and deeper euphotic layer (Moore *et al.*, 1998; Partensky *et al.*, 1999a). Our results generally showed that in the investigated microbial community autotrophic component was dominant over the heterotrophic component during the winter season, while dominance of heterotrophic component in the microbial community was observed during the warmer seasons. Further, within the prokaryotic community heterotrophic prokaryotes were mostly dominant throughout the studied area. It is also important to point out that autotrophic prokaryotic community was mostly dominated by the *Synechococcus* biomass, and it was also observed that the biomass of *Prochlorococcus* was higher in the open sea area in comparison with the coastal site (Figure 8).

Owing to the ability to analyze around ten thousand cells in few minutes, flow cytometry can really reduce the time needed for determination of microbial abundances and offer new insights into the structure and functioning of microbial communities that can not be obtained with conventional epifluorescence microscopy.

The future research of microbial communities in the Adriatic Sea, in addition to the characterisation of the microbial community by analysing endogenous fluorescence (chlorophyll and phicoerythrin fluorescence) and exogenous fluorescence (DNA dyes), should also introduce the methods of single cell analysis by cytometry. Introduction of activity probes, nucleic acid probes and immunofluorescent probes will expand the knowledge about functioning within the specific communities and between different ones.

4. Conclusions

In conclusion, the results reported herewith show a significant relationship between epifluorescence microscopy and flow cytometry, but coefficients of variation were considerably lower for bacterial counts estimated by flow cytometry than epifluorescence microscopy. Generally, the use of flow cytometry in marine microbiology reduces the processing time of the sample and increases the number of processed samples. Also, the use of this method provides more information about microbial community members, especially for *Prochlorococcus*, HNA and LNA bacterial groups (cells are not visible by epifluorescence microscopy). Thanks to flow cytometry, first data for abundances of *Prochlorococcus*, HNA and LNA bacteria were published, and this method increases the knowledge about microbial community members and their relationships in the Adriatic Sea.

5. Acknowledgments

This research was supported by the Croatian Ministry of Science, Education and Sport as part of the research program 'Role of plankton communities in the energy and matter flow in the Adriatic Sea '(project no 001-0013077-0845). Also thank Olja Vidjak and Marin Ordulj to help.

6. References

Agawin, N.S.R., Duarte, C.M. and S. Agustí. 1998. Growth and abundance of *Synechococcus* sp. in a Mediterranean Bay: seasonality and relationship with temperature. *Mar. Ecol. Prog. Ser.* 170: 45–53.

Agawin, N.S.R., Duarte, C.M. and S. Agustí. 2000. Nutrient and temperature control of the contribution of picoplankton to phytoplankton biomass and production. Limnol. Oceanogr. 45: 591–600.

Allman, R., R. Manchee and D. Lloyd. 1993. Flow cytometric analysis of heterogeneousbacterial populations. In 27-47. *Flow cytometry in microbiology*. D. Lloyd (ed.). pp. Springer-Verlag, London, United Kingdom.

Andrade, L., A.M.Gonzales, C.E. Rezende, M. Suzuki, J.L. Valentin and R. Paranhos. 2007. Distribution of HNA and LNA bacterial groups in the Southwest Atlantic Ocean. Braz. J. Microbiol. 38: 330-336.

Azam, F. and R.E. Hodson. 1977. Size distribution and activity of marine microheterotrophs. Limnol. Oceanogr. 22: 492–501.

Bernardi-Aubry, F., F. Acri, M. Bastianini, A. Pugnetti, and G. Socal. 2006. Picophytoplankton contribution to phytoplankton community structure in the Gulf of Venice (NW Adriatic Sea). International Review of Hydrobiology. 91: 51–70.

Buck, K.R., F.P. Chavez and L. Campbell. 1996. Basin-wide distributions of living carbon components and the inverted trophic pyramid of the central gyre of the North Atlantic Ocean, summer 1993. Aquat. Microb. Ecol. 10: 283-298.

Burkill, P.H. 1987. Analytical flow cytometry and its application to marine microbial ecology. IN: *Microbes in the sea*. M. A. Sleigh (Ed.). pp.139-166. J. Wiley & Sns, Chichester, W. Sussex (England).

Callieri, C. and J. C: Stockner. 2002. Freshwater autotrophic picoplankton: a review. J. Limnol. 61: 1–14.

Calvo-Díaz, A. and X.A.G. Morán. 2006. Seasonal dynamics of picoplankton in shelf waters of the southern Bay of Biscay. Aquat. Microb. Ecol. 42: 159–174.

Chisholm, S.W., R.J. Olson, E.R. Zettler, J.B. Waterbury, R. Goericke and N. Welschmeyer. 1988. A novel free-living prochlorophyte occurs at high cell concentrations in the oceanic euphotic zone. *Nature*. 334: 340–343.

Christaki, U., A. Giannakourou, F. Van Wambeke and G. Grégori. 2001. Nanoflagellate predation on auto- and heterotrophic picoplankton in the oligotrophic Mediterranean Sea. J. Plankton Res. 23 : 1297-1310.

Christaki, U., C. Courties, H. Karayanni, A. Giannakourou, C. Maravelias, K.A. Kormas and P. Lebaron. 2002. Dynamic characteristics of *Prochlorococcus* and *Synechococcus* consumption by bacterivorous nanoflagellates. Microb. Ecol. 43: 341-352.

Cole, J.J., S. Findlay and M.L. Pace. 1988. Bacterial production in fresh and saltwater ecosystems: a cross-system overview.Mar. Ecol. Prog. Ser.43: 1–10.

Collier, J. L. and L. Campbell. 1999. Flow cytometry in molecular aquatic ecology. Hydrobiologia. 401:33–53.

Cotner, J.B. and B. A. Biddanda. 2002. Small players, large role: microbial influence on auto-heterotrophic coupling and biogeochemical processes in aquatic ecosystems. Ecosystems. 5: 105–121.

Darzynkiewicz, Z. and Crissman, H.A.: Preface. 1990. In: *Methods in Cell Biology* Vol. 33. Flow Cytometry. Z. Darzynkiewicz and H.A. Crissman, (eds.). pp, 15-17. Academic Press. New York.

Davey, H., and D. Kell. 1996. Flow cytometry and cell sorting of heterogeneous microbial populations: the importance of single-cell analysis. Microbiol. Rev. 60: 641-696.

Ducklow, H.W., D.A. Purdie, P.J.L. Williams and J.M. Davis. 1986. Bacterioplankton: A sink for carbon in a coastal marine plancton community. Science. 232: 865–867.

Fouchet, P., C. Jayat, Y. Hechard, M.H. Ratinaud, and G. Frelat. 1993. Recent advances in flow cytometry in fundamental and applied microbiology. Biochem. Cell Biol. 78: 95–109.

Fuks, D., J. Radić, T. Radić, M. Najdek, M. Blažina, D. Degobbis and N. Smodlaka. 2005. Relationships between heterotrophic bacteria and cyanobacteria in the northern Adriatic in relation to the mucilage phenomenon. Sci. Total Environ. 353: 178-188.

Garczarek, L., A. Dufresne, S. Rousvoal, N.J. West, S. Mazard, D. marie, H. Claustre, P. Raimbault, A.F.Post, D.J.Scanlan and F. Partensky. 2007. High vertical and low horizontal diversity of *Prochlorococcus* in the Mediterranean Sea in summer. FEMS Microbiol. Ecol. 60: 189-206.

Gasol, J.M. and X.A.G. Morán. 1999. Effects of filtration on bacterial activity and picoplankton community structure as assessed by flow cytometry. Aquat. Microb. Ecol. 16: 251–264.

Gasol, J.M., U.L. Zweifel, F. Peters, J.A. Furhman and Å. Hagström. 1999. Significance of size and nucleic acid content heterogeneity as assessed by flow cytometry in natural planktonic bacteria. Appl. Environ. Microbiol. 65: 4475–4483.

Guillou, L., S. Jacquet, M.J. Chretiennot-Dinet and D. Vaulot. 2001. Grazing impact of two heterotrophic flagellates on *Prochlorococcus* and *Synechococcus*. Aquat. Microb. Ecol. 26: 201–207.

Hobbie, J.E., R.J. Daley and S. Jasper. 1977. Use of nucleopore filters for counting bacteria by epifluorescence microscopy. Appl.Environ.Microbiol.33: 1225-1228.

Jiao, N.Z., Y.H. Yang, H. Koshikawa and M. Watanabe. 2002. Influence of hydrographic conditions on picoplankton distribution in the East China Sea. *Aquat. Microb. Ecol.* 30: 37-48.

Joachimsthal, E.L., V. Ivanov, J-H. Tay and S.T-L. Tay. 2003. Flow cytometry and conventional enumeration of microorganisms in ships' ballast water and marine samples. Mar.Poll.Bul. 46: 308-313.

Jochem, F.J. 2001. Morphology and DNA content of bacterioplankton in the northern Gulf of Mexico: analysis by epifluorescence microscopy and flow cytometry. Aquat. Microb. Ecol. 25: 179-194.

Jochem, F.J., P.J. Lavrentyev and M.R. First. 2004. Growth and grazing rates of bacteria groups with different apparent DNA content in the Gulf of Mexico, Mar. Biol. 145: 1213–1225.

Krstulović, N. 1992. Bacterial biomass and production rates in the central Adriatic. Acta Adriat. 33: 49-65.

Krstulović, N., T. Pucher-Petković and M. Šolić. 1995. The relation between bacterioplankton and phytoplankton production in the mid Adriatic Sea. Aquat. Microb. Ecol. 9: 41-45.

Krstulović, N., M. Šolić and I. Marasović. 1997. Relationship between bacteria, phytoplankton and heterotrophic nanoflagellates along the trophic gradient. Helgöland. Meeresuntersuch. 51: 433-443.

Lebaron, P., M. Troussellier and P. Got. 1993. Accuracy and precision of epifluorescence microscopy count for direct estimates of bacterial numbers. J.Microbiol.Meth.19: 89-94.

Lebaron, P., N. Parthuisot and P.Catala. 1998. Comparison of blue nucleic acid dyes for flow cytometric enumeration of bacteria in aquatic systems. Appl.Environ.Microbiol. 64: 1725-1730.

Li, W.K.W., T. Zohary, Z. Yacobi and A.M. Wood. 1993: Ultraphytoplankton in the eastern Mediterranean Sea: towards deriving phytoplankton biomass from flow cytometric measurements of abundance, fluorescence and light scatter. Mar. Ecol. Prog. Ser. 102: 79–87.

Li, W.K.W., J.F. Jellett and P.M. Dickie. 1995. DNA distribution in planktonic bacteria stained with TOTO or TO-PRO. Limnol. Oceanog. 40: 1485-1495.

López-Lozano, A., J. Diez, S. El Alaoui, C. Moreno-Vivián and J.M. García-Fernández. 2002. Nitrate is reduced by heterotrophic bacteria but not transferred to *Prochlorococcus* non axenic cultures. FEMS Microb. Ecol .41: 151–160.

Marie, D., D. Vaulot and F. Partensky. 1996. Application of the novel nucleic acid dyes YOYO-1, YO-PRO-1, and PicoGreen for flow cytometric analysis of marine prokaryotes. Appl.Environ.Microbiol .62: 1649-1655.

Marie, D., F. Partensky, S. Jacquet and D. Vaulot. 1997. Enumeration and cell cycle analysis of natural populations of marine picoplankton by flow cytometry using the nucleic acid stain SYBR Green I. Appl. Environ. Microb. 63: 186-193.

Marasović, I. i sur. 2006. *Biološke osobine* pp. 68-81. u Kušpilić. G. i sur. Kontrola kakvoće obalnog mora (Projekt Vir-Konavle 2005). Studije i elaborati Instituta za oceanografiju i ribarstvo, Split.

Martin, V. 1997. Etude par cytometrie en flux de la distribution des populations phytoplanctoniques en Mediterranée. Mise en relation avec la production metabolique de CO2 et comparaison avec le golfe du Saint-Laurent. Thesis: Université de la Mediterranée. 250 p.

Monger, B.C. and M. R.Landry. 1993. Flow cytometric analysis of marine bacteria with Hoechst 33342. Appl.Environ.Microbiol. 59: 905-911.

Moore, L.R., G. Rocap, and S.W. Chisholm. 1998. Physiology and molecular phylogeny of coexisting *Prochlorococcus* ecotypes. Nature. 393: 464-467.

Moore, L.R., A.F. Post, G. Rocap and S.W. Chisholm. 2002. Utilization of Different Nitrogen Sources by the Marine Cyanobacteria *Prochlorococcus* and *Synechococcus*. Limnol. Oceanogr. 47: 989-996.

Neuer, S. 1992. Growth dynamics of marine *Synechococcus* spp in the Gulf of Alaska. Mar. Ecol. Prog. Ser. 83: 251-262.

Ninčević Gladan, Ž., I. Marasović, G. Kušpilić, N. Krstulović, M. Šolić and S. Šestanović. 2006. Abundance and composition of picoplankton in the mid Adriatic Sea. Acta Adriat. 47: 127-140.

Olson, R.J. S.W. Chisholm, E.R. Zettler and E.V. Armbrust. 1990. Pigments, Size, and Distribution of *Synechococcus* in the North Atlantic and Pacific Oceans. Limnol. Oceanogr. 35: 45-58.

Olson, R.J., S.W. Chisholm, E.R. Zettler and E.V. Armbrust. 1988. Analysis of *Synechococcus* pigment types in the sea using single and dual beam flow cytometry. Deep Sea Res. 35: 425-440.

Pan, L.A., L.H. Zhang, J. Zhang, J.M. Gasol and M.Chao. 2005. On-board flow cytometric observation of picoplankton community structure in the East China Sea during the fall of different years. FEMS Microb. Ecol. 52: 243–253.

Pan, L.A., J. Zhang and L.H. Zhang. 2007. Picophytoplankton, nanophytoplankton, heterotrohpic bacteria and viruses in the Changjiang Estuary and adjacent coastal waters. J. Plankton Res. 29: 187-197.

Paoli, A. and P. Del Negro. 2006. Bacterial abundances in the Gulf of Trieste waters from 1993 to 2004. Biol. Mar. Medit. 13: 141–148.

Partensky, F., J. Blanchot, and D. Vaulot. 1999a. Differential distribution and ecology of *Prochlorococcus* and *Synechococcus* in oceanic waters: a review. Bull. Inst. Oceanogr. Monaco Numero Spec. 19: 431-449.

Partensky, F., W.R. Hess and D.Vaulot. 1999b. *Prochlorococcus*, a marine photosynthetic prokaryote of global significance. *Microb. Mol. Biol. Rev.* 63: 106–127.

Porter, K.G. and Y.S. Feig. 1980. The use of DAPI for identifying and counting aquatic microflora. Limnol.Oceanol. 25: 943-948.

Porter, J., D. Deere, M. Hardman, C. Edwards and R. Pickup. 1997. Go with the flow: use of flow cytometry in environmental microbiology. FEMS Microbiol. Ecol. 24: 93–101.

Radić, T., T. Šilović, D. Šantić, D. Fuks and M. Mičić. 2009. Preliminary flow cytometric analyses of phototrophic pico-and nanoplankton communities in the Northern Adriatic. Fresen. Environ. Bull. 18: 715-724.

Raven, J.A. 1986. Physiological consequences of extremely small size for autotrophic organisms in the sea. In: Photosyntetic picoplankton. Pp. 1-70. Platt T, Li WKW (eds) Can. Bull. Fish. Aquat. Sci. 214.

Shapiro, L.P, and E.M. Haugen. 1988. Seasonal distribution and tolerance of *Synechococcus* in Boothbay harbor, maine. Estuar. Coast. Shelf. Sci. 26:517-525.

Sieracki, M.E., E.M. Haugen and T.L. Cucci. 1995.Overestimation of heterotrophic bacteria in the Sargasso Sea. Direct evidence by flow and imaging cytometry. Deep-Sea Res. Part I 42: 1399-1409.

Shapiro, H. M. 1995. Practical flow cytometry, 3rd ed. Wiley-Liss, New York, N.Y.

Sommaruga, R., J.S. Hofer, L. Alonso-Sáez and J.M. Gasol. 2005. Differential sunlight sensitivity of picophytoplankton from surface Mediterranean coastal waters. Appl. Environ. Microbiol. 71:2157-2157.

Šantić, D., N. Krstulović and M. Šolić. 2007. Comparison of flow cytometric and epifluorescent counting methods for marine heterotrophic bacteria. Acta Adriatic. 48: 107-114.

Šantić, D., N. Krstulović, M. Šolić, Mladen and G. Kušpilić, 2011. Distribution of *Synechococcus* and *Prochlorococcus* in the central Adriatic Sea. Acta Adriatic. 52 : 101-113.

Šolić, M., N. Krstulović and S. Šestanović. 2001. The roles of predation, substrate suply and temperature in controlling bacterial abundance : interaction between spatial and seasonal scale. Acta Adriat. 42: 35-48.

Šolić, M., N. Krstulović, I.Vilibić, G. Kušpilić S. Šestanović, D. Šantić and M. Ordulj. 2008. The role of water mass dynamics in controlling bacterial abundance and production in the middle Adriatic Sea. Mar. Environ. Res. 65: 388-404.

Šolić, M., N. Krstulović, I. Vilibić, N. Bojanić, G. Kušpilić, S. Šestanović, D. Šantić and M. Ordulj. 2009. Variability in the bottom-up and top-down control of bacteria on trophic and temporal scale in the middle Adriatic Sea. Aquat. Microb. Ecol. 58: 15–29.

Šolić, M., N. Krstulović, G. Kušpilić, Ž. Ninčević Gladan, N. Bojanić, S. Šestanović, D. Šantić and M. Ordulj. 2010.Changes in microbial food web structure in response to changed environmental trophic status: A case study of the Vranjic Basin (Adriatic Sea). Mar. Environ. Res.70: 239-249.

Troussellier, M., C. Courties and A. Vaquer. 1993. Recent applications of flow cytometry in aquatic microbial ecology. Biol. Cell. 78: 111–121.

Uysal, Z. and İ. Köksalan. 2006. The annual cycle of *Synechococcus* (cyanobacteria) in the northern Levantine Basin shelf waters (Eastern Mediterranean). Mar. Ecol. 27:187–197.

Vaquer, A., M. Troussellier, C. Courties and B. Bibent, 1996: Standing stock and dynamics of picophytoplankton in the Thau Lagoon (northwest Mediterranean coast). Limnol. Oceanogr. 41: 1821–1828.

Vaulot D., F. Partensky, J. Neveux., R.F.C. Mantoura and C. Llewellyn. 1990. Winter presence of prochlorophytes in surface waters of the northwestern Mediteranean Sea. Limnol. Oceanogr. 35: 1156-1164.

Vaulot, D. and F.Partensky. 1992. Cell cycle distributions of prochlorophytes in the North Western Mediterranean Sea. Deep Sea Res. 39: 727-742.

Viličić, D., M. Kuzmić, S. Bosak, T. Šilović, E. Hrustić and Z. Burić. 2009. Distribution of phytoplankton along the thermohaline gradient in the north-eastern Adriatic channel; winter aspect. Oceanologya. 51: 495-513.

Waterbury, J.B., S.W. Watson, F.W. Valois and D.G. Franks. 1986b. "Biological and ecological characterization of the marine unicellular cyanobacterium *Synechococcus*". Can. J. Fish. Aquat. Sci. 214: 71–120.

Wehr, J. D. 1993. Effects of experimental manipulations of light and phosphorus supply on competition among picoplankton and nanoplankton in an oligotrophic lake. Can. J. Fish. Aquat. Sci.50: 936–945.

Worden, A.Z., J.K Nolan and B. Palenik. 2004. Assessing the dynamics and ecology of marine picophytoplankton: the importance of the eukaryotic component. Limnol. Oceanogr. 49: 168–179.

Zhang, Y., N.Z. Jiao and N. Hong. 2008. Comparative study of picoplankton biomass and community structure in different provinces from Subarctic to Subtropical oceans. Deep-Sea Res. Part II. 55: 1605- 1614.

Zubkov, M.V., B.M. Fuchs, P.H. Burkill and R. Amann. 2001a. Comparison of cellular and biomass specific activities of dominant bacterioplankton groups in stratified waters of the Celtic Sea. Appl. Environ. Microbiol. 67: 5210–5218.

Zweifel, U. L. and Å. Hagström. 1995. Total counts of marine bacteria include a large fraction of non-nucleoid-containing bacteria (ghosts). Appl. Environ. Microbiol. 61: 2180-2185.

3

Flow Cytometry as a Powerful Tool for Monitoring Microbial Population Dynamics in Sludge

Audrey Prorot, Philippe Chazal and Patrick Leprat
Groupement de Recherche Eau Sol et Environnement (GRESE), Université de Limoges, France

1. Introduction

Flow cytometry is a technology that simultaneously measures and analyses multiple physical characteristics of single particles, usually cells, as they flow in a fluid stream through a beam of light. The properties measured include a particle's relative size (represented by forward angle light scatter), relative granularity or internal complexity (represented by right-angle scatter), and relative fluorescence intensity. These characteristics are determined using an optical-to-electronic coupling system which records how the cell or particle scatters incident laser light and emits fluorescence. A wide range of dyes, which may bind or intercalate with different cellular components, can be used as labels for applications in a number of fields, including molecular biology, immunology, plant biology, marine biology and environmental microbiology. Interest in rapid methods and automation for prokaryotic cell studies in environmental microbiology has been growing over the past few years.

There are several available methods for the detection and enumeration of microorganisms in raw and processed environmental samples. Culture techniques are the most common, but a major disadvantage of these is their failure to isolate viable but nonculturable organisms (Davey & Kell, 1996). Actually, in both natural samples and axenic cultures in the laboratory, there is clear evidence of the presence of intermediate cell states which remain undetectable by classical methods (Kell *et al.*, 1998). In recent years, this fact has generated a great confusion in the scientific community as to the concept of cell viability. The reality is that the absence of colonies on solid media does not necessarily mean that cells are dead at the time of sampling (Nebe-von-Caron *et al.*, 2000).

Various other methods have been developed in order to investigate the problems associated with culture-based detection systems. Among these methods, flow cytometry has become a valuable tool for rapidly enumerating microorganisms and allowing the detection and discrimination of viable culturable, viable nonculturable and nonviable organisms. There is also the possibility that numerous (or even rare) microbial cells could be detected against a background of other bacteria or nonbacterial particles by combining flow cytometry and specific fluorescent probes. In this case, the objective is to label cells with different structural properties or else differing in their activity or functionality.

Since the practical and accurate microbial assessment of environmental systems is predicated on the detection and quantification of various microbial parameters in complex matrices, flow cytometry represents an accurate tool in environmental microbiology and in particular for bioprocesses monitoring.

Considerable research has been devoted over recent decades to the optimisation and control of biological wastewater treatment processes. Many treatment processes have been studied so as to increase the methane potential of sludge with a rate-limiting hydrolysis stage of organic matter associated with microbial cells. Although a great deal of information about sludge minimisation processes is currently available in WWTP (i.e., sonication, ozonation or thermal treatment), little data is available as to its fundamental mechanisms, especially microbial changes.

The most common parameter used for quantifying activated sludge is the content of suspended solids, expressed as Total Suspended Solids (TSSs) or Volatile Suspended Solids (VSSs). However, VSSs do not coincide with the effective bacterial biomass in activated sludge because they also include endogenous biomass (the residue produced by bacterial death and lysis) and organic non-biotic particulate matter fed into the plant with the influent wastewater (Foladori *et al.*, 2010a). On the one hand, the bacterial biomass in activated sludge is generally estimated by theoretical calculations based on substrate mass balances using kinetic and stoichiometric parameters (Henze, 2000). On the other hand, knowledge of the amount of bacterial biomass and the physiological state of microorganisms in an activated sludge system represents key parameters for understanding the processes, kinetics and dynamics of substrate removal (Foladori *et al.*, 2010b).

Early investigations which aimed to recover bacteria from activated sludge for quantification were based on cultivation methods. For a long time, no routine methods have been proposed to rapidly quantify the bacterial biomass in activated sludge and wastewater. To obtain a more accurate view of bacterial populations, the application of *in situ* techniques or direct molecular approaches are needed (Foladori *et al.*, 2010b). With regard to the recovery of bacteria from complex matrices such as sludge in order to count them, sonication has been proposed in several studies so as to disaggregate activated sludge flocs while maintaining cell viability (Falcioni *et al.*, 2006a;Foladori *et al.*, 2007;Foladori *et al.*, 2007 and Foladori *et al.*, 2010a) or to induce cell lysis and bacteria inactivation (Zhang *et al.*, 2007). In the same manner, the characterisation of the impact of enhanced hydrolysis by the pre-treatments mentioned above (sonication, ozonation and thermal treatment) in terms of microbial activity (active cells able to convert organic matter) and viability (cell lysis with the resulting release of intracellular material) remain fundamental for sludge reduction optimisation (Prorot *et al.*, 2011).

The procedure recently developed by Ziglio *et al.* (2002) to disaggregate sludge flocs before staining (with dyes), and flow cytometry analysis has demonstrated that fluorescent dyes combined with this technique can be a valuable tool for the assessment of the viability and activity of an activated sludge mixed-bacterial population. These studies indicated that flow cytometry allows a rapid and accurate quantification of the total bacterial population, including the viable nonculturable fraction, and consequently that flow cytometry represents an appropriate tool for activated sludge investigations.

This review seeks to highlight the interest of the technique of flow cytometry for quantitative and qualitative bacterial biomass monitoring in activated or anaerobic sludge.

In the first part, we review the basic principles of flow cytometry and its use in different areas in environmental microbiology. As cells differ in their metabolic or physiological states, we presented the flow cytometry potentialities in order to allow for the detection of different subpopulations according to their structural or physiological parameters. We describe the strategies used for cell detection (scattering and fluorescence signals) and the cellular targets associated with fluorescent probes which are currently used in assays related to microbial assessment in environmental systems, and especially those related to sludge investigations. The second part is devoted to a discussion of the concept of cell viability and functionality, with a detailed review of the different intermediate physiological states between cellular life and death. Next, a concise revision concerning the most recent applications of flow cytometry related to cell analyses and quantification in sludge processes is presented. Finally, a general conclusion provides an overview of the main perspectives related to this powerful technique for the sludge treatment process.

2. Flow cytometry technique

Flow cytometry is a quantitative technology for the rapid individual analysis of large numbers of cells in a mixture, using light scattering and fluorescence measurements. The power of this method lies both in the wide range of cellular parameters that can be determined and in its ability to obtain information on how these parameters are distributed in the cell population.

2.1 Basic principles

Flow cytometry uses the principles of light scattering, light excitation and the emission of fluorochrome molecules to generate specific multi-parameter data from particles and cells within the size range of 0.5 um to 40 um diameter. A common flow cytometer is formed by several basic units (Díaz *et al.*, 2010): a light source (lasers are most often used), a flow cell and hydraulic fluidic system, several optical filters to select specific wavelengths, a group of photodiodes or photomultiplier tubes to detect the signals of interest and, finally, a data processing unit (Figure 1).

Light scattering occurs when a particle or a cell deflects incident laser light. The extent to which this occurs depends on the physical properties of a cell, namely its size and internal complexity. Factors that affect light scattering are the cell membrane, the nucleus and any granular material inside the cell. Cell shape and surface topography also contribute to the total light scatter. The forward scatter light (FSC - light scatter at low angles) provides information on cell size, although there is no direct correlation between size and FSC (Julià *et al.*, 2000). Light scattered in an orthogonal direction can also be collected by a different detector (a side scatter or SSC detector), which provides information about granularity and cell morphology.

The most common type of quantitative analysis using flow cytometry data involves creating a histogram of fluorescence events to count the number of cells with the attached probe. This effectively creates a set of data which gives a ratio of the cells in a population with a particular structural parameter or else with a specific functional property. Except for fluorescence naturally produced by some intracellular compounds, fluorescence signals are generally produced consecutive to the staining of sample-containing cells with dyes related to structural or functional parameters as physiological probes. These dyes are specifically bound and - after excitation with the laser beams - fluoresce, giving quantitative information on the respective cell parameters.

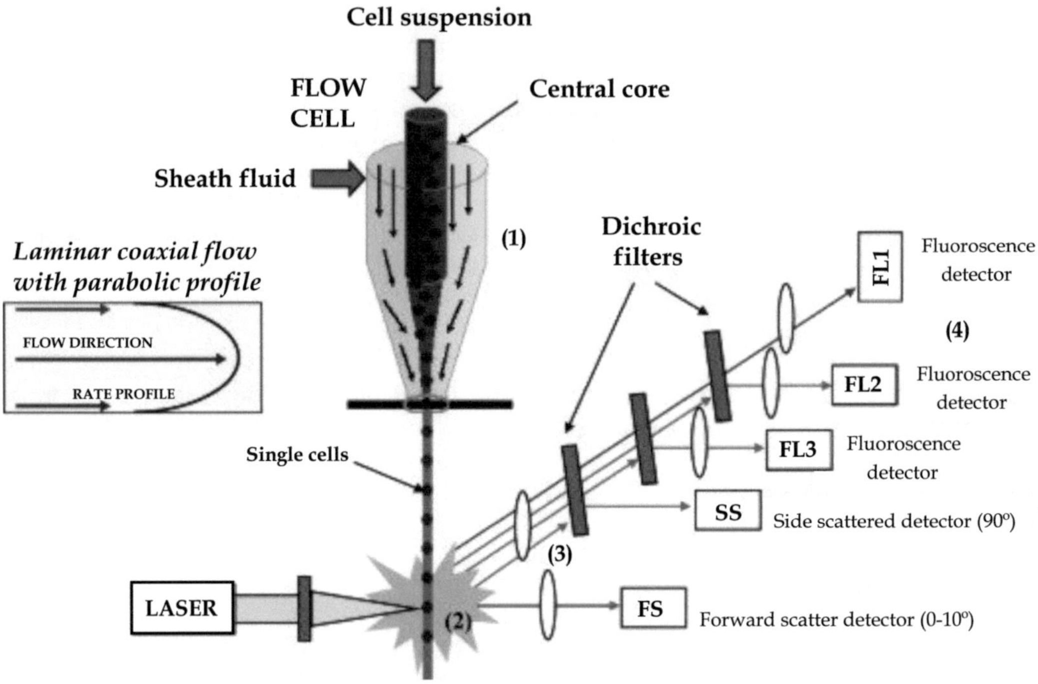

Fig. 1. Scheme of and principles behind a typical flow cytometer (from (Díaz *et al.*, 2010): the cell suspension or mixture containing cells is hydro-dynamically focused in a sheath fluid before passing excitation sources, such as laser beams. The combined flow is reduced in diameter, forcing the cells into the centre of the stream (1). These cells are aligned to pass, single file, through a laser beam and impact with the laser in a confined site, emitting different signals related to diverse cell parameters (2). For each cell or particle, a multi-parametric analysis is made using a combination of dyes which have different properties and subcellular specificities. The emitted and scattered light resulting from the cell-laser intersection are divided into appropriate colours using a group of wavelength-selective mirrors and filters (3). The signals are collected by the detection system, which is formed by a collection of photodiodes, two scattering and different fluorescence (FL1, FL2, FL3) detectors (4). Finally, signals are sent to a computer, thereby obtaining a representation of the distribution of the population with respect to the different parameters

The intensity of the optical signals generated (scattering and/or fluorescence signals) is therefore correlated to structural and/or functional cell parameters (Davey & Kell, 1996). A combination of light-scattering and fluorescence measurements on stained or unstained cells allows for the detection of multiple cellular parameters. Depending on the dye used, many of these measurements can be done simultaneously on the same cells. The scatter and fluorescence signals detected can be combined in various ways to allow for the detection of subpopulations (Comas-Riu & Rius, 2009). This contrasts with spectrophotometry, in which the percentage of the absorption and transmission of specific wavelengths of light is measured for a bulk volume of the sample.

2.2 Cell parameter measurements

Flow cytometric assays have been developed to determine both cellular characteristics (such as size, membrane potential and intracellular pH) and the levels of cellular components (such as DNA, protein or surface receptors). Flow cytometry is generally used in microbial cell analysis for rapid counting, the study of heterogeneous bacterial populations, strain improvement in industrial microbiology, and in order to sort bacteria for further molecular analysis (Díaz *et al.*, 2010);(Müller & Nebe-von-Caron, 2010)(Müller *et al.*, 2010)(Comas-Riu & Rius, 2009). In microbiological applications using one or several dyes, the main objective is the labelling of cells with different structural properties or differing in their activity or functionality (Díaz *et al.*, 2010)(Achilles *et al.*, 2006).

Measurements that reveal the heterogeneous distribution in bacterial cell populations are important for bioprocesses because they describe the population better than the average values obtained from traditional techniques (Rieseberg *et al.*, 2001), and consequently they provide a valuable tool for bioprocess design and control (Díaz *et al.*, 2010). Although many different measurements are possible, only those most related to the study of microbial population dynamics in environmental and water systems will now be discussed. An earlier review has already summarised the flow cytometry potentialities for single-cell analysis in environmental microbiology (Czechowska & Johnson, 2008).

Actually, the data mainly sought in environmental microbiology has been focused on the analysis of the physiological state of bacteria in different microbial ecosystems, including sludge. Plate-culturing techniques only reveal a small proportion (viable and cultivable bacteria) of the total microbial population. This can be explained mainly by the inability of microorganisms that are either stressed or which have entered into a non-cultivable state to growth on conventional plating techniques (Giraffa, 2004)(Lahtinen *et al.*, 2005). One promising tool of flow cytometry consists of characterising and distinguishing different the physiological states of microorganisms at the single-cell level (Joux & Lebaron, 2000) (Nebe-von-Caron *et al.*, 2000). The ability of flow cytometry to distinguish between different physiological states is important for assessing the growth of microorganisms in oligotrophic environments (Berney *et al.*, 2007), the survival of pathogenic microorganisms (Vital *et al.*, 2007) and the effects of bactericidal treatments or different environmental stresses on microbial activity (Prorot *et al.*, 2008)(Ziglio *et al.*, 2002)(Foladori *et al.*, 2010a)(Booth, Ian R, 2002). When employed in conjunction with fluorescent dyes, flow cytometry is able to measure various biological parameters (i.e., nucleic acid content, metabolic activity, enzyme activity and membrane integrity), allowing the detection of microorganisms at viable, viable but non-cultivable (or intermediate) and non-viable states (Joux & Lebaron, 2000)(Walberg *et al.*, 1999).

One widely-used strategy for analysing viable and dead bacterial cells in environmental samples was done on the basis of membrane integrity, coupling a cell-impermeant dye - such as propidium iodide - and a cell-permeant dye, like most of the SYTO family or SYBR (Berney *et al.*, 2007)(Ziglio *et al.*, 2002). Dyes from the SYTO family and propidium iodide are nucleic acid-binding probes and are, with others, well described.

In this approach, all cells are supposed to incorporate SYTO and fluoresce green. Only dead or damaged cells (considered as associated with the loss of cell membrane integrity) are permeable for propidium iodide, and the cells thus fluoresce red (Czechowska & Johnson, 2008). Thanks to this approach, the transition phases between viable and non-viable states have been observed for different microbial ecosystems (e.g., when bacterial cells in drinking water are irradiated by UVA) (Berney *et al.*, 2007). In this case, cells in intermediate states displayed high levels of both green and red fluorescence. For this purpose, Molecular Probes Inc. (Leiden, The Netherlands) has developed a fluorescent stain - the LIVE/DEAD BacLight™ bacterial viability kit - which is composed of SYTO9™ and propidium iodide. This last dye can also be used alone to assess membrane integrity (Shi *et al.*, 2008).

Another method is proposed to deduce cellular activity from the amount of nucleic acid within the cell (Kleinsteuber *et al.*, 2006)(Servais *et al.*, 2003). However, this method is based on the use of a nucleic acid binding fluorescent dye that has been recently critically discussed by (Bouvier *et al.*, 2007). From a wide range of environmental communities, they have demonstrated that nucleic acid contents do not necessary correlate with differences in metabolic activity. The use of the redox dye 5-cyano-2,3ditolyl tetrazolium chloride (CTC) is also available for discriminating between active (respiring cells) and non-active (non-respiring cells) populations of microorganisms, although this technique does not always show consistent results (Longnecker *et al.*, 2005;Czechowska & Johnson, 2008).

The uptake of a growth substrate by a cell represents the first step of metabolism. Therefore, fluorescently marked substrates can be used to obtain information on either substrate transport mechanisms, enzyme activity or the viability of cells (Sträuber & Müller, 2010). For example, the non-fluorescent esterase substrate fluorescein di-acetate (FDA) is cleaved by esterases in viable cells, releasing fluorescein which stains the cells green. FDA could ideally be used in combination with propidium, which stains non-viable cells red (Veal *et al.*, 2000).

3. Cell viability and functionality

3.1 Cell viability and physiological target sites

The impact of micro-organisms on the environment has been widely investigated via studies based on the growth characteristics of viable cells, and on the related consequences of microbial proliferation. Bacteria were the most extensively studied, using quantitative methods set on the determination of the number of colony-forming units. If the plate count methods could not be used, because of a wide variety of reasons (unknown growth requirements, auxotrophic micro-organisms, etc.), cultures in liquid media followed by a statistical treatment of values could lead to interesting interpretations, although with much less accuracy than those obtained with Petri plates.

However, cells which are unable to cultivate may possess basic metabolic capacities which could influence the environment accordingly (Sträuber & Müller, 2010). Furthermore, and in a theoretical sense, attention should be paid to dead cells resulting from severe - and thus irreversible - structural damage. Dead cells may release numerous molecules, ranging from small-sized ones to macromolecules. They may induce the cryptic growth of other living cells or act as chelating agents, and the listing of such possible forms of interference is far from exhaustive.

FCM was first applied to eukaryotic cells, but in the late 1970s this technology began to be used for the study of prokaryotic cells (mostly bacteria) (Steen *et al.*, 1982; Allman *et al.*, 1992) and yeasts (Scheper *et al.*, 1987). FCM gained interest with its application to industrial microbial processes (Díaz *et al.*, 2010). Other fields of application have appeared to be of interest, such as the optimisation of SRP (sludge reduction processes) (Prorot *et al.*, 2008; Prorot *et al.*, 2011).

The development of fields of application for FCM was accompanied with research seeking a better understanding of cellular bacterial viability. Apart from irreversibly dead cells, the main cellular states were commonly sorted into two classes: viable and able to cultivate cells and viable but unable to cultivate cells.

This classification into three groups (irreversibly dead, cultivable, viable but non-cultivable cells) could be improved by taking into account various intermediate states, and especially those concerning viable but non-cultivable cells. This requires the fixing beforehand of an adequate definition of cellular viability. The viability of a cell is its capacity to live. We chose, as point of departure, the definition back by a high degree of scientific authority, namely the NASA definition (definition 1) (Joyce *et al.*, 1994):

(Definition 1) "Life is a self-sustained chemical system capable of undergoing Darwinian evolution"

The publication of this definition aroused numerous amendments aiming to approach it in a more precise way at the level of the cell. Luisi (1998) proposed several interesting amendments based on various points of view. The first definition emanates from the point of view of the biochemist (definition 2):

(Definition 2) "a system which is spatially defined by a semipermeable compartment of its own making and which is self-sustaining by transforming external energy/nutrients by its own process of components production"

Considering the geneticist's view, the same author in the same paper proposed definition 3:

(Definition 3) "a system which is self-sustaining by utilising external energy/nutrients owing to its internal process of components production and coupled to the medium via adaptive changes which persist during the time history of the system"

At present, no definitive definition has met with general approval. Some attempts have been made to investigate the different states of bacterial viability. The existence of three bacterial viability states was admitted by Barer (1997):

1. dead cells
2. viable but non-cultivable cells (VBNC)
3. colony-forming cells

Bogosian (2001) investigated the intermediate cellular state(s) of VBNC cells. This author discussed works relating the (weakly) possible resuscitation of injured bacteria exhibiting the characteristics of VBNCs for a long time before their resuscitation by using appropriate techniques. The need for a better understanding of such intermediate cellular states appeared after the work of several authors who developed cytological methods for investigating them and who provided interesting data concerning these states (Czechowska & Johnson, 2008; Sträuber & Müller, 2010).

Thus we proposed a definition based on and adapted from the former definitions in order to improve the classification of the various states of cellular life, by taking into account the "intermediate viability states" (concerning the VBNCs). This approach is referred to by definition 4.

(Definition 4) "Cellular viability is the property of any system bounded by a semipermeable membrane of its own manufacturing and potentially capable of auto-speaking, of reproducing almost as before by making its own constituents from energy and\or from outer (foreign) elements and to evolve according to its environment"

Accordingly, we admitted that a bacterium could be classified as viable if the following criteria were satisfied:

1. maintenance of membrane integrity (structure and functions)
2. normal gene expression, protein synthesis and division (scissiparity) control
3. maintenance of metabolic activity (for both catabolism and anabolism)

We hypothesised the existence of five physiological states according to environmental conditions (varying from the worst to the most favourable ones for the cell):

State 1: corresponds to the worst one (irreversible damage). Different states evolve up to the most favourable one (state 5, or standard cell growth, allowing colony formation). The originality of the classification lies in the appearance of new intermediate states (3 and 4):(

State 3: this state corresponds to wounded cells but differs from state 2, because they can resuscitate under well-defined conditions

State 4: this state corresponds to endospores. Endospores can form colonies when inoculated in favorable growth media. Nevertheless endospores cannot be classified within state 5, because typical bacteria of state 5 form colonies originating from viable vegetative cells (the physiology of which greatly differing from the endospores one)

Additional comments should be made in order to complete the data provided by Table 1.

State 1: This state should correspond to cells which were in contact with harsh physico-chemical conditions, for instance after a Ultra High Temperature (UHT) thermal treatment as generally proceeds in the food industry (135°-150° for 15 seconds). The cellular corpses may be observed via microscopy, but no detectable sign of life can be determined (e.g., enzymatic activities). Extreme pH values, violent osmotic shock or starvation conditions can also lead to death or the appearance of such a physiological state.

The influence of dead microbial cells should not be underestimated, because they can provide nutrients for the growth of other bacteria inoculated in the medium after the physico-chemical conditions return to acceptable levels. Some dead cell components can also interfere with biofilms' evolution. Working in the field of bacterial adhesion, Mai-Prochnow *et al.* (2004) studied the development of the multicellular biofilm of *Pseudomonas tunicata* They discovered a novel 190-kDa autotoxic protein produced by this Pseudomonas, designated AlpP. They found that this protein was involved in the killing of the biofilm and its detachment. An Δ*AlpP* mutant derivative of *P. tunicata* was generated, and this mutant did not show cell death during biofilm development. Thus, (MaiProchnow *et al.*, 2004) proposed that AlpP-mediated cell death plays an important role in the development of the multicellular biofilm of *P. tunicata* and the subsequent dispersal of surviving cells within the marine environment.

State	State characteristics	Examples of causes of such damages	Some effects on the environment
1	Irreversible death, cells still observable using microscopy. No sign of any biological activity is detectable (e.g., residual enzymatic activity). Loss of membrane integrity.	Excessive physico-chemical parameters values (temperature, pH, ionic strength, etc.), the action of drugs, chemical effectors, radiations, biological inhibitors, prolonged starvation, etc.	No biological activity is detected. Nevertheless, chemicals of a biological origin may interfere. The presence of dead cell components (EPS) can favour biofilm formation. They can also provide nutrients for further cryptic growth.
2	Wounded cell, possibility of repair(s) allowing survival, membrane integrity remains intact, but the cell is non-cultivable.	The same as above but to a much lower extent.	Resting cells with their effects remaining to be determined. In addition to the potential role of chemicals as nutrients and/or biofilms' starters, some residual enzymatic activities to be determined could influence the environment (for instance oxidation or reduction processes).
3	Wounded cell, possibility of repair(s) allowing survival. Physiological state close to state 2. Regrowth might be possible, but under well-defined conditions and after a long "lag phase".	The same type as above (state 2).	Some pathogenic bacteria lose their capacity for growth after a prolonged starvation period in a media poor in nutrients. After re-inoculation in living organisms, pathogenicity reappears after a period of time, which can be of a great magnitude.
4	Wounded cells, possibility of repair(s), growth possible when conditions are favourable. After adaptation, the characteristics of survivors appear to be identical to the ones of the initial cells. This is the case of so-called "spores forming cells"	Intermediate between the conditions of states 1 and 2.	Regrowth of pathogens in products which are badly sterilised.
5	Viable cells, cultivable (colony-forming).	These are the standard colony forming units on Petri plates, or else cultivable in adequate liquid media	The usual effects of living bacteria (positive or negative for the environment).

Table 1. The different physiological bacterial cellular states

State 2: A recent paper by Ben Said *et al.* (2010) provides an excellent example of this category. They irradiated a strain of E. coli with UV. They noted a 99.99% decrease of viable cells (colony forming units) from 45 mJ/cm^2. In studying the potential evolution of the cells' viability, they employed a useful tool : the Qb phage (RNA). They checked the lytic effect of this phage on the population before and after irradiation (doses higher than 45 mJ/cm^2 were investigated up to 120 mJ/cm^2). They studied the P'/P_0 ratio as a function of the irradiation dose (0 for the blank and from 45 to 120 mJ/cm^2 irradiation doses). P' was the Qb phage units number after 18 hours of incubation at 37°C, and P_0 was the initiated free-phage concentration at time 0.

At time 0 (UV dose = 0), this ratio was close to 10^4. At 45 mJ/cm^2 the ration fell to 10^3, whereas a 99.99% decrease of viable cells was determined. The presence of 0.01% residual cultivable cells could not justify by itself the P'/Po ration value (10^3) if only viable and cultivable cells would allow the phage's growth. This showed that, even if the major part of the bacterial population was killed by UV, the dead cells could nevertheless induce Qb phage replication. This also showed that UV did not integrally destroy any "vital" function of *Escherichia coli* cells..The ones implied in phage multiplication would have been affected to a low extent or just preserved. For higher UV doses, the P'/P_0 ration proportionally decreased as a function of the UV dose, and at 120 mJ/cm^2 the ratio was still around 10^1. This showed that much higher UV doses appeared to be required in order to really affect the major vital functions of the cells.

Qb phage replication depends, at first, on its fixation on the cell membrane. For a second time, the RNA has to cross over the membrane to reach the cytoplasm. Once in the cytoplasm replication of Qb phage only occurs if intact or repaired components of the host cells are available. This experiment proved that the membrane's integrity was persistent and a major part of the cellular components remained active, whereas cellular division could not occur.

The authors hypothesised that the transformation of vegetative cells into VBNC could be a strategy developed by the cell in order to survive the action of UV.

State 3: This state is related to bacteria which were in contact with unfavourable growth conditions that greatly affected cellular viability, but which were able to give rise to colonies on Petri plates when treated adequately. The word "resuscitation" was often cited to describe this phenomenon. (Steinert *et al.*, 1997; Whitesides & Oliver, 1997). Steinert *et al.*.) (1997) studied *Legionella pneumophila,* an aquatic bacterium responsible for Legionnaire's disease in humans. The legionellae usually parasitise free-living amoebae which provide the accurate environment for the proliferation of these bacteria. When starved (inoculation in low nutrient media), *L. pneumophila* can enter into a VBNC state. These authors inoculated sterilised tap water by a suspension of *L. pneumophila* at 10^4 cells/ml. After 125 days of incubation in tap water, no colony-forming unit appeared on the routine plating media. Counts were made in parallel using the Acridine Orange Direct Count (AODC) method and hybridisation with 16S rRNA-targeted oligonucleotide probes: cells were still detectable.

After this incubation period, cells of *Acanthamoeba castellanii* were added. This led to the "resuscitation" of *L. pneumophila* cells that became cultivable. This tended to show that during the starvation period, the damage that affected the cell was reversible, at least for these latter cells and that the amoeba provided enough elements for reversing the VBNC state. The notion of a survival strategy could be implied in this phenomenon.

A similar phenomenon was evidenced for *Vibrio vulnificus*, a human pathogen responsible for wound infections often leading to septicaemia. For *V. vulnificus*, the VBNC state can be induced by incubation at temperatures below 10°C. Whitesides & Oliver (1997) studied the reversibility of this phenomenon for the latter bacterium. Cells were incubated at 5°C for several days. The total counts were determined via AODC and made-viable CFU by the routine plate count method. Starting from a population of 10^7 viable cells/ml, no CFU occurred after 4 days of incubation, whereas the AODC did not show any significant decrease of the total count. At day 4, the medium was placed for 24h at c.a. 22°C. On day 5 (24h temperature upshift) the CFU value was close to approximately 2.10^6 CFU/ml, apparently showing a "resuscitation" phenomenon. Once more, the damage affecting cells placed at a low temperature could be partially repaired by the temperature upshift described here.

State 4: Bacterial endospores give rise to vegetative cells able to form colonies, but the procedure implied in the "daughter" cells' formation greatly differs from that implied by standard bacterial division. In addition, the structure of the mother cell completely differs from that of the daughter vegetative cells. Furthermore, both sporulation and germination appear as real physiological crises, lasting a relatively long time (10-12 hours) and generally accompanied with the production of highly pathogenic toxins.

The aptitude of bacterial endospores to give rise to viable, cultivable but structurally different cells does not make it possible to classify according to the three previous groups. This validates the existence of a separate state, referred to as State 4 and different from State 5 described below.

State 5: The bacteria are able to form colonies on Petri plates. Their growth in liquid media is accompanied with an increase of optical density (shape, morphology and constitution are identical for "daughter" and "mother" cells. Mutation phenomena are not discussed here). The optimal viability criteria of bacteria of State 5 are those previously noted:

1. maintenance of membrane integrity (structure and functions)
2. normal genes expression, proteins synthesis and division (scissiparity) control
3. maintenance of metabolic activity (for both catabolism and anabolism)

3.2 Fluorescent dyes

There are dozens of Fluorochromes which can aid flow cytometry studies and their number is constantly increasing. The aim of this chapter is not to study them all but rather to show the diversity of dye/cell interactions and the variety of information available according to the type of fluorochrome employed.

Table 2 summarises the properties and the mode of interaction of some of the most commonly used fluorochromes. We classified them into three groups according to the nature of their interactions with cells:

Interactions with nucleic acids. This can provide information about the nuclear content and state of the cell. A given dye can provide indirect information about the physiological state of a given bacterium. For instance, propidium iodide - which binds to DNA or RNA - is normally excluded from healthy cells, being a membrane impermeant. However, if the membrane has been damaged or altered it can more easily cross the latter and stain intracellular components.

Dye	Structure	λ_{em} (nm) and λ_{ex}(nm)	References	Mode of action
Interactions with nucleic acids				
DAPI 4',6'-diamidino-2-phénylindole	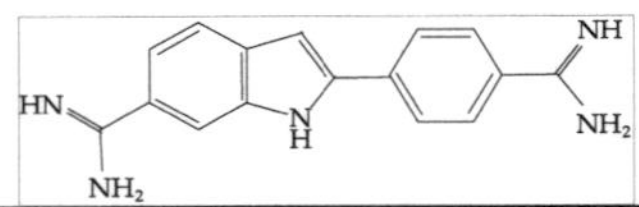	451 357	Kapuscinski (1995) Zink *et al.* (2003)	Binds strongly to A-T rich regions in DNA
Propidium iodide 3,8-diamino-5-[3-(diethylmethylammonio)propyl]-6-phenylphenantridinium diiodide	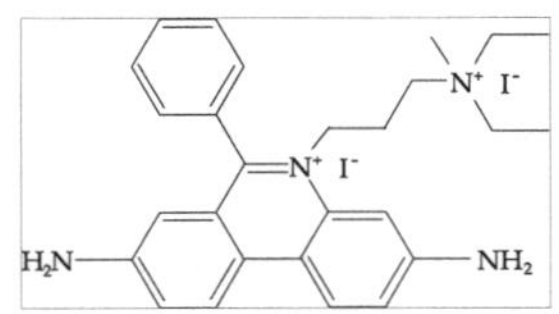	631 370/560	Lecoeur (2002) Moore *et al.* (1998) Jones & Kniss (1987)	Binds to DNA by intercalating between the bases with little or no sequence preference. Also binds to RNA, necessitating its treatment with nucleases so as to distinguish between RNA and DNA staining. Membrane impermeant
Ethidium bromide 3,8-Diamino-5-ethyl-6-phenylphenanthridinium bromide	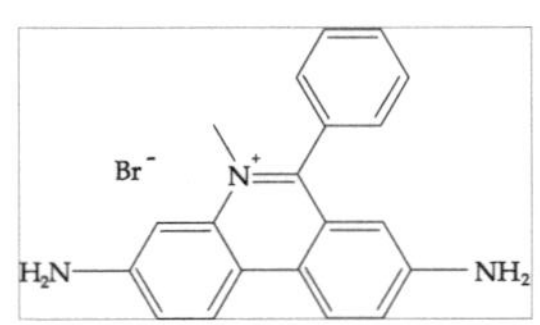	622 370/530	Ohta *et al.* (2001)	Ethidium bromide is a large, flat basic molecule which looks like a DNA base pair. its chemical structure allows it to intercalate into a DNA strand.

Table 2. Continues on next page

Dye	Structure	λ_{em} (nm) and λ_{ex}(nm)	References	Mode of action
Interactions with nucleic acids				
Hoechst 33342, 33258, 34580 Bisbenzimides derivatives	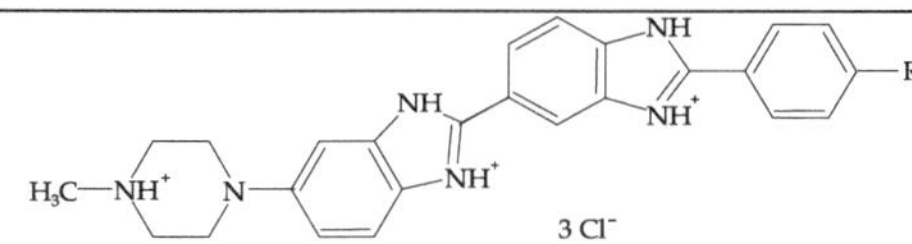 33342, R = - CH_2CH_3 / 33258, R = -OH / 34580, R = -$N(CH_3)_2$	402 For 33342 365 For 33342	Latt & Stetten (1976) Allen *et al.* (2001) Portugal & Waring (1988)	Binds strongly to A-T rich regions in DNA
SYBR green [2-[N-(3-dimethylaminopropyl)- N-propylamino]-4-[2,3-dihydro-3-methyl-(benzo-1,3-thiazol-2-yl)-methylidene]-1-phenyl-quinolinium	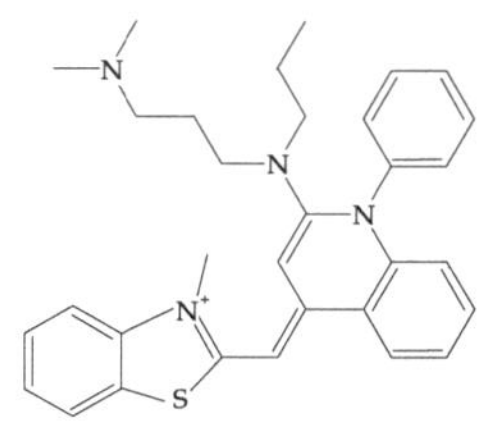	520 497	Ohta *et al.* (2001) Bachoon *et al.* (2001) Kiltie & Ryan (1997)	SYBR Green binds to any type of double stranded DNA. High sensitivity
7-AAD 7 amino-actinomycin D	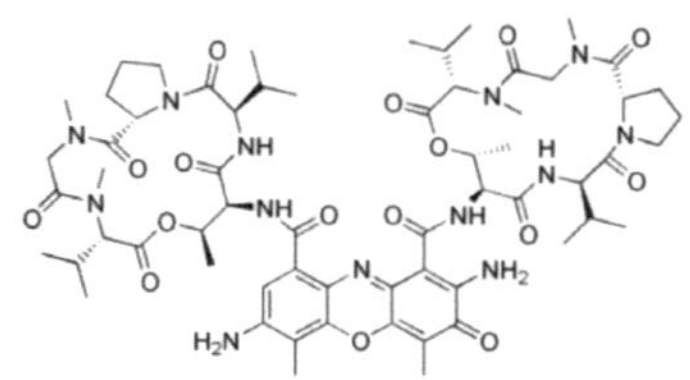	650 488	Schmid *et al.* (1992)	7-AAD intercalates in double-stranded DNA, with a high affinity for GC-rich regions. It is excluded by viable cells but can penetrate cell membranes of dying or dead cells.

Table 2. Continues on next page

Dye	Structure	λ_{em} (nm) and λ_{ex}(nm)	References	Mode of action
Intracellular calcium indicators				
Fura Red Glycine,N-[2-[(acetyloxy)methoxy]-2-oxoethyl]-N-[5-[2-[2-[bis[2-[(acetyloxy)methoxy]-2-oxoethyl]amino]-5-methylphenoxy]ethoxy]-2-[(5-oxo-2-thioxo-4-imidazolidinylidene)methyl]-6-benzofuranyl]-,(acetyloxy)methyl ester	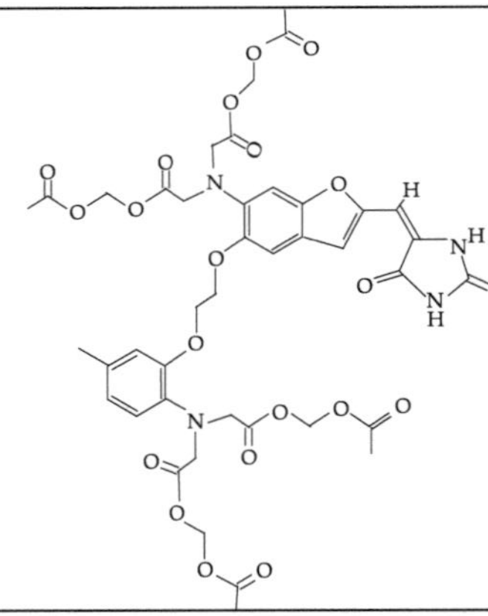	660 450/500	Kurebayashi *et al.* (1993) Novak & Rabinovitch (1994)	This dye is labelled as cell permeant
Fluo-3 1-[2-Amino-5-(2,7-dichloro-6-hydroxy-3-oxo-3H-xanthen-9-yl)]-2-(2 -amino-5 -methylphenoxy)ethane-N,N,N,N -tetraacetic Acid Pentaacetoxymethyl Ester	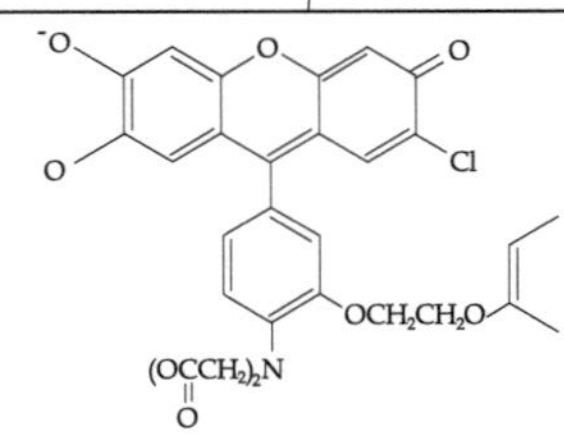	526 506	Merritt *et al.* (1990) Caputo & Bolaños (1994)	Fluo-3 is membrane-permeant Fluo-3 is essentially non-fluorescent, unless it binds to Ca2+

Table 2. Continues on next page

Dye	Structure	λ_{em} (nm) and λ_{ex}(nm)	References	Mode of action
Miscellaneous indicators				
SNARF 1 ® (seminaphtorhodafluor-1-acetoxymethylester	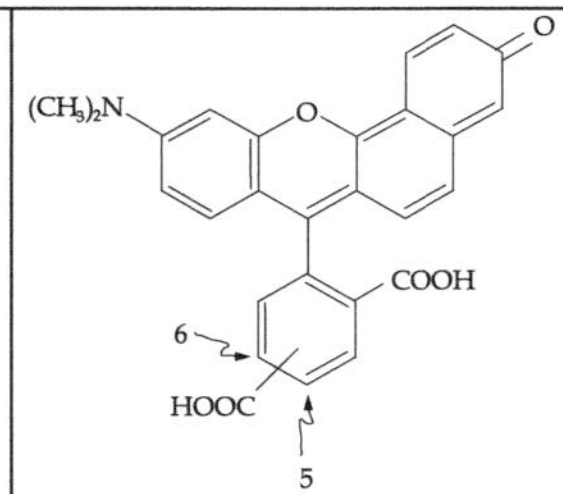	580/630 488	Wieder *et al.*, 1993 Ribou *et al.*, 2002	SNARF -1 is a long-wavelength fluorescent pHindicator developed by Molecular Probes
BCECF-AM 2',7'-bis-(2-carboxyethyl)-5-(and-6)-carboxyfluorescein, acetoxymethyl ester	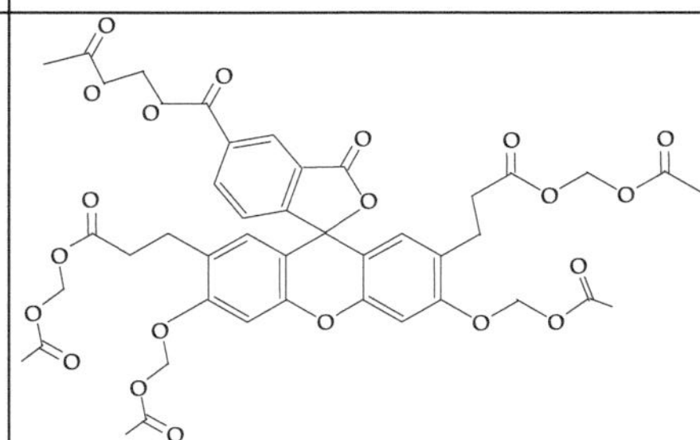	530 440	Ozkan & Mutharasan, 2002 Dascalu *et al.*, 1992	BCECF AM is non-fluorescent. Its conversion to fluorescent BCECF via the action of intracellular esterases can be used as an indicator of cell viability.
Cascade blue	Cascade Blue acetyl azide is the amine-reactive derivative of the trademarked and patented sulphonated pyrene that Molecular Probes uses to prepare its Cascade Blue dye–labelled proteins	423 399	Whitaker *et al.*, 1991	The membrane-impermeant Cascade Blue acetyl azide may be useful for identifying proteins located on extracellular cell surfaces.

Table 2.

Calcium flow indicators. For instance, Ca^{2+} has important roles in bacterial cell differentiation, such as the sporulation of *Bacillus* (Herbaud *et al.*, 1998).

Miscellaneous dyes. This group gathers together dyes able to provide interesting information covering a wide range of physiological properties, for instance intracellular pH, the presence or absence of specific enzymatic activities, etc., which are related to the metabolic activity of a given cell.

Each dye has to be chosen according to the type of answer expected, and several of them may be used to improve our understanding of the cellular state of a given bacterium.

New techniques allowed the attachment of fluorochromes to antibodies. This research is under development for finer cytological approaches (both on and inside the cell) as well as specific applications, such as the research of pathogens in the food industry (Comas-Riu & Rius, 2009).

4. Applications of FCM to sludge samples analyses

4.1 General considerations: Sludge matrix composition

In biological wastewater treatment systems, most of the microorganisms are present in the form of microbial aggregates, such as sludge flocs. Basic floc formation is due to a growth-form of many species of natural bacteria. Floc-forming species share the characteristics of the formation of an extracellular polysaccharide layer, also termed glycocalyx. This material - which consists of polysaccharides, proteins and sometimes cellulose fibrils - "cements" the bacteria together to form a floc. Floc formation occurs at lower growth rates and at lower nutrient levels, essentially starvation or stationary growth conditions. The size of activated sludge flocs ranges from very small aggregates of only a few cells (few µm) to large flocs of more than 1 mm. In most activated sludges, the flocs are typically 10 to 100 µm in diameter, relatively strong and not easy to break apart (Figure 2).

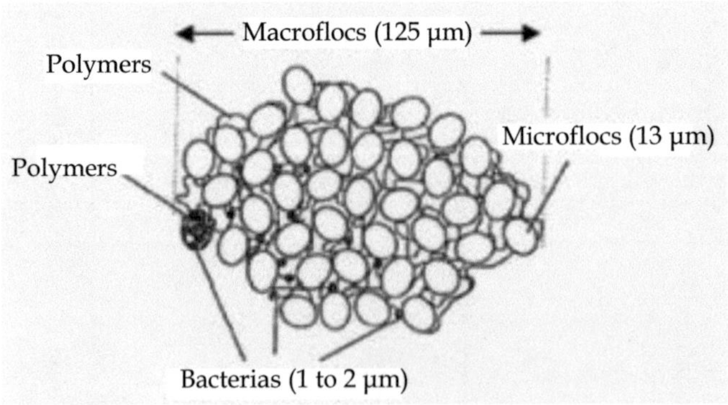

Fig. 2. Schematic representation of activated sludge flocs and their typical size (Jorand *et al.*, 1995)

An activated sludge floc consists of many different components: bacterial cells, various types of extracellular polymeric substances (EPS), adsorbed organic matter, organic fibres, and inorganic compounds (Figure 3). This basic composition is common to all flocs, but the relative proportion of the components and the exact types of chemical compounds or types of microorganisms vary from plant to plant. The organic matter is usually the largest fraction of the dry matter weight of sludge (60 to 80%) whereas the inorganic fraction (ions adsorbed in the EPS matrix, attached minerals, etc.,) is much less abundant. The EPS matrix consists of various macromolecules, such as proteins, polysaccharides, nucleic acids, humic substances, various heteropolymers and lipids. The macromolecules are partly exopolymers produced by bacterial activity and lysis and hydrolysis products, but they are also adsorbed from the wastewater (Wilén *et al.*, 2003).

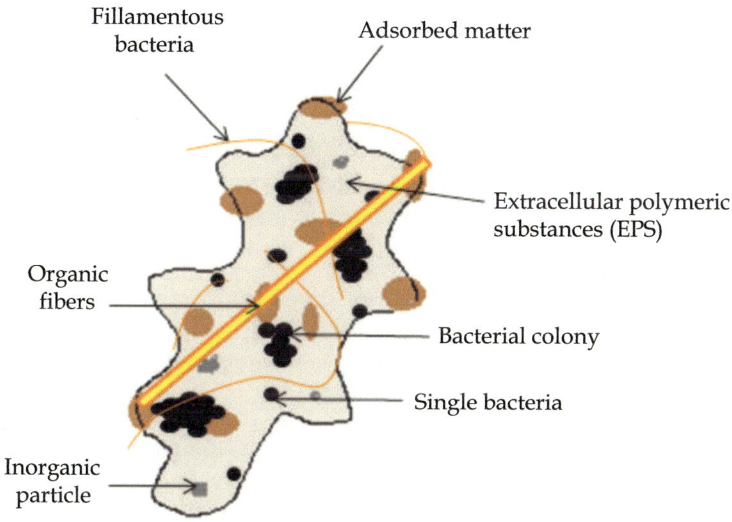

Fig. 3. Schematic illustration of the constituents of activated sludge flocs

It is important to note that polysaccharides - which are assumed to be an important part of bacterial exopolymers - are not present in large amounts in typical sludge flocs (Frolund *et al.*, 1996). Instead, proteins seem to act as the most important "glue" component. The exact function of the large protein pool is not well understood, but exo-enzymatic activity is present (Frolund *et al.*, 1995). Humic substances can form a large fraction in those systems in which they are present in the wastewater and in which the sludge is old. The amount of the extracted EPS and its components and the ratio between each EPS constituent vary, depending on the sample source, the extraction technique and also on the analytical method. While implementing analytical methods for measuring EPS constituents, it is important to know whether they have a high sensitivity to the compound and a low sensitivity to interfering substances (Raunkjaer *et al.*, 1994). The most doubt when choosing the correct analytical method seem to arise with regard to proteins and saccharides.

Thus, only a minor part of organic matter represents the living cells of a biomass. The bacteria can be single, growing in microcolonies or else growing as filaments (Figure 3), but the majority of bacteria grow in aggregates which provide a number of advantages for them when compared to suspended growth. In particular, the presence of EPS components ensures a well-buffered local chemical environment that provides a substrate and important ions, and protection against predators and toxic compounds (Lazarova & Manem, 1995). Furthermore, close proximity to other cells improves interspecies substrates and gene transfer. Considerable effort has been made in recent years in gaining an understanding about the most important mechanisms controlling the floc structure and biofilm formation. This has been supported by the development of various tools, such as light microscopy, epifluorescence microscopy and confocal laser scanning microscopy for *in situ* studies.

4.2 Disruption procedure

As previously described, in activated sludge samples the major fraction of bacterial cells is attached to aggregates, and this represents a problem for microbiological analysis by flow cytometry. Cytometric analysis requires an homogeneous cell suspension and so the detachment of bacteria from flocs is required (Falcioni *et al.*, 2006b) since in FCM, individual particles are analysed; i.e., for free-living bacteria the properties of single cells are measured (Figure 1).Therefore, cells within activated-sludge flocs cannot reasonably be identified by FCM without an appropriate disruption procedure (Wallner *et al.*, 1995). A fundamental difficulty in efficiently dissociating bacteria from flocculated clumps lies in the balance between using procedures which are hard enough to achieve near-complete detachment and the concomitant risk of cell disruption.

There is no agreement as to which procedure gives the best results with which type of substratum, but different methodologies can be found in the literature, mainly based on chemical (detergent) (Duhamel *et al.*, 2008) or physical treatments (mechanical or ultrasonication) (Ziglio *et al.*, 2002; Foladori *et al.*, 2010b).

Recently, Duhamel *et al.* (2008) developed a method for analysing phosphatase activity in aquatic bacteria at the single cell level using flow cytometry. In this study, the most efficient means for disaggregating/separating bacterial cell clumps was obtained by incubating the sample for 30 min with Tween 80 (10 mg l^{-1}, final concentration). Lake samples were chemically treated after cell staining with the substrate ELF-97 [2-(59-chloro-29-phosphoryloxyphenyl)-6-chloro-4-(3H)-quinazolinone] -phosphate (ELF-P) and centrifugation or filtration in order to concentrate cells. Microscopic inspection confirmed that the Tween 80 treatment was efficient at separating the cell clumps. The number of free bacteria and aggregates increased significantly with the addition of Tween 80, up to a final concentration of 10 mg l^{-1}. On the contrary, sonication in a water bath did not generate any increase in the free/attached ratio. Even worse, it led to a significant decrease in total bacteria counts and gave an increase in the filter background.

Buesing & Gessner (2002) tested the effect of 4 detachment instruments (an ultrasonic probe, an ultrasonic bath, an Ultra-Turrax tissue homogeniser and a Stomacher 80 laboratory blender) on the release of bacteria associated with leaf litter, sediment and epiphytic biofilms from a natural aquatic system. They concluded that relatively harsh extraction procedures with an ultrasonic probe turned out to be most appropriate for organic materials, such as decaying leaves and epiphytic biofilms, whereas a more gentle treatment with a Stomacher laboratory blender was preferable for mineral sediment particles.

Ziglio *et al.* (2002) developed a procedure for disaggregating sludge flocs before dye staining and cytometric analysis. The developed procedure, based on mechanical disaggregation (Ultra Turrax), allows a high recovery of bacteria with high accuracy and repeatability, and minimising the damage to the cells' suspension obtained from the disaggregation of the flocs.

In another study, Falcioni *et al.* (2006) compared two different instruments and techniques: sonication and mechanical treatment, in terms of the total detached bacteria number and cell viability. These authors concluded that the treatments used were quite satisfactory, although a complete detachment without bacterial cell death seemed unlikely to be achieved. Although the maximum detachment value was obtained by sonication, mechanical treatment, even if a little bit lower in terms of detachment, showed a good linearity in its results without cell damages, so it could be an alternative method for disaggregating sludge flocs. In addition, they concluded that a combination of the two treatments showed a higher efficiency in terms of bacteria detachment compared with the single treatment with respect to cell viability.

More recently, Foladori *et al.* (2007) also compared mechanical treatment and ultrasonication as pre-treatments for disaggregate activated sludge flocs, with the aim of obtaining a suspension mostly made up of free single cells. According to this study, the pre-treatment based on ultrasonication was more effective than mechanical treatment (after ultrasonication, the maximum range of viable cells was 3.2 times higher than after mechanical treatment). In order to investigate eventual losses in bacterial viability after ultrasonication and mechanical treatment, the ratio of dead/viable free cells was evaluated, and it was found that it did not change significantly for increasing specific energy during sonication or for mechanical treatment times below 20 min.

To conclude this part, it appears that it is not possible to apply a standardised method as a sample preparation before flow cytometric analysis. There is no agreement on which procedure gives the best results with which type of substratum. This is particularly true if activated sludge is considered due to its variable composition and variable floc structure, having different shapes, a different porosity, and irregular boundaries and sizes, ranging widely from a few microns (small clumps of microbial cells) to several hundred microns (Figure2).

4.3 Specific applications to the sludge treatment processes

Conventional municipal sewage treatment plants utilise mechanical and biological processes to treat wastewater. The activated sludge process is the most widely used for biological waste water treatment in the world, but it results in the generation of a considerable amount of excess sludge that has to be disposed of (Pérez-Elvira *et al.*, 2006). The cost of the excess sludge treatment and disposal can represent up to 60% of the total operating costs. The main alternative methods for sludge disposal in the EU are landfill, land application and incineration, accounting for nearly 90% of total sludge production in the EU. The land application of sewage sludge is restricted to prevent health risks to people and livestock due to potentially toxic elements in the sewage sludge, i.e., heavy metals, pathogens and persisting organic pollutants (Wei *et al.*, 2003). Therefore, current legal constraints, rising costs and public sensitivity towards sewage sludge disposal necessitate the development of strategies for the reduction and minimisation of excess sludge production. Reducing sludge production in waste water treatment instead of post-treating the sludge that is produced appears to be an ideal solution to this issue, because the problem would be treated at its roots (Pérez-Elvira *et al.*, 2006). The biological sludge production in conventional wastewater treatment plants can be minimised in a number of ways. There is a large number of different processes by which sludge reduction can be achieved, but most of these alternative technologies involve a disintegration of the organic sludge matrix ("solubilisation") in order to improve its further biodegradation (the concept of "solubilisation" and subsequent cryptic growth)(Camacho *et al.*, 2005).

Sewage sludge disintegration during hydrolysis treatment can be defined as the destruction of sludge by external forces. These forces can be physical, chemical or biological in nature. A result of the disintegration process is numerous changes to a sludge's properties, which can be grouped into three main categories (Müller *et al.*, 2004):

- the destruction of floc structures and the disruption of cells
- the release of soluble substances and fine particles
- biochemical processes

Floc destruction and cell disruption will lead to many changes in a sludge's characteristics and the result is an accelerated and enhanced degradation of the organic fraction of the solid phase. The applied stress during the disintegration causes the destruction of floc structures within the sludge and/or leads to the break-up of microorganisms. If the energy input is increased, the first result is a drastic decrease in particle sizes within the sludge. The destruction of floc structures is the main reason for this phenomenon. The disruption of microorganisms is not so easily determined by the analysis of particle size because disrupted cell walls and the original cells are of a similar size (Müller *et al.*, 2004). For this reason, the use of FCM - which allows a rapid and accurate quantification of the total bacterial population - could provide very specific and useful information about the physiological state of bacteria, including cell disruption (Prorot *et al.*, 2008)) during sludge hydrolysis treatment.

Foladori *et al.* (2007) investigated the effect of the sonication treatment on the viability of bacteria present at different points in a WWTP using FCM after fluorescent nucleic acid staining (SYBR-Green and propidium iodide). In particular, they investigated the effects of sonication on mixed populations of microorganisms in raw wastewater and activated sludge, with particular attention paid to the viability and disruption of bacteria. They concluded that in activated sludge samples, low levels of specific ultrasonic energy (Es) produced a prevalent disaggregation of flocs releasing single cells in the bulk liquid, while the disruption of the bacteria was induced only by very high levels of Es (Es>120 kJ L-1).

Prorot *et al.* (2008) assessed the possibility of using FCM to evaluate the physiological state changes of bacteria occurring during sludge thermal treatment. To this end, they stained bacteria with CTC and SYTOX green was used to evaluate biological cell activity and the viability of cell types contained in the activated sludge. The monitoring of cell activity and viability was performed using FCM analysis both before and after the thermal treatment of the activated sludge. Their results indicated an increase in the number of permeabilised cells and a decrease in the number of active cells, and hence the potential of FCM to successfully evaluate the physiological heterogeneity of an activated sludge bacterial population. The same methodology was used by (Salsabil *et al.*, 2009) to investigate cell lysis after activated sludge treatment using sonication. The use of FCM has shown that this sludge treatment did not lead to cell lysis and, therefore, that the origin of soluble organic matter was essentially extracellular (PEC).

Recently, Foladori *et al.* (2010) analysed how sludge reduction technologies (ultrasonication, high pressure homogenisation, thermal treatment and ozonation) affect the integrity and permeabilisation of bacterial cells in sludge using FCM after a double fluorescent DNA-staining with SYBR-Green and propidium iodide. Whereas the damage to cells increased for increasing levels of applied energy irrespective of the technology, this methodology allowed them to identify different mechanisms of cell disruption depending on the treatment applied.

Finally, Prorot *et al.* (2011) investigated chemical, physical and biological effects of thermal treatment using a multi-parametric approach. In order to clarify the relationship between sludge reduction efficiency and both chemical and biological modifications, the effects of thermal treatment on activated sludge were investigated by combining the monitoring of cell lysis using flow cytometry (FCM), organic matter solubilisation, floc structure and biodegradability. This complete investigation underlines the necessity to combine all parameters, i.e. chemical, physical and biological effects in order to understand and improve the reduction of sludge production during waste water treatment processes.

5. Conclusion

The improvement of control strategies and process optimisation in biotechnology requires the application of analytical methods which allow for the rapid evaluation of metabolic activities and cell viability in environmental processes. Among the many microbiological methods, FCM stands out for its accuracy, speed and the option of sorting components of interest. Nevertheless, the first point that should be taken care of is that there may remain some bias in specific counts by FCM due to the difficulty of achieve complete disaggregation in flocs without the destruction of a fraction of the microbial cells. The design and commercialisation of new cell probes could clearly improve the understanding of individual cells in environmental processes. For instance, the use of fluorochromes bound to specific antibodies could provide interesting information both on and inside the cell. Finally, the potential of FCM for microbiology is still a long way away from being fully utilised. Because each method (culture-dependent methods, PCR, microscopy and FCM) has various advantages and limitations, a combination of methods might be the most reasonable way to achieve a better understanding of microbial life, especially in the environmental field.

6. References

Achilles, J., Harms, H. & Müller, S. (2006). Analysis of living S. cerevisiae cell states—A three color approach. *Cytometry Part A* 69A(3), 173-177.

Allen, S., Sotos, J., Sylte, M. J. & Czuprynski, C. J. (2001). Use of Hoechst 33342 Staining To Detect Apoptotic Changes in Bovine Mononuclear Phagocytes Infected with Mycobacterium avium subsp. paratuberculosis. *Clin. Diagn. Lab. Immunol.* 8(2), 460-464.

Allman, R., Hann, A. C., Manchee, R. & Lloyd, D. (1992). Characterization of bacteria by multiparameter flow cytometry. *Journal of Applied Microbiology* 73(5), 438-444.

Bachoon, D. S., Otero, E. & Hodson, R. E. (2001). Effects of humic substances on fluorometric DNA quantification and DNA hybridization. *Journal of Microbiological Methods* 47(1), 73-82.

Barer, M. R. (1997). Viable but non-culturable and dormant bacteria: time to resolve an oxymoron and a misnomer? *Journal of Medical Microbiology* 46(8), 629 -631.

Ben Said, M., Masahiro, O. & Hassen, A. (2010). Detection of viable but non cultivable Escherichia coli after UV irradiation using a lytic Qβ phage. 60(1), 121-127.

Berney, M., Hammes, F., Bosshard, F., Weilenmann, H.-U. & Egli, T. (2007). Assessment and Interpretation of Bacterial Viability by Using the LIVE/DEAD BacLight Kit in Combination with Flow Cytometry. *Appl. Environ. Microbiol.* 73(10), 3283-3290.

Bogosian, G. (2001). A matter of bacterial life and death. *EMBO Reports* 2, 770-774.

Booth, Ian R, B., Ian R (2002). Stress and the single cell: Intrapopulation diversity is a mechanism to ensure survival upon exposure to stress. *International Journal of Food Microbiology* 78(1-2), 19-30.

Bouvier, T., Del Giorgio, P. A. & Gasol, J. M. (2007). A comparative study of the cytometric characteristics of High and Low nucleic-acid bacterioplankton cells from different aquatic ecosystems. *Environmental Microbiology* 9(8), 2050-2066.

Buesing, N. & Gessner, M. O. (2002). Comparison of detachment procedures for direct counts of bacteria associated with sediment particles, plant litter and epiphytic biofilms. *Aquatic Microbial Ecology* 27(1), 29-36.

Camacho, P., Ginestet, P. & Audic, J.-M. (2005). Understanding the mechanisms of thermal disintegrating treatment in the reduction of sludge production. *Water Science and Technology: A Journal of the International Association on Water Pollution Research* 52(10-11), 235-245.

Caputo, C. & Bolaños, P. (1994). Fluo-3 signals associated with potassium contractures in single amphibian muscle fibres. *The Journal of Physiology* 481(Pt 1), 119-128.

Comas-Riu, J. & Rius, N. (2009). Flow cytometry applications in the food industry. *Journal of Industrial Microbiology and Biotechnology* 36(8), 999-1011.

Czechowska, K. & Johnson, D. R. (2008). Use of flow cytometric methods for single-cell analysis in environmental microbiology. *Current Opinion in Microbiology* 11(3), 205-212.

Dascalu, A., Nevo, Z. & Korenstein, R. (1992). Hyperosmotic activation of the Na(+)-H+ exchanger in a rat bone cell line: temperature dependence and activation pathways. *The Journal of Physiology* 456(1), 503-518.

Davey, H. M. & Kell, D. B. (1996). Flow cytometry and cell sorting of heterogeneous microbial populations: the importance of single-cell analyses. *Microbiological Reviews* 60(4), 641-696.

Díaz, M., Herrero, M., García, L. A. & Quirós, C. (2010). Application of flow cytometry to industrial microbial bioprocesses. *Biochemical Engineering Journal* 48(3), 385-407.

Duhamel, S., Gregori, G., Van Wambeke, F., Mauriac, R. & Nedoma, J. (2008). A method for analysing phosphatase activity in aquatic bacteria at the single cell level using flow cytometry. *Journal of Microbiological Methods* 75(2), 269-278.

Falcioni, T., Manti, A., Boi, P., Canonico, B., Balsamo, M. & Papa, S. (2006a). Comparison of disruption procedures for enumeration of activated sludge floc bacteria by flow cytometry. *Cytometry Part B: Clinical Cytometry* 70B(3), 149-153.

Falcioni, T., Manti, A., Boi, P., Canonico, B., Balsamo, M. & Papa, S. (2006b). Comparison of disruption procedures for enumeration of activated sludge floc bacteria by flow cytometry. *Cytometry Part B: Clinical Cytometry* 70B(3), 149-153.

Foladori, P., Bruni, L., Tamburini, S. & Ziglio, G. (2010a). Direct quantification of bacterial biomass in influent, effluent and activated sludge of wastewater treatment plants by using flow cytometry. *Water Research* 44(13), 3807-3818.

Foladori, P., Laura, B., Gianni, A. & Giuliano, Z. (2007). Effects of sonication on bacteria viability in wastewater treatment plants evaluated by flow cytometry—Fecal indicators, wastewater and activated sludge. *Water Research* 41(1), 235-243.

Foladori, P., Tamburini, S. & Bruni, L. (2010b). Bacteria permeabilization and disruption caused by sludge reduction technologies evaluated by flow cytometry. *Water Research* 44(17), 4888-4899.

Frolund, B., Griebe, T. & Nielsen, P. H. (1995). Enzymatic activity in the activated-sludge floc matrix. *Applied Microbiology and Biotechnology* 43, 755-761.

Frolund, B., Palmgren, R., Keiding, K. & Nielsen, P. H. (1996). Extraction of extracellular polymers from activated sludge using a cation exchange resin. *Water Research* 30(8), 1749-1758.

Giraffa (2004). Studying the dynamics of microbial populations during food fermentation. *FEMS Microbiology Reviews* 28(2), 251-260.

Henze, M. (2000). *Activated sludge models ASM1, ASM2, ASM2d and ASM3*. IWA Publishing. ISBN 9781900222242.

Herbaud, M. L., Guiseppi, A., Denizot, F., Haiech, J. & Kilhoffer, M. C. (1998). Calcium signalling in Bacillus subtilis. *Biochimica Et Biophysica Acta* 1448(2), 212-226.

Jones, K. H. & Kniss, D. A. (1987). Propidium iodide as a nuclear counterstain for immunofluorescence studies on cells in culture. *Journal of Histochemistry & Cytochemistry* 35(1), 123 -125.

Jorand, F., Zartarian, F., Thomas, F., Block, J. C., Bottero, J. Y., Villemin, G., Urbain, V. & Manem, J. (1995). Chemical and structural (2D) linkage between bacteria within activated sludge flocs. *Water Research* 29(7), 1639-1647.

Joux, F. & Lebaron, P. (2000). Use of fluorescent probes to assess physiological functions of bacteriaat single-cell level. *Microbes and Infection* 2(12), 1523-1535.

Julià, O., Comas, J. & Vives-Rego, J. (2000). Second-order functions are the simplest correlations between flow cytometric light scatter and bacterial diameter. *Journal of Microbiological Methods* 40(1), 57-61.

Kapuscinski, J. (1995). DAPI: a DNA-specific fluorescent probe. *Biotechnic & Histochemistry: Official Publication of the Biological Stain Commission* 70(5), 220-233.

Kell, D. B., Kaprelyants, A. S., Weichart, D. H., Harwood, C. R. & Barer, M. R. (1998). Viability and activity in readily culturable bacteria: a review and discussion of the practical issues. *Antonie Van Leeuwenhoek* 73(2), 169-187.

Kiltie, A. E. & Ryan, A. J. (1997). SYBR Green I staining of pulsed field agarose gels is a sensitive and inexpensive way of quantitating DNA double-strand breaks in mammalian cells. *Nucleic Acids Research* 25(14), 2945 -2946.

Kleinsteuber, S., Riis, V., Fetzer, I., Harms, H. & Muller, S. (2006). Population Dynamics within a Microbial Consortium during Growth on Diesel Fuel in Saline Environments. *Appl. Environ. Microbiol.* 72(5), 3531-3542.

Kurebayashi, N., Harkins, A. B. & Baylor, S. M. (1993). Use of fura red as an intracellular calcium indicator in frog skeletal muscle fibers. *Biophysical Journal* 64(6), 1934-1960.

Lahtinen, S. J., Gueimonde, M., Ouwehand, A. C., Reinikainen, J. P. & Salminen, S. J. (2005). Probiotic Bacteria May Become Dormant during Storage. *Applied and Environmental Microbiology* 71(3), 1662-1663.

Latt, S. A. & Stetten, G. (1976). Spectral studies on 33258 Hoechst and related bisbenzimidazole dyes useful for fluorescent detection of deoxyribonucleic acid synthesis. *Journal of Histochemistry & Cytochemistry* 24(1), 24 -33.

Lazarova, V. & Manem, J. (1995). Biofilm characterization and activity analysis in water and wastewater treatment. *Water Research* 29(10), 2227-2245.

Lecoeur, Hervé (2002). Nuclear Apoptosis Detection by Flow Cytometry: Influence of Endogenous Endonucleases. *Experimental Cell Research* 277(1), 1-14.

Longnecker, K., Sherr, B. F. & Sherr, E. B. (2005). Activity and phylogenetic diversity of bacterial cells with high and low nucleic acid content and electron transport system activity in an upwelling ecosystem. *Applied and Environmental Microbiology* 71(12), 7737-7749.

Luisi, P. L. (1998). About various definitions of life. *Origins of Life and Evolution of the Biosphere: The Journal of the International Society for the Study of the Origin of Life* 28(4-6), 613-622.

Mai-Prochnow, A., Evans, F., Dalisay-Saludes, D., Stelzer, S., Egan, S., James, S., Webb, J. S. & Kjelleberg, S. (2004). Biofilm Development and Cell Death in the Marine Bacterium Pseudoalteromonas tunicata. *Appl. Environ. Microbiol.* 70(6), 3232-3238.

Merritt, J. E., McCarthy, S. A., Davies, M. P. & Moores, K. E. (1990). Use of fluo-3 to measure cytosolic Ca2+ in platelets and neutrophils. Loading cells with the dye, calibration of traces, measurements in the presence of plasma, and buffering of cytosolic Ca2+. *Biochemical Journal* 269(2), 513-519.

Moore, A., Donahue, C. J., Bauer, K. D. & Mather, J. P. (1998). Chapter 15 Simultaneous Measurement of Cell Cycle and Apoptotic Cell Death. *Animal Cell Culture Methods.* pp 265-278. Academic Press. ISBN 0091-679X.

Müller, J. A., Winter, A. & Strünkmann, G. (2004). Investigation and assessment of sludge pre-treatment processes. *Water Science and Technology: A Journal of the International Association on Water Pollution Research* 49(10), 97-104.

Müller, S. & Nebe-von-Caron, G. (2010). Functional single-cell analyses: flow cytometry and cell sorting of microbial populations and communities. *FEMS Microbiology Reviews* 34(4), 554-587.

Müller, S., Harms, H. & Bley, T. (2010). Origin and analysis of microbial population heterogeneity in bioprocesses. *Current Opinion in Biotechnology* 21(1), 100-113.

Nebe-von-Caron, G., Stephens, P. ., Hewitt, C. ., Powell, J. . & Badley, R. . (2000). Analysis of bacterial function by multi-colour fluorescence flow cytometry and single cell sorting. *Journal of Microbiological Methods* 42(1), 97-114.

Novak, E. J. & Rabinovitch, P. S. (1994). Improved sensitivity in flow cytometric intracellular ionized calcium measurement using fluo-3/Fura Red fluorescence ratios. *Cytometry* 17(2), 135-141.

Ohta, T., Tokishita, S.-ichi & Yamagata, H. (2001). Ethidium bromide and SYBR Green I enhance the genotoxicity of UV-irradiation and chemical mutagens in E. coli. *Mutation Research/Genetic Toxicology and Environmental Mutagenesis* 492(1-2), 91-97.

Ozkan, P. & Mutharasan, R. (2002). A rapid method for measuring intracellular pH using BCECF-AM. *Biochimica et Biophysica Acta (BBA) - General Subjects* 1572(1), 143-148.

Pérez-Elvira, S. I., Nieto Diez, P. & Fdz-Polanco, F. (2006). Sludge minimisation technologies. *Reviews in Environmental Science and Bio/Technology* 5, 375-398.

Portugal, J. & Waring, M. J. (1988). Assignment of DNA binding sites for 4',6-diamidine-2-phenylindole and bisbenzimide (Hoechst 33258). A comparative footprinting study. *Biochimica et Biophysica Acta (BBA) - Gene Structure and Expression* 949(2), 158-168.

Prorot, A., Eskicioglu, C., Droste, R., Dagot, C. & Leprat, P. (2008). Assessment of physiological state of microorganisms in activated sludge with flow cytometry: application for monitoring sludge production minimization. *Journal of Industrial Microbiology & Biotechnology* 35, 1261-1268.

Prorot, A., Julien, L., Christophe, D. & Patrick, L. (2011). Sludge disintegration during heat treatment at low temperature: A better understanding of involved mechanisms with a multiparametric approach. *Biochemical Engineering Journal* 54(3), 178-184.

Raunkjaer, K., Hvitved-Jacobsen, T. & Nielsen, P. H. (1994). Measurement of pools of protein, carbohydrate and lipid in domestic wastewater. *Water Research* 28(2), 251-262.

Ribou, A.-C., Vigo, J. & Salmon, J.-M. (2002). C-SNARF-1 as a Fluorescent Probe for pH Measurements in Living Cells: Two-Wavelength-Ratio Method versus Whole-Spectral-Resolution Method. *J. Chem. Educ.* 79(12), 1471.

Rieseberg, M., Kasper, C., Reardon, K. F. & Scheper, T. (2001). Flow cytometry in biotechnology. *Applied Microbiology and Biotechnology* 56, 350-360.

Salsabil, M. R., Prorot, A., Casellas, M. & Dagot, C. (2009). Pre-treatment of activated sludge: Effect of sonication on aerobic and anaerobic digestibility. *Chemical Engineering Journal* 148(2-3), 327-335.

Scheper, T., Hoffmann, H. & Schügerl, K. (1987). Flow cytometric studies during culture of Saccharomyces cerevisiae. *Enzyme and Microbial Technology* 9(7), 399-405.

Schmid, I., Krall, W. J., Uittenbogaart, C. H., Braun, J. & Giorgi, J. V. (1992). Dead cell discrimination with 7-amino-actinomcin D in combination with dual color immunofluorescence in single laser flow cytometry. *Cytometry* 13(2), 204-208.

Servais, P., Casamayor, E. O., Courties, C., Catala, P., Parthuisot, N. & Lebaron, P. (2003). Activity and diversity of bacterial cells with high and low nucleic acid content. *Aquatic Microbial Ecology* 33(1), 41-51.

Shi, L., Müller, S., Harms, H. & Wick, L. Y. (2008). Effect of electrokinetic transport on the vulnerability of PAH-degrading bacteria in a model aquifer. *Environmental Geochemistry and Health* 30, 177-182.

Steen, H. B., Boye, E., Skarstad, K., Bloom, B., Godal, T. & Mustafa, S. (1982). Applications of flow cytometry on bacteria: Cell cycle kinetics, drug effects, and quantitation of antibody binding. *Cytometry* 2(4), 249-257.

Steinert, M., Emody, L., Amann, R. & Hacker, J. (1997). Resuscitation of viable but nonculturable Legionella pneumophila Philadelphia JR32 by Acanthamoeba castellanii. *Appl. Environ. Microbiol.* 63(5), 2047-2053.

Sträuber, H. & Müller, S. (2010). Viability states of bacteria--specific mechanisms of selected probes. *Cytometry. Part A: The Journal of the International Society for Analytical Cytology* 77(7), 623-634.

Veal, D. A., Deere, D., Ferrari, B., Piper, J. & Attfield, P. V. (2000). Fluorescence staining and flow cytometry for monitoring microbial cells. *Journal of Immunological Methods* 243(1-2), 191-210.

Vital, M., Füchslin, H. P., Hammes, F. & Egli, T. (2007). Growth of Vibrio cholerae O1 Ogawa Eltor in freshwater. *Microbiology* 153(7), 1993 -2001.

Walberg, M., Gaustad, P. & Steen, H. B. (1999). Uptake kinetics of nucleic acid targeting dyes inS. aureus, E. faecalis andB. cereus: a flow cytometric study. *Journal of Microbiological Methods* 35(2), 167-176.

Wallner, G., Erhart, R. & Amann, R. (1995). Flow cytometric analysis of activated sludge with rRNA-targeted probes. *Appl. Environ. Microbiol.* 61(5), 1859-1866.

Wei, Y., Van Houten, R. T., Borger, A. R., Eikelboom, D. H. & Fan, Y. (2003). Minimization of excess sludge production for biological wastewater treatment. *Water Research* 37(18), 4453-4467.

Whitaker, J. E., Haugland, R. P. & Prendergast, F. G. (1991). Spectral and photophysical studies of benzo[c]xanthene dyes: Dual emission pH sensors. *Analytical Biochemistry* 194(2), 330-344.

Whitesides, M. & Oliver, J. (1997). Resuscitation of Vibrio vulnificus from the Viable but Nonculturable State. *Appl. Environ. Microbiol.* 63(3), 1002-1005.

Wieder, E. D., Hang, H. & Fox, M. H. (1993). Measurement of intracellular pH using flow cytometry with carboxy-SNARF-1. *Cytometry* 14(8), 916-921.

Wilén, B.-M., Jin, B. & Lant, P. (2003). The influence of key chemical constituents in activated sludge on surface and flocculating properties. *Water Research* 37(9), 2127-2139.

Zhang, P., Zhang, G. & Wang, W. (2007). Ultrasonic treatment of biological sludge: Floc disintegration, cell lysis and inactivation. *Bioresource Technology* 98(1), 207-210.

Ziglio, G., Andreottola, G., Barbesti, S., Boschetti, G., Bruni, L., Foladori, P. & Villa, R. (2002). Assessment of activated sludge viability with flow cytometry. *Water Research* 36(2), 460-468.

Zink, D., Sadoni, N. & Stelzer, E. (2003). Visualizing chromatin and chromosomes in living cells. *Methods* 29(1), 42-50.

4

Flow Cytometry Applications in Food Safety Studies

Antonello Paparella, Annalisa Serio and Clemencia Chaves López
Dipartimento di Scienze degli Alimenti, Università degli Studi di Teramo, Mosciano Stazione TE, Italy

1. Introduction

Flow cytometry (FC) is a technique for the rapid analysis of multiple parameters of individual cells. One of the limitations of conventional methods for the analysis of cell populations is the determination of a single value for each cell parameter, which is considered representative of the whole cell population. In contrast, FC aims to obtain segregated data, corresponding to different cell subpopulations. In flow cytometers, single cells or particles pass through a light source in a directed fluid stream, and the interaction of the individual cells with the light source can be recorded and analysed, using the principles of light scattering, light excitation and the emission from fluorescent stains. Thus, the data obtained can provide useful information on the distribution of specific characteristics in cell populations.

Although FC has been primarily used for the analysis of mammalian cells, it has indeed important applications in many areas of food microbiology. One of the strengths of FC is the ability to analyse cells rapidly and individually, which can be notably useful to evaluate the distribution of a property or properties in microbial populations, as well as to detect specific microorganisms by conjugating antibodies with fluorochromes. However, the early applications of this technique in food microbiology were hampered by the small size of microbial cells and the difficulty in discriminating the debris. Not only are bacteria one thousandth smaller than mammalian cells, but they also occur in samples that may show a high level of background fluorescence.

These problems can be successfully managed using modern flow cytometers and specific protocols. Developments in fluidics, light sources and optics allow magnifying the optical signals obtained from bacterial cells, while discrimination of different cell components can be achieved using fluorescent labels. In this way, the size range of detectable particles and the possible applications have grown considerably, ranging from zooplankton to single molecules (Cram, 2002). Thus, FC methods are widely used in many areas of microbiology, from protozoology to virology. Whilst the advantages in microbial ecology (Bergquist et al., 2009; Steen, 2000; Wang et al., 2010) and single-cell physiology (Berney et al., 2008; Quirós et al., 2007) are well documented, specific applications in the field of food pathogens can be considered more recent and particularly interesting.

A flow cytometer consists of five integrated systems: a light source (typically laser or a mercury lamp), optical filters for different wavelength detection, light detectors (photodiodes or photomultiplier tubes) for signal detection and amplification, the flow chamber, and a data processing unit. The sample cells or particles, delivered into a laminar flow, intersect the light source one at a time in the interrogation point. In most flow cytometers, the pneumatic system injects the sample stream into a sheath fluid (*hydrodynamic focusing*), and light detectors detect the resulting scatter and fluorescence.

Forward scatter is the amount of light that is scattered in the forward direction, which can be considered proportional to the size of the cell. The obscuration bar, placed between the light source and the forward scatter detector, allows detecting the scattering light as each particle passes through the interrogation point; in this way, the forward scatter detector converts intensity into voltage and provides information on the size of the particles.

Side scatter is the light scattered to the side, which is affected by several parameters such as surface structure, particle size and particle morphology (Mourant et al., 1998). Side scatter is focused through a lens system and is collected by the side scatter detector, which is usually placed at 90 degrees from light source direction.

Specific cell components can be selectively determined by measuring the intrinsic fluorescence of some compounds or staining the cells with fluorescent dyes. Fluorescence signals travel along the same path as side scatter, being directed through different filters and mirrors to reach a series of detectors for different wavelength ranges.

Fluorescent labelling is commonly used to discriminate different microbial cell types in FC assays. Generic dyes can be utilized to detect cell components or particular biological activities, as well as to discriminate cells from debris. In addition, staining protocols have been developed for specific applications in food microbiology. For example, different fluorogenic substrates can be selected to label microbial cells according to expression of specific enzyme activities; the application of many fluorescent dyes for microbiological analyses has been reviewed by Davey & Kell (1996), Attfield et al. (1999), Veal et al. (2000), Comas-Riu & Rius (2009), and Sträuber & Müller (2010). In particular, the use of esterified fluorochromes is now a routine procedure in food microbiology, to gain information on viability and vitality of cells (Breeuwer et al., 1994). These fluorochromes become fluorescent only after cleaving by intracellular enzymes, and this leads to cell fluorescence if intact membranes retain the fluorescent product. Therefore, these methods provide important information on different cellular functions such as esterase activity and membrane integrity.

On the other hand, *Fluorescence In Situ Hybridization* (FISH) methods discriminate specific nucleic acid sequences inside intact cells (Delong et al, 1989), thus labelling cells according to phylogeny (*phylogenetic labelling*); a combination of CARD-FISH (*Catalyzed Reporter Deposition*) and FC has recently been proposed for bacterial cell quantification within natural microbial communities. Finally, fluorescent antibodies can label microorganisms according to expression of selected antigens (*immunological labelling*), even when high levels of contaminating molecules are present (Veal et al., 2000).

Fluorescence and scatter data, amplified by photomultipliers, are processed by the data processing unit, and the results are combined in different ways to highlight discrimination of subpopulations. In most cases, two-dimensional dot plots and two-colour dot plots are used to represent cytometric data, e.g. combining forward scatter and side scatter, or two different dyes (Nebe-von-Caron et al., 2000); moreover, the data can be processed by multiparameter analysis and suitable graphic methods can be used to improve extraction of information (Davey et al., 1999).

Some specialized flow cytometers are equipped with *Fluorescence-Activated Cell Sorting* or FACS (Battye et al., 2000). This technology allows separating specific cell subpopulations for further analyses such as proteomics or downstream genomics. Most sorters use a droplet formation device, which breaks the sample stream into droplets by means of a vibrating piezoelectric crystal inside the flow chamber. Droplets containing segregated cells pass through a high-voltage electrical field and are collected into different vessels. Droplet cell sorters can sort thousands of cells per second, while simple sorters have a capacity of hundreds of cells per second.

The applications of FC and cell sorting in food safety studies include the study of viable but not culturable cells (VNC), the recovery of rare mutants, and the isolation of slow-growing pathogens from mixed microbial communities (Katsuragi & Tani, 2000).

This chapter reviews the applications of FC in food safety studies, with particular emphasis on foodborne pathogens. Compared to other reviews (Alvarez-Barrientos et al., 2000; Bergquist et al., 2009; Davey & Kell, 1996; Vives-Rego at al., 2000), we analyse the recent developments of FC in the field of foodborne pathogens and point out the possible perspectives in food safety studies.

2. Cellular measurements in food microbiology

2.1 Physiological state of microorganisms

The physiological state of microorganisms influences their ability to survive and grow in foods. In recent years, remarkable progress has been made in the design of rapid methods for determining viability and growth of microbial living cells. In fact, the rapid and specific detection of microorganisms is a challenge in food safety studies, particularly in presence of complex indigenous communities or subpopulations varying in viability, activity and physiological state (Hammes & Egli, 2010). On the other hand, measurements of microbial growth are useful to test antimicrobial substances, as well as to evaluate the efficacy of sanitization and food processing methods, in order to provide information in making decisions on the microbiological safety of foods.

Although viability and culturability are key concepts in food microbiology, the use of these words in scientific literature has often been confusing. The following definitions have been proposed by Paparella et al. (2008):

- **viable cells**, able to reproduce themselves, having both metabolic activity and membrane integrity;
- **vital cells**, which are living cells that do not necessarily show their reproductive activity on growth media;
- **viable but not culturable cells**, which are metabolically active, but do not form colonies on non-selective growth media and can remain in this state for more than a year;
- **sublethally stressed cells**, which do not show any viability loss, but reduce or arrest their growth rate;

- **injured cells**, whose growth is impaired due to damage to cellular components;
- **inactivated cells** (dead cells), which are not able to resume growth when they are inoculated into media that would normally support their growth.

FC is used in food microbiology to provide real time counting of microorganisms, to gather information on the physiological state of individual cells and heterogeneous microbial populations, to detect and identify specific microorganisms, and to sort cells for further analyses. These measurements can be performed using fluorescent dyes aimed at specific cellular targets such as DNA, enzyme activities, internal pH, or cytoplasmic membrane. Fluorescent or fluorogenic dyes are frequently used as indicators for the following cellular functions: (a) membrane integrity; (b) bacterial respiration; (c) membrane potential or (d) intracellular enzyme activity.

2.2 Membrane integrity

Microbial viability can be monitored by FC using the cell capacity to maintain an effective barrier to external media. This approach promotes a better understanding of cellular injury sites and compromised metabolic activities, based on the real time assessment of the viability of the single cells. In a healthy cell, the cytoplasmic membrane allows selective communication with its immediate environment by means of passive and active transport systems. Cells with a damaged membrane cannot sustain any electrochemical gradient and are normally classified as dead cells.

FC can be used to estimate cell membrane integrity, by staining cells with fluorescent dyes that can cross intact cytoplasmic membranes. Therefore, dyes that are normally cell impermeable and have specific intracellular binding sites, can be used to measure membrane integrity. In particular, membrane integrity can be detected by dye exclusion or dye retention. For example, propidium iodide (PI) or ethidium bromide (EB) are exclusion dyes; being positively charged, they bind nucleic acids but cannot cross an intact cytoplasmic membrane. Following the loss of membrane integrity, PI diffuses and intercalates into DNA or RNA, staining cells with a red fluorescence emission. Different dyes, like the cell-impermeant SYTOX® family, have been used to detect nucleic acids in bacteria having a lower DNA content. Moreover, 7-aminoactinomycin D (7-AAD) is a useful alternative to PI, which can penetrate only into dead cells with compromised membrane integrity; this dye is preferable as a viability marker when fluorescein isothiocyanate (FITC) and phyco-erythrin (PE) are used to label surface antigens (Schmid et al., 1992).

2.3 Membrane potential

Membrane potential ($\Delta\Psi$) is considered an early indicator of cell damage. In fact, an electrical potential difference drives and regulates secondary ion and solute transfer across the membrane. Membrane potential, together with the pH difference between the inside and the outside of the cell (ΔpH), constitutes the proton motive force (Michels & Bakker, 1985; Richard & Foster, 2004). As cell wall damage and cell death cause membrane depolarization, $\Delta\Psi$ reflects both the physical integrity of cytoplasmic membranes (viability indicator) and the activity of energetic metabolism (physiological indicator). $\Delta\Psi$ can be detected with membrane potential sensitive dyes such as the anionic lipophilic dye bis-(1,3-dibutylbarbituric acid) trimethine oxonol, named DiBAC$_4$(3). This dye has only a low binding affinity for intact membranes and is limited to the outer regions of the cell membrane in living bacteria. Therefore, $DiBAC_4(3)$ is excluded by live polarized cells, because they are negatively charged in the interior, while it enters into depolarized cells and binds to lipid rich surfaces resulting in bright green fluorescence. In Gram-negative bacteria, a possible problem for measurement of the membrane potential, is that the proper distribution of the membrane potential probes is sometimes hindered by the low permeability of the outer membrane (Breeuwer & Abee, 2004). Although the addition of EDTA or EGTA can favour permeabilization of the outer membrane, such treatments may obviously influence cell viability. Finally, rhodamine 123, a cationic lipophilic dye that partitions into the low electrochemical potential of mitochondrial membranes, can be used to evaluate the functional status of mitochondria in eukaryotic cells.

2.4 Intracellular enzyme activities

Intracellular enzyme activities, and in particular esterase and dehydrogenase activity, provide important information on the metabolic state of microbial cells. A number of esterase substrates have been evaluated on several organisms. The measure of esterase activity can be assessed by dye retention methods that use non-fluorescent cell-permeant esterase substrates as fluorescein diacetate (FDA), carboxyfluorescein diacetate (cFDA), or chemChrome B (Joux & Lebaron, 2000). cFDA is a lipophilic, non-fluorescent precursor that readily diffuses across the cell membranes; once inside the cell, it is converted by nonspecific esterases to a membrane-impermeant fluorescent compound, carboxyfluorescein (cF), resulting in fluorescein accumulation over time. Retention of the dye by the cell, by its electrical charge and polarity, indicates membrane integrity and functional cytoplasmic enzymes, while dead cells do not stain because they lack enzyme activity, and therefore cF diffuses freely through the damaged membranes.

Moreover, the reduction of tetrazolium salts has been widely used as a measure of dehydrogenase activity and cell viability. Tetrazolium salts act as artificial acceptors of electrons and therefore have become an indicator also referred to as the activity of the electron transport system (Lew et al., 2010). In particular, 5-cyano-2,3-ditolyl tetrazolium chloride (CTC) is reduced by electron transfer from the respiratory chain with formation of a water-insoluble red fluorescent intracellular formazan. The reduction of CTC in a cell is considered as an indicator of microbial respiratory activity in environment (Rezaeinejad & Ivanov, 2011).

2.5 Intracellular pH

Intracellular pH affects a wide range of cellular processes and functions such as control of DNA synthesis, cellular proliferation, protein synthesis rate and glycolyis/gluconeogenesis, by governing the uptake of nutrients. As a result, it is regulated within a narrow range by a variety of transport proteins that transfer ions across the cellular membrane. It is believed that viable cells need to maintain a transmembrane pH gradient with their intracellular pH above the acidic extracellular pH; failure to maintain intracellular pH homeostasis indicates that the bacterial cell is severely stressed, and ultimately leads to a loss of cell viability (Kastbjerg et al., 2009). Thus, intracellular pH can also be used as an indicator of the physiological state and metabolic activity of cultivated cells, and as a measure of viability. The fluorescent dyes used for intracellular pH measurements should be non-toxic and should have a pK_a within the physiological range (6.8 and 7.4), to allow detection of small pH changes; clearly, they should have excitation and emission wavelengths suitable for detection by FC. In particular, a variety of fluorogenic esterase substrates like 2',7'-bis-carboxyethyl-5,6-carboxyluorescein (BCECF-AM), calcein-AM, and various fluorescein diacetate derivatives are available for measurement of intracellular pH.

3. Application of flow cytometry to viability assessment and cell counting

3.1 Plate count and rapid methods

Stress responses are of particular importance to food pathogens, as they are commonly exposed to a number of stressors during processing such as heating, freezing, pH changes, high osmotic pressure, oxidative stress, chemical preservatives and biopreservatives. Many studies have highlighted the substantial impact of microbial stress on cell growth probability and showed that the proportion of growing cells is dependent on the stress encountered (Dupont & Augustin, 2009; Vermeulen et al., 2007). The ability to distinguish among different physiological states is especially important in assessing survival and growth of pathogenic microorganisms. Furthermore, accurate measurement of biomass concentration is necessary if informed decisions on process control are to be made, because process performance will largely depend on cell number and individual cell physiological states (Hewitt & Nebe-Von-Caron, 2001).

Microbiological analysis of foods is normally performed by colony counting on agar plates. In plate count method, the time needed for the formation of visible colonies is relatively long, from 20-24 hours for the fast-growing organisms to a week for some slow-growing bacteria. In addition, this method lacks in sensitivity, in particular in traditional fermented foods, and it reveals only a part of the population, as a number of novel microorganisms are not culturable in common media. Moreover, this method is heavily dependent on the physiological status of microorganisms. In fact, bacteria may exist in an eclipsed state, defined as viable but not culturable; in VNC condition, cells are metabolically active, do not form colonies on non-selective growth media and can remain in this state for more than a year (Roszak & Colwell, 1984). The VNC state is only one of the possible microbial responses to stress conditions. Indeed, microorganisms may also become sublethally stressed cells when they are exposed to detrimental nutritional conditions, toxic chemicals and sub-optimal physical conditions (Neidhardt & VanBogelen, 2000), which adversely affect growth without impairing survival.

Despite these limitations, plate count method remains the gold standard in food microbiology. Several rapid methods have been developed for the microbiological analysis of foods, based on direct microscopic examination, optical density, dry-cell-weight or capacitance. However, many of these techniques show significant limitations that hamper their potential application in food safety studies. For example, optical density and dry-cell-weight cannot assess cell viability and are unable to distinguish different cell types. Capacitance methods rely on the measurement of the capacitance generated in an intact cell when passing through an electrical field; although there is a good linear correlation between optical density and capacitance for high biomass concentrations, problems occur when biomass concentrations are low or the ionic strength of the medium is high (Hewitt & Nebe-Von-Caron, 2001). Moreover, capacitance does not provide information on the physiological state of the cells after chemical or physical stresses.

To estimate microbial population density and viability, fluorescence microscopy has been successfully used. In this method, microorganisms are stained with acridine dyes to differentially label viable and non-viable cells, which are enumerated using fluorescence microscopy. In particular, *Direct Epifluorescent Filter Technique* (DEFT) has been used for many years for direct quantification of microbial load in a variety of applications. The major advantages of this technique are: the very short time required for determination of microbial numbers and the elimination of overnight incubation. Active and non active cells can be distinguished by the different reaction of the dye with nucleic acids, with viable microorganisms resulting in an orange and orange-yellow fluorescence under illumination with blue light at 450-490 nm, related with the high RNA content present in the active cells (Kroll, 1995). Conversely, nonviable microorganisms show green fluorescence and are not counted, since this fluorescence is correlated to the presence of DNA.

Although DEFT it is a relatively rapid and sensitive method, acridine dyes react indiscriminately with organic material, and interference from preservatives such as sorbic acid has been reported; moreover, foods with high fat content are not suitable for DEFT analysis (Kroll, 1995). These substances which often interfere with the outcome of the microbiological analysis, are also considered an important reason for requiring enrichment and isolation steps before the use of highly specific assays such as ELISA methods and PCR (Tortorello & Stewart, 1994).

3.2 Flow cytometric assessment of microbial viability and cell number

To overcome the limitations and drawbacks of the rapid methods, FC in combination with selected fluorescent probes has been adapted for cell counting and for the analysis of the viability, metabolic state and antigenic markers of food microorganisms (Barker et al., 1997; Boulos et al., 1999; Bolter et al., 2002; Buyanovsky et al., 1982; Comas-Riu & Rius, 2009; Davey & Kell, 1996;). FC measurements are made very rapidly on a large number of individual cells and give objective and accurate results. In fact, using fluorescent dyes with defined cellular targets along with suitable staining strategies, it is possible to separately examine specific cellular metabolic activities and their relative changes after food processing treatments. Compared with direct microscopic examination, FC is more than four times faster (3–5 min per sample compared to >20 min per sample) and more accurate (<5% standard deviation compared to >10%) (Wang et al., 2010).

In FC, discrimination of different cell types and cell counting are mostly performed using fluorescent labelling. The choice of the fluorescent dye, aimed to stain biologic material or respond to biological activities, is of paramount importance to achieve a reliable assessment of microbial viability (Berney, et al. 2006; Freese, et al. 2006; Nebe-von-Caron, et al. 2000). Viable cells are normally labelled with cationic dyes, whilst lipophilic anionic dyes stain non-viable cells. In multi-colour fluorescence FC, two fluorescent probes are combined to obtain simultaneous detection of viable and non-viable microorganisms, e.g. PI and cFDA, or the permeant SYTO 9 (green) and the non-permeant PI.

Discrimination between intact and permeable cells by FC and fluorescent stains has been used in many studies on bacteria and yeasts in synthetic media, as well as in real systems. This approach has provided additional insights into the subtle changes of cellular events induced by food processing, which were not explicitly assessable by culture techniques.

Evidence of the advantages of FC is given by the advances achieved in particular areas of food microbiology such as the research on lactic acid bacteria, where this method was proved to be a powerful and sensitive tool for assessment of the cell viability and stability (Ben Amor et al., 2002; Bunthof et al, 2001). In particular, multiparametric FC, using multiple stains, was used successfully to differentiate lactic acid bacteria according to their susceptibility to freezing and frozen storage (Rault et al., 2007), as well as to resistance to host biological barriers such as gastric acid and bile (Breeuwer & Abee, 2000; Papadimitriou et al., 2006).

Cell counting and viability assessment, performed by FC, offers the advantage of process optimization according to the meaningful changes in FC observations, and provides important information on the mechanism of action of food processing treatments (Kennedy et al., 2011). For example, FC investigations on the mode of action of high hydrostatic pressure processing (HPP) and thermal treatments on *Lactobacillus rhamnosus* GG (LGG) and *Bacillus subtilis* pointed out significant differences between the treatments. In fact, these studies showed that heat inactivation was closely related to membrane disintegration, while pressure inactivation involved the damage of cellular transport system on dye accumulating cells (Ananta et al 2002; Doherty et al., 2010; Shen et al., 2009).

Moreover, multiparametric FC can highlight differences in the impact of processing treatments on the individual cells of microbial populations. Ritz et al. (2002), evaluating the effects of HPP on *Listeria monocytogenes*, observed that some of the pressurised cells had a membrane potential halfway between those of untreated and pressurised cells; this intermediate physiological state could be reversible in presence of a residual metabolic activity. On the other hand, results obtained by FC on a stressed *Aeromonas hydrophila* population at increasing concentrations of NaCl at different temperatures, evidenced the occurrence of stressed cells that maintained metabolic activity although they were not able to form colonies on agar plates, especially at 6% NaCl (Pianetti et al., 2008).

In other studies on the impact of food processing on microbial populations, performed by FC, no evidence of sublethal injury was observed even when low number of viable cells survived (Uyttendaele et al., 2008).

Very recently, FC was used to detect the changes in microbial populations after exposure to ultraviolet radiation (Schenk et al., 2011). The profiles obtained using double staining techniques indicated that UV radiation produced significant damage in cytoplasmic membrane integrity and in cellular enzyme activity of *Escherichia coli* and *Saccharomyces cerevisiae*. *Listeria innocua* was the most resistant to UV-C radiation, with a VNC subpopulation due to membrane rupture.

FC has also been useful to identify markers for the transition between lag and growth phase in *Bacillus cereus* after exposure to near growth boundary acid stress for both strong and weak organic acids. In fact, the change in the signal of selected probes (cFDA, PI, C12-resazurin and DiOC2(3)) was useful to detect esterase activity and electron transport chain activity, marking the exit from lag phase (Biesta-Peters et al., 2011).

Although multiparametric FC analysis is useful to determine the physiological state of the cells, it may overestimate microbial viability. Furthermore, FC requires the preparation of single cell suspensions because the presence of cell aggregates would provide a single cumulative signal, thus decreasing accuracy and producing misleading results (Nebe-von-Caron et al., 2000). However, this problem has been solved by means of sonication (Falcioni et al., 2006).

4. Detection of foodborne pathogens

4.1 Overview of pathogens detection and identification

Identification of pathogens is important in many scientific fields, especially in medicine and in food and environmental safety. As early detection of pathogens is often crucial, FC is a method of great interest, both in terms of rapidity and in potential automation. Researchers have shown a great interest in the application of FC in research on foodborne pathogens, as indicated by the increasing number of published papers in recent years (Table 1).

Pathogens detection by means of classical methods requires specific media, often with added antibiotics and supplements. This condition implies to know exactly the type of microorganism that has to be searched and its nutritional and environmental requirements. Moreover, pathogens often occur at low numbers, and therefore can usually be detected after pre-enrichment and selective enrichment, which are time-consuming.

One of the most important limits of classical plating methods is underestimation of unculturable cells. VNC pathogens are a critical issue in food safety studies, because they can retain their pathogenic potential without being detectable with classical plating methods. In addition, some slow-growing pathogens (e.g. mycobacteria) can require a very long time (even several days) to be isolated and counted on agar plates.

FC is a culture-independent technique, and therefore it has the great advantage of detecting microorganisms without the need of cultivation. The short time required for each analysis enables a near real-time pathogen detection in food samples. In general, FC exploits the different cell wall characteristics of bacteria to discriminate Gram-positives from Gram-negatives, thus providing information on **Gram staining**.

In Gram-negatives, the lipopolysaccharide outer membrane acts as an efficient permeability barrier to lipophilic molecules, and therefore to many dyes. Several approaches have been proposed to overcome this problem. Shapiro (2003) proposed the use of 1,11,3,3,31,31-hexamethylindodicarbocyanine iodide ($DiIC_1(5)$), EDTA and carbonyl cyanide 3-chlorophenylhydrazone (CCCP): $DiIC_1(5)$ is a membrane potential marker, EDTA is used to permeabilize the outer membrane to the entrance of dyes, and CCCP is a proton ionophore which reduces membrane potential to zero. Combining these stains, it was possible to correctly determine the Gram staining of many bacteria, including pathogens such as *Staphylococcus aureus, Streptococcus pyogenes, Klebsiella pneumoniae, Pseudomonas aeruginosa* and *Salmonella* Typhimurium.

FC is also useful for **pathogen identification and fingerprinting** in mixed populations, using fluorescent labelled DNA probes specific for 16S rRNA (Valdivia & Falkow, 1998). For example, Lange et al. (1997) used rRNA probes to determine *Pseudomonas* species among other airborne contaminants. In fact, FC can analyse large volumes of food samples, and ribosomes are normally present in thousand copies in cells; hence, enough target sequences are available even without amplification. However, it is necessary to possess sequence information for bacteria identification, to develop the specific oligonucleotide probes, and for this reason some novel pathogens might remain undetected.

Microorganism	Probe	Aim of the study	References
Bacillus cereus	MitoSOX, SYTOX green, CYTO 9 and Carboxyfluorescein diacetate	Evaluation of responses to heat stress exposure	Mols et al., 2011
	Carboxyfluorescein diacetate, Propidium iodide, C12 Resazurin, 3,3′-Diethyloxacarbocyanine iodide	Evaluation of cells after exposure to near-growth-boundary acid stress, and markers for the transition between lag phase and growth	Biesta-Peters et al., 2011
	SYTO 9, Propidium iodide and Carboxyfluorescein diacetate	Evaluation of the effect of simulated cooking temperatures and times on endospores	Cronin & Wilkinson, 2008
	$DiOC_2(3)$	Evaluation of the antimicrobial activity of valinomycin and cereulide	Tempelaars et al., 2011
	3′-(p-Hydroxyphenyl) fluorescein	Evaluation of acid stress resistance	Mols et al., 2010
Escherichia coli	SYTO 9, Propidium iodide, $DiOC_2(3)$	Evaluation of growth and recovery rates in simulated food processing treatment	Kennedy et al., 2011
	Propidium iodide and Acridine orange	Evaluation of the effect of high-pressure carbon dioxide (HPCD)	Liao et al., 2011
	Propidium iodide and SYTO 9	Assessment of the effectiveness of disinfection on the amount of viable bacteria in water distribution	Berney et al., 2007
Escherichia coli 0157:H7	SYTO 9, SYTO 13, SYTO 17, SYTO 40 and Propidium iodide	Detection of viable but non culturable (VNC) and viable-culturable (VC)	Khan et al., 2010
	Dihydrorhodamine 123 (DHR 123)	Study of the differential effects of oxidative stress using tea polyphenols	Cui et al., 2012
	5-Cyano-2,3-ditolyl tetrazolium chloride (CTC), Fluorescein isothiocyanate-labelled antibodies	Detection of respiring *E. coli* O157:H7 in apple juice, milk and ground beef	Yamaguchi et al., 2003
Listeria monocytogenes	Propidium iodide and Carboxyfluorescein diacetate	Effects of oregano, thyme and cinnamon essential oils on membrane and metabolic activity	Paparella et al., 2008

Table 1. (continues on next page)

Microorganism	Probe	Aim of the study	References
	Propidium iodide, $DiBAC_4(3)$ and Carboxyfluorescein diacetate	Evaluation of the damage of *Listeria monocytogenes* cells treated by high pressure for 10 min at 400 MPa in pH 5.6 citrate buffer	Ritz et al., 2001
	Propidium iodide and Carboxyfluorescein diacetate	Assessment of the effect caused by the single treatment of nisin and mangainin II amide	Ueckert et al., 1998
	Dead/Live *Bac*light Bacterial Viability Kit™	Assessment of the antimicrobial activity of the bacteriocin leucocin B-TA11a	Swarts et al., 1998
Pseudomonas aeruginosa	SYTO 9, SYTO 13, SYTO 17, SYTO 40 and Propidium iodide	Detection of viable but non culturable (VNC) and viable-culturable (VC)	Khan et al., 2010
	Dihydrorhodamine 123	Study of the differential effects of oxidative stress using tea polyphenols	Cui et al., 2012
Salmonella enterica serovar Typhimurium	SYTO 9, SYTO 13, SYTO 17, SYTO 40 and Propidium iodide	Detection of viable but non culturable (VNC) and viable-culturable (VC)	Khan et al., 2010
	Propidium iodide and SYTO 9	Assessment of the effectiveness of disinfection methods in water distribution systems	Berney et al., 2007
	Fluorescein isothiocyanate (FITC)-labelled antibody and Ethidium bromide	Detection in dairy products	McClelland & Pinder, 1994a
Staphylococcus aureus	SYTO 9, Propidium iodide and $DiOC_2(3)$	Evaluation of growth and recovery rates in simulated food processing treatment	Kennedy et al., 2011
	Dihydrorhodamine 123	Study on the differential effects of oxidative stress using tea polyphenols	Cui et al., 2012

Table 1. (continued) Examples of studies on foodborne pathogens, performed by flow cytometry

Several research groups performed DNA fragment analysis by means of FC measurements. In particular, Kim et al. (1999) stained restriction fragments with a fluorescent intercalating dye that stoichiometrically binds to DNA; the amount of dye bound is therefore directly proportional to fragment length. Bacterial species discrimination is possible analysing DNA restriction fragments by FC, following a procedure similar to *Pulsed Field Gel Electrophoresis* (PFGE).

Unique peak patterns were obtained for each bacterial species, which could be identified by comparing the fragment pattern with data from a fingerprinting library, with sizes from FC being in good agreement with sizes obtained by PFGE. This approach has some advantages with respect to PFGE, both in terms of shorter time of analysis, and in amount of DNA to be used. The FC method is effective but still hardworking, since requires DNA extraction. Some issues still have to be improved, beginning from rapid DNA extraction. Some authors (Suda & Leitch, 2010) highlighted as cytosolic compounds can act as staining inhibitors, therefore affecting the stoichiometry of fluorochromes binding to DNA and the accuracy of genome size estimation. Therefore, it would be necessary to stabilize the DNA-fluorochrome complex or to protect DNA from staining inhibitors. Another useful method for pathogen identification takes advantage of autofluorescence of cellular components such as flavins, pigments, pyridines and aromatic amino acids, for discrimination among bacterial species (Valdivia & Falkow, 1998).

Another important application is **pathogen detection and counting** (Comas-Riu & Rius, 2009), where fluorescent staining has been widely used, obtaining strong signals and high specificity, even though antibodies and oligonucleotide applications are still limited when looking for many pathogenic strains or species at the same time. Salzmann et al. (1975) proposed a procedure for cell characterization without labelling, and later other authors demonstrated the feasibility of this method. In particular, Rajwa et al. (2008) unequivocally identified different bacterial strains, detecting signals of several light scattering angles. The choice of angles was determined by the fact that, as mentioned above, scattered light in the forward region first of all depends on refractive index and cell size, while side-scatter depends on the granularity of cellular structures and cell morphology. By using a classic flow cytometer with a compact enhanced scatter detector and Support Vector Machine (SVM)-based algorithms, only five angles of scatter and axial light loss were sufficient to identify *Escherichia coli, Listeria innocua, Bacillus subtilis* and *Enterococcus faecalis* with a success rate between 68 and 99%. However, also this method cannot be used when the characteristics of the bioparticles to be analyzed are completely unknown, since different bacteria would presumably occupy the same measurement space.

4.2 Microbial interactions

In nature, microbes do not normally grow as planktonic single cells, but often interact in structured communities (i.e. biofilms), which affect individual cell behaviour. In particular, cells respond to environmental stimuli and to signals of neighbouring cells (Müller & Davey, 2009). This aspect is particularly important for pathogens, since interactions among cells could somehow influence the development of infection.

Moreover, cells react to environmental stressors, modifying their pathogenic potential. Bacterial interaction and quorum sensing regulate virulence factors expression and also sporulation (Shapiro, 2003). Bacterial endospores can maintain a dormant condition for long periods with little or no metabolic activity, being resistant to thermal treatments and chemical preserving agents, commonly applied to food products. FC allows to distinguish between live and dead endospores on the basis of their scatter (Comas-Riu & Rius, 2009; Stopa, 2000) or in combination with nucleic acid stain (Comas-Riu & Vives Rego, 2002).

FC combined with image analysis provides new effective tools in studying individual cells and microbial interactions. Héchard et al. (1992) used FC to monitor interactions between

Listeria monocytogenes and an anti-*Listeria* bacteriocin producer, belonging to *Leuconostoc* genus. Instead, Valdivia and Falkow (1996) applied FC and GFP (green fluorescent protein) to study bacteria and yeasts, with special attention to bacterial virulence genes. GFP is a protein that exhibits a green fluorescence when exposed to blue light; as this fluorescence is intrinsic to the protein and does not require substrates or enzymes, it is widely used to investigate protein localization. GFP is also a reliable reporter of gene expression in individual cells when fluorescence is measured by FC.

To study pathogen interaction with the target host cells, many authors labelled bacterial surfaces with fluorescent dyes such as fluorescein isothiocyanate, lucifer yellow or lipophilic dyes (Valdivia & Falkow, 1998). Pathogen cells were then incubated with host cells and fluorescence was measured by FC. This method is very effective, quite simple, rapid and quantitative, since fluorescence intensity is proportional to the degree of pathogen association with host cells (Valdivia and Falkow, 1998). Finally, the capacity to perform the analysis without requiring microbial growth is particularly useful for fastidious pathogens (Dhandayuthapani et al., 1995).

4.3 Pathogen detection in food microbiology

Fluorescent labelled antibodies can be used for species-specific detection of pathogens in solutions, drinking water and foods. In an early study performed by FC in water samples, Tyndall et al. (1985) used fluorescein isothiocyanate-labelled antibodies and propidium iodide to detect *Legionella* spp. in cooling towers. *Legionella pneumophila* lives in water and is the etiologic agent of legionellosis. The major problem regarding water samples is that microorganisms are very diluted, and therefore a preliminary step of sample concentration is usually required. In that study, FC could detect the microorganism rapidly, even in unconcentrated samples.

Other authors (Tanaka et al., 2000) used a FC method to detect viable *E. coli* O157 in river water, combining fluorescent antibody staining and direct viable count, after incubation of cells with nutrients and quinolone antibiotics to prevent cell division and elongate nutrient-responsive cells (Kogure et al., 1979). Since the method requires some hours to elongate viable cells, the same authors proposed a procedure based on fluorescent antibody staining with cFDA and PI to detect esterase-active *E. coli* O157 cells in river water (Yamaguchi et al, 1997).

Due to their structure and composition, foods are very complex substrates for microbial detection by means of FC. In fact, pectins, proteins and lipids can interfere with analysis, requiring additional treatments of the sample. Gunasekera et al. (2000) reported the results of *Escherichia coli* and *Staphylococcus aureus* detection in milk, and pointed out the need of a preliminary treatment with proteinase K or savinase for UHT milk, and with savinase and Triton X-100 for raw milk.

Yamaguchi et al. (2003) developed a rapid method for *E. coli* O157:H7 detection in foods, based on fluorescein isothiocyanate-labelled specific antibodies. In apple juice, it was necessary to reduce background noise from non-bacterial particles, by means of repeated centrifugation steps, whereas a pretreatment with proteinase and Triton X-100 was necessary for milk, to reduce matrix interactions and to resolve signals from bacterial cells and from other particles, obtaining an excellent cell recovery. In solid food samples such as ground beef, several centrifugations at different speeds were needed to remove non-bacterial particles; however, only a poor recovery was reached, and detection limit was above 10^3 cells/g, which can be too high for pathogens. In any case, FC analysis required much less time than microscopy to enumerate cells (2-3 hours).

Donnelly et al. (1988) used FC with fluorescent antibodies to detect *Listeria monocytogenes* in milk, and obtained 6% false-positive results and 0.53% false-negatives, compared with culture methods.

Assunção et al. (2007) applied FC to mycoplasmas detection in goat milk. Mycoplasmas isolation by means of culture techniques requires several days and is labour demanding. As these microorganisms are slow-growing, additional problems can occur due to fast-growing contaminants. By staining milk samples with the cell-permeant DNA-fluorochrome Sybr green I, mycoplasmas were distinguished from milk debris and from *Staphylococcus aureus* cells, with a detection limit of 10^3-10^4 cells/ml. A similar detection limit (10^3 cells/ml) was found for *Salmonella* detection in eggs and milk, which is quite high in comparison with standard methods, able to detect 1 cell/25g (McClelland & Pinder, 1994 a,b). However, after enrichment in broth, FC sensitivity was strongly increased, reaching values below 1 cell/ml.

Ultimately, the advantages of FC with respect to conventional laboratory techniques are not only specificity and rapidity, but also a good correlation between FC enumeration and plate count in unprocessed food samples; however, as we show later on in this chapter, the correlation was different in other studies carried out on processed foods, mainly due to the presence of VNC cells. On the other hand, some problems still have to be solved, to eliminate or at least to reduce matrix interactions, to increase sensitivity, and to improve discrimination among different species.

5. Commercial probes

To reduce the time required for sample preparation and the quantity of reagents, many commercial kits have been developed. In particular, Molecular Probes (Invitrogen Life Technologies) has developed specific kits for cell viability assessment, cell counting and bacterial gram staining.

5.1 Cell viability

LIVE/DEAD® *Bac*Light™ Bacterial Viability Kit (Molecular Probes, Invitrogen Life Technologies) is the best-known commercial probe for viability assessment. Two different nucleic acid-binding stains, SYTO 9 and propidium iodide, are used for a rapid discrimination between live bacteria with intact cytoplasmic membrane, and dead bacteria with compromised membranes. Membrane-permeant SYTO 9 labels live bacteria with green fluorescence, while membrane-impermeant propidium iodide labels membrane-compromised bacteria with red fluorescence.

This probe is reliable and easy to use, and yields both viable and total count in one step. Moreover, the stains are supplied dry, without any harmful solvent, do not require refrigeration, and are chemically stable even in poor conditions. Probably, the most important advantage is that the reagents are simultaneously added to bacterial suspensions, then an incubation step of 5-10 minutes is necessary; as no washing is required, the total analysis time is strongly reduced. The results are easily acquirable, since the background remains virtually non-fluorescent and the contrast degree between green and red fluorescence is high (Comas-Riu & Rius, 2009). Leuko et al. (2004) evidenced the high sensitivity and the robustness of this probe in extreme environments (e.g. hypersaline samples), and suggested a possible application for life detection in extraterrestrial halites.

However, under certain conditions, bacteria with compromised membranes may recover and reproduce, though they may be revealed as dead in the assay. In the meantime, bacteria with intact membranes and therefore scored as alive, may be unable to reproduce in nutrient medium (Boulos et al., 1999).

LIVE/DEAD® *Funga*Light™ Yeast Viability Kit (Molecular Probes, Invitrogen Life Technologies) works on the same basis of *Bac*Light, discriminating yeast cells with intact or damaged membranes by means of SYTO 9 and propidium iodide. *Funga*Light CFDA AM/ Propidium iodide yeast vitality kit exploits the cell-permeant dye 5-carboxyfluorescein diacetate acetoxymethyl ester (CFDA AM) instead of SYTO 9, in combination with propidium iodide, to evaluate the viability of yeast cells by FC or microscopy. Esterase-active yeasts with intact cell membranes stain fluorescent green, while cells with damaged membranes stain fluorescent red.

Other kits measure bacterial cells vitality by means of CCCP (sodium azide carbonyl cyanide 3-chlorophenylhydrazone), which marks reductase activity in Gram-positive and Gram-negative bacteria in *Bac*Light™ RedoxSensor™ Green Vitality Kit, and CTC (5-cyano-2,3-ditolyltetrazolium chloride), able to evaluate respiratory activity in *Bac*Light™ RedoxSensor™ CTC Vitality Kit (Molecular Probes, Invitrogen Life Technologies).

Bacterial oxidation–reduction activity is an informative parameter for measuring cell vitality. The RedoxSensor™ green reagent penetrates both Gram-positive and Gram-negative bacteria, although differences in signal intensity may be observed based upon cell wall characteristics. In presence of reduction activity, the RedoxSensor™ green reagent produces a green-fluorescent signal in 10 minutes. This kit is useful for measuring the effects of antimicrobial agents and for monitoring cultures in fermenters.

By using *Bac*Light™ RedoxSensor™ CTC Vitality Kit, respiring cells will absorb and reduce CTC into formazan, that is insoluble and red-fluorescent. Non-respiring and slow-respiring cells cause a lower reduction of CTC, and consequently produce less fluorescent product, giving a semiquantitative estimation. This kit has been used for the determination of respiring *Escherichia coli* in foods (Yamaguchi et al., 2003).

Finally, *Bac*Light™ Bacterial Membrane Potential kit contains $DiOC_2$, which exhibits green fluorescence at low concentrations in all bacterial cells, but becomes more concentrated in cells which maintain a membrane fluorescence and shows a shift of fluorescence emission towards red.

5.2 Cell counting

Conventional direct-count assays of bacterial viability are based on metabolic characteristics or membrane integrity. Both factors could give uncertain results, because of different growth and staining conditions. In addition, marked differences exist among many bacterial genera, in terms of morphology and physiology, so that a universally applicable assay is difficult to be obtained. For this reason, LIVE/DEAD® *Bac*Light™ Bacterial Counting and Viability Kit (Molecular Probes, Invitrogen Life Technologies) has been developed, to count live and dead bacteria even in mixed populations. Based on SYTO 9 and propidium iodide, the kit contains a calibrated suspension of polystyrene microspheres as a standard for the volume of suspension analysed. Size and fluorescence of these beads have been chosen to be easily distinguished from stained bacteria. A fixed number of microsphere is added to the sample before the FC analysis, and the number of live and dead bacteria can be determined from the ratio bacteria events/microsphere events in the cytogram.

*Bac*Light™ RedoxSensor™ CTC Vitality Kit (Molecular Probes, Invitrogen Life Technologies), previously described, is also useful to detect the respiratory activity of many bacterial populations. In this kit, the contextual presence of SYTO 24 and DAPI facilitate the differentiation of cells from debris and the calculation of total cell numbers.

As far as commercial flow cytometers are concerned, BactoScan™ (Foss) has become very popular in the milk industry worldwide. This instrument is widely used for total count assessment in milk, and has become the industrial standard for payment purposes. The major problems of FC analysis of milk, which are bacteria clusters and interference with milk components, have been solved by using a mechanical pretreatment of the sample. In this way, reliable results are obtained in less than nine minutes, at a capacity of up to 150 milk samples per hour.

5.3 Gram staining

Classical techniques for Gram staining require cell fixation. Some kits suitable for FC have been developed aimed at reducing the labour and the time required for samples preparation (fixing, washing, etc.). The LIVE® *Bac*Light™ Bacterial Gram Stain Kit contains the green-fluorescent SYTO 9 and the red-fluorescent hexidium iodide nucleic acid stains. The two dyes differ in their spectral characteristics: Gram-positives fluoresce red-orange, while Gram-negatives fluoresce green. The kit gives the possibility to stain also mixed bacterial populations, and results can be obtained by FC or by any fluorescence microscope.

6. Antimicrobial susceptibility testing

6.1 Conventional methods

Besides detection and identification, the evaluation of antimicrobial susceptibility is an essential step in pathogen diagnostics, to select the therapeutic options.

Many methods are available for **antimicrobial susceptibility testing** (AST) such as disk diffusion and E-test, based on the same principle, broth or agar dilution test, breakpoint tests, and so on. These methods generally require an incubation time of about 18-24 hours to obtain the final results. Moreover, they are subjected to several sources of error, and therefore the correct performance of ASTs requires strict adherence to standardized protocols regarding culture medium, inoculum size, and preparation and incubation conditions. Generally, MIC (Minimal Inhibitory Concentrations) values are determined, not always corresponding to MBC, which is the Minimal Bactericidal Concentration. In addition, a phenomenon known as postantibiotic effect, which is a transient inhibition of bacterial growth after drug removal, following exposure to an antimicrobial agent (Bigger,

1944), often remains unconsidered. The same happens also for subinhibitory concentration effects, which is rarely determined, since this kind of analysis is tedious and time-consuming (Álvarez-Barrientos et al., 2000).

Together with rapid detection and identification, also rapid susceptibility testing has a relevant clinical impact, especially for severe infections. In particular, the emergence of new pathogens and the increasing antibacterial drug resistance justify the need for rapid diagnostics.

6.2 Early flow cytometry applications

In the last decades automated systems have been developed to obtain AST results in few hours instead of 24 hours, as for traditional methods. However, several rapid methods provide information only on the average behaviour of bacterial populations and not on individual cells, which can be very heterogeneous in terms of age, growth rate and metabolism (Gant et al., 1993). This issue is particularly important, since antimicrobial susceptibility may be strongly influenced by individual growth rate and physiological state. Although cell age can be almost synchronized in laboratory conditions, individual differences are very common *in vivo*.

To solve this problem, many researchers have proposed the application of FC in ASTs. At the beginning of 1980s, it was proved (Steen et al., 1982) that the antimicrobial effect of rifampin could be detected by measuring light scattering and DNA content after only 10 minutes of drug incubation. Cohen & Sahar (1989) used FC (light scatter and ethidium fluorescence) to identify and determine susceptibility to amikacin of bacteria from body fluids and exudates, in only one hour. However, in these studies, drug concentrations exceeded the MIC values of the tested microorganisms (Walberg et al., 1997). The effect of beta-lactams, even at sub-MIC concentrations, on *E. coli* DNA content was detected after 30 minutes of incubation (Martinez et al., 1982).

A different approach was applied by Durodie et al. (1995), who used the protein content/forward scatter ratio plotted as a function of time, as a reliable and sensitive indicator of the effect of several drugs (amoxicillin, mecillinam, chloramphenicol, ciprofloxacin and trimethoprim) at the sub-MIC value on *E. coli* cells. Although the ratio would theoretically appear more suitable for the detection of antibiotics affecting cell size or protein metabolism, it appeared to be valid for all the compounds studied, regardless the mode of action.

Gant et al. (1993) clearly demonstrated how the exposure of *E. coli* to several antibiotics with different mechanisms of action gave specific cytometer profiles. By staining cells with PI and measuring forward and side light scatter and fluorescence data by means of a FACScan flow cytometer, different three-dimensional patterns of events were obtained for gentamicin (active on ribosome and indirectly on cell membrane), ciprofloxacin (which inhibits DNA gyrase), and β-lactams (specifically acting on cell wall). PI intake indicates cell damage or defective outer membrane repair, and therefore it is more appropriate than ethidium bromide in FC evaluation of drugs susceptibility.

Other AST probes belong to the carbocyanine group. Carbocyanine dyes are positively charged and accumulate inside the cell; they give a measure of membrane depolarization, decreasing the fluorescence signal produced. Cells respond to different environmental conditions increasing or decreasing their membrane potential; cell death and/or membrane damage usually causes a collapse of the electrical potential. The dye [$DiOC_5(3)$] (3,3'-dipentyloxacarbocyanine iodide), previously used for measuring membrane potential in mammalian cells, was also employed to assess *Staphylococcus aureus* susceptibility to penicillin G and oxacillin (Ordóñez & Wehman, 1993). Results were obtained in only 90 minutes after antibiotic exposure, and were comparable to those obtained by conventional susceptibility tests.

Rhodamine 123 and $DiBAC_4(3)$ [bis (1,3-dibutylbarbituric acid) trimethine oxonol] are other membrane potential probes used in AST applications. In particular, rhodamine 123 is a cationic lipophilic dye, not taken up by Gram-negative bacteria and therefore used only for Gram-positives. It accumulates in cytosol of cells with an active transmembrane potential. On the contrary, oxonols are anionic lipophilic dyes that enter the cells with depolarized plasma membranes and bind to lipid-rich intracellular components. In this case, fluorescence-emitting cells have a low membrane potential; as membrane potential decreases, oxonol fluorescence intensity becomes higher. Moreover, differently from cationic dyes, anionic dyes are non-toxic for microorganisms, and thus can be successfully used in viability studies after exposure to antimicrobials. Another important advantage of oxonol is that it can be added directly to the culture in broth, avoiding pretreatment steps that may alter bacteria reactions or interfere with the antimicrobial effect (Álvarez-Barrientos et al., 2000). Mason et al (1995) used oxonol in studies on gentamicin and ciprofloxacin action, while Suller et al. (1997) chose this probe for a rapid determination of antibiotic susceptibility of methicillin-resistant *Staphylococcus aureus*.

Mortimer et al. (2000) compared three nucleic acid binding probes, and in detail PI, TO-PRO-1 and SYTOX green, to detect antibiotic-induced injury in *E. coli* cells. TO-PRO-1 is a cyanine dye, generally used as DNA electrophoresis stain that can be useful as viability probe. SYTOX green is also a cyanine dye, which emits a strong fluorescence when bound to nucleic acid. All three dyes were able to detect antimicrobial activity; the intensity of fluorescence was related to the antibiotic mechanism of action, with small or no changes for cells treated with molecules acting on nucleic acid synthesis. Furthermore, in this case cell-associated fluorescence did not relate to results obtained by plate count. Therefore, although FC offers important insight into antimicrobial mechanism of action, the results are not always comparable with standard plate methods.

According to Gauthier et al. (2002), the agreement between FC results and microdilution and broth dilution tests was generally good or perfect for nine antibiotics tested on control strains and urinary tracts isolates (including *Escherichia coli, Enterococcus faecalis, Staphylococcus aureus* and *S. epidermidis*), but norfloxacin, nitrifurantoin and tetracycline gave high percentage (65%) of discrepancies.

Together with SYTOX green, also SYTO 13 and SYTO 17, both labelling nucleic acids, were successfully used in FC studies (Comas & Vives-Rego, 1997), but other authors (Lebaron et al., 1998) noticed that their binding sites could be degraded or modified in cells during a starvation period, suggesting a similar problem in presence of antimicrobials targeted at nucleic acids.

Other authors (Novo et al., 2000) pointed out that, although FC is a sensitive tool in monitoring dynamic cellular events, a single parameter would not be sufficient to determine the sensitivity to many different antimicrobial molecules. Therefore they proposed the contextual evaluation of membrane potential, membrane permeability and particle-counts of antibiotic treated and untreated *S. aureus* and *Micrococcus luteus* cells. Together with TO-PRO-3 and PI (membrane permeability indicators), the authors also used diethyloxacarbocyanine $DiOC_2(3)$ and $DiBAC_4(3)$ (membrane potential sensitive dyes), CCCP and valinomycin (ionophores), while bacterial count was calculated adding polystyrene beads to the sample at known concentration.

6.3 Recent developments

An innovative approach to improve FC efficiency in AST has been recently proposed by Mi-Leong et al. (2007). Antimicrobial testing of *Orientia tsutsugamushi* (a pathogen causing scrub typhus) by classical methods is not standardized, since viable cells are required and, as well as for other *Rickettsia* spp., intracellular pathogens require slow, labour-intensive and very expensive analysis. The authors used a monoclonal antibody to increase FC sensitivity in measuring cells growth.

FC is also useful for AST of *Mycobacterium tuberculosis*, and allows working with heat-killed cells, thus reducing health risks for operators. However, the method has to be improved, since poor correlation with traditional methods has been reported (Govender et a., 2010).

In a recent paper (Chau et al., 2011), FC and confocal microscopy were used to study the effect of daptomycin and telavancin, whose mechanism of action is still not completely clarified, on enterococci susceptible or resistant to vancomycin. This approach was useful in determining the drugs effect, and the physiological and morphological response of *E. faecalis* strains to cell wall-active antibiotics.

Due to the importance of antibiotic susceptibility determination, it is necessary to simplify cells preparation and reduce analysis time. Walberg et al. (1997) demonstrated the efficacy of cold-shock permeabilization (in PBS with EDTA and azide), which eliminates cell washing and reduce sample preparation time to less than five minutes. The results were comparable to ethanol fixation used in preparing cells for AST, although it was not applicable to cells exposed to gentamicin. Following this method, the total time of the analysis was less than one hour.

Several companies have developed new products to rapidly perform AST by FC. For example, *Bac*Light™ (Molecular Probes, Invitrogen Life Technologies) has been used to study the antimicrobial effect of vancomycin on *Enterococcus faecalis* and *E. faecium*, by measuring fluorescence changes due to dead cells within three hours of incubation with antibiotic (Álvarez-Barrientos et al., 2000). Bio-Rad has developed a Flow Cytometric Antimicrobial Susceptibility Test (FAST kit), which does not rely on growth inhibition but on the rapid detection of the antimicrobial effect measured by a couple of fluorescent probes. Besides identifying susceptible and resistant microbes, FAST System could also be used to determine antimicrobial kinetics, synergy and dose response effects, with a good analytical performance. A Finnish research group (Jalava-Karvinen et al., 2009) has developed a fast method (BIS point method), based on FC immunophenotyping of phagocytes, able to discriminate between bacterial and viral infections in one hour. It is not always easy to distinguish between bacterial and viral infections on the basis of clinical symptoms, but the correct diagnosis is fundamental to start the appropriate therapy in short times. This fast method may prevent delay of therapy and inappropriate antibiotic treatments.

In conclusion, FC can be successfully used in AST, and is labour saving and often safer with respect to conventional methods. In addition, one of the most significant advantages of FC is the ability to point out microbial heterogeneity in response to antimicrobial agents. This is a fundamental issue in clinical microbiology, considering the possible presence of subpopulations less susceptible to drugs. Indeed, these features could be useful in food safety studies, to test susceptibility to chemical and physical agents or biopreservatives, and evaluate their mechanism of action.

7. Applications to food preservation/biopreservation

7.1 Definitions

Traditional food preservation technologies for pathogen control in foods rely on heat treatments, modifications of water activity and/or pH, addition of chemical preservatives, and control of storage temperature. In recent years, as a result of the consumer demand for minimally processed products, other technologies are emerging as alternatives for shelf-life extension and pathogen control, e.g. high pressure processing (HPP), pulsed electric fields (PEF), and ultraviolet light. Furthermore, the expanding interest in the green image of the food product promotes new preservation technologies, based on the use of natural compounds, which are commonly known as biopreservation technologies.

Biopreservation aims to prevent the contamination and growth of undesired microorganisms in foods, by addition of: a) antimicrobial compounds, naturally present in foods; b) antimicrobial compounds, produced in foods after physical or chemical stimulation, or after protective cultures addition (Stiles, 1996). This goal ought to be achieved without changing the sensory properties of the product (Holzapfel et al., 1995). In particular, food surface treatments with essential oils and plant extracts have been proposed for pathogen decontamination and/or control in packaging environments and clean rooms (Paparella et al., 2006).

7.2 Conventional preservation technologies

The ability of FC to discriminate different subpopulations on the basis of physiological characteristics of individual cells is particularly useful to assess the effects of preservation treatments on microbial survival. In fact, the success of most preservation technologies relies on ensuring metabolic exhaustion (Lee, 2004); as microbial stress reaction usually involves energy consumption, reduction of energy availability is considered a primary goal in food preservation.

The responses of *E. coli*, *L. monocytogenes* and *S. aureus* to various **stressors**, simulating food processing treatments, have recently been studied by Kennedy et al. (2011) by means of FC and FACS. The latter technique allowed to sort individual cells exposed to different stressors onto agar media, in order to evaluate growth under standard plating conditions. Stressors with the highest impact on plate count also showed the greatest effects on cell membrane integrity and membrane potential. However, treatments that impaired membrane permeability did not show necessarily a comparable impact on membrane potential. Moreover, the outcome of this study points out the complexity of the relationship between cytometric profiles and traditional plate count methods; in fact, cells with extensive damaged membranes were able to grow on agar plates, whereas in some cases the staining procedure rendered cells incapable of growth on solid media. For this reason, further protocol developments are needed for microbiological applications, to correlate FACS-generated results with microbial viability.

Traditionally, the methods used to assess the performance of conventional food preservation technologies are based on the enumeration of viable cells using a standard plating technique. However, FC is emerging as a useful tool for the evaluation of the antimicrobial effects of preservation treatments. For example, the effects of **osmotic shock** on *Escherichia coli* and *Staphylococcus aureus*, after exposure to NaCl and sucrose, have been tested by FC, using the fluorochromes SYTO 13 and calcein (Comas-Riu & Vives-Rego, 1999); in this study, calcein proved to be a good marker for esterase activity in *Staphylococcus aureus*, whereas SYTO 13 was an efficient marker for plate counts.

FC is also considered a valuable tool for evaluating the effects of **heat treatments** by determining the percentages of dead, living and metabolically inactive cells (Comas & Vives-Rego, 1998). In fact, quantification of viability beyond the traditional plating methods is deemed advisable not only in minimally processed foods, but also in conventional heat treatments. The bactericidal effects of different heat treatments have been demonstrated by FC (Kennedy et al., 2011), and heat treated samples have also been used as control populations in FC studies (Paparella et al., 2008; Boudhid et al., 2010).

Moreover, a flow cytometric assay has been successfully used to evaluate the efficacy of heat shock treatments (30 min at 70°C) on *Legionella* strains in hospital water systems, where the mean percentage of viable cells and VNC cells varied from 4.6% to 71.7% (Allegra et al., 2011).

The heat stress response of *Bacillus cereus* has been recently studied by FC (Mols et al., 2011); by using the fluorescent probe MitoSOX, the authors confirmed the formation of superoxide in the cells after exposure to heat, and suggested that superoxide can play a role in the death of this microbial species during heat treatments. These findings correlate well with those reported by Cronin & Wilkinson (2008), who observed an increasing proportion of membrane-damaged endospores of *Bacillus cereus*, with increasing heat treatment.

In *Bacillus cereus*, the **acid stress** response at pH values ranging from pH 5.4 to pH 4.4 with HCl, was studied by Mols et al. (2010). FC analysis, after staining with the hydroxyl (OH·) and peroxynitrite (ONOO(-))-specific fluorescent probe 3'-(p-hydroxyphenyl) fluorescein (HPF), showed excessive radical formation in cells exposed to bactericidal conditions, suggesting an acid-induced malfunctioning of cellular processes that lead to cell death.

7.3 Non-conventional preservation technologies

Multiparameter FC has also been applied in food safety studies on **pressure-assisted thermal sterilization**, to analyse the physiological response of sporeformers to thermal inactivation and high pressure. Mathys et al. (2007) treated spores of *Bacillus licheniformis* by heat-only at 121 °C, by high pressure at 150 MPa (37 °C), or by a combined high pressure and heat treatment at 600 MPa and 77 °C, and then dual stained the samples with the fluorescent dyes SYTO 16 and propidium iodide (PI). For pressure treated spores, but not heat-only treated spores, four distinct subpopulations were discriminated; in this respect, the authors suggested a three step model of inactivation involving a germination step following hydrolysis of the spore cortex, an unknown step, and finally an inactivation step with physical compromise of the inner membrane.

Likewise, FC methods have been developed to determine the germination rate of sporeformers. Cronin and Wilkinson (2007) stained *Bacillus cereus* endospores with SYTO 9 alone or cFDA, together with Hoechst 33342, after arresting germination at defined stages. FC was able to estimate the percentage of germinating and outgrowing endospores; in this study, cFDA/Hoechst 33342 staining was effective to measure overall germination rate, while SYTO 9 was useful to quantify ungerminated, germinating and outgrowing spores.

The efficacy of heat treatments can also be improved by **ultrasound-assisted thermal processing** (*thermosonication*), especially to minimize the undesired effects of conventional heat treatments on food quality. The bactericidal effect of thermosonication is affected by ultrasound amplitude, external static pressure, temperature, pH, and substrate composition (Sala et al., 1995; Pagán et al., 1999). The impact of high-intensity ultrasound treatments (20 kHz; 17.6 W) on *Escherichia coli* cells was evaluated by Ananta et al. (2005), comparing FC results with plate count data. Although plate count results indicated a marked decrease of viability (D-value: 8.3 min), PI intake data showed that only a small proportion of cells lost membrane integrity upon exposure to ultrasound for up to 20 minutes. Comparing cFDA and PI intake, the authors assumed that ultrasound induced damage on the lipopolysaccharide layer of the outer membrane of *E. coli*, as cFDA penetration apparently occurred without any cytoplasmic membrane integrity loss (PI negative). Based on these results, one interesting consideration is the possibility to combine ultrasound processing with biopreservatives, whose bactericidal activity is reduced by the presence of an intact outer membrane in Gram-negatives.

The resistance of microorganisms to **high pressure processing** (HPP) has been evaluated by FC methods. In HPP, one of the major problems is the possible underestimation of the number of viable cells that will grow during product shelf-life.

Ritz et al. (2001) used FC to evaluate the cellular damage on *Listeria monocytogenes* cells treated by high pressure for 10 min at 400 MPa in pH 5.6 citrate buffer. While no cell growth was observed after 48 hours on plate count agar, FC data obtained after staining with cFDA, PI and $DiBAC_4$, revealed that cellular morphology was not really affected. In fact, cFDA intake indicated a dramatic decrease of esterase activity in treated cells, although such activity was not completely obliterated, and membrane integrity (PI) and membrane potential ($DiBAC_4$) were not evenly distributed across the cellular population. $DiBAC_4$ probes, in combination with LIVE/DEAD® *Bac*Light™ viability kit, were found to be good indicators of the viability of *E. coli* cells after long-term starvation (Rezaeinejad & Ivanov, 2011).

7.4 Biopreservation with essential oils and plant extracts

Finally, the antibacterial activity of **essential oils (EOs) in biopreservation** strategies has been investigated by FC. The unprecedented interest in this specific application of FC is proved by the increasing number of published papers after 2008. In fact, the use of FC methods to evaluate the antibacterial activity of biopreserving agents can be considered a new approach, as the first documented application on food pathogens was published by Paparella et al. in 2008. Recently, FC has also been employed to evaluate the antifungal activity of coriander EO (Silva et al., 2011a) and lavender EO (Zuzarte et al., 2011) for the clinical treatment of fungal diseases. Nguefack et al. (2004) had used FC to estimate cell membrane permeability in *Listeria innocua* treated with three EOs at two concentrations. In their study, the EOs (*Cymbopogon citratus*, *Ocimum gratissimum* and *Thymus vulgaris*) were emulsified using 5% (v/v) Tagat V20 in PBS, and added to *L. innocua* suspension, stained with cFDA. The treated cells were incubated at 37°C, and the fluorescence intensity was measured by FC after 0-90 min. The fluorescence intensity of the cells exposed to EOs decreased faster than non-exposed cells, and this result was assumed to be due to cytoplasmic membrane permeabilization with cFDA leakage. However, FC data showed a reverse order of activity for the EOs compared with the diffusion assay, with *C. citratus* being more active than *T. vulgaris* and *O. gratissimum*.

Paparella et al. (2008) used FC to evaluate the physiological behaviour of *L. monocytogenes* after exposure to cinnamon, thyme and oregano EOs applied alone and in combination with NaCl. The EOs were emulsified with 1% Tween 80, sterilized by filtration, and added to vials containing PBS to obtain different final concentrations, ranging from 0.02 to 0.50 % EO. After treatments, the cells were harvested by centrifugation, washed twice with PBS, and resuspended in PBS, to remove the EO. After double staining with PI and cFDA, three cell subpopulations were identified: PI positive, cFDA positive, and PI and cFDA positive, representing dead, viable and injured cells, respectively. Figure 1 illustrates the shifts in cell subpopulations of *L. monocytogenes* at increasing EOs concentrations: starting from Gate 4 (cFDA positive), they move to Gate 2 (cFDA and PI positive) to reach Gate 1 (PI positive) and finally Gate 3 (low fluorescence, most likely representing lysed cells).

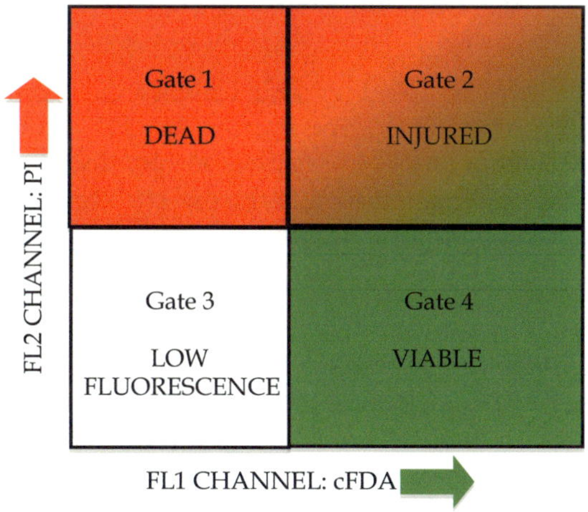

Fig. 1. Microbial subpopulations, after exposure to essential oils, evaluated by flow cytometry (dyes: carboxyfluorescein diacetate cFDA; propidium iodide PI)

According to FC results, membrane disintegration seemed to be the primary inactivation mechanism of oregano and thyme EOs, while a different mechanism of action was apparently involved in cinnamon EO treatments, with a lower activity and a minimal membrane damage. The outcome of this study also suggested that NaCl addition promoted membrane disintegration (PI positivity); the authors proposed that NaCl could increase vapour pressure and favour interaction between cell membrane and EOs, with a higher impact on membrane integrity.

Similar results were obtained by Muñoz et al. (2009), after treatment of *L. monocytogenes* with one extract of oregano EO. Viability evaluation, carried out by dual staining with PI and SYTO 9, revealed that live cell percentage decreased with exposure time, while the percentage of compromised cells remained constant and dead cells increased. Just as observed by Paparella et al. (2008) for cinnamon EO, in this study the comparison between plate count results and FC data suggested the presence of a viable but not culturable subpopulation, which was able to retain SYTO 9 but could not grow on Triptic Soy Broth containing Yeast Extract (TSBYE).

Evidence of VNC cells after EO treatments was found by Bouhdid et al. (2010), by using FC to investigate the mechanisms of action of cinnamon EO in *Pseudomonas aeruginosa* and *Staphylococcus aureus* cells. In this study, the authors compared the results obtained by plate counts, potassium leakage, transmission electron microscopy, and FC after staining with PI, CTC (metabolic activity) and bis-oxonol (membrane potential). Important differences in the effects of cinnamon EO in *P. aeruginosa* and *S. aureus* were observed, but in both cases membrane integrity did not appear to be the first target. In *P. aeruginosa*, cell death followed the decrease of respiratory activity, as indicated by the collapse of membrane potential, the loss of membrane-selective permeability, and PI accumulation. On the other hand, the antimicrobial activity against *S. aureus* was characterized by a marked decrease of metabolic activity and replication capacity, with cells entering a VNC state. On the basis of these findings, the activity of cinnamon EO against *S. aureus* appears to be due to the effects on membrane permeability, and namely to an increase of permeability to small ions like potassium; this membrane alteration impaired enzymatic activity but was not sufficient to allow PI intake.

The effect of rosemary EO on morphology and viability of *S. aureus* was investigated by Jiang et al. (2011), by comparing FC performed by PI staining, with Atomic Force Microscopy (AFM). The number of PI-positive events increased with increasing EO concentration, and AFM imaging revealed that the cell surface first became depressed, then the cell wall and cell membrane were damaged, and finally the cell was completely destroyed.

Membrane damage was also found to be the possible mechanism of action of coriander EO, in a recent FC study carried out by Silva et al. (2011b) on different Gram-positive and Gram-negative bacteria. This EO exerted bactericidal activity against all tested strains, with the exception of *Bacillus cereus* and *Enterococcus faecalis*. In sensitive strains, the antibacterial activity was indicated by PI incorporation and coexistent loss of other physiological functions such as membrane potential, efflux activity and respiratory activity.

Very recently, Cui et al. (2012) coupled FC and AFM to study morphological alterations in different microbial species, treated with a green tea polyphenol (EGCG) at sub-minimum inhibitory concentration. The comparison between FC data and AFM results showed an induced aggregation effect in *Staphylococcus aureus* and *Staphylococcus mutans*, and perforations in *Pseudomonas aeruginosa* and *Escherichia coli* O157:H7, with oxidative stress being confirmed by FC in Gram-negatives.

8. Conclusions

FC is a powerful technique that has a great potential in food safety studies. The single-cell nature of this method makes it ideal for pathogen detection in food samples, where a complex microbial community is exposed to combinations of stressors.

Many areas of the food industry are highly automated, and require on-line monitoring of microbial parameters. This is particularly important in the manufacturing of perishable foods and beverages, where traditional methods have limited advantages. In fact, the use of FC is widespread in the milk industry for payment purposes, but would also provide relevant benefits for pathogen detection in other sectors, e.g. fresh-cut vegetables and fruits, raw meats, and seafood.

One of the reasons often cited as to why FC is not extensively used for routine microbiological analysis in the food industry is the cost of instrumentation and the need for specialized staff. Developments in optics and electronics, and possibly a market expansion, might open up new perspectives for applications both in quality control and in research and development.

In fact, FC can be considered a very versatile technique, which would be suitable to obtain real-time results in HACCP monitoring activities. In this respect, the main limitation is that plate count is still considered the gold standard for food producers, being the base for official analytical methods and microbiological criteria. However, researchers are investigating the reasons of the bias between the methods, and will presumably contribute to a better correlation between results.

Research and development is a new area of application for FC methods. Actually, product development projects are very labour-intensive but have to be performed in a short time, to keep up with a changing market. Therefore, FC is an ideal candidate for validation of new antimicrobial strategies in food formulations, as well as in disinfection and decontamination. Finally, together with other real-time devices (e.g. biosensors), FC might be able to offer new insight into process control, in particular in defining the set points of preserving and biopreserving technologies, to improve food safety.

9. References

Allegra S., Grattard F., Girardot F., Riffard S., Pozzetto B. & Berthelot P. (2011). Longitudinal evaluation of the efficacy of heat treatment procedures against *Legionella* spp. in hospital water systems by using a flow cytometric assay. *Applied and Environmental Microbiology* 77(4): 1268-1275.

Álvarez-Barrientos A., Arroyo J., Cantón R., Nombela C. & Sánchez-Pérez M. (2000). Applications of flow cytometry to clinical microbiology. *Clinical Microbiology Reviews* 13(2): 167-195.

Ananta E., Heinz V. & Knorr D. (2004). Assessment of high pressure induced damage on *Lactobacillus rhamnosus* GG by flow cytometry. *Food Microbiology* 21: 567–577.

Ananta E., Voigt D., Zenker M., Heinz V. & Knorr D. (2005). Cellular injuries upon exposure of *Escherichia coli* and *Lactobacillus rhamnosus* to high-intensity ultrasound. *Journal of Applied Microbiology* 99: 271-278.

Assunção P., Davey H.M., Rosales R.S., Antunes N.T., de la Fe C., Ramirez A.S., Ruiz de Galarreta C.M. & Poveda J.B. (2007). Detection of mycoplasmas in goat milk by flow cytometry. *Cytometry part A* 71A: 1034-1038.

Attfield P., Gunasekera T., Boyd A., Deere D. & Veal D. (1999). Applications of flow cytometry to microbiology of food and beverage industries. *Australasian Biotechnology* 9: 159-166.

Battye F.L., Light A. & Tarlinton D.M. (2000). Single cell sorting and cloning. *Journal of Immunological Methods* 243: 25-32.

Ben Amor K., Breeuwer P., Verbaarschot P., Rombouts F.M., Akkermans A.D.L., De Vos W.M. & Abee T. (2002). Multiparametric flow cytometry and cell sorting for the assessment of viable, injured, and dead *Bifidobacterium* cells during bile salt stress. *Applied and Environmental Microbiology* 68(11): 5209-5216.

Berney M., Weilenmann H.U. & Egli T. (2006). Flow-cytometric study of vital cellular functions in *Escherichia coli* during solar disinfection (SODIS). *Microbiology* 152: 1719–1729.

Berney M., Hammes F., Bosshard F., Weilenmann H.U. & Egli T. (2007). Assessment and interpretation of bacterial viability by using the LIVE/DEAD BacLight Kit in combination with flow cytometry. *Applied and Environmental Microbiology* 73(10): 3283-3290.

Berney M., Vital M., Hülshoff I., Weilenmann H.U., Egli T. & Hammes F. (2008). Rapid, cultivation-independent assessment of microbial viability in drinking water. *Water Research* 42(14): 4010-4018.

Bergquist P.L., Hardiman E.M., Ferrari B.C. & Winsley T. (2009). Applications of flow cytometry in environmental microbiology and biotechnology. *Extremophiles* 13: 389-401.

Biesta-Peters E.G., Mols M., Reij M. W. & Abee T. (2011). Physiological parameters of *Bacillus cereus* marking the end of acid-induced lag phases. *International Journal of Food Microbiology* 148: 42–47.

Bigger J.W. (1944). The bactericidal action of penicillin on *Staphylococcus pyogenes. Irish Journal of Medical Science* 227: 533-568.

Bouhdid S., Abrini J., Amensour M., Zhiri A., Espuny M.J. & Manresa A. (2010). Functional and ultrastructural changes in *Pseudomonas aeruginosa* and *Staphylococcus aureus* cells induced by *Cinnamonum verum* essential oil. *Journal of Applied Microbiology* 109: 1139-1149.

Boulos L., Prévost M., Barbeau B., Coallier J. & Desjardins R. (1999). LIVE/DEAD® BacLight™: application of a new rapid staining method for direct enumeration of viable and total bacteria in drinking water. *Journal of Microbiological Methods* 37: 77–86.

Breeuwer P., Drocourt J.L., Rombouts F.M. & Abee T. (1994). Energy dependent, carrier-mediated extrusion of carboxyfluorescein from *Saccharomyces cerevisiae* allows rapid assessment of cell viability by flow cytometry. *Applied Environmental Microbiology* 60: 1467-1472.

Breeuwer P. & Abee, T. (2000). Assessment of viability of microorganisms employing fluorescence techniques. *International Journal of Food Microbiology* 55: 193–200.

Breeuwer P. & Abee T. (2004). Assessment of the membrane potential, intracellular pH and respiration of bacteria employing fluorescence techniques. In: *Molecular Microbial*

Ecology Manual Kowalchuk G. A., De Bruijn F. J. Head I.M., Akkermans A.D. & van Elsas J.D. (Eds)., pp. 1563–1579, Springer. ISBN 978-1-4020-4860-9.

Bunthof C. J., Bloemen K., Breeuwer P., Rombouts F.M. & Abee T. (2001). Flow cytometric assessment of viability of lactic acid bacteria. *Applied and Environmental Microbiology* 67(5): 2326–2335.

Chau F., Lefort A., Benadda S., Dubée V. & Fantin B. (2011). Flow cytometry as a tool to determine the effects of cell wall-active antibiotics on vancomycin -susceptible and -resistant *Enterococcus faecalis* strains. *Antimicrobial agents and chemotherapy* 55(1): 395-398.

Chen S., Ferguson L.R., Shu Q. & Garg S. (2011). The application of flow cytometry to the characterisation of a probiotic strain *Lactobacillus reuteri* DPC16 and the evaluation of sugar preservatives for its lyophilisation. *LWT Food Science and technology* 44: 1973-1879.

Comas J. & Vives-Rego J. (1997). Assessment of the effects of gramicidin, formaldehyde and surfactants on *Escherichia coli* by flow cytometry using nucleic acid and membrane potential dyes. *Cytometry* 29: 58-64.

Comas J. & Vives-Rego J. (1998). Enumeration, viability and heterogeneity in *Staphylococcus aureus* cultures by flow cytometry. *Journal of Microbiological Methods* 32: 45-53.

Comas-Riu J. & Vives-Rego J. (1999). Use of calcein and SYTO-13 to assess cell cycle phases and osmotic shock effects on *Escherichia coli* and *Staphylococcus aureus* by flow cytometry. *Journal of Microbiological Methods* (34): 215-221.

Comas-Riu J. & Vives-Rego J. (2002). Cytometric monitoring growth, sporogenesis and spore cell sorting in *Paenibacillus polymyxa* (formerly *Bacillus polymyxa*). *Journal of Applied Microbiology* 92: 475-481.

Comas-Riu J. & Rius N. (2009). Flow cytometry applications in the food industry. *Journal of Industrial Microbiology and Biotechnology* 36: 999-1011.

Cram L.S. (2002). Flow cytometry, an overview. *Methods in Cell Science* 24: 1-9.

Cronin U.P. & Wilkinson M.G. (2007). The use of flow cytometry to study the germination of *Bacillus cereus* endospores. *Cytometry* Part A 71A: 143-153.

Cronin, U.P. & Wilkinson, M.G. (2008). *Bacillus cereus* endospores exhibit a heterogeneous response to heat treatment and low-temperature storage. *Food Microbiology* 25(2): 235–243.

Cui Y., Oh Y.J., Lim J., Youn M., Lee I., Pak H.K., Park W., Jo W., & Park S. (2012). AFM study of the differential inhibitory effects of the green tea polyphenol b (-)-epigallocatechin-3-gallate (EGCG) against Gram-positive and Gram-negative bacteria. *Food Microbiology* 29(1): 80-87.

Davey H.M. (2002). Flow cytometric techniques for the detection of microorganisms. *Methods in Cell Science* 24: 91-97.

Davey H.M., Jones A., Shaw A.D., Kell D.B. (1999). Variable selection and multivariate methods for the identification of microorganisms by flow cytometry. *Cytometry* 35: 162-168.

Davey H.M. & Kell D.B. (1996). Flow cytometry and cell sorting of heterogeneous microbial populations: the importance of single-cell analyses. *Microbiological Reviews* 60: 641-696.

Delong E.F., Wickham G.S. & Pace N.R. (1989). Phylogenetic stains - ribosomal RNA-based probes for the identification of single cells. *Science* 243: 1360-1363.

Dhandayuthapani S, Via L.E., Thomas C.A., Horowitz P.M., Deretic D. & Deretic V. (1995). Green fluorescent protein as a marker for gene expression and cell biology of mycobacterial interactions with macrophages. *Molecular microbiology* 17: 901-912.

Doherty S.B., Wang L., Ross R.P., Stanton C., Fitzgerald G.F. & Brodkorb A. (2010). Use of viability staining in combination with flow cytometry for rapid viability assessment of *Lactobacillus rhamnosus* GG in complex protein matrices. *Journal of Microbiological Methods* 82: 301-310.

Donnelly C.W., Baigent G.J. & Briggs E.H. (1988). Flow cytometry for automated analysis of milk containing *Listeria monocytogenes*. *Journal of the Association of Official Analytical Chemistry* 71: 655-658.

Dupont C. & Augustin J. C. (2009). Influence of stress on single-cell lag time and growth probability for *Listeria monocytogenes* in Half Fraser Broth. *Applied and Environmental Microbiology* 75(10): 3069-3076.

Durodie J., Coleman K., Simpson I.N., Loughborough S.H. & Winstanley D.W. (1995). Rapid detection of antimicrobial activity using flow cytometry. *Cytometry* 21: 374-377.

Falcioni T., Manti A., Boi P., Canonico B., Balsamo M. & Papa S. (2006). Comparison of disruption procedures for enumeration of activated sludge floc bacteria by flow cytometry. *Cytometry* Part B 70B: 149-153.

Freese H.M., Karsten U. & Schumann R. (2006). Bacterial abundance, activity, and viability in the eutrophic River Warnow, Northeast Germany. *Microbial Ecology* 51: 117–127.

Gant V.A., Warnes G., Phillips I. & Savidge G.F. (1993). The application of flow cytometry to the study of bacterial responses to antibiotics. *Journal of Medical Microbiology* 39: 147-154.

Gauthier C., St-Pierre Y. & Villemur R. (2002). Rapid antimicrobial susceptibility testing of urinary tract isolates and samples by flow cytometry. *Journal of Medical Microbiology* 51: 192-200.

Govender S., du Plessis S.J., van de Venter M. & Hayes C. (2010). Antibiotic susceptibility of multi-drug resistant *Mycobacterium tuberculosis* using flow cytometry. *Medical Technology SA* 24(2): 25-28.

Gunasekera T.S., Attfield P.V. & Veal D.A. (2000). A flow cytometry method for rapid detection and enumeration of total bacteria in milk. *Applied and Environmental Microbiology* 66(3): 1228-1232.

Hammes F. & Egli T. (2010). Cytometric methods for measuring bacteria in water: advantages, pitfalls and applications *Analytical and Bioanalytical Chemistry* 397(3): 1083-1095.

Héchard Y., Jayat C., Letellier F., Julien R., Cenatiempo Y. & Ratinaud M.H. (1992). On-line visualization of the competitive behavior of antagonistic bacteria. *Applied and Environmental Microbiology* 58(11): 3784-3786.

Hewitt C. J & Nebe-von-Caron G. (2001). An industrial application of multiparameter flow cytometry: assessment of cell physiological state and its application to the study of microbial fermentations. *Cytometry* 44: 179–187.

Holzapfel W.H., Geisen R. & Schillinger U. (1995). Biological preservation of foods with reference to protective cultures, bacteriocins and food-grade enzymes. *International Journal of Food Microbiology* 24: 343-362.

Jalava-Karvinen P., Hohenthal U., Laitinen I., Kotilainen P., Rajamäki A., Nikoskelainen J., Lilius E.M. & Nuutila J. (2009). Simultaneous quantitative analysis of FcγRI (CD64) and CR1 (CD35) on neutrophils in distinguishing between bacterial infections, viral infections, and inflammatory diseases. *Clinical Immunology* 133(3): 314–323.

Jiang Y., Wu N., Fu Y.J., Wang W., Luo M., Zhao C.J., Zu Y.G., Liu X.L. (2011). Chemical composition and antimicrobial activity of the essential oil of Rosemary. *Environmental Toxicology and Pharmacology* 32: 63-68.

Kaprelyants A.S., Mukamolova G.V., Davey H.M. & Kell D.B. (1996). Quantitative analysis of the physiological heterogeneity within starved cultures of *Micrococcus luteus* by flow cytometry and cell sorting. *Applied and Environmental Microbiology* 62(4): 1311–1316.

Kastbjerg V.G., Nielsen D.S., Arneborg N. & Gram L. (2009). Response of *Listeria monocytogenes* to disinfection stress at the single-cell and population levels as monitored by intracellular pH measurements and viable-cell counts. *Applied Environmental Microbiology* 75(13): 4550–4556.

Katsuragi T. & Tani Y.(2000). Screening for microorganisms with specific characteristics by flow cytometry and single-cell sorting. *Journal of Bioscience and Bioengineering* 89: 217-222.

Kennedy D., Cronin U.P. & Wilkinson M.G. (2011). Responses of *Escherichia coli, Listeria monocytogenes,* and *Staphylococcus aureus* to simulated food processing treatments, determined using Fluorescence-Activated Cell Sorting and plate counting. *Applied and Environmental Microbiology* 77 (13): 4657-4668.

Khan M.M., Pyle B.H. & Camper A.K. (2010). Specific and rapid enumeration of viable but non culturable and viable-culturable gram-negative bacteria by using flow cytometry. *Applied and Environmental Microbiology* 76(15): 5088-5096.

Kim Y., Jett J.H., Larson E.J., Penttila J.R., Marrone B.L. & Keller R.A. (1999). Bacterial fingerprinting by flow cytometry: bacterial species discrimination. *Cytometry* 36: 324-332.

Kogure K., Simidu U. & Taga N. (1979). A tentative direct microscopic method for counting living marine bacteria. *Canadian Journal of Microbiology* 25(3): 5415-420.

Lange J.L., Thorne P.S. & Lynch N. (1997). Application of flow cytometry and fluorescent *in situ* hybridization for assessment of exposures to airborne bacteria. *Applied and Environmental Microbiology* 63(4): 1557-1563.

Lebaron P., Catala P. & Parthuisot N. (1998). Effectiveness of SYTOX green stain for bacterial viability assessment. *Applied and Environmental Microbiology* 64(7): 2697-2700.

Lee S.Y. (2004). Microbial safety of pickled fruits and vegetables and hurdle technology. *Internet Journal of Food Safety* 4: 21-32.

Leuko S., Legat A., Fendrihan S. & Stan-Lotter H. (2004). Evaluation of the LIVE/DEAD BacLight kit for detection of extremophilic Archaea and visualization of microorganisms in environmental hypersaline samples. *Applied Environmental Microbiology* 70(11): 6884–6886.

Lew S., Lew M., Mieszczyński T. & Szarek J. (2010). Selected fluorescent techniques for identification of the physiological state of individual water and soil bacterial cells. *Folia Microbiologica* 55(2): 107–118.

Liao H., Zhang F., Hu X. & Liao X (2011). Effects of high-pressure carbon dioxide on proteins and DNA in *Escherichia coli*. *Microbiology* 157(3): 709-720.

Manti A., Boi P., Amalfitano S., Puddu A. & Papa S. (2011). Experimental improvements in combining CARD-FISH and flow cytometry for bacterial cell quantification. *Journal of Microbiological Methods,* doi:10.1016/j.mimet.2011.09.003

Martinez O.V., Gratzner H.G., Malinin T.I. & Ingram M. (1982). The effect of some β- lactam antibiotics on *E. coli* studied by flow cytometry. *Cytometry* 3: 129-133.

Mason D.J., Allman R., Stark J.M. & Lloyd D (1995). The application of flow cytometry to the estimation of bacterial antibiotic susceptibility. *Journal of Antimicrobial Chemotherapy* 36: 441-443

Mathys A., Chapman B., Bull M., Heinz V. & Knorr D. (2007). Flow cytometric assessment of *Bacillus* spore response to high pressure and heat. *Innovative Food Science and Emerging Technologies* 8: 519-527.

McClelland R.G. & Pinder A.C. (1994a). Detection of *Salmonella typhimurium* in dairy products with flow cytometry and monoclonal antibodies. *Applied Environmental Microbiology* 60(12): 4255-4262.

McClelland R.G. & Pinder A.C. (1994b). Detection of low levels of specific *Salmonella* species by fluorescent antibodies and FC. *Journal of Applied Bacteriology* 77: 440-447.

Michels M. & Bakker. E.P. (1985). Generation of a large, protonophore-sensitive proton motive force and pH difference in the acidophilic bacteria *Thermoplasma acidophilum* and *Bacillus acidocaldarius. Journal of Bacteriology* 161: 231–237.

Mi-Jeong K., Mee-Kyung K. & Jae-Sung K (2007). Improved antibiotic susceptibility test of *Orientia tsutsugamushi* by FC using a monoclonal antibody. *Journal of Korean Medical Science* 22: 1-6.

Mols M., van Kranenburg R., van Melis C.C. Moezelaar R., and Abee T. (2010). Analysis of acid-stressed *Bacillus cereus* reveals a major oxidative response and inactivation-associated radical formation. *Environmental Microbiology* 12 (4): 873-885.

Mols M., Ceragioli M. & Abee T. (2011). Heat stress lead to superoxide formation in *Bacillus cereus* detected using the fluorescent probe MitoSOX. *International Journal of Food Microbiology* 151: 119-122.

Mourant J.R., Freyer J.P., Hielscher A.H., Eick A.A., Shen D. & Johnson T.M. (1998). Mechanisms of light scattering from biological cells relevant to noninvasive optical-tissue diagnostics. *Applied Optics* 37(16): 3586-3593.

Müller S. & Davey H. (2009). Recent advances in the analysis of individual microbial cells. *Cytometry part A* 75A: 83-85.

Muñoz M., Guevara L., Palop A., Tabera J. & Fernández P.S. (2009). Determination of the effect of plant essential oils obtained by supercritical fluid extraction on the growth and viability of *Listeria monocytogenes* in broth and food systems using flow cytometry. *LWT – Food Science and Technology* 42: 220-227.

Nebe-von-Caron G., Stephens P.J., Hewitt C.J., Powell J.R. & Badley R.A. (2000). Analysis of bacterial function by multi-colour fluorescence flow cytometry and single cell sorting. *Journal of Microbiological Methods* 42: 97–114.

Neidhardt F.C., VanBogelen R.A. (2000). Proteomic analysis of bacterial stress response. In: *Bacterial stress responses,* Storz G. & Hengge-Aronis R. (Eds.), pp. 445–452, ASM Press. ISBN 978-1-55581-621-6, Washington D.C.

Nguefack J., Budde B.B. & Jakobsen M. (2004). Five essential oils from aromatic plants of Cameroon: their antibacterial activity and ability to permeabilize the cytoplasmic membrane of *Listeria innocua* examined by flow cytometry. *Letters in Applied Microbiology* 39: 395-400.

Nocker A., Caspers M., Esveld-Amanatidou A., van der Vossen J., Schuren F., Montijn R. & Kort R. (2011). Multiparameter viability assay for stress profiling applied to the food pathogen *Listeria monocytogenes* F2365. *Applied and Environmental Microbiology* 77(18): 6433-6440.

Novo D.J., Perlmutter N.G., Hunt R.H. & Shapiro H.M. (2000). Multiparameter flow cytometric analysis of antibiotic effects on membrane potential, membrane permeability and bacterial counts of *Staphylococcus aureus* and *Micrococcus luteus*. *Antimicrobial agents and chemotherapy* 44(4): 827-834.

Ordóñez J.V & Wehman N.W. (1993). Rapid flow cytometric antibiotic susceptibility assay for *Staphylococcus aureus*. *Cytometry* 14: 811-818.

Pagán R., Mañas P., Raso J. & Condón S. (1999). Bacterial resistance to ultrasonic waves under pressure at nonlethal (manosonication) and lethal (thermomanosonication) temperatures. *Applied and Environmental Microbiology* 65(1): 297-300.

Papadimitriou K., Pratsinis H., Nebe-von-Caron G., Kletsas D. & Tsakalidou E. (2006). Rapid assessment of the physiological status of *Streptococcus macedonicus* by flow cytometry and fluorescence probes. *International Journal of Food Microbiology* 111: 197-205.

Paparella A., Taccogna L., Chaves López C., Serio A., Di Berardo L. & Suzzi G. (2006). Food biopreservation in clean rooms. *Italian Journal of Food Science,* special issue Convegno Nazionale: Aspetti microbiologici degli alimenti confezionati, 43-52.

Paparella A., Taccogna L., Aguzzi I., Chaves López C., Serio A., Marsilio F. & Suzzi G. (2008). Flow cytometric assessment of the antimicrobial activity of essential oils against *Listeria monocytogenes*. *Food Control* 19: 1174-1182.

Pianetti A., Manti A., Boi P., Citterio B., Sabatini L., Papa S., Bruno M., Rocchi L. & Bruscolini F. (2008). Determination of viability of *Aeromonas hydrophila* in increasing concentrations of sodium chloride at different temperatures by flow cytometry and plate count technique. *International Journal of Food Microbiology* 127: 252-260.

Quirós C., Herrero M., García L.A. & Díaz M. (2007). Application of flow cytometry to segregated kinetic modelling based on the physiological states of microorganisms. *Applied and Environmental Microbiology* 73(12): 3993-4000.

Rajwa B., Venkatapathi M., Ragheb K., Banada P.P., Hirleman E.D., Lary T. & Robinson J.P. (2008). Automated classification of bacterial particles in flow by multiangle scatter measurement and support vector machine classifier. *Cytometry part A* 73A: 369-379.

Rault A., Béal C., Ghorbal S., Ogier J-C. & Bouix M. (2007). Multiparametric flow cytometry allows rapid assessment and comparison of lactic acid bacteria viability after freezing and during frozen storage. *Cryobiology* 55: 35–43.

Rezaeinejad S. & Ivanov V. (2011). Heterogeneity of *Escherichia coli* population by respiratory activity and membrane potential of cells during growth and long-term starvation. *Microbiological Research* 166: 129-135.

Richard H. & Foster. J.W. (2004). *Escherichia coli* glutamate- and arginine-dependent acid resistance systems increase internal pH and reverse transmembrane potential. *Journal of Bacteriology* 186: 6032–6041.

Ritz M., Tholozan J.L., Federighi M. & Pilet M.F. (2001). Morphological and physiological characteristics of *Listeria monocytogenes* subjected to high hydrostatic pressure. *Applied and Environmental Microbiology* 67(5): 2240-2247.

Roszak D.B., Grimes D.J. & Colwell, R.R. (1984). Viable but nonrecoverable stage of *Salmonella enteritidis* in acquatic systems. *Canadian Journal of Microbiology* 30: 334–338.

Sala F.J., Burgos J., Condón S., López P. & Raso J. (1995). Effect of heat and ultrasound on microorganisms and enzymes. In: *New Methods of Food Preservation*, Gould G.W. (Ed.), pp. 176-204, Blackie Academic & Professional London, ISBN: 0- 8342-1341-9, UK.

Salzmann G.C., Crowell J.M. & Mullaney P.F. (1975). Flow-system multi-angle light-scattering instrument for biological cell characterization. *Journal of the Optical Society of America* 24: 284-291.

Schenk M., Raffellini S., Guerrero S., Blanco G.A. & Alzamora S.M. (2011). Inactivation of *Escherichia coli, Listeria innocua* and *Saccharomyces cerevisiae* by UV-C light: Study of cell injury by flow cytometry. *LWT - Food Science and Technology* 44: 191-198.

Schmid I., Krall W.J., Uittenbogaart C.H., Braun J. & Giorgi J.V. (1992). Dead cell discrimination with 7-amino-actinomycin D in combination with dual color immunofluorescence in single laser flow cytometry. *Cytometry* 13: 204-208.

Shapiro H.M. (2003). *Practical Flow Cytometry* (fourth edition). Wiley-Liss, ISBN: 9780471411253, Hoboken, New Jersey.

Shen T., Bos A.P. & Brul, S. (2009). Assessing freeze–thaw and high pressure low temperature induced damage to *Bacillus subtilis* cells with flow cytometry. *Innovative Food Science and Emerging Technologies* 10: 9–15.

Silva F., Ferreira S., Duarte A., Mendonça D.I. & Domingues F.C. (2011a). Antifungal activity of *Coriandrum sativum* essential oil, its mode of action against *Candida* species and potential synergism with amphotericin B. *Phytomedicine* doi: 10.1016/j.phymed.2011.06.033.

Silva F., Ferreira S., Queiroz J.A. & Domingues F.C. (2011b). Coriander (*Coriandrum sativum* L.) essential oil: its antibacterial activity and mode of action evaluated by flow cytometry. *Journal of Medical Microbiology* 60: 1479-1486.

Steen H.B. (2000). Flow cytometry of bacteria: glimpses from the past with a view to the future. *Journal of Microbiological Methods* 42: 65-74.

Steen H.B., Boye E., Skarstad K., Bloom B., Godal T. & Mustafa S. (1982). Applications of flow cytometry on bacteria: Cell cycle kinetics, drug effects and quantitation of antibody binding. *Cytometry* 2, 249-257.

Stiles, M.E. (1996). Biopreservation by lactic acid bacteria. *Antonie van Leeuwenhoek* 70: 331-345.

Stopa P.J. (2000). The flow cytometry of *Bacillus anthracis* spores revisited. *Cytometry* 41: 2327-2440.

Sträuber H. & Müller S. (2010). Viability states of bacteria - specific mechanisms of selected probes. *Cytometry Part A* 77A: 623-634.

Suda J. & Leitch I.J. (2010). The quest for suitable reference standards in genome size research. *Cytometry part A* 77A: 717-720.

Sueller M.T.E., Stark J.M. & Lloyd D. (1997). A flow cytometric study of antibiotic-induced damage and evaluation as a rapid antibiotic susceptibility test for methicillin-resistant *Staphylococcus aureus*. *Journal of Antimicrobial Chemotherapy* 40: 77-83.

Swarts A.J., Hastings J.W., Roberts R.F. & von Holy A. (1998). Flow cytometry demonstrates bacteriocin-induced injury to *Listeria monocytogenes*. *Current Microbiology* 36(5): 266–270.

Tanaka Y., Yamaguchi N. & Nasu M. (2000). Viability of *Escherichia coli* O157:H7 in natural river water determined by the use of flow cytometry. *Journal of Applied Microbiology* 88: 228-236.

Tempelaars M.H., Rodrigues S. & Abee, T. (2011). Comparative analysis of antimicrobial activities of valinomycin and cereulide, the *Bacillus cereus* emetic toxin. *Applied and Environmental Microbiology*. 77(8): 2755-2762.

Tortorello M.L. & Stewart D.S. (1994). Antibody-Direct Epifluorescent Filter Technique for Rapid, Direct Enumeration of *Escherichia coli* 0157:H7 in Beef. *Applied and Environmental Microbiology* 60(10): 3553-3559.

Tyndall R.L., Hand Jr. R.E., Mann R.C:, Evans C. & Jeringen R. (1985). Application of flow cytometry to detection and characterization of *Legionella* spp. *Applied and Environmental Microbiology* 49(4): 852-857.

Ueckert J.E., ter Steeg P.F. & Coote, P.J. (1998). Synergistic antibacterial action of heat in combination with nisin and magainin II amide. *Journal of Applied Microbiology* 85(3): 487-494

Uyttendaele M., Rajkovic A., Van Houteghem N., Boon N., Thas O., Debevere J. & Devlieghere F. (2008). Multi-method approach indicates no presence of sub-lethally injured *Listeria monocytogenes* cells after mild heat treatment. *International Journal of Food Microbiology* 123: 262–268.

Valdivia R.H. & Falkow S. (1996). Bacterial genetics by flow cytometry; rapid isolation of *Salmonella typhimurium* acid-inducible promoters by differential fluorescence induction. *Molecular Microbiology* 22: 367-378.

Valdivia R.H. & Falkow S. (1998). Flow cytometry and bacterial pathogenesis. *Current Opinion in Microbiology* 1: 359-363.

Valdivia R.H., Hromockyj A.E., Monack D., Ramakrishnan L. & Falkow S. (1996). Application for green fluorescent protein (GFP) in the study of host-pathogen interactions. *Gene* 173: 47-52.

Veal D.A., Deere D., Ferrari B., Piper J. & Attfield P.V. (2000). Fluorescence staining and flow cytometry for monitoring microbial cells. *Journal of Immunological Methods* 243: 191-210.

Vermeulen A., Gysemans K.P.M., Bernaerts K., Geeraerd A.H., Van Impe J.F., Debevere J. & Devlieghere F. (2007). Influence of pH, water activity and acetic acid concentration on *Listeria monocytogenes* at 7°C: data collection for the development of a growth/no growth model. *International Journal of Food Microbiology* 114: 332-341.

Vives-Rego J., Lebaron P. & Nebe-von-Caron G. (2000). Current and future applications of flow cytometry in aquatic microbiology. *FEMS Microbiology Reviews* 24(4): 429-448.

Walberg M., Gaustad P. & Steen H.B., (1997). Rapid assessment of ceftazidime, ciprofloxacin and gentamicin susceptibility in exponentially-growing *E. coli* cells by means of flow cytometry. *Cytometry* 27: 169-178.

Wang Y., Hammes F., De Roy K., Verstraete W. & Boon N. (2010). Past, present and future applications of flow cytometry in aquatic microbiology. *Trends in Biotechnology* 28: 416-424.

Yamaguchi N. & Nasu M. (1997). Flow cytometric analysis of bacterial respiratory and enzymatic activity in the natural aquatic environment. *Journal of Applied Microbiology* 83: 43-52.

Yamaguchi N., Sasada M., Yamanaka M. & Nasu M. (2003). Rapid detection of respiring *Escherichia coli* O157:H7 in apple juice, milk and ground beef by flow cytometry. *Cytometry part A* 54A: 27-35.

Zuzarte M., Gonçalves M.J., Cavaleiro C., Canhoto J., Vale-Silva L., Silva M.J., Pinto E. & Salgueiro L. (2011). Chemical composition and antifungal activity of the essential oils of *Lavandula viridis* L'Hér. *Journal of Medical Microbiology* 60: 612-618.

5

Estimation of Nuclear DNA Content and Determination of Ploidy Level in Tunisian Populations of *Atriplex halimus* L. by Flow Cytometry

Kheiria Hcini[1], David J. Walker[2], Elena González[3], Nora Frayssinet[4], Enrique Correal[2] and Sadok Bouzid[1]
[1]*Faculté des Sciences de Tunis, Département des Sciences Biologiques, Tunis,*
[2]*Instituto Murciano de Investigación y Desarrollo Agrario y Alimentario (IMIDA), C/Mayor, s/n 30150 La Alberca, Murcia,*
[3]*Facultad de Ciencias Exactas y Naturales, UNPSJB – Comodoro Rivadavia,*
[4]*Facultad de Agronomía, Universidad de Buenos Aires, Buenos Aires,*
[1]*Tunisia*
[2]*Spain*
[3,4]*Argentina*

1. Introduction

The genus *Atriplex* (Chenopodiaceae) contains various species distinguishable by different morphology, biological cycles and ecological adaptations (Le Houérou, 1992). Because of their favorable crude protein content, many species of *Atriplex* are excellent livestock fodder during of season periods when grasses are low in feed value. *Atriplex*, as well as other shrub species, are important components of arid land vegetation (Haddioui & Baaziz, 2001). Chenopodiaceae are known as a plant family with many special ecological adaptations, enabling them to grow on very special stands (Freitas, 1993).Among the species of *Atriplex* in North Africa, *Atriplex halimus* L. (Chenopodiaceae) is an important high-protein livestock forage plant in arid and semi-arid zones of North Africa. It is particularly well-adapted to arid and salt-affected areas (Le Houérou, 1992). This species is interesting because of its tolerance to environmental stresses, its use as a fodder shrub for livestock in low rainfall Mediterranean areas (Le Houérou 1992; Cibilis et al. 1998; Zervoudakis et al. 1998; Haddioui & Baaziz, 2001) and its value as a promising forage plant for large-scale plantings (Valderrábano et al. 1996). Considerable variability has been described within *A. halimus* L., at both the morphological and isozyme polymorphism levels (Franclet & Le Houérou, 1971; Le Houérou 1992; Haddioui & Baaziz, 2001). Abbad et al. (2003) reported that the differences in leaf morphology among populations from geographically-distant sites were apparently under genetic control. Based on differences in habit, plant size, leaf shape and fruit morphology, *A. halimus* has been divided into two subspecies: *halimus* and *schweinfurthii* (Franclet & Le Houérou, 1971; Le Houérou, 1992). The two sub-species show relatively large levels of morphological variability. The base chromosome number in the genus *Atriplex* is x = 9 (Nobs, 1975; McArthur & Sanderson, 1984) with variable ploidy levels occurring in several species. The subspecies are based on differences in morphology, with respect to habit, size, leaf shape and fruit morphology. However the existence of intermediate morphotypes complicates the designation of plants as one or the other subspecies (David et al. 2005).

Description and Conservation of *A. halimus* L. genetic resources seem particularly important for the rehabilitation of disturbed areas by salt and low rainfall. There is little literature concerning nuclear DNA content and ploidy levels in *A. halimus* L. The evaluation of genomic size and ploidy levels while determining its nuclear DNA content by flow cytometry is necessary.

In nature, considerable variation in nuclear DNA content occurs both within and among plant species. Manipulation of ploidy level is an important tool for plant breeding in a number of crops. Flow cytometry is increasingly employed as the method of choice for determination of nuclear DNA content and ploidy level in plants (Galbraith et al. 1997). Flow cytometry is a technique which permits rapid estimation of nuclear DNA content (Doležel, 1991) and has been already found very useful in plant taxonomy to screen ploidy levels and to determine genome size (Doležel, 1997).

The method is based on the isolation of single cells or nuclei in suspension and on the staining of nuclei with DNA fluorochromes. The fluorescence emitted from each nucleus is then quantified using a flow cytometer. Although the method was originally developed for the analysis of humain and animal cells, it is now widely used also for plants (Galbraith et al. 1989; Doležel, 1991). Fluorochromes currently used for flow cytometric estimation of DNA content can be broadly classified into two groups: stains that intercalate with double stranded nucleic acids and include ethidium bromide (EB) and propidium iodide (PI); and dyes and drugs that show a base preference and include Hoechst 33258 (H33258), 4′,6-diamidino-2-phenylindole (DAPI), mithramycin (MI), chromomycin A3 (CH), and olivomycin (OL). As flow cytometry provides only relative values, comparison with a reference standard having a known DNA content is necessary to determine picogram quantities of DNA. To make such a comparison valid, emitted fluorescence must be proportional to nuclear DNA content both in a reference standard and in the sample (Doležel et al. 1992).

Flow cytometry is used widely for determining amounts of nuclear DNA content. It can also be used to determine (DNA) ploidy (Lysák & Doležel, 1998; Emshwiller, 2002), although cytological studies are required for confirmation (Bennett et al. 2000). This protocol showed to be convenient (sample preparation is easy), rapid (several hundreds of samples can be analysed in one working day), it does not require dividing cells, it is non-destructive (one sample can be prepared, e.g., from a few milligrams of leaf tissue), and can detect mixoploidy. Therefore the method is used in different areas ranging from basic research to plant breeding and production.

The aim of this work was to evaluate the use of flow cytometry as a quick, reliable tool to determine ploidy level and estimated nuclear DNA content of populations of *A. halimus* L. from different sites in Tunisia. This would allow elucidation of the relationships between ploidy, subspecies, morphology and edapho-climatic conditions for this important shrub.

2. Materials and methods

2.1 Plant material

Plants from nine populations of *A. halimus* were analysed: seven populations from Tunisia (Gabès, Médenine, Tataouine, Monastir, Tunis, Sidi Bouzid and Kairouan) and two populations which preliminary analyses had shown to be diploid (2n = 2x = 18) (Cala Tarida Spain) and tetraploid (2n = 4x =36) (Eraclea, Italy), respectively. Details of the original locations of these populations are given in Table 1.

Population	Position	Altitude (m asl)	Mean temperature (°C)		Annual precipitation (minus evapotranspiration, for populations Cala Tarida and Eraclea) (mm)
			Max. in hottest month	Min. in coldest month	
Gabes	33°54′ N, 10°06′ E	4	32.5	5.8	193
Kairouain	35°41′ N, 10°06′ E	60	37.6	4.4	321
Médenine	33°21′ N, 10°29′ E	116	36.7	6.2	195
Monastir	35°47′ N, 10°50′ E	2	33.4	9.2	383
Sidi- Bouzid	35°04′ N, 09°37′ E	354	37.8	5.0	237
Tataouine	35°50′ N, 10°28′ E	215	37.9	4.7	107
Tunis	36°51′ N, 10°19′ E	3	32.5	5.6	473
CalaTarida	38°56′ N, 01°14′ E	4	30.2	8.9	493-849 = -356
Eraclea	37°24′ N, 13°21′ E	120	29.0	8.1	560-878 = -318

Table 1. Description of the original locations of the populations of *A. halimus* L

2.2 Flow cytometry

Plants were grown from seeds in a peat-soil mixture, in a greenhouse, for 4 weeks (Figure 1). For most populations, four plants were analysed. For Tataouine and Tunis, due to poor germination, only three and two plants, respectively, were analysed. For each plant, one measurement was conducted in each analysis; an analysis being performed on four different days to give 16 measurements per population (12 and 8 for Tataouine and Tunis, respectively).

Flow cytometric estimation of nuclear DNA content was performed with a Partec PA II flow cytometer, using Propidium Iodide (PI) as the fuorescent stain. Samples of growing leaf tissue of *A. halimus* and tomato (*Lycopersicon esculentum* Mill., cv. Stupicke polni) (20 mg

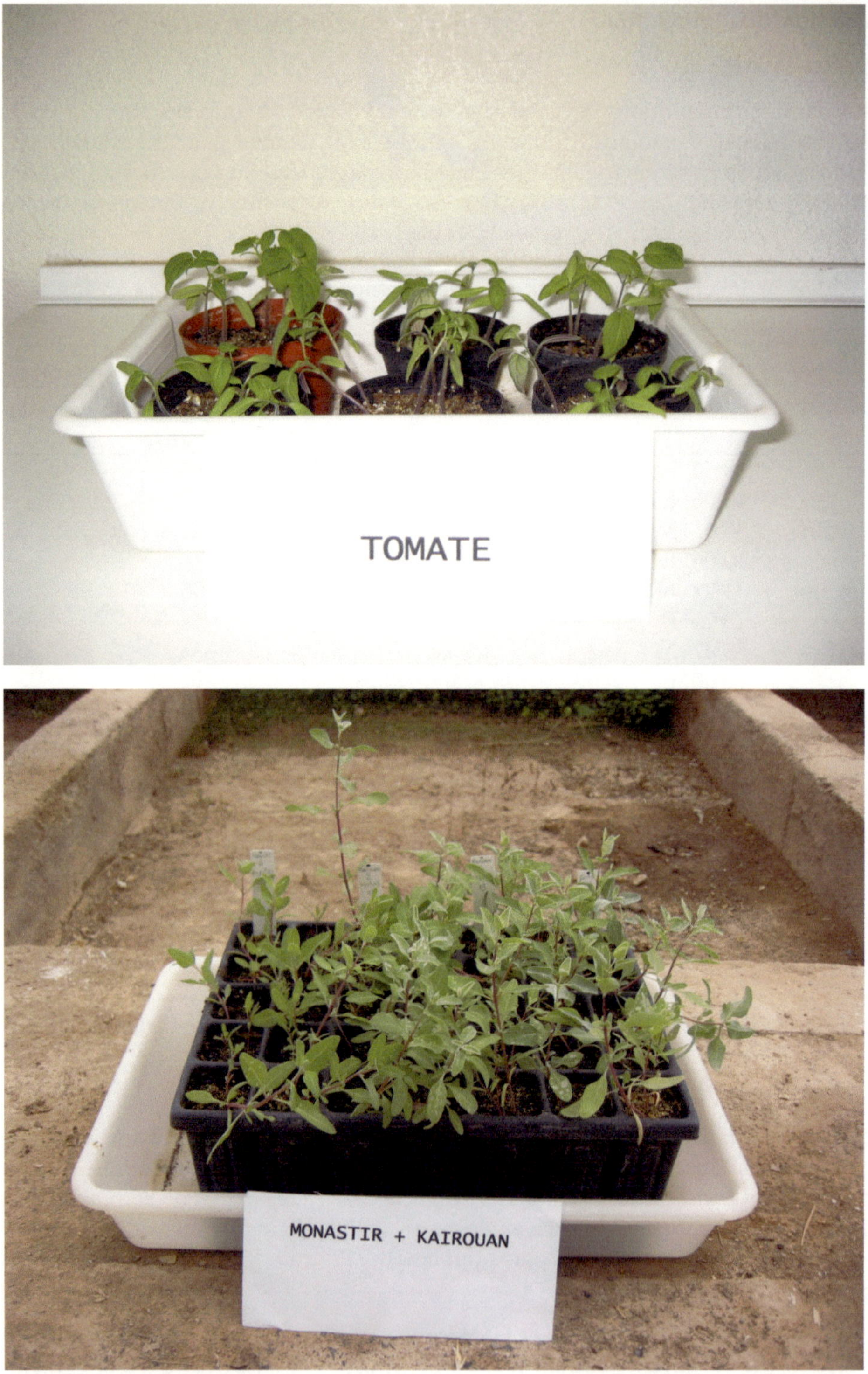

Fig. 1. Plants used for measurements

fresh weight each) were prepared together. This tomato cultivar was chosen as the internal standard because of the similarity of its 2C nuclear DNA content (1.96 pg; Doležel et al. 1992) to that of *A. halimus*. Leaf material was chopped with a razor blade for 30–60 s, in a plastic Petri dish containing 0.4 ml of extraction buffer (Partec CyStain PI Absolute P Nuclei Extraction Buffer; Partec GMBH, Münster, Germany). To arrive at the DNA histograms, the resulting extract was passed through a 30 µm filter into a 3.5 ml plastic tube, to which was then added 1.6 ml of Partec CyStain PI Absolute P Staining Buffer, to give final PI and RNase concentrations of 6.3 µg ml^{-1} and 5.0 µg ml^{-1}, respectively. Samples were kept in the dark for 30 min before analysis by fow cytometry.

All stages of the extraction and staining were per formed at 4 °C. For cytometry, 20 mW argon ion laser light source (488 nm wavelength) (Model PS9600, LG-Laser Technologies GmbH, Kle-inosthein, Germany) and RG 590 long pass filter were employed (Figure 2). The precision and linearity of the flow cytometer were checked on a daily basis using 3 µm calibration beads (Partec). The gain of the instrument was adjusted so that the peak representing the G_0/G_1 nuclei of the internal standard was positioned on channel 100. At least 5000 nuclei were analysed in each sample. *A. halimus* nuclear DNA was estimated by the internal standard method, using the ratio of the *A. halimus*: tomato G_0/G_1 peak positions. The 2C nuclear DNA content of the unknown sample was calculated according to a formula: Sample 2C DNA content = (sample peak mean/standard peak mean) x 2C DNA content of standard (Doležel, 1997). The equivalent number of base pairs was calculated assuming that 1 pg DNA = 965 Mbp (Bennett et al. 2000).

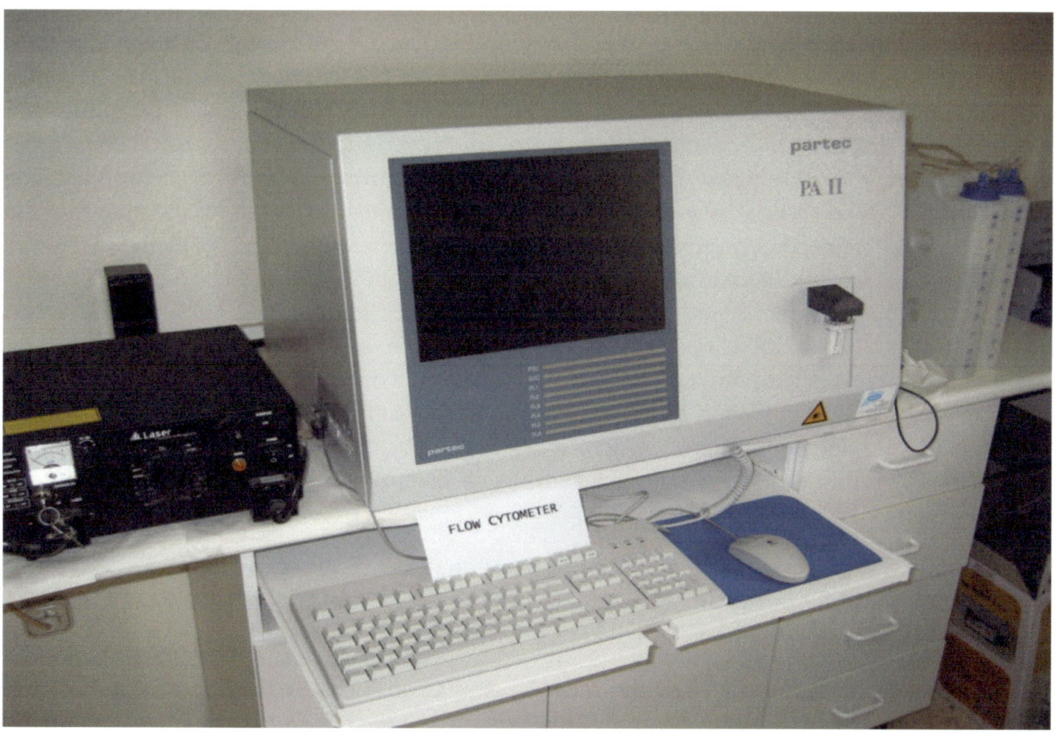

Fig. 2. Flow cytometer used for estimation of nuclear DNA content

2.3 Chromosome counts

Seeds of the Tunisian populations Gabès, Tataouine, Monastir, Sidi Bouzid and Kairouan, and of the populations Cala Tarida and Eraclea, were sown in Petri dishes, on paper towels wetted with tap water. Root tips from 100 germinated seeds per plant (1–3 plants per population) were pre-treated with 8 hydroxyquinoline (2 mM) for 5 h at 4 °C, and fixed in 3:1 ethanol:acetic acid solution. The tissue was macerated for 45 min at 37 °C, with a mixture of cellulase and pectinase (10%) in a 10 mM sodium citrate buffer (pH 4.6). Feulgen stain was applied, followed by acetic-hematoxylin (Nuňez, 1968). At least five slides were observed for each seedling, using a Zeiss ST16 microscope.

2.4 Statistical analyses

A general Model analysis was used to determine the effect of population on nuclear DNA content. To determine whether mean values differed significantly ($p < 5$), the Student-Newman–Keuls test was used. These tests were performed using SPSS software, version 11.0. Log- transformation of values was not necessary since Cochran's C test ($p = 0.396$) and Bartlett's test ($p = 0.094$) showed that variance did not differ significantly between populations.

3. Results

3.1 Flow cytometry

Using flow cytometry, the genome size of any species can be estimated after simultaneous measurements of the fluorescence of stained nuclei of the species and of the reference standard with known DNA content. Flow cytometry is a technique which permits rapid estimation of nuclear DNA content. Because of its speed, precision and convenience, this method of analysis of nuclear DNA content finds an enormous number of applications which cover basic research, breeding and production. The results obtained indicate that the technique might greatly simplify the analysis of plant genomes at the molecular level.We have estimated nuclear DNA content in nine populations of *A. halimus* L., two DNA ploidy levels were found: diploid and tetraploid. With respect to nuclear DNA, the 2C DNA content of population Cala Tarida was estimated to be 2.41pg. As expected, tetraploid populations had approximately two times higher DNA content, ranging from 4.918 pg in Tataouine to 4.972 pg in Gabes, but without statistically-significant differences among them ($p > 0.05$). The two populations which were not subjected to chromosome counting, Médenine and Tunis, had the mean nuclear DNA content of 4.950 and 4.970 pg, respectively, showing them to be tetraploid.

Representative histograms of the flow cytometric analyses of all populations are shown in Figures 3,4,5,6 and Figure 7. The coefficient of variation (= (100 standard deviation)/mean) values of *A. halimus* G_0/G_1 peaks ranged from 1.5 to 4.4%.

We can observe other peaks than the ones labeled G_0G_1, Because homogenization of the plant tissue produces debris that interferes with the detection and measurement of the isolated nuclei.

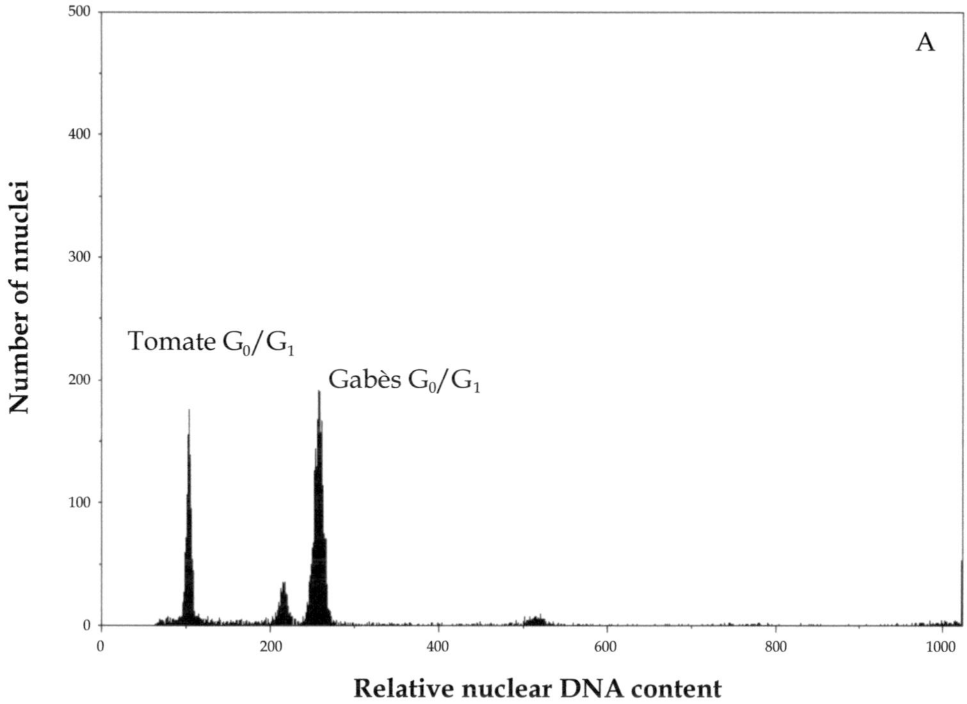

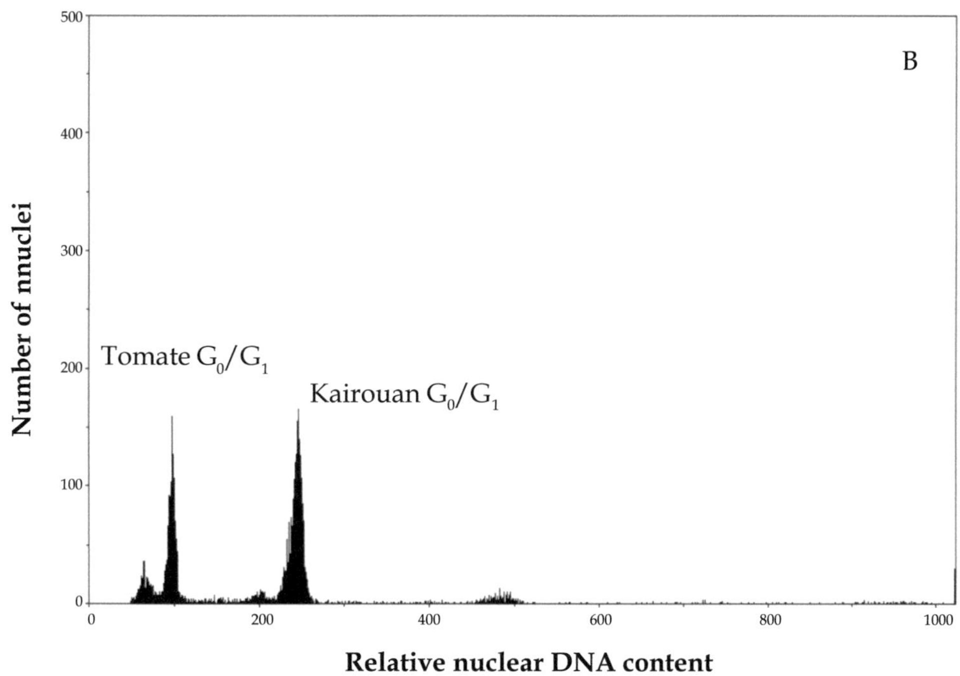

Fig. 3. Flow cytometric analyses of *A. halimus* L. : (A) Gabès, (B) Kairouan (Tunisia) populations

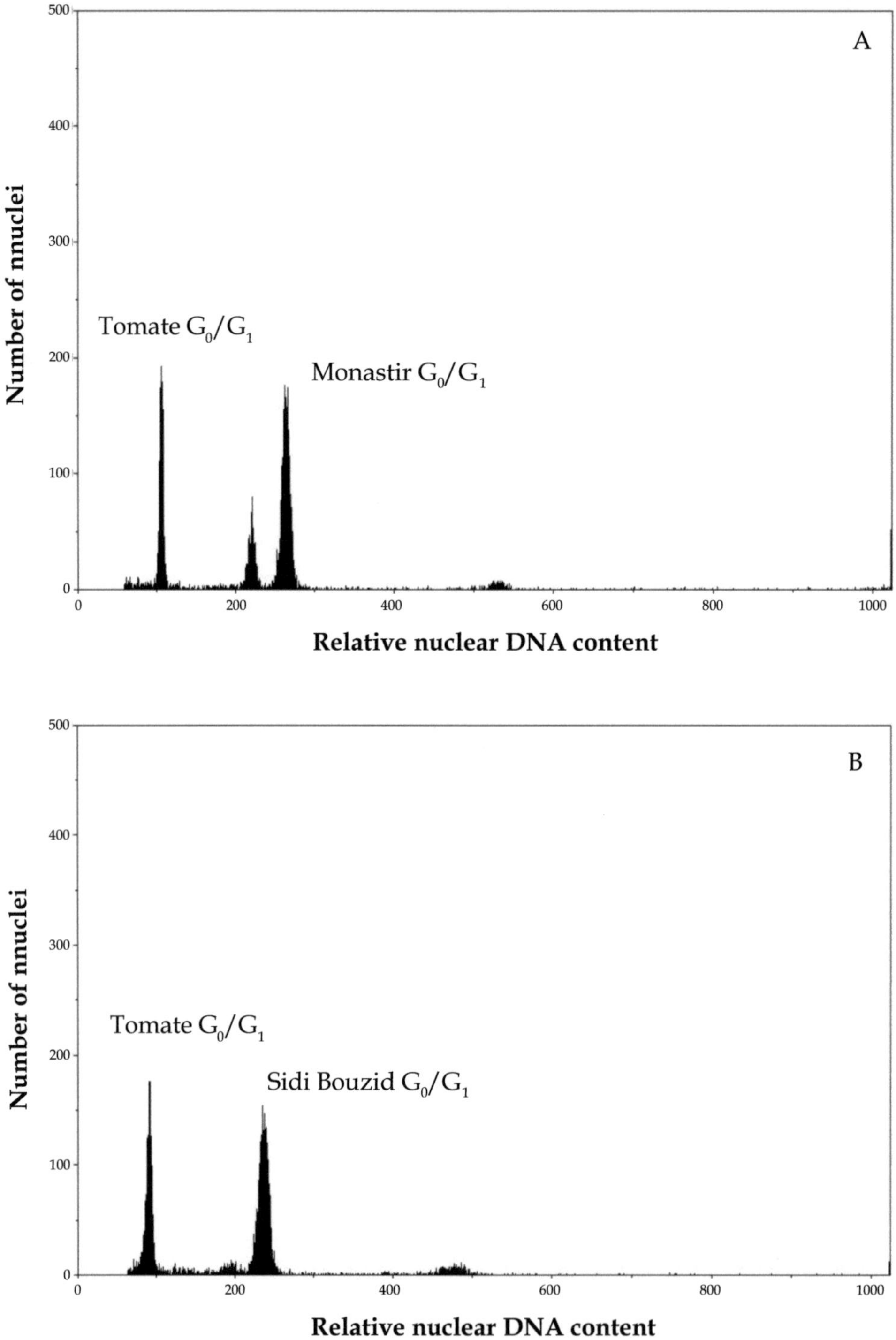

Fig. 4. Flow cytometric analyses of *A. halimus* L. : (A) Monastir, (B) Sidi Bouzid (Tunisia) populations

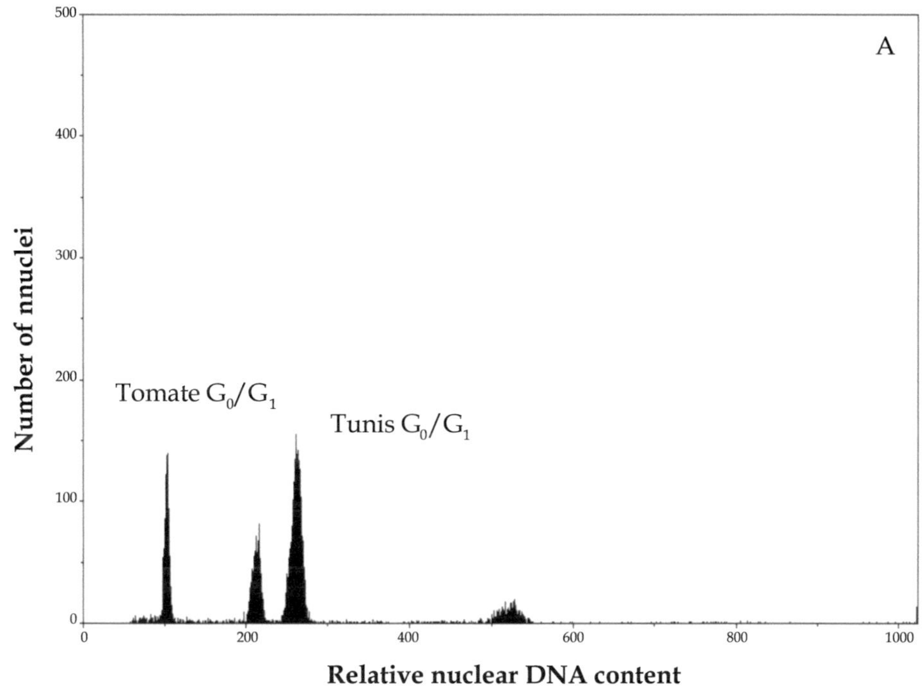

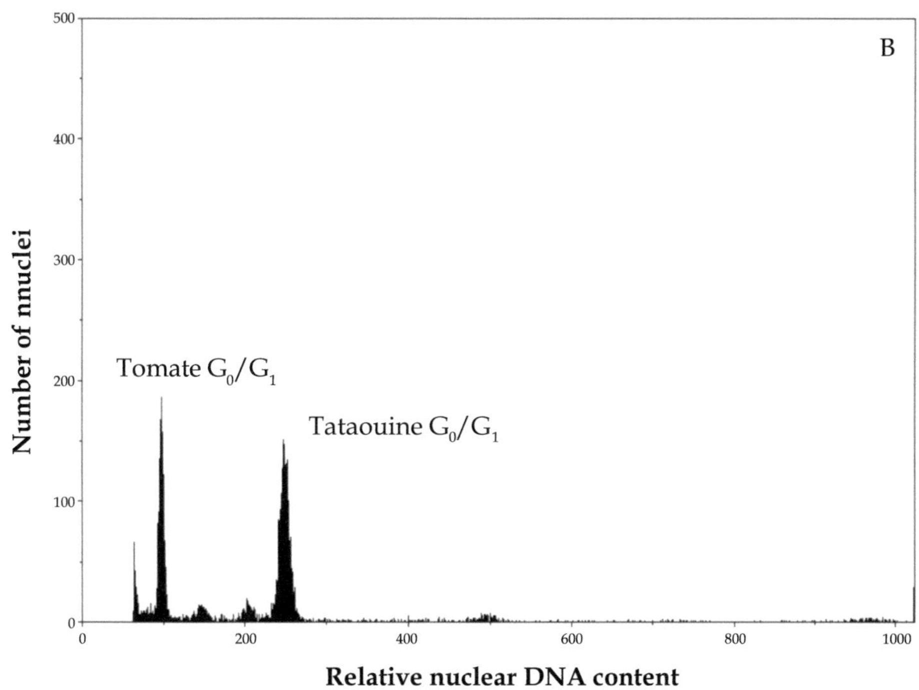

Fig. 5. Flow cytometric analyses of *A. halimus* L. : (A) Tunis, (B) Tataouine (Tunisia) populations

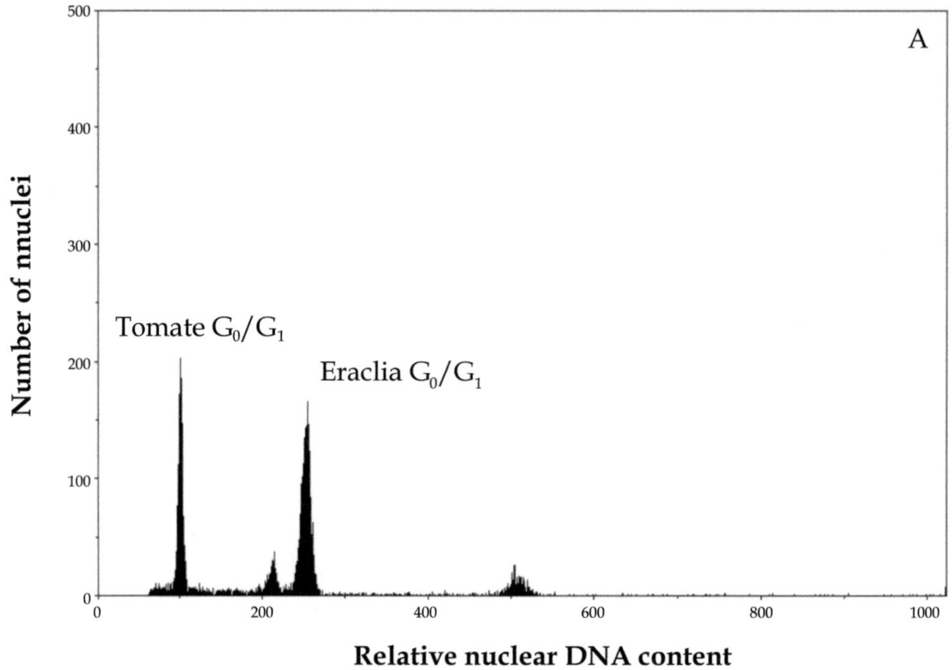

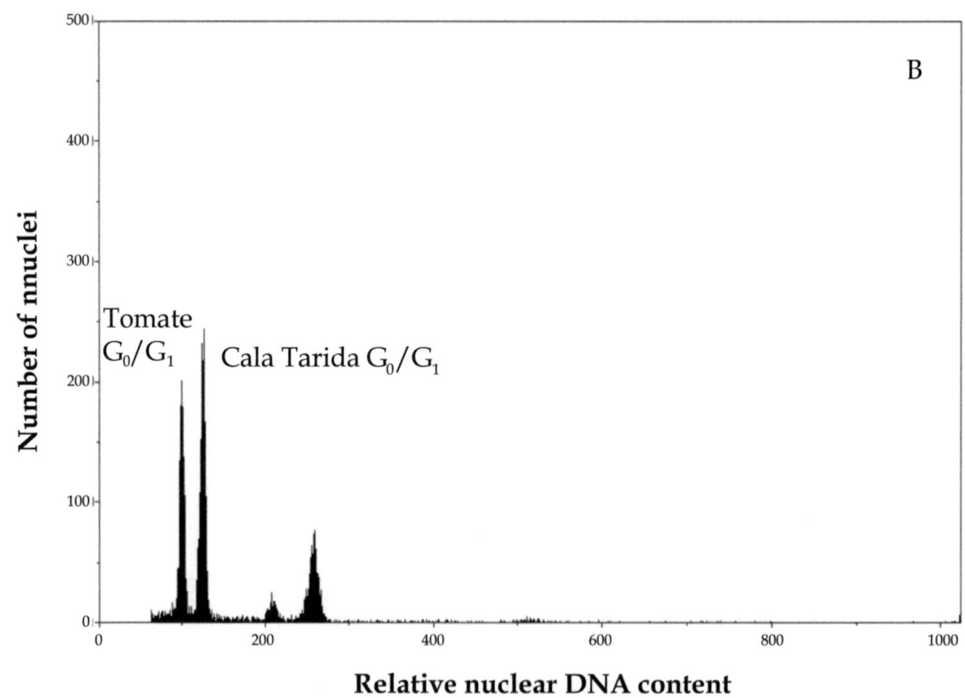

Fig. 6. Flow cytometric analyses of *A. halimus* L. : (A) Eraclia, (Italy) (B) (Cala tarida (Spain) populations

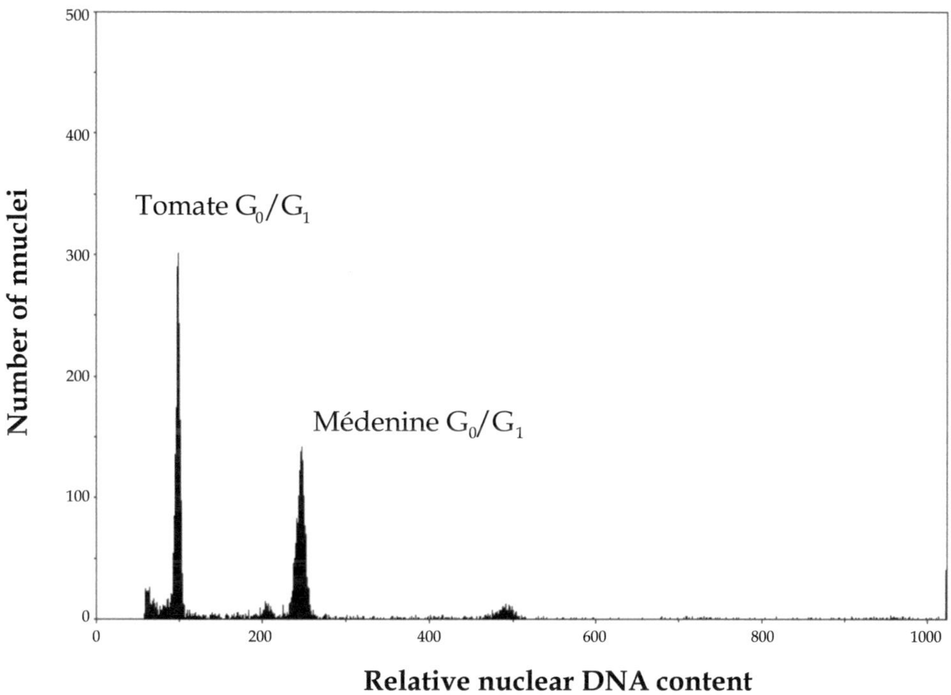

Fig. 7. Flow cytometric analyses of *A. halimus* L.: Médenine (Tunisia) population

The results of nuclear DNA content analysis are shown in Table 2. The mean 2C DNA content of the diploid population Cala Tarida was 2.412 pg. As expected, tetraploid populations had approximately two times higher DNA content, ranging from 4.918 pg in Tataouine to 4.972 pg in Gabès, but without statistically-significant differences among them (p >0.05).

Population	2C nuclear DNA content (pg)		1C genome size (Mpb)
	Mean	s.d.	
Tunis	4.970	0.095	2398
Monastir	4.958	0.104	2392
Kairouan	4.961	0.113	2394
Sidi Bouzid	4.950	0.106	2388
Gabes	4.972	0.135	2399
Medenine	4.950	0.116	2388
Tataouine	4.918	0.110	2373
Eraclea	4.967	0.098	2397
Cala Tarida	2.412	0.051	1164

Table 2. Estimated of nuclear DNA (2C) amounts (pg) ± s.d. (n = 8_16) for the studied populations of *A. halimus* L. General Linear Model analysis gave an F value of 1013.4 (p <0.001) for the population effect on nuclear DNA content. Sub-groups not sharing a common letter differ significantly (p <0.001), according to the Student-Newman–Keuls test

3.2 Chromosome counts

The chromosome numbers in the *A. halimus* L. populations studied are shown in table 3. For the Tunisian populations and the population from Eraclea (Italy), the chromosome number in a somatic metaphase nucleus was observed to be 36. Thus, since the base chromosome number in the genus Atriplex is x = 9 (Nobs 1975), these populations are tetraploid (2n = 4x = 36). The Cala Tarida population (Spain) was diploid (2n = 2x = 18).

Population	Chromosome number (2n)
Tunis	n.d.[a]
Monastir	36
Kairouan	36
Sidi Bouzid	36
Gabes	36
Medenine	n.d
Tataouine	36
Eraclea	36
Cala Tarida	18

[a]n.d., not determined.

Table 3. Estimated somatic chromosome number for the studied populations of *A. halimus* L

4. Discussion

An efficient method for the determination of the ploidy level is described, based on a measurement of the DNA content of interphase nuclei by flow cytometry. Both individual plants as well as plant populations can be used to obtain the desired DNA-histograms (De Laat et al. 1987).This can provide a diagnostic tool for separating the subspecies in cases where the morphological observation in inconclusive. Flow cytometry has been recognized as being superior to microscopic chromosome counts for a number of reasons. With recent technical improvements in modern flow cytometers, it is now a matter of days instead of months for researcher to become confident with the technique. Leaf material can collected at any growth stage, leaving tha plant alive, and only small amount of living material is necessary (Galbraith et al. 1997). The method was found to be reliable and highly sensitive for detecting small differences in DNA content (Lysák et al. 2000).

Ploidy determination using flow cytometry reduces the need for many morphological measurements and chromosome counts, and flow cytometry can be used on seedlings or mature plants with rapid, reliable results. The success of flow cytomery in distinguishing between species that differ in ploidy level is important for breedings programs (Stacy et al. 2002). Compared to conventional chromosome counting flow cytometry turned out to be highly competetive in terms of simplicity, accuracy and costs.

Polyploidy, which is known to occur in numerous dryland shrubs, is present in one third of the known *Atriplex* species (Stutz 1989). Polyploidy is one of the most important mechanisms in plant evolution. About 30-35% of phanerogamous species are polyploid. The ploidy levels frequently identified are tetraploid and hexaploid (Bouharmont, 1976). Within the genus *Atriplex*, the diploid state has been found in 26 species recorded in California

(Nobs, 1975) and 27 endemic species in Australia (Nobs, 1979). More recently, meiotic chromosome counts of n = 9 (2n = 18) have been determined from wild plants of *Atriplex* (Subgenus Theleophyton) *billardierei* gathered in New Zealand and on Chatham Island (De Lang et al., 1997). The existence of polyploidy has been found in *Atriplex canescens* (Stutz et al., 1975; McArthur, 1977; Sanderson and Stutz, 1994), in *A. tridentata* (Stutz et al., 1979), in *A. confertifolia* (Stutz et al., 1983; Sanderson et al., 1990). Considerable variability has been described within *A. halimus*, at both the morphological and isozyme polymorphism levels (Franclet & Le Houérou, 1971; Le Houérou, 1992; Abbad et al., 2003). Differences in floral sex ratio (male/female flowers), floral architecture and other vegetative and fruit morphological characteristics, related to population and growth conditions, have been reported recently (Abbad et al., 2003; Hcini et al., 2003; Talamali et al., 2003).

With respect to their morphology, the tetraploid populations from Tunisia and Italy studied here correspond to ssp. schweinfurthii, whilst the diploid Cala Tarida has a ssp. *halimus* morphology: ssp. *halimus* having a more erect habit, smaller in size (0.5–2.0 m height compared to 1.0– 3.0 m for schweinfurthii), shorter fruit-bearing branches (0.2–0.5 m compared to 0.5–1.0 m) and less-markedly-toothed fruit valves (Franclet & Le Houérou, 1971; Le Houérou, 1992). Franclet & Le Houérou (1971) & Le Houérou (1992) divided *A. halimus* into two subspecies: *halimus* and *schweinfurthii*. This was based on differences in morphology, with respect to habit, size, leaf shape and fruit morphology. Regarding distribution, ssp. *halimus* generally grows in higher-rainfall (>400 mm year_1) zones, in western Mediterranean areas such as France and Spain and on Atlantic coasts, whilst ssp. *schweinfurthii* is adapted to arid zones (100–400 mm rainfall period 1000–500 BC (Le Houérou, 1981); ssp. *schweinfurthii* may have subsequently populated such areas.

According to Le Houérou (2000), both subspecies are extremely heterogeneous in terms of their morphology, ecology, productivity and palatability to herbivores. However, ssp. *halimus* predominates in semi-arid to subhumid areas and has a higher leaf: shoot ratio than ssp. *schweinfurthii*, which is better adapted to arid environments but is less productive in terms of browsing biomass. The high levels of variability observed may be required to maintain plasticity in a highly fluctuating and diverse environment like Mediterranean Basin. Another reason for the higher intrapopulational variation of ssp *schweinfurthii* could be its polyploid character. According to Soltis & Soltis (2000), polyploids, both individuals and populations, maintain higher levels of heterozygosity than do their diploid progenitors. Moreover, most polyploids may have a much better adaptability to diverse ecosystems, which may contribute to their success in nature. This is illustrated in the case of ssp. *schweinfurthii*, by its much bigger distribution area than ssp. *halimus* and by its presence in very contrasting biotopes.

To our knowledge, this is the first report on genome size estimation in the Tunisian populations of *A. halimus* L. compared to a known range of genome size in plants (Bennet et al. 1997), the *Atriplex* specie should be considered taxa with a small size genome. Haddioui & Baaziz (2001), studying isozyme polymorphism in Moroccan populations of *A. halimus* (presumably tetraploid), found a relatively high degree of genetic diversity, predominantly due to within-population diversity, with between-population variation accounting for only 8%. These authors attributed this to the highly-outbreeding nature of *A. halimus*. The greater genetic heterozygosity of polyploids, at both individual and population levels, may give them a selective advantage in unstable environments (Sanderson et al., 1989; Soltis & Soltis,

2000). In the current work, we found no significant differences among plants within populations with respect to nuclear DNA content.

5. Conclusion

The Tunisian populations originated from widely-separated sites of contrasting climatic conditions plus a population from Eraclea, Sicily (Italy), were tetraploid (2n = 4x = 36) whereas a population from Cala Tarida, Ibiza (Spain) was diploid (2n = 2x = 18). With respect to nuclear DNA, the 2C DNA content of population Cala Tarida was estimated to be 2.41 pg. There was no significant difference among the tetraploid populations (or among plants within populations), whose 2C DNA content ranged from 4.92 to 4.97 pg. The present study clearly shows that the precision and rapidity of flow cytometric estimation of nuclear DNA content makes the method very attractive for estimation of genome size both in animal and plant species. This protocol showed to be convenient (sample preparation is easy), rapid (several hundreds of samples can be analysed in one working day), it does not require dividing cells, it is non-destructive (one sample can be prepared, e.g., from a few milligrams of leaf tissue), and can detected mixoploidy. Therefore the method is used in different areas ranging from basic research to plant breeding and production. On the other hand, determination of nuclear DNA content showed that certain populations with morphologies intermediate between those considered typical of ssp. *halimus* and *schweinfurthii* were tetraploid. This kind of approach, together with studies of morphology and isoenzyme polymorphism, as well as molecular techniques could be employed on a wider (and more detailed) geographical scale to ascertain the phylogenetic relationships within the species.

6. Acknowledgment

Seeds of tomato cv. Stupicke polni were supplied by Dr. J. Doležel (Laboratory of Molecular Cytogenetics and Cytometry, Institute of Experimental Botany, Olomouc, Czech Republic). We Thank P. Dutuit, M. Bounejmate, M. Forty, L. Stringi, H.N. Le Houérou, A. robeldo and I. Delgado for the Seed samples of *Atriplex halimus* L. from Morroco, Algeria, France and Spain. This work was funded by the European Union (DG12, INCO programme ERB 3514 IC18-CT98-0390), by the Consejería de Agricultura y Medioambiente de la Región de Murcia, and by F.S.T. of Tunisia.

7. References

Abbad, A., Cherkaoui, M. & Benchaabane, A. (2003). Morphology and allozyme variability of three natural populations of *Atriplex halimus* L. *Ecologica Mediterranea,*Vol. 29, pp. 99-109.

Bennet, M.D., Cox, A.V. and Leitch, I.J. (1997). Angiosperm DNA C-values database. http://www.rbgkew.org.uk/cval/database1.html.

Bennett, M.D., Bhandol, P. & Leitch I.J. (2000). Nuclear DNA amounts in Angiosperms and their modern uses new estimates. *Annals of Botany,* Vol. 86, pp. 859-909.

Bouharmont, J. (1976). Cytotaxonomie. Université Catholique de Louvain, Faculté des Sciences, Louvain-la-Neuve.

Cibilis, A.F., Swift, D.M. and Mcarthur, E.D. (1998). Plant-herbivory interactions in *Atriplex*: current state of knowledge. USDA Forest Service General Technical Report, Vol. 14, pp. 1-29.

David, J.W., Immaculda, M., Elena, G., Nora, F. & Enrique, C. (2005). Determination of ploidy and nuclear DNA content in populations of *Atriplex halimus* (Chenopodiaceae). *Botanical Journal of the Linnean Society*, Vol. 147, pp. 441-448.

De Laat, A.M.M, Gôhde,W. & Vogelzang, M.J.D.C.(1987). Determination of ploidy of single plants and plant populations by flow cytometry. *Plant Breed.* Vol. 99, pp. 303-307.

De Lange, P.J., Murray, B.J. & Crowcroft, G.M. (1997). Chromosome number of New Zealand specimens of *Atriplex billardierei*, Chenopodiaceae. *New Zealand J. Bot.*, Vol. 35, pp. 129-131.

Doležel, J. (1991). Flow cytometric analysis of nuclear DNA content in higher plants. *Phytochem. Anal.*, Vol. 2, pp. 143-154.

Doležel, J. (1997). Application of flow cytometry for study of plant genomes. *J. Appl. Genet.*, Vol. 38, pp. 285-302.

Doležel, J., Sgorbati S. & Lucretti, S. (1992). Comparison of three DNA fluorochromes for flow cytometric estimation of nuclear DNA content in plants. *Physiologia Plantarum*, Vol. 85, pp. 625-631.

Emshiller, E. (2002). Ploidy levels among species in the' Oxalis tuberose alliance' as inferred by flow cytometry. *Annals of Botany*, Vol. 89, pp. 741-735.

Franclet, A. & Le Houérou, H.N. (1971). Les Atriplex en Tunisie et en Afrique du Nord. Food and Agriculture Organization, Rome.

Freitas, H. & Breckle, S.W. (1993). Accumulation of nitrate in bladder hairs of Atriplex species. *Plant Physiol. Biochem.*, Vol. 31, pp. 887-892.

Galbraith, D.W. (1989). Analysis of higher plants by flow cytometry and cell sorting. *Int. Rev. Cytol.* Vol. 116, pp. 165-228.

Galbraith D.W., Lambert G.M, Macas J. & Doležel J. 1997. Analysis of nuclear DNA content and ploidy in higher plants. Current Protocols in Cytometry: 7.6.1-7.6.22.

Haddioui, A. & Baaziz, M. (2001). Genetic diversity of natural populations of Atriplex halimus L. in Morocco: An isoenzyme-based overview. *Euphytica*, Vol. 121, pp. 99-106.

Hcini, K., Ben Farhat, M., Harzallah, H. & Bouzid, S. (2003). Contribution à l'étude du polymorphisme chez dix populations naturelles d'Atriplex halimus L. en Tunisie. *Bull. Soc. Sci. Nat. de Tunisie,* Vol. 30, pp. 69-78.

Le Houérou, H.N. (1981). Impact of man and his animals on Mediterranean vegetation. In: di Castri F., Goodall D.W. and Specht R.L. (eds), Ecosystems of the world. 11. Mediterranean-type shrublands, Elsevier, Amsterdam, pp. 479-521.

Le Houerou, H.N. (1992). The role of saltbushes (Atriplex spp.) in arid land rehabilitation in the Mediterranean Basin. *A review. Agrofor. Syst.*, Vol. 18, pp. 107-148.

Le Houérou, H.N. (2000). Utilization of fodder trees and shrubs in the arid and semiarid zones of west Asia and North Africa. *Arid soil Research and Rehabilitation*, Vol. 14, pp. 101-135.

Lysák, M.A., Rostková, A., Dixon, J.M., Rossi, G. & Doležel, J. (2000). Limited genome size variation in *Sesleria albicans*. *Annals of Botany*, Vol. 86, pp. 399-403.

McArthur, E.D. (1977). Environmentally induced changes of sex expression in Atriplex canescens. *Heredity* , Vol. 38, pp. 97-103.

McAthur, E.D. & Sanderson, S.C. (1984). Distribution, systematics and evolution of Chenopodiaceae: an overview. USDA *Forest Service General technical report*, Vol. 172, pp. 14-24.

Nobs, M.A. (1975). Chromosome numbers in Atriplex. Carnegie Institute of Washington yearbook. Vol. 74: 762.

Nobs, M.A. (1979). Chromosome numbers in Australian species of Atriplex. Carnegie Institue of Washington Year Book. Vol. 78, pp 164-169.

Nuñez, O. (1968). A acetic-hematoxylin squash method for small chromosomes. Caryologia Vol. 21, pp. 115-119.

Sanderson, S.C. & Stutz, H.C. (1994). High chromosome numbers in Mojavean and Sonoran desert *Atriplex canescens* (Chenopodiaceae). *Amer. J. Bot.*, Vol. 81, pp. 1045-1053.

Sanderson, S.C., McArthur, E.D. & Stutz, H.C. (1989). A relationship between polyploidy and habitat in western shrub species. *USDA Forest Service General Technical Report*, Vol. 256, pp. 23-30.

Sanderson,S.C., Stutz, H.C. & McArthur, E.D. (1990). Geographic differentiation in Atriplex confertifolia. *Amer. J. Bot.*, Vol. 77, pp. 490-498.

Soltis, P.E. & Soltis, D.E. (2000). The role of genetic and genomic attributes in the success of polyploids. Proceedings of the National Academy of Sciences U.S.A., Vol. 97, pp. 7051-7057.

Stacy, A. B., Karen, A. P., & William, A. M. (2002). Ploidy determination in Agrotis using flow Cytometry and Morphological traits. *Crop Science,* vol. 42 pp

Stutz, H.C. & Sanderson, S.C. (1983). Evolutionary studies of Atriplex: chromosome races of A. confertifolia (Shadscale). *Amer. J. Bot.*, Vol. 77, pp. 490-498.

Stutz, H.C., Melby, J.M. & Livingston, G.K. (1975). Evolutionary studies of Atriplex: a relic gigas diploid population of Atriplex canescens. *Amer. J. Bot.*, Vol. 62, pp. 236-245.

Stutz, H.C., Pope, C.L. & Sandeson, S.C. (1979). Evolutionary studies of Atriplex: adaptive products from the natural hybrid, 6n *A. tiendatata* x 4n *A. canescens*. *Amer. J. Bot.*, Vol. 66, pp. 1181-1193.

Talamali, A., Bajji, M., Le Thomas, A., Kinet, J.M. & Dutuit P. (2003). Flower architecture and sex determination: how does Atriplex halimus play with floral morphogenesis and sex genes? *New Phytologist,* Vol. 157, pp. 105-113.

Valderrábano, J., Muñoz, F. & Delgado, I. (1996). Browsing ability and utilization by sheep and goats of *Atriplex halimus* L. shrubs. *Small Ruminant Research*, Vol. 19, pp. 131-136.

Zervoudakis, G., Angelopoulos, K., Salahas, G., Georgiou, C.D., (1998). Differences in cold inactivation of phospho-enolpyruvate carboxylase among C4 species: The effect of pH and of enzyme concentration. *Photosynthetica*, Vol.35, pp. 169-175.

6

Yeast Cell Death During the Drying and Rehydration Process

Boris Rodríguez-Porrata[1], Didac Carmona-Gutierrez[2], Gema López-Matínez[1], Angela Reisenbichler[2], Maria Bauer[2], Frank Madeo[2] and Ricardo Cordero-Otero[1]
[1]*Dep. Biochemestry and Biotechnology, University Rovira i Virgili,*
[2]*Institute of Molecular Biosciences, University of Graz,*
[1]*Spain*
[2]*Austria*

1. Introduction

Dehydration and rehydration stress (DRS) is a serious problem affecting plants, animals and humans and much research has been devoted to the subject over the years. Attempts to enhance the desiccation tolerance of cells first focused on plant cells and seeds of agricultural significance, as the availability of water is one of the main parameters that limits plant productivity (Bartels et al., 2001). More recently, lyophilisation and other dehydration-based technologies have been explored by a number of groups for the purpose of cell and tissue preservation (Liang et al., 2002; Wolkers et al., 2002; Elliott et al., 2006). Furthermore, active dry yeast is commonly used in the food industry for the production of beer, wine and bread. *Saccharomyces cerevisiae*, in addition to being an excellent model for the study of eukaryotic cells, is an ideal starting point for deciphering DRS response mechanisms due to its anhydrobiotic qualities. The transformation of yeast cells from the state of vital activity to that of anhydrobiosis as a result of cell desiccation is followed by a period of suspended animation, and the subsequent recovery of metabolic functions. To understand what yeasts do, we must address controversial issues such as cell age, longevity, the structural and biochemical properties of anhydrous cytoplasm, and metabolic stasis (Beker & Rapoport, 1987). The resulting damage may be classified into damage of different macromolecules, structures, organelles, and defensive intracellular reactions. Membrane changes are especially interesting (Rapoport et al., 1994). Increased plasma permeability or rehydration has been proposed as the main cause of cell death during dehydration. In fact, the increase and decrease of osmotic pressure causes the leakage of nucleotides, ions and other soluble cell components into the surrounding medium (Attfield et al., 2000). The highly dynamic lipid bilayer of the plasma membrane is known to undergo phase transitions during dehydration (Laroche et al., 2005) and rehydration (Crowe et al., 1992). These phase transitions of some phospholipids in the membrane may be the cause of membrane rupture or changes in permeability (Laroche et al., 2003). Other authors suggest that the formation of endovesicles during dehydration leads to plasma membrane lysis during osmotic expansion when the cells are rehydrated (Mille et al., 2003). Yeast cells can recover faster or slower depending on the culture conditions (Anand & Brown, 1968; Rodríguez-Porrata et al., 2011) and/or rehydration conditions (Poirier et al., 1999; Rodríguez-Porrata et al., 2008). Despite the accumulated knowledge about the structural changes and the mechanical damage to cells during DRS, little is known about the molecular mechanisms involved in yeast cell death under these stressful conditions. In recent years, it has become clear that yeast can succumb to cell death, exhibiting typical apoptotic markers (Ludovico et al., 2001; Madeo et al., 1997, Madeo et al., 1999). Moreover, the yeast genome codes for many proteins of the basic molecular machinery responsible for cell death, including orthologues of caspases (Madeo et al., 2002), AIF (Wissing et al., 2004), and yeast EndoG (NUC1) (Büttner, et al., 2007). In addition, programmed death in yeast has been linked to complex apoptotic scenarios such as mitochondrial fragmentation (Fannjiang et al., 2004), cytochrome c release (Ludovico et al., 2002), and aging (Fabrizio et al., 2004; Herker et al., 2004; Laun et al., 2001). Notably, histone H2B phosphorylation, which is considered to be a universal prerequisite for apoptosis execution (Cheung et al., 2003), was shown to be necessary for cell-death induction upon oxidative stress in yeast (Ahn et al., 2005). Recently, yeast apoptosis research has begun to resolve the complex interplay of mitochondrial cell death mediators. It is becoming increasingly clear that the connection between mitochondrial respiration and apoptosis is intricate, as suppression of respiration can either be beneficial or detrimental to the cell, depending greatly on the apoptotic scenario (Eisenberg et al., 2007). It is not likely by chance that nature has coupled pro-apoptotic potential to many molecules that have a genuine function in the respiratory chain of healthy cells, such as cytochrome *c*, AIF (**a**poptosis-**i**nducing **f**actor) or AMID (**a**poptosis-inducing factor-homologous **m**itochondrion-associated **i**nducer of **d**eath). By simply changing the location from mitochondria, the daytime place of action, to the cytosol, cell death is executed in a redundant, highly effective manner. As a result, the permeabilisation of the mitochondrial outer membrane is probably the point of no return in cell death execution and thus an excellent target for clinical manipulations of apoptosis (Galluzzi et al., 2006) and perhaps even necrosis (Golstein & Kroemer, 2006).

Here, we identified a group of mitochondrial knockout mutants (Δ*Aif1*, Δ*Cpr3*, Δ*Nuc1*, and Δ*Qcr7)* as hyper-tolerant to dehydration stress. Yeast cells were analysed for apoptotic hallmarks. DHE staining revealed that during dehydration and rehydration, the wild type showed enhanced ROS production compared to the mutants. Additionally, Annexin V/PI double staining indicated that, after the imposition of stress, the wild type culture also contains an elevated percentage of necrotic and late apoptotic/secondary necrotic cells. Further tests using the strains Δ*oxa1*, Δ*mgm1*, and Δ*yac1* suggested that cell death during dehydration stress is neither caspase nor respiratory dependent.

2. Materials and methods

2.1 Strains and growth conditions

Table 1 summarises the yeast strains used in this study. The single null mutant collection of strains and the reference strain, all in the BY4742 genetic background, were purchased from EUROSCARF (Frankfurt, Germany). Yeast strains were grown in shake flasks (150 rpm) in SC media containing 0.17% yeast nitrogen base supplied by Difco, 2% glucose, 0.5% $(NH_4)_2SO_4$ and 25 mg l^{-1} uracil, 84 mg l^{-1} leucine, and 42 mg l^{-1} lysine, and histidine. The desiccation-rehydration process and the determination of yeast viability were performed as described in Rodríguez et al. (2011).

2.2 Determination of yeast viability

Yeast cells were cultivated in SC medium until the stationary phase and then some of the culture was transferred to a 12-well plate in the presence of trehalose at 10% W/V of the final concentration. Half of the cell suspension was transferred to another 12-well plate for drying. The cells in the second plate were air-dried at 28°C for 24 hours. They were then rehydrated with sterile water at 37°C for 30 minutes. To calculate cell survival, the cell cultures were diluted and cell concentration was determined with a CASY cell counter and aliquots containing 500 cells, which were spread onto YPD agar medium using a Whitley Automatic Spiral Plater furnished by AES Laboratoire (France). The number of colonies was determined after two days at 28°C. The CFU were quantified using a Lemnatec Microbiology-Colony-Counter and processed with ProtoCOL SR/HR counting system software version 1.27, supplied by Symbiosis (Cambridge, UK). After the colonies were counted, the percentage of viability was determined by means of a simple calculation.

2.3 Tests for apoptotic markers

Dihydroethidium (DHE) staining was performed with approximately $5 \cdot 10^6$ cells per experiment, which were washed with PBS (pH 7.0) and resuspended with 250 ml of 2.5 mg$\cdot$ml^{-1} DHE/PBS. After 5 min dark incubation at 25°C, the cells were washed with 250 ml PBS prior to both microscopic and flowcytometric evaluation. Each double Annexin V fluorescein and propidium iodide (PI) staining was carried out with $2 \cdot 10^7$ yeast cells washed with 500 ml sorbitol buffer (1.2 M sorbitol, 0.5 mM $MgCl_2$, 35 mM potassium phosphate, pH 6.8). The resuspended cells in 330 ml sorbitol buffer were incubated with 2.5µl Lyticase and 15 µl beta-glucuronidase/arylsulfatase (Roche) for 1 h at 28°C. After this treatment the cells became spheroblasts, so the centrifugation and resuspension steps were very brief. The cells were harvested, washed again in 500 ml sorbitol buffer, and suspended in incubation buffer (10 mM HEPES, 140 mM NaCl, 5 mM $CaCl_2$ at pH7.4) containing 0.6 M sorbitol. Then, 3 µl Annexin V acquired from Roche and 3 µl PI (100µg$\cdot$ml^{-1} in H_2O) were added and the cells were dark incubated for 20 min at 25°C. After adding 500 µl incubation buffer containing 0.6 M sorbitol the cells were ready to be analysed with the flowcytometer using 488 nm excitation and a 515 nm bandpass filter for fluorescein detection and a >560 nm filter for PI detection. TUNEL staining was performed as previously described in the literature (Büttner *et al.*, 2007). To determine frequencies of morphological phenotypes revealed by TUNEL, DHE- and Annexin V/PI double staining, at least 300 cells of three independent experiments were evaluated using flowcytometry and BD FACSDiva software.

2.4 Microscopy

Cultures of the strains were grown to the stationary phase in SC medium. The cells were washed with 1 x PBS buffer (pH 7.4) and fixed with 70% ethanol for 10 min at R.T. Images were taken using an Olympus model BH-2RFCA fluorescence microscope, an Olympus model c35AD-4 digital camera, and Metamorph® software provided by Soft Imaging System GmbH.

2.5 Statistical analyses

The results were statistically analysed by one-way ANOVA and the Scheffé test from the statistical software package SPSS 15.1. Statistical significance was set at $P<0.05$.

3. Results

3.1 Drying and rehydration stress compromises yeast survival

To study the molecular response to drying and rehydration stress (DRS) in yeast, we analysed the viability of the complete EUROSCARF collection of *Saccharomyces cerevisiae* upon DRS. This collection comprises a total of 4794 mutants, each deleted in one of the non-essential genes. While viability in the wild-type reference strain BY4742 was approximately 40%, we detected a group of around 100 deletion mutants with viability of less than 10%. Figure 1 shows the functional distribution of the corresponding genes ranked according to their relative abundance. Pathways involving protein synthesis and the biogenesis of cellular components occurred more frequently, while pathways connected to cell fate, cellular rescue and environment interaction were the least abundant. Furthermore, we detected a group of 12 deletion mutants with viability values higher than those of the reference strain.

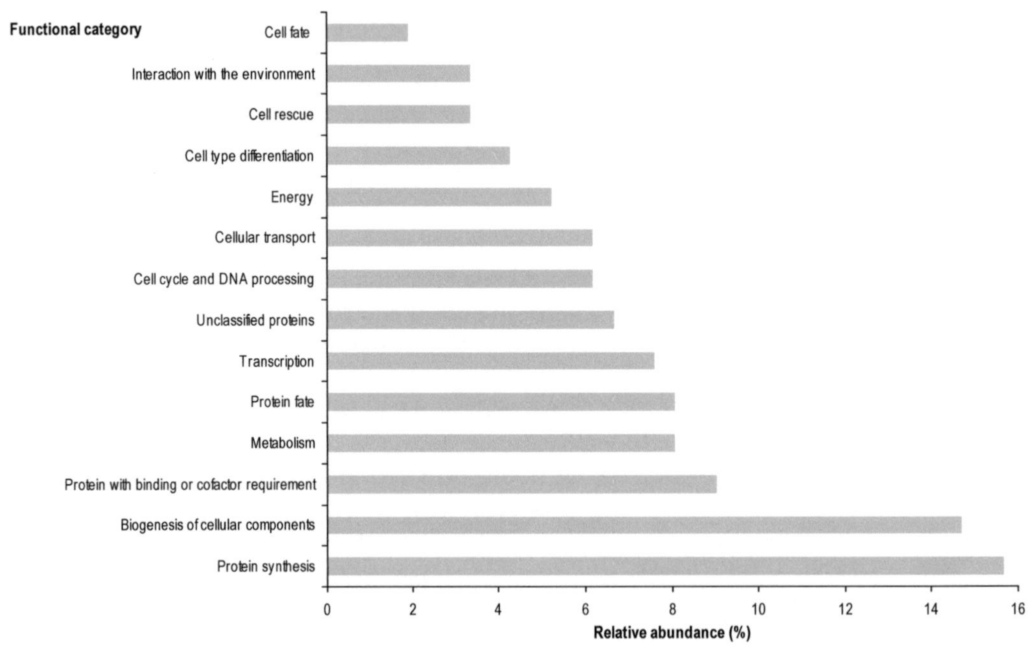

Fig. 1. Distribution of functional classes of 112 EUROSCARF deletion mutants showing less than 10% viability after drying and rehydration stress

3.2 Several mutants can rescue cell death upon rehydration stress

Among the 12 mutants that showed enhanced cell viability after dehydration stress, some are directly connected to programmed cell death (PCD). Figure 2 represents the fold increase in viability of some mutants deleted in genes closely linked to PCD. Interestingly, the knockouts with viabilities higher than the reference strain BY4742 lack the mitochondrial genes *AIF1*, *CPR3* and *NUC1* (2-fold increase in viability) and *QCR7* (3-fold increase). *CPR3* encodes for a yeast homologue of cyclophilin D (Dolinski et al., 1997), which is a peptidyl-prolyl isomerase located within the mitochondrial matrix and which is a component of mPTP, along with adenine nucleotide translocator (ANT) and the voltage-dependent anion transporter (VDAC). Cyclophilin D is thought to facilitate a calcium-triggered conformational change in the ANT mitochondrial permeability transition associated with mitochondrial swelling, outer membrane rupture, and the release of apoptotic mediators (Halestrap, 2005). Cyclophilin D has previously been implicated in both necrosis and apoptosis programmes (Halestrap, 2005; Schneider, 2005). Cpr3p has been reported to be central to the PCD process induced by Cu in *S. cerevisiae* (Liang & Zhou, 2007). MPTP has been shown to be a key component of necrotic cell death caused by calcium overload and oxidative stress and does not usually play much of a role in apoptosis (Crompton et al., 1988). The release of proteins from the compartment between the two mitochondrial membranes, of which citochrome C is the major player, triggers apoptosis in many cells through the caspase pathway. However, many researchers argue that this is unlikely because it would disrupt the production of ATP, which is required in the apoptosis process. This is supported by results obtained with cyclophilin D knockout mice in which the extensive apoptosis involved in development was not affected by the loss of cyclophilin D (Nakagawa et al., 2005). *AIF1* encodes for Aif1p, a homologue of the mammalian Apoptosis-Inducing Factor (AIF). Aif1p is a flavoprotein with NADH oxidase activity and contains a mitochondrial localisation sequence in the NH_2 terminus and a nuclear localisation sequence in the COOH terminus, as well as a putative DNA binding domain composed of positively charged amino acids (Wu et al., 2002). Upon the induction of apoptosis, Aif1p translocates to the nucleus, where it leads to chromatin condensation and DNA degradation (Susin et al., 1999; Madeo et al., 1999). It has recently been shown that chronological aging is a physiological trigger for apoptosis in yeast (Herker et al., 2004). The release of Aif1p from mitochondria may be subordinated to earlier caspase activation, supporting the notion that caspases and Aif1p may be engaged in cooperative or redundant pathways and they are activated by the same apoptotic stimulus (Arnoult et al., 2003; Madeo et al., 2002). *NUC1* encodes for the major mitochondrial nuclease and has RNAse and DNA endo- and exonucleolytic activities. Nuc1p plays a role in mitochondrial recombination, apoptosis and the maintenance of polyploidy. Nuc1p and mammalian mitochondrial nuclease EndoG share well preserved residues in the catalytically active site, suggesting that both belong to the large family of DNA/RNA nonspecific bba-Me-finger nucleases (Schafer et al., 2004). Upon the induction of apoptosis, the translocation of mammalian EndoG to the nucleus coincides with large-scale DNA fragmentation (Li et al., 2001; Parrish et al., 2001). EndoG may have a genuine vital function in addition to its pro-apoptotic function, which plays a role in cell proliferation and replication, as has in fact been suggested by other authors (Huang et al., 2006). The last mutated strain showing enhanced viability after the dehydration and rehydration process lacks *QCR7*, which is associated with Qcr8p and cytochrome *b*, both constituents of one of the sub-complexes of the mitochondrial inner membrane electron transport chain of the yeast cytochrome bc_1. The existence of this sub-complex has been proposed on the basis of the finding that the deletion of any one of these three genes leads to the disappearance of the other two subunits, and because the Qcr7p N-terminal was shown to stabilise the central core of the cytochrome bc_1 complex (Zara et al.,

2004; Lee et al., 2001). Furthermore, the *Δqcr7* strain does not continue the PDC process induced by Cu in *S. cerevisiae* (Liang & Zhou, 2007).

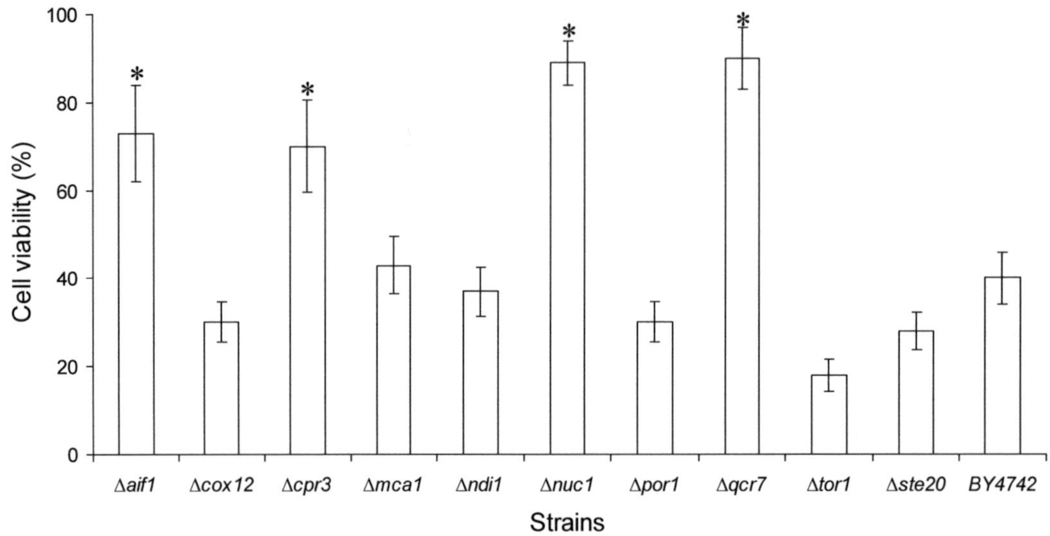

Fig. 2. Effect of deletion of genes linked to cell death mechanisms in cell viability after stress imposition. Values shown are means of n=3 independent samples ±SD. *Significant differences ($p \leq 0.05$) to BY4742 strain

Among the mutants evaluated and those deleted in genes closely linked to PCD, only four showed enhanced cell viability after the imposition of stress. We wanted to ascertain whether the higher viability rate for these four strains under dehydration stress could be due to differences in the apoptotic hallmark profile.

3.3 Dehydration survival is associated with diminished apoptosis and necrosis

We characterised the mode of cell death accompanying DRS by performing various assays using flowcytometry to quantify apoptotic and necrotic markers. The conversion of dihydroethidium (DHE) to fluorescent ethidium was used to visualise the accumulation of reactive oxygen species (ROS). DNA fragmentation was detected using TUNEL staining. Furthermore, Annexin V/propidium iodide (PI) co-staining was used to quantify the externalisation of phosphatidylserine, an early apoptotic event, and membrane permeabilisation, which is indicative for necrotic death. This staining allows a distinction to be made between early apoptotic (Annexin V positive, PI negative), late apoptotic (Annexin V positive, PI positive), and necrotic (Annexin V negative, PI positive) death. Figure 3 shows the results obtained for the apoptotic hallmarks of the BY4742, *Δaif1, Δcpr3, Δnuc1*, and *Δqcr7* strains before dehydration (BD) and after rehydration (AR), respectively. All strains began with comparable ROS levels before dehydration (Fig. 3-B). However, after rehydration, the *Δaif1, Δcpr3, Δnuc1* and *Δqcr7* strains show an approximate 20% reduction in ROS accumulation compared to the BY4742 strain. These reduced ROS levels in the mutated strains during stress imposition are accompanied by an increase in both early apoptotic and late apoptotic cell populations (Fig. 3 C-D), even when before the imposition of stress the

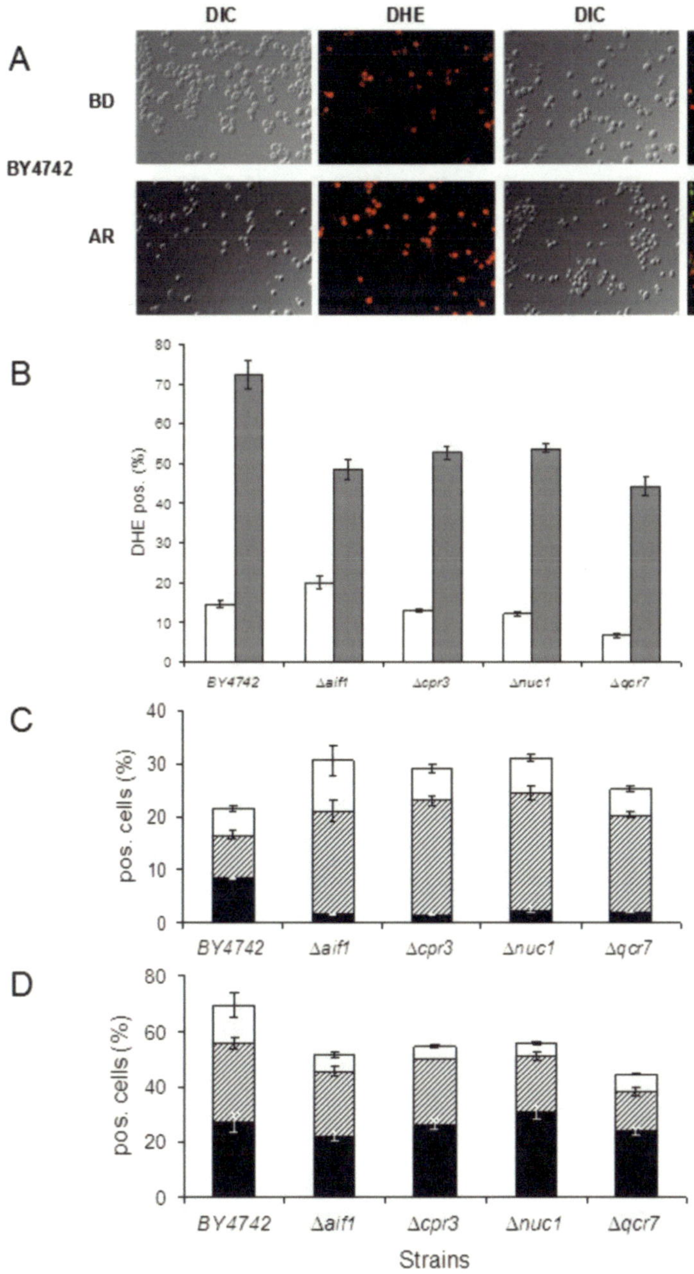

Fig. 3. Deletion of mitochondrial cell death genes prevents necrotic cell death. (A) These pictures are a representative example of fluorescence microscopy of DHE-, and AnnexinV/PI-costaining of before dehydration (BD) and after rehydration (AR) of the same BY4742 cell samples. (B) Level of ROS-accumulating cells using DHE-staining before drying (white bars) and after rehydration (grey bars). Quantification of stained cells before (C) and after (D) stress imposition: V^-/PI^+ □, V^+/PI^+ ▒, and V^+/PI^- ■. In each experiment, $3 \cdot 10^4$ cells were evaluated using flowcytometry. DIC, differential interference contrast; DHE pos., DHE-positive cells

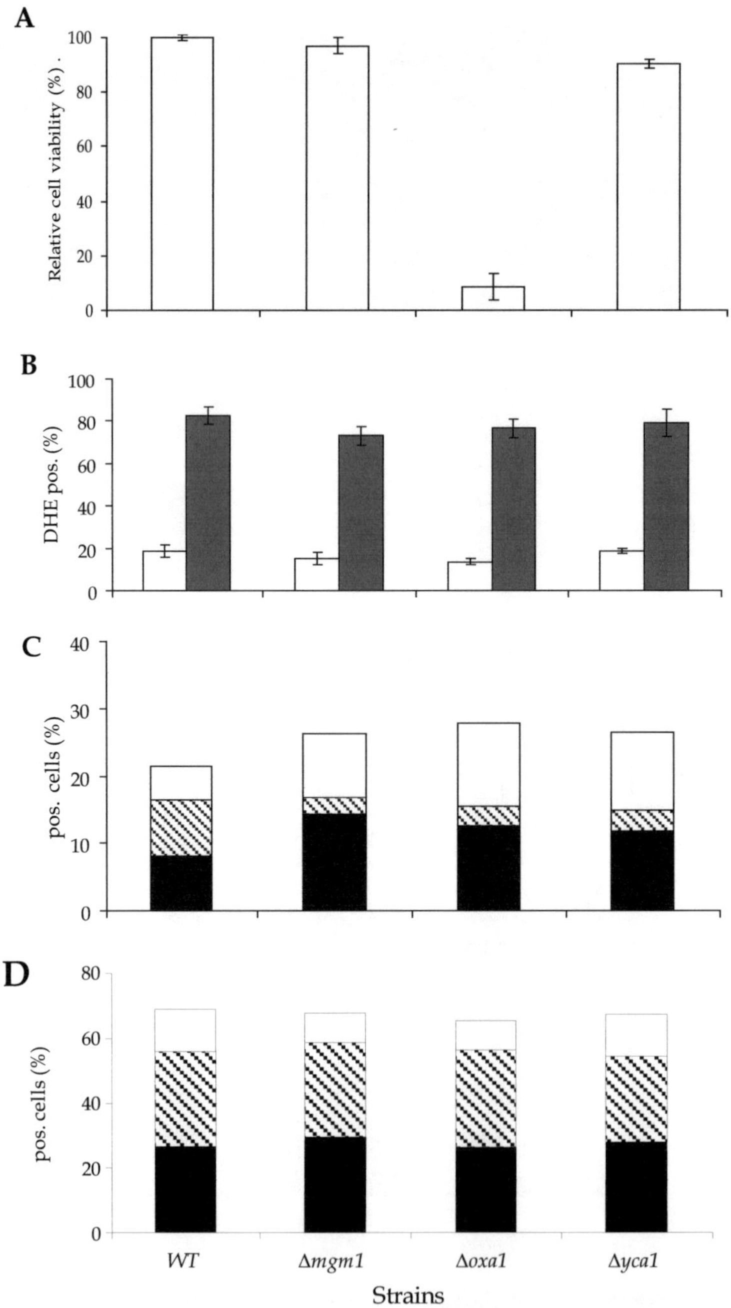

Fig. 4. Dehydration stress characterisation of respiratory deficient strains. (A) The scale of relative viability (%) indicates the percentage of experimental values for the different strains relative to the highest viability for *S. cereviciae*. (B) ROS accumulating cells before dehydration (white bars) and after rehydration (grey bars). V^-/PI^+ □, V^+/PI^+ ▒, and V^+/PI^- ■ stained cells before (C) and after (D) stress imposition. Values shown are means of *n*=3 independent samples ±SD

mutants showed 8% less early apoptotic and 10% more late apoptotic cells than BY4742. However, after stress imposition cell necrosis and late apoptotic populations were reduced in Δ strains by 17% and 10%, respectively. This result suggests that the aforementioned improved viability upon the absence of these genes corresponds to a prevention of necrosis and apoptosis under dehydration stress.

3.4 Respiration deficiency is not responsible for cell death prevention

Among the deleted mitochondrial strains, which provide resistance upon DRS, *QCR7* is essential to respiratory activity. We therefore evaluated two further respiratory deficient strains in order to rule out an effect due to loss of respiratory capacity. We chose the Δ*mgm1* and Δ*oxa1* mutants, which lack respiratory growth and have significantly different viability values after dehydration stress (40% and 5% respectively) (Fig. 4-A). Neither Δ*mgm1* nor Δ*oxa1* showed reduced ROS levels compared to the wild type (Fig. 4-B).

The analysis of apoptotic and necrotic markers further showed no significant differences in DNA fragmentation, phosphatidylserine externalisation or loss of cell integrity after rehydration (Fig. 4 C-D). Thus, we might suggest that the observed reduction in the apoptotic and necrotic populations for the Δ*aif1*, Δ*cpr3*, Δ*nuc1* and Δ*qcr7* strains after DRS is independent of respiration capacity.

3.5 Reduction of apoptotic and necrotic cell populations is caspase-independent

We tested the Δ*yca1* strain to determine whether cell death was associated with the caspase pathway in our stress evaluation. The *S. cerevisiae YCA1* gene encodes for a metacaspase that is involved in yeast apoptosis in response to multiple stimuli, such as cell aging, oxidative stress, etc. (Herker et al., 2004; Madeo et al., 2002). The Δ*yca1* strain does not show improved survival or reduced ROS levels compared to BY4742 after stress imposition (Fig. 4-A and -B). Furthermore, the analysis of apoptotic and necrotic markers also revealed no significant differences to the reference strain in DNA fragmentation, phosphatidylserine externalisation or loss of cell integrity after rehydration (Fig. 4-C and -D). This result supports the suggestion that the reduction in the apoptotic and necrotic populations observed during dehydration stress does not involve the metacaspase pathway.

Strain	Genotype	Source
BY4742	*MATa his3Δ1 leu2Δ0 lys2Δ0 ura3Δ0*	EUROSCARF
Δ*aif1*	*MATa his3Δ1 leu2Δ0 lys2Δ0 ura3Δ0 aif1::kanMX4*	EUROSCARF
Δ*cox12*	*MATa his3Δ1 leu2Δ0 lys2Δ0 ura3Δ0 cox12::kanMX4*	EUROSCARF
Δ*cpr3*	*MATa his3Δ1 leu2Δ0 lys2Δ0 ura3Δ0 cpr3::kanMX4*	EUROSCARF
Δ*mca1*	*MATa his3Δ1 leu2Δ0 lys2Δ0 ura3Δ0 mca1::kanMX4*	EUROSCARF
Δ*ndi1*	*MATa his3Δ1 leu2Δ0 lys2Δ0 ura3Δ0 ndi1::kanMX4*	EUROSCARF
Δ*nuc1*	*MATa his3Δ1 leu2Δ0 lys2Δ0 ura3Δ0 nuc1::kanMX4*	EUROSCARF
Δ*por1*	*MATa his3Δ1 leu2Δ0 lys2Δ0 ura3Δ0 por1::kanMX4*	EUROSCARF
Δ*qcr7*	*MATa his3Δ1 leu2Δ0 lys2Δ0 ura3Δ0 qcr7 ::kanMX4*	EUROSCARF
Δ*tor1*	*MATa his3Δ1 leu2Δ0 lys2Δ0 ura3Δ0 tor1::kanMX4*	EUROSCARF
Δ*ste20*	*MATa his3Δ1 leu2Δ0 lys2Δ0 ura3Δ0 ste20::kanMX4*	EUROSCARF
Δ*yca1*	*MATa his3Δ1 leu2Δ0 lys2Δ0 ura3Δ0 yca1::kanMX4*	EUROSCARF
Δ*oxa1*	*MATa his3Δ1 leu2Δ0 lys2Δ0 ura3Δ0 oxa1::kanMX4*	EUROSCARF
Δ*mgm1*	*MATa his3Δ1 leu2Δ0 lys2Δ0 ura3Δ0 mgm1::kanMX4*	EUROSCARF

Table 1. Yeasts strains used in this study

4. Discussion and conclusions

Dehydration and rehydration stress (DRS) is of great interest in the food industry. For example, the rehydration of active dry wine yeast probably represents one of the most critical phases in the entire winemaking process. Only proper rehydration can ensure the viability of healthy cells which lead to efficient fermentation. Dehydration causes a rapid efflux of water through the cell membrane, resulting in the collapse of the cytoskeleton. This dry state has a deleterious effect on yeast cell physiology by altering the structure and function of the vacuole, and the integrity and functionality of nuclear and cell membranes (Walker and van Dijck, 2006). The liquid-crystalline phase transition experienced by both dry membranes and lipid bi-layers during rehydration leads to changes in their permeability (Crowe et al., 1992, 1998). In fact, dehydrated yeast has been shown to lose up to 30% of soluble cell compounds when rehydrated, thus proving the loss of cell membrane functionality (Beker et al., 1984; Rapoport et al., 1994; Rodríguez-Porrata et al., 2008). The yeast *S. cerevisiae* is one of the few organisms capable of resisting these complex changes, which may allow it to overcome the multifaceted stress of the desiccation-rehydration process. However, in this study we found that only approximately 40% of BY4742 cells are able to generate a colony in rich medium after DRS. We systematically analysed the viability of the complete EUROSCARF collection of *S. cerevisiae* upon DRS and detected a series of knockouts displaying increased viability compared to the reference strain. Interestingly, among them were the *AIF1*, *CPR3* and *NUC1* deleted mutants, all genes directly involved in yeast apoptosis and necrosis, and coding for mitochondrial proteins (Büttner et al., 2007; Madeo et al., 1999; Halestrap, 2005). Of note, the lack of an additional mitochondrial protein, Qcr7p (the subunit 7 of the ubiquinol cytochrome-bc_1 reductase complex), also provided resistance upon DRS. Beyond their importance in energy metabolism, mitochondria have emerged as crucial organelles in PCD control (Kroemer, 2002). Like mammals, yeast also bears mitochondrially dictated cell death pathways (Eisenberg et al., 2007). For instance, Aif1p and Nuc1p are caspase-independent pro-death mitochondrial factors that upon various stresses translocate from mitochondria to the nucleus to facilitate degradation of nuclear DNA (Wissing et al., 2004; Liang et al., 2008). Therefore, the lethal function of Aif1p has been shown to depend on the yeast homologue of cyclophilin A (Cande et al., 2004; Herker, 2004). However, until now there has been no direct mention of a link between Aif1p and Cpr3p. Our experiments suggest that Aif1p and Crp3p as well as Nuc1p are activated upon DRS. In addition, we show that they perform their lethal activity in a caspase-independent manner since metacaspase deficiency did not prevent DRS-mediated cell death. Importantly, mitochondria is a major source for reactive oxygen species (ROS), which play a central role in mediating yeast cell death (Mazzoni et al., 2003; Weinberger et al., 2003). The bulk of mitochondrial ROS generation occurs as a by-product of respiration in the electron transport chain (ETC), where Q-cytochrome c oxireductase (complex III) acts as a source of ROS (Cadenas et al., 2000; Turrens, 2003; Dröse, et al., 2008). In keeping with this, the deletion of *QCR7*, which derives in disassembly from complex III, reveals lower levels of ROS before and more markedly after the imposition of DRS. This effect, however, does not seem to rely solely on respiratory disruption, as other respiration deficient mutants did not show any rescuing effect. The molecular significance of Qcr7p in cell death will need to be further clarified in future studies. Interestingly, our results show that DRS mediates a type of death which combines both apoptosis and necrosis. The enhanced viability of the different deletion mutants is thereby accompanied by a reduction in both apoptotic and necrotic markers. In fact, death mediated by mammalian AIF, cyclophilin D and endonuclease G has been described as including both types of death depending on the scenario (Madeo et al., 1999; Halestrap, 2005; Schneider, 2005; Büttner et al., 2006). It is thus possible that DRS activates both types of death in yeast which the proteins we describe are able to execute in parallel or in series.

In conclusion, based on our results we suggest that under DRS cell death is closely linked to molecular pathways that induce death by apoptosis and necrosis in a caspase- and respiratory-independent way, with DRS being dependent, at least partially, on mitochondrial death. The study of yeast genes involved in PCD under these stress conditions provides the opportunity to gain new insight into the mechanistic pathways behind DRS in high eukaryotic cells and the resulting pathologies in a legitimate PCD model organism. Additionally, it allows new cell death based strategies to be established in order to address the difficulties arising from DRS in any industry using dry yeast.

5. Acknowledgements

This work was supported by grant AGL2009-07933/FEDER from the Spanish *Ministerio de Ciencia e Innovación*.

6. References

Ahn, S.H.; Cheung, W.L.; Hsu, J.Y.; Diaz, R.L.; Smith, M.M. & Allis, C.D. (2005). Sterile 20 kinase phosphorylates histone H2B at serine 10 during hydrogen peroxide-induced apoptosis in S. cerevisiae. Cell 120: 25–36.

Anand; J.C. & Brown, A.D. (1968) Growth rate patterns of the so-called osmophilic and non-osmophilic yeasts in solutions of polyethylene glycol. Journal Gen Microbiol 52: 205–212.

Arnoult, D.; Gaume, B.; Karbowski, M.; Sharpe, J.C.; Cecconi, F. & Youle, R.J. (2003) Mitochondrial release of AIF and EndoG requires caspase activation downstream of Bax/Bak-mediated permeabilization. EMBO J 22: 4385-4399.

Attfield; P.V.; Veal, D. A.; van Rooijen, R. & Bell, P.J.L. (2000) Use of flow cytometry to monitor cell damage and predict fermentation activity of dried yeasts. J Appl Microbiol 89: 207-214.

Bartels, D. & Salamini, F. (2001) Desiccation tolerance in the resurrection plant Craterostigma plantagineum. A contribution to the study of drought tolerance at the molecular level. Plant Physiol 127:1346–1353.

Beker, M.J.; Blumbergs, J.E.; Ventina, E.J. & Rapoport , A.I. (1984) Characteristic of cellular membranes at rehydration of dehydrated yeast Saccharomyces cerevisiae. Eur J. Appl Microbiol Biotechnol 19:347: 352.

Beker, M.J. & Rapoport, A.I. (1987) Conservation of yeasts by dehydration. Adv Biochem Eng/Biotechnol 35: 127–171.

Büttner, S.; Eisenberg, T.; Herker, E.; Carmona-Gutierrez, D.; Kroemer, G. & Madeo, F. (2006) Why yeast cells can undergo apoptosis: death in times of peace, love, and war. J Cell Biol 175: 521-525.

Büttner, S.; Eisenberg, T.; Carmona-Gutierrez, D.; Ruli, D.; Knauer, H.; Ruckenstuhl, Ch.; Sigrist, C.; Wissing, S.; Kollroser, M.; Fröhlich, K.-U.; Sigrist, S. & Frank Madeo, F.

(2007) Endonuclease G regulates budding yeast life and death. Mol Cell 2007; 25:233-46.
Cadenas, E. & Davies, K.J. (2000) Mitochondrial free radical generation, oxidative stress, and aging. Free Radic Biol Med 29: 222-230.
Cande, C.; Vahsen, N.; Garrido, C. & Kroemer, G. (2004) Apoptosis-inducing factor (AIF): caspase-independent after all. Cell Death Differ 11: 591-595.
Cheung, W.L.; Ajiro, K.; Samejima, K.; Kloc, M.; Cheung, P.; Mizzen, C.A.; Beeser, A.; Etkin, L.D.; Chernoff, J.; Earnshaw, W.C. & Allis, C.D. (2003) Apoptotic phosphorylation of histone H2B is mediated by mammalian sterile twenty kinase. Cell 113: 507-517.
Crompton, M. & Costi, A. (1988) Kinetic evidence for a heart mitochondrial pore activated by Ca2+, inorganic phosphate and oxidative stress. A potential mechanism for mitochondrial dysfunction during cellular Ca2+ overload. *Eur J Biochem* 178: 489–501.
Crowe, J.H.; Hoekstra, F.A. & Crowe, L.M. (1992) Anhydrobiosis. Annu Rev Physiol 54: 579–599.
Crowe, J.H.; Carpenter, J.F. & Crowe, L.M. (1998) The role of vitrification in anhydrobiosis. Annu Rev Physiol 60: 73–103.
Dolinski, K.; Muir, R.S.; Cardenas, M.E. & Heitman, J. (1997) All cyclophilins and FK506 binding proteins are, individually and collectively, dispensable for viability in Saccharomyces cerevisiae. *Proc Natl Acad Sci USA* 94: 13093–13098.
Dröse, S. & Brandt, U. (2008) The Mechanism of Mitochondrial Superoxide Production by the Cytochrome bc_1 Complex. J Biol Chem 283: 21649–21654.
Eisenberg, T.; Buttner S.; Kroemer G. & Madeo, F. (2007) The mitochondrial pathway in yeast apoptosis. Apoptosis 12: 1011-23.
Elliott, G.D.; Liu, X.H.; Cusick, J.L.; Menze, M.; Vincent, J.; Witt, T.; Hand, S.; & Toner, M. (2006) Trehalose uptake through P2X7 purinergic channels provides dehydration protection. *Cryobiol* 52: 114-127.
Fabrizio, P.; Battistella, L.; Vardavas, R.; Gattazzo, C.; Liou, L.L.; Diaspro, A.; Dossen, J.W.; Gralla, E.B. & Longo, V.D. (2004). Superoxide is a mediator of an altruistic aging program in Saccharomyces cerevisiae. J Cell Biol 166: 1055–1067.
Fannjiang, Y.; Cheng, W.C.; Lee, S.J.; Qi, B.; Pevsner, J.; McCaffery, J.M.; Hill, R.B.; Basañez G. & Hardwick, J.M. (2004) Mitochondrial fission proteins regulate programmed cell death in yeast. Genes Dev 18: 2785-2797.
Galluzzi, L.; Larochette, N.; Zamzami, N. & Kroemer, G. (2006) Mitochondria as therapeutic targets for cancer chemotherapy. Oncogene 25: 4812–4830.
Golstein, P. & Kroemer, G. (2006) Cell death by necrosis: towards a molecular definition. Trends Biochem Sci 32: 37-43.
Halestrap, A. (2005). Biochemistry: a pore way to die. Nature 434: 578–579.
Heller, M.C.; Carpenter, J.F. & Randolph, T.W. (1997) Manipulation of lyophilization-induced phase separation: implications for pharmaceutical proteins. Biotechnol Prog 13: 590–596.
Herker, E.; Jungwirth, H.; Lehmann, K.A.; Maldener, C.; Frohlich, K.U.; Wissing, S.; Buttner, S.; Fehr, M.; Sigrist, S. & Madeo, F. (2004). Chronological aging leads to apoptosis in yeast. J. Cell Biol 164: 501–507.
Huang, K.-J.; Ku, C.-C. & Lehman, I.R (2006) Endonuclease G: A role for the enzyme in recombination and cellular proliferation. Proc. Natl. Acad. Sci. USA 103: 8995-9000.

Kroemer, G. (2002) Introduction: mitochondrial control of apoptosis. Biochimie 84: 103-104.

Laroche, C. & Gervais, P. (2003) Achievement of rapid osmotic dehydration at specific temperatures could maintain high Saccharomyces cerevisiae viability. Appl Microbiol Biotechnol 60: 743–747.

Laroche, C.; Simonin, H.; Beney, L. & Gervais, P. (2005) Phase transition as a function of osmotic pressure in S. cerevisiae whole cells, membrane extracts and phospholipid mixtures. Biochim Biophys Acta 1669: 8–16.

Laun, P.; Pichova, A. & Madeo. F. (2001) Aged mother cells of Saccharomyces cerevisiae show markers of oxidative stress and apoptosis. Mol Microbiol 39: 1166-73.

Lee, S.Y.; Hunte, C.; Malaney, S. & Robinson, B.H. (2001) The N-terminus of the Qcr7 protein of the cytochrome bc_1 complex in S. cerevisiae may be involved in facilitating stability of the subcomplex with the Qcr8 protein and cytochrome b. Arch Biochem Biophys 393: 215-221.

Li, L.Y.; Luo, X. & Wang, X. (2001) Endonuclease G is an apoptotic DNase when released from mitochondria. Nature 412: 95–99.

Liang, Y.H. & Sun, W.Q. (2002) Rate of dehydration and cumulative stress interacted to modulate desiccation tolerance of recalcitrant cocoa and ginkgo embryonic tissues. Plant Physiol 12: 1323–1331.

Liang, Q. & Zhou, B. (2007) Copper and manganese induce yeast apoptosis via different pathways. Mol Biol Cell 18: 4741-4749.

Liang, Q.; Li, W. & Zhou, B.(2008) Caspase-independent apoptosis in yeast. BBA 1783: 1311–1319.

Ludovico, P.; Sousa, M.J.; Silva, M.T.; Leao, C. & Corte-Real, M. (2001). Saccharomyces cerevisiae commits to a programmed cell death process in response to acetic acid. Microbiol 147: 2409–2415.

Ludovico, P.; Rodrígues, F.; Almeida, A.; Silva, M.T.; Barrientos, A. & Corte-Real, M. (2002). Cytochrome c release and mitochondria involvement in programmed cell death induced by acetic acid in Saccharomyces cerevisiae. Mol Biol Cell 13: 2598–2606.

Madeo, F.; Frohlich, E. & Frohlich, K.U. (1997). A yeast mutant showing diagnostic markers of early and late apoptosis. J Cell Biol 139: 729–734.

Madeo, F.; Frohlich, E.; Ligr, M.; Grey, M.; Sigrist, S.J.; Wolf, D.H. & Frohlich, K.U. (1999). Oxygen stress: a regulator of apoptosis in yeast. J Cell Biol 145: 757–767.

Madeo, F.; Herker, E.; Maldener, C.; Wissing, S.; Lachelt, S.; Herlan, M.; Fehr, M.; Lauber, K.; Sigrist, S.J.; Wesselborg, S.; & Frohlich, K.U. (2002). A caspase-related protease regulates apoptosis in yeast. Mol Cell 9: 911–917.

Mazzoni, C.; Mancini, P.; Verdone, L.; Madeo, F.; Serafini, A.; Herker, E. & Falcone, C. (2003) A truncated form of KlLsm4p and the absence of factors involved in mRNA decapping trigger apoptosis in yeast. Mol Biol Cell 14: 721–729.

Mille, Y.; Beney, L. & Gervais, P. (2003) Magnitude and kinetics of rehydration influence the viability of dehydrated E. coli K-12. Biotechnol Bioeng 83: 578–582.

Nakagawa, T.; Shimizu, S.; Watanabe, T.; Yamaguchi, O.; Otsu, K.; Yamagata, H.; Inohara, H.; Kubo, T. & Tsujimoto, Y. (2005) Cyclophilin D-dependent mitochondrial permeability transition regulates some necrotic but not apoptotic cell death. Nature 434: 652– 658.

Parrish, J.; Li, L.; Klotz, K.; Ledwich, D.; Wang, X. & Xue, D. (2001) Mitochondrial endonuclease G is important for apoptosis in C. elegans. Nature 412: 90–94.

Poirier, I.; Maréchal, P.A.; Richard, S. & Gervais, P. (1999) Saccharomyces cerevisiae is strongly dependant on rehydration kinetics and the temperature of dried cells. J Applied Microbiol 86: 87–92.

Rapoport, A.I.; Khrustaleva, G.; Chamanis, Ya. & Beker M.E. (1994) Yeast Anhydrobiosis: Permeability of the Plasma Membrane. Microbiol 64: 229-232.

Rodríguez-Porrata, B.; Novo, M.; Guillamón, J.; Rozès, N.; Mas, A. & Cordero-Otero, R. (2008) Vitality enhancement of the rehydrated active dry wine yeast. Int J Food Microbiol 126: 116-122.

Rodríguez-Porrata, B.; Lopez, G.; Redón, M.; Sancho, M.; Rozès, N.; Mas, A. & Cordero-Otero, R. (2011) Effect of lipids on the desiccation tolerance of yeasts. W J Microbiol Biotech 27: 75-83.

Schafer, P.; Scholz, S.R.; Gimadutdinow, O.; Cymerman, I.A.; Bujnicki, J.M.; Ruiz-Carrillo, A.; Pingoud, A. & Meiss, G. (2004). Structural and functional characterization of mitochondrial EndoG, a sugar non-specific nuclease which plays an important role during apoptosis. J. Mol. Biol. 338: 217–228.

Schneider, M.D. & Cyclophilin, D. (2005) Knocking on death's door. *Sci. STKE*. Vol. 2005, Issue 287, p.p.26

Susin, S.A.; Lorenzo H.K.; Zamzami,N.; Marzo, I.; Snow, B.E.; Brothers, G.M.; Mangion, J.; Jacotot, E.; Costantini, P. & Loeffler, M. (1999) Molecular characterization of mitochondrial apoptosis-inducing factor. *Nature* 397: 441–446.

Turrens, J.F. (2003) Mitochondrial formation of reactive oxygen species. *J. Physiol.* 555: 335–344.

Walker, G.M. & van Dijck, P. (2006) Physiological and molecular responses of yeasts to the environment. In: Querol, A., Fleet, G.H. (Eds.), Yeasts in Food and Beverages. The Yeast Handbook. Springer-Verlag, Berlin Heidelberg, pp. 111–152.

Weinberger, M.; Ramachandran, L. & Burhans, W.C. (2003) Apoptosis in yeasts. IUBMB Life. 55: 467–472.

Wissing, S.; Ludovico, P.; Herker, E.; Buttner, S.; Engelhardt, S.M; Decker, T.; Link, A.; Proksch, A.; Rodrigues, F. & Corte-Real, M. (2004). An AIF orthologue regulates apoptosis in yeast. J. Cell Biol.166: 969–974.

Wolkers, W.F.; Walker, N.J. & Tamari, Y. (2002) Towards a clinical application of freeze-dried human platelets. Cell Preserv Technol 1:175–188.

Wu, M.; Xu, L.G.; Li, X.; Zhai, Z. & Shu H.B. (2002) AMID, an apoptosis-inducing factorhomologous mitochondrion-associated protein, induces caspase-independent apoptosis. J Biol Chem 277:25617-25623.

Zara, V.; Palmisano, L, & Conte, B.L. (2004) Further insights into the assembly of the yeast cytochrome bc_1 complex based on analysis based on single and double deletion mutants lacking supernumerary subunits and cytochrome b. Eur J Biochem 271:1209-1218.

7

Use of Flow Cytometry in the *In Vitro* and *In Vivo* Analysis of Tolerance/Anergy Induction by Immunocamouflage

Duncheng Wang, Wendy M. Toyofuku, Dana L. Kyluik and Mark D. Scott
Canadian Blood Services and The Department of Pathology and Laboratory Medicine and Centre for Blood Research at The University of British Columbia
Canada

1. Introduction

Organ and tissue transplantations (including blood transfusions) are a critical care component for many life-threatening diseases. In transfusion and transplantation medicine, the concept of "self" is of crucial importance. Immunological "self" in transfusion medicine is primarily mediated by the ABO/RhD blood group antigens, though several hundred blood groups exist that can cause problems especially in the chronically transfused patient. For most other tissues, "self" is imparted by the major histocompatibility complex (MHC) proteins which provide a means for identifying, targeting and eliminating foreign (allorecognition) or diseased cells while preserving normal tissue. If the differences between donor and recipient occur only at minor MHC molecules (or non-ABO blood group antigens) or the transplanted antigens are only weakly antigenic or immunogenic, successful engraftment may result. In contrast, if significant differences in the exceedingly polymorphic MHC loci are present, or other highly antigenic (*e.g.,* ABO) or immunogenic antigens are present, allorecognition of the donor tissue occurs leading to rejection. Importantly, while rejection may be manifested as either Host versus Graft or Graft versus Host Disease (HVGD and GVHD, respectively), both are mediated by T lymphocyte (T cell) activation, differentiation and proliferation consequent to allorecognition. [Cote *et al.*, 2001] In this chapter, we will demonstrate how we have utilized flow cytometry to measure the induction of tolerance and/or anergy by polymer-mediated immunocamouflage using *in vitro* and *in vivo* models of allorecognition.

2. Allorecognition and allorejection

In HVGD, the host *(i.e.,* recipient) immune system recognizes (allorecognition) and rejects the allograft.[Li *et al.*, 2011, Dallman, 2001, Suthanthiran & Strom, 1995] Three major patterns of rejection can be identified based on the rapidity of graft injury: hyperacute (minutes to hours), acute (days to weeks) and chronic (weeks to years). [Goldstein, 2011, Battaglia, 2010, Weigt *et al.*, 2010] In hyperacute rejection not all parts of the graft are actively attacked. The primary site of injury is typically the vascular endothelium which can exhibit the ABO blood group antigens as well as MHC class I antigens. Damage is initiated by the binding of complement fixing antibodies, complement activation, platelet aggregation, graft thrombosis, lytic damage, release of pro-inflammatory complement components (C3a and C5a) and leukocyte recruitment. These events result in the microvascular occlusion and the rapid loss of graft viability. Because hyperacute rejection occurs rapidly, few if any effective therapies for its prevention currently exist. Thus, many patients cannot be transplanted due to ABO-incompatibility or the presence of preformed anti-HLA antibodies. In contrast to hyperacute rejection, acute and chronic rejection are primarily cell mediated and initiated by T cell activation in context of mismatched MHC. Because of its central role, T cells have been the traditional focus of immunosuppressive drugs such as cyclosporin A. [Abadja *et al.*, 2009, Bonnotte *et al.*, 1996, Noris *et al.*, 2007]

GVHD is, essentially, a special category of HVGD.[Devetten & Vose, 2004] In GVHD, immunologically competent T cells, or their precursors, are transfused or transplanted into immunocompromised recipients. GVHD occurs most commonly in the setting of allogeneic bone marrow transplantation, but may also follow transfusion of whole blood into immunocompromised individuals and even some immunocompetent individuals. [Kleinman *et al.*, 2003] While both CD4+ (helper) and CD8+ (cytotoxic) T cells play a role in mediating tissue rejection in HVGD and GVHD, previous studies have found that depletion of MHC class II-recognizing CD4+ T cells to be most effective in preventing rejection.[Noris *et al.*, 2007] The MHC disparity between the donor and recipient induces the direct activation, differentiation and proliferation of either the recipient's (HVGD) or donor (GVHD) naïve T cells into effector subsets. Moreover, with regards to GVHD, surprisingly few T cells are necessary to induce a fatal outcome. Animal models suggest that as few as 10^7 donor lymphocytes/kg of recipient weight are sufficient to induce GVHD; though the degree of host immunosuppression and the overall disparity of the HLA antigens will exert a significant effect on the probability of GVHD induction.

The risk of donor tissue rejection (and to a lesser extent GVHD) has severely impacted the advancement of transplantation medicine. To counter these risks, pharmacologic interventions have been employed. Indeed, over the last 40 years, the significant improvements in transplantation success have been achieved primarily through immunosuppressive drugs that attenuate chronic tissue rejection. Because of the central importance of the T cell in graft rejection, thes pharmacological approaches have almost exclusively targeted T cell activation or proliferation (Figure 1A). [Allison, 2000] Perhaps the most prominent of these drugs has been cyclosporin, which blocks activation of resting T cells by inhibiting the signaling pathway necessary for the transcription of interleukin (IL)-2 and the high affinity IL-2 receptor. As a consequence, production of both IL-2 and its receptor are significantly diminished, thus removing the autocrine and paracrine stimulation necessary for T cell proliferation. Unfortunately, these drugs are nondiscriminatory and target not only the alloreactive, but all T cell proliferation leading to the induction of a general, non-selective, immunosuppressive state that is linked to both a chronic susceptibility to infective agents and an increased cancer risk. Moreover, even with pharmacologic intervention, long-term graft (as well as patient) survival is often problematic. In part, graft failure is a side effect of the immunosuppressive therapy as current pharmacologic agents exert both organ specific and systemic toxicity.

Hence, both HVGD and GVHD are T cell-mediated events that require antigenic recognition of the foreign tissue and the elicitation of a T cell-mediated immune response. These effector

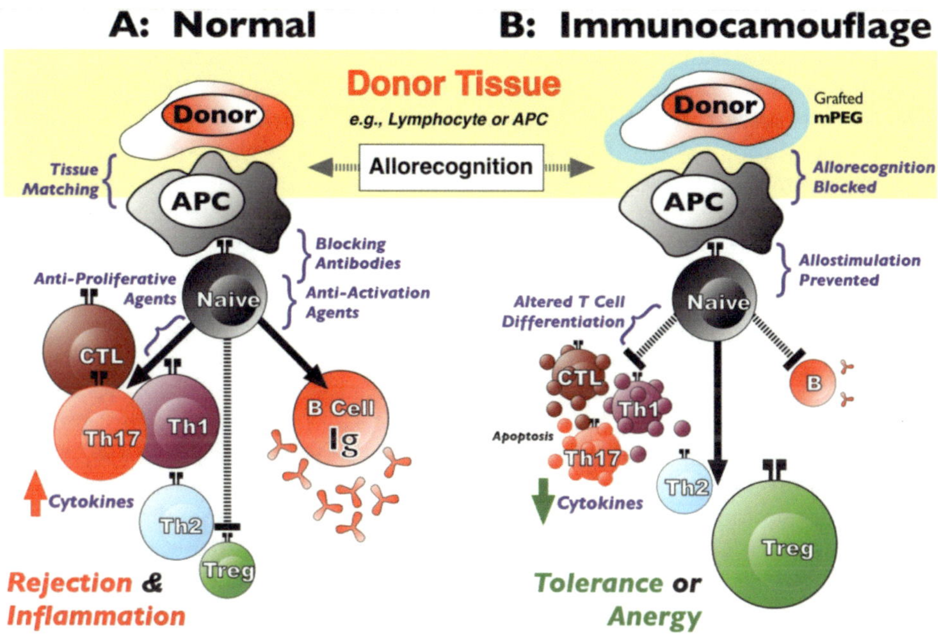

Fig. 1. Immune modulation via pharmacologic and immunocamouflage therapy. Panel A: Current pharmacologic therapy almost exclusively targets T cell activation and proliferation consequent to allorecognition. Response to non-self is in large part mediated by cell-cell interactions between Antigen Presenting Cells (APC; *e.g.*, dendritic cells) and naïve T cells. This cell-cell interaction is characterized by essential adhesion, allorecognition and co-stimulation events. Consequent to allorecognition, a proliferation of pro-inflammatory T cells (*e.g.*, CTL, Th17, Th1 populations) and decrease in regulatory T cells (Treg) is observed. Current therapeutic agents are primarily cytotoxic agents preventing T cell activation (*e.g.*, cyclosporine and rapamycin) or T cell proliferation (*e.g.*, methotrexate, corticosteroids and azathioprine). Additionally some blocking antibodies have been investigated. Panel B: In contrast, immunocamouflage of donor cells results in the disruption of the essential cell-cell interactions decreasing T cell proliferation and altering differentiation patterns (decreased Th17 and increased Tregs). In aggregate, these polymer induced changes induces a tolerogenic/anergic state both *in vitro* and *in vivo*. Size of T cell population denotes increase or decrease in number. Size of B cell indicates antibody response. Modified from: Wang *et al.* (2011). [Wang *et al.*, 2011]

cells arise via differentiation and proliferation of naïve T cells into proinflammatory and cytotoxic subsets (*e.g.*, Th17, Th1, CTL). While a number of different approaches to reduce the risk of tissue rejection are currently being examined, these strategies are, typically, unilaterally targeted to specific components of the allorecipient's T cell activation/ proliferation pathway (Figure 1A). These include blocking monoclonal antibodies directed against the TCR, CD4, co-stimulatory ligands and receptors, adhesion molecules, and cytokine receptors. Some of these approaches have undergone clinical testing (*e.g.*, Anti-CD3 monoclonal antibodies) and demonstrated some promising effects. However, concurrent with the anti-rejection efficacy, these agents have been plagued by both significant toxicity and an inability to adequately eliminate or inhibit reactive T cells. Hence, these approaches are not commonly used at most transplant institutions. Clinical trials have also tested the use of pharmacological inhibitors of T cell proliferation and differentiation. Antiproliferative agents such as azathioprine and methotrexate interfere with cellular functions by limiting the metabolites necessary for DNA synthesis (Figure 1). However, these compounds also demonstrate significant toxicity to organs characterized by high proliferation rates (*e.g.*, gastrointestinal tract) and/or drug metabolism (liver), thus limiting their practical application.

Consequently, novel approaches that effectively attenuate the risk of HVGD/GVHD and directly target the difficult challenges of the inherent antigenicity and immunogenicity of human (and possibly xenogeneic) donor tissues would be of significant value to transplantation medicine. Biologically, the most attractive strategy to improve donor tissue engraftment and to simultaneously reduce drug toxicity, would be to induce immune tolerance and/or anergy in the recipient's immune system thereby negating the need for toxic immunosuppressive pharmacologic agents. Tolerance may be viewed as a relatively specific non-responsiveness to a unique antigen while anergy is a more broad-spectrum attenuation of the immune response. As with cell-mediated rejection, tolerance and anergy are also mediated by a T cells subset (T regulatory cells; Tregs). [Muller *et al.*, 2011]

3. Immunocamouflage: Concept and mechanism of action

To prevent allorecognition and alloimmunization, our laboratory has pioneered the 'immunocamouflage' of donor cells and tissues (Figure 1B). [Bradley *et al.*, 2002, Bradley & Scott, 2004, Chen & Scott, 2001, Chen & Scott, 2003, Le & Scott, 2010, McCoy & Scott, 2005, Murad *et al.*, 1999a, Murad *et al.*, 1999b, Rossi *et al.*, 2010a, Rossi *et al.*, 2010b, Scott *et al.*, 2003, Scott *et al.*, 1997, Sutton & Scott, 2010] The immunocamouflage of cells and tissues is created by the covalent grafting of safe, non-toxic and low-immunogenic biocompatible polymers such as methoxypoly(ethylene glycol, PEGylation) and hyperbranched polyglycerols (HPG) to the surface of cells. The efficacy of immunocamouflage is dependent upon both the density and depth (*i.e.*, thickness) of the polymer layer. As shown in Figure 2, a rigid linear molecules lacks any significant radius of gyration (R_g; space filling) resulting in a poor or absent camouflaging (*a,b*) of the membrane antigens. In contrast, polymers with either high intra-chain flexibility (*e.g.*, methoxypoly(ethylene glycol); mPEG; *c,d*) or inherent density (*e.g.*, hyperbranched polyglycerols; HPG; *e*) exhibit either a significant radius of gyration (mPEG) or space filling capacity (HPG). Thus, while mPEG is a linear molecule, its high degree of intra-chain flexibility (due to the repeating, highly mobile, ethoxy units) gives rise to its expansive Rg. Moreover, due to its hydroscopic nature, the heavily hydrated polymer is able to sterically occlude a large three dimensional volume (Figure 2). Consequent to the space filling capacity of mPEG, the immunocamouflage of surface membrane proteins and carbohydrates (potential antigenic sites) occurs. In addition, the mPEG coating obscures the inherent electrical charge associated with surface proteins since the charged molecules become buried beneath the viscous, hydrated, neutral PEG layer thus further diminishing the antigenic/immunologic character of the cell surface. [Bradley *et al.*, 2002, Bradley & Scott, 2004, Le & Scott, 2010] As denoted in Figure 2, the longer the mPEG polymer chain the larger the membrane surface area covered by this steric shield (c, d and stippled area). In contrast to the flexible linear mPEG, HPG molecules are highly branched structures that exhibit limited flexibility but, due to its extensive branching, create a dense steric shield (Figure 2e). [Rossi *et al.*, 2010a, Rossi *et al.*, 2010b]

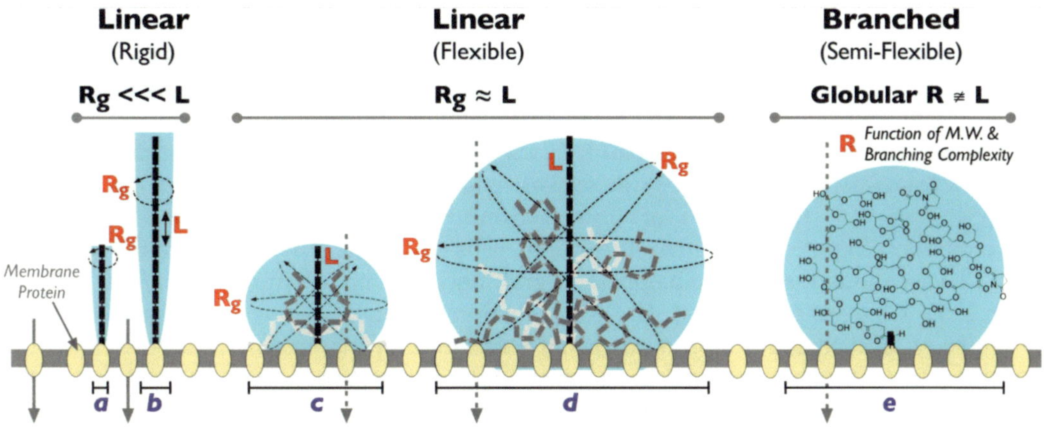

Fig. 2. Immunocamouflage of cells is produced via the grafting of polymers to membrane proteins. The linear flexible molecule and branched, semi-flexible, grafted polymers creates a steric barrier preventing the approach and binding of proteins (*e.g.*, antibodies) and cells (*e.g.*, APC or T cells) but along for metabolite (dashed arrows; *e.g.*, glucose) uptake. In contrast, rigid linear polymers produce a minimal steric barrier. Some polymers, such as mPEG, also very effectively camouflage membrane surface charge. Result present in this chapter all refer to methoxy(polyethylene glycol) [mPEG], a linear flexible polymer (*c, d*). L=polymer length as denoted by molecular weight while R_g is the radius of gyration

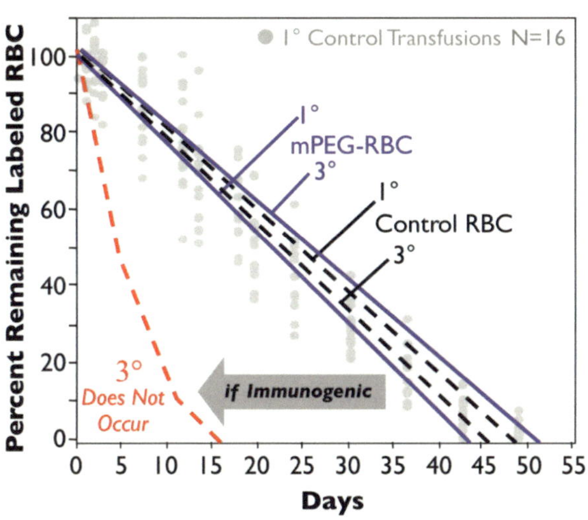

Fig. 3. Immuno-camouflage of murine RBC with mPEG (SVAmPEG; 20 kDa) results in normal *in vivo* survival. Donor RBC survival was measured via flow cytometry and detection of a fluorescent marker (PKH-26) inserted into the RBC membrane via a lipid tail. The theoretical effect of the production of anti-mPEG antibodies is shown by the red dashed line representing a tertiary transfusion of modified RBC

Previous studies in our laboratory on red blood cells, lymphocytes, pancreatic islets and viral models have demonstrated that the immunocamouflage of tissues is effective, reproducible and does not impair tissue function. [Bradley *et al.*, 2002, Bradley & Scott, 2004,

Chen & Scott, 2001, Chen & Scott, 2003, Le & Scott, 2010, McCoy & Scott, 2005, Murad *et al.*, 1999a, Murad *et al.*, 1999b, Rossi *et al.*, 2010a, Rossi *et al.*, 2010b, Scott *et al.*, 2003, Scott *et al.*, 1997, Sutton & Scott, 2010] For example, the PEGylated red blood cell function (*i.e.*, O_2 delivery and cellular deformability) were unaffected by the grafted polymer and exhibited normal *in vivo* circulation and lifespan (~50 day) in a murine transfusion model even after repeated transfusions (Figure 3). With relevance to tissue transplantation, our studies have demonstrated that transfusion of immunocamouflaged allogeneic murine splenocytes prevents allorecognition by either the donor cells (*e.g.*, Transfusion-Associated Graft vs. Host Disease model) or the recipients (*e.g.*, graft rejection model) immune system. [Chen & Scott 2003, Chen & Scott 2006] The loss of allorecognition is not accompanied by any systemic or local toxicity. More surprisingly, recent adoptive transfer studies within our laboratory using a murine model have demonstrated that immunocamouflaged leukocytes may be able to induce long-lasting systemic immunotolerance. [Wang *et al.*, 2011] An important and exceptionally powerful tool in assessing the efficacy of immunocamouflage in both *in vitro* and *in vivo* modeling systems has been flow cytometry.

4. Assessing polymer-mediated immunomodulation by flow cytometry: T cell camouflage, differentiation and proliferation

Flow cytometry is essential in characterizing both *in vitro* and *in vivo* immunological response including cell proliferation (CSFE staining and murine H2 determination), cytokine expression (cytometric bead array), intra-cellular signaling cascades, lymphocyte differentiation (*e.g.*, Tregs and Th17 cells) and *in vivo* cell trafficking (*e.g.*, thymus, spleen, lymph node and blood). Indeed, as will be shown in this chapter, flow cytometry is an exceptionally powerful tool in investigating the induction of tolerance and/or anergy in experimental models.

Mechanistically, allorecognition requires multiple sustained interactions between the donor and recipient tissues for the activation, differentiation and proliferation of alloresponsive T cell to occur. These interactions, involving both external receptor-ligand interactions and intracellular signalling cascades fall within three general categories: 1) cell:cell adhesion events; 2) allorecognition; and 3) costimulation. [Chen & Scott, 2001, Murad *et al.*, 1999a] Blockade or attenuation of any (or all) of these events will reduce allorecognition and allograft rejection. The *in vitro* and *in vivo* effects of polymer-mediated immunocamouflage on these essential events are readily measured via flow cytometry.

4.1 Immunocamouflage of membrane markers

Multiple receptor-ligand interactions (encompassing adhesion, allorecognition and costimulation pathways) between the T cell and APC are essential for successful allostimulation. The membrane proteins involved in these cell:cell events have been well characterized over the last several years and often targeted by experimental therapies. Importantly, the efficacy of immunocamouflage can be readily assessed by the literal camouflage of these markers using flow cytometry.

Previously, we investigated the efficacy of immunocamouflage in a murine model of transfusion-associated graft versus host disease (TA-GVHD). [Chen & Scott, 2003, Chen & Scott, 2006] Using this model, flow cytometric analysis demonstrated that polymer grafting significantly camouflaged membrane proteins involved in adhesion, allorecognition and co-stimulation events. As shown in Table 1, the immunocamouflage of allogeneic donor lymphocytes resulted in the efficient camouflage of donor leukocyte membrane markers. These membrane proteins are still present on the surface of the allogeneic leukocytes but are camouflaged by the grafted polymer from detection by anti-marker antibodies. Consequent to the polymer-mediated camouflage, signal transduction is block or significantly attenuated.

mM mPEG	Polymer *m.w.*	CD3ε	T cell receptor	CD11a	MHC Class II	CD4	CD25	CD28
0	-	100%	100%	100%	100%	100%	100%	100%
0.6	5 kDa	59*	20*	49*	100	75	ND	64*
	20 kDa	73*	14*	53*	100	84	67*	35*
1.2	5 kDa	53*	11*	39*	100	65*	62*	31*
	20 kDa	27*	2*	26*	45*	53*	67*	30*
2.4	5 kDa	38*	7*	30*	59*	7*	12*	31*
	20 kDa	3*	5*	7*	8*	3*	67*	40*

Table 1. The covalent grafting of mPEG to membrane proteins results in the global camouflage of multiple proteins crucial for effective allorecognition of foreign tissue. Values shown are "Percent Positive Cells" relative to the unmodified control (=100%). Results shown are the mean of a minimum of 3 independent experiments. * $p < 0.01$ compared to unmodified controls

4.2 Effect of immunocamouflage on cytokine-chemokine release

Consequent to the camouflage of the receptor-ligands necessary for alloresponsiveness, a dramatic reduction in cytokine/chemokine release is observed. Flow cytometry provides a valuable tool for the simultaneous measurement of cytokine (signalling molecules integral to the immune response) production, T cell proliferation and differentiation. Historically, cytokines were commonly measured using enzyme-linked immunosorbent assays (ELISA or EIA); a relatively low throughput system. Flow cytometry has greatly increased both the speed and sensitivity of cytokine measurements both *in vitro* and *in vivo*. One of the most powerful flow cytometric tools in this regard is the BD™ Cytometric Bead Array (CBA; BD™ Biosciences, San Diego, CA). There are significant advantages for using the CBA versus ELISA. The CBA Array system is a multiplex quantitive assay requiring fewer sample dilutions and utilizing a single set of standards to generate a standard curve for each analyte. Moreover, the throughput of the CBA is significantly greater than ELISA (*e.g.*, 1/2 day for the CBA Array versus 2-3 days for ELISA).

The CBA system is a multiplexed bead based immunoassay used to simultaneously quantitate multiple soluble cytokines within a single sample by fluorescence-based emission. This assay allows multiple simultaneous cytokine determinations in serum, plasma, cell lysates or tissue culture supernatants. As shown in Figure 4, each sample preparation can contain multiple bead populations, each with distinct fluorescence intensity. Each of these bead populations (capture beads) are coated with an antibody for a specific cytokine and essentially mimics an individually coated well in an ELISA plate. The capture beads are mixed with the sample of interest (standard or experimental sample) and a PE-conjugated detection antibody to form a sandwich complex and resolved using the FL3 or FL4 channel. The data is analyzed using specific software (FCAP Array™ and BD CBA™ analysis software; BD Biosicences, San Diego, CA and Soft Flow Inc, St. Louis Park, MN) to provide a quantitative value for the selected cytokines.

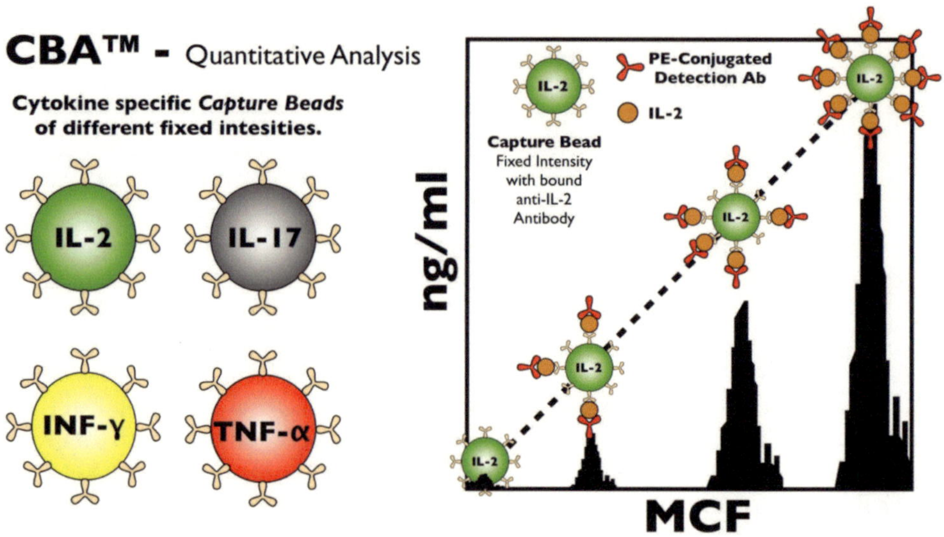

Fig. 4. Quantitative Cytometric Bead Array™. Capture beads are conjugated to analyte specific antibodies (*e.g.*, anti-Il-2, Il-17, INF-γ or TNF-α as shown). Each bead has a different fluorescent intensity allowing for analyate discrimination

For our experiments, a BD™ CBA Human Th1/Th2 Cytokine Kit (Catalog No. 550749) and Murine Th1/Th2 Cytokine Kit (Catalog No. 551287) were utilized to determine the effects of immunocamouflage on allorecognition *in vitro* and *in vivo*. For *in vitro* human or mouse studies, cell culture supernatants were collected and stored at -80°C prior to analysis. For flow cytometric analysis samples were incubated with desired detection kit (*e.g.*, Th1/Th2) capture beads and a PE-conjugated detection antibody and aquired using a BD FACSCaliburTM flow cytometer and the Cell Quest Pro Software. Cytokine protein levels were analyzed using the BD™ Cytometric Bead Array and FCAP Array™ analysis software (BD Biosicences, San Diego, CA and Soft Flow Inc, St. Louis Park, MN).

As demonstrated in Figure 5, resting human PBMC, as well as resting PEGylated PBMC, expressed little detectable IL-2, TNF-α or INF-γ. [Wang *et al.*, 2011] However, when two disparate populations (two-way mixed lymphocyte reaction; 2-way MLR) of PBMC are mixed together, allorecognition occurs resulting in very significant increases in these cytokines. In stark contrast to the positive control MLR, the PEGylation of either donor population results in an immunoquiescent state characterized by baseline (*i.e.*, resting PBMC) levels of these cytokines. Also shown in Figure 5 is a diagrammatic presentation of how the capture beads detect cytokine levels of the control and PEGylated MLR.

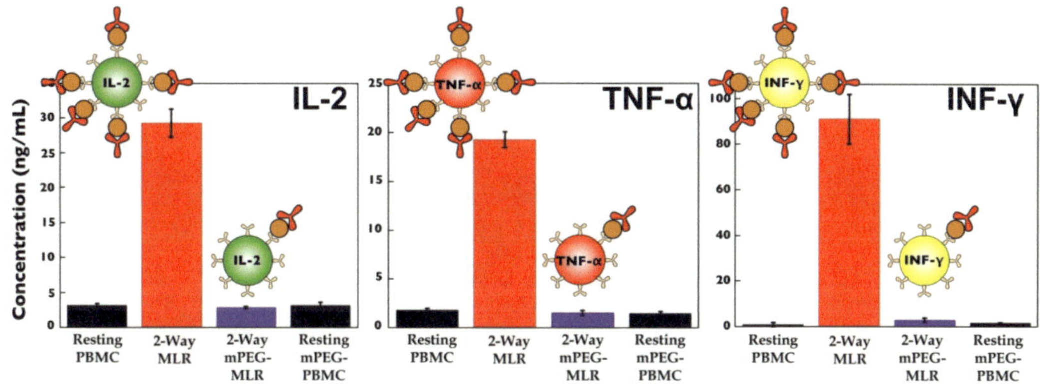

Fig. 5. Effect of immunocamouflage on cytokine secretion as measured by flow cytometry using the BD Cytometric Bead Array™ (CBA). Also shown is a diagrammatic representation of the capture beads and bound analayte for the control 2-way MLR and mPEG 2-way MLR. Modified from Wang *et al.* (2011). [Wang et al., 2011]

4.3 Effect of immunocamouflage on *In Vitro* and *In Vivo* T cell proliferation and differentiation

For decades, ^{3}H-thymidine incorporation was the standard for measuring cell proliferation in MLRs. While highly useful *in vitro*, this methodology is less useful *in vivo*. Moreover, radionucleotides bring additional regulatory burden to research laboratories. Hence, alternative approaches for measuring proliferation have been developed. Multiple flow cytometric tools are available for this purpose. Perhaps the most common of these flow methodologies is a dye dilution assay utilizing carboxyfluorescein succinimidyl ester (CFSE). Importantly, the CFSE assay is a valuable tool for both *in vitro* and *in vivo* proliferation assays.

CFSE was originally developed to label lymphocytes and track their *in vivo* migration over several months. [Weston & Parish, 1990] Subsequent studies demonstrated its utility in measuring lymphocyte proliferation both *in vitro* and *in vivo* consequent to the progressive dilution of CFSE fluorescence within daughter cells following each cell division. For cell staining, carboxyfluorescein diacetate succinimidyl ester (CFDA-SE; a non-fluorescent precursor to CFSE), a highly cell permeable compound, is added to a cell population (*e.g.*, human PBMC or murine splenocytes) where it enters the cytoplasm of cells. Within the cell, intracellular esterases remove the acetate groups present on CFDA-SE and convert the molecule to the fluorescent ester, CFSE. The CFSE molecule is permanently retained within cells due to its covalent coupling to intracellular molecules via its succinimidyl group. The CSFE signal is extremely stable allowing for long-term studies and is not transferred to adjacent cells. However, upon allostimulation (or mitogen challenge) and proliferation, the CFSE dye is evenly diluted between the daughter cells and continues to be diluted with subsequent proliferation of these cells (Figure 6). With optimal labelling, 7-8 cell divisions can be identified before the CFSE fluorescence is indistinguishable from backgound autofluorescence. Thus, this assay thereby provides significant quantitative data as to the percentage of alloresponsive cells within a population as well as the degree of proliferation over a course of several days to weeks.

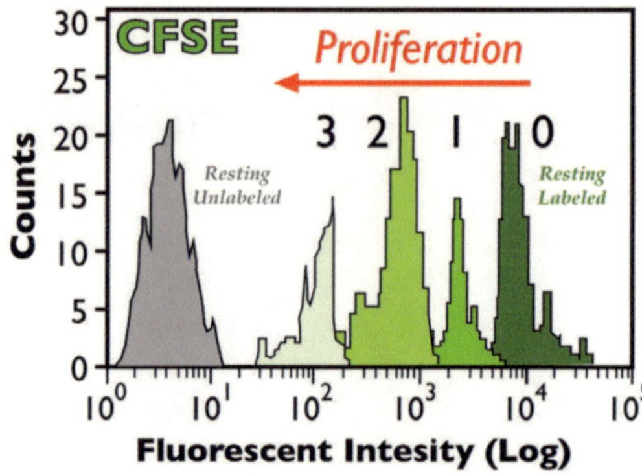

Fig. 6. Flow cytometric analysis of intracellular CFSE can be used to measure cell proliferation based on dye-dilution within the daughter cells (0-4). CFSE can be used both *in vitro* and *in vivo* where it can also be used to investigate cell trafficking. The grey peak represents unlabeled cells

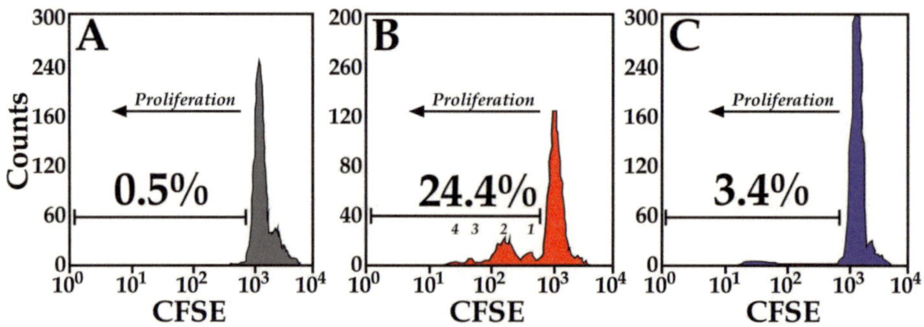

Fig. 7. Proliferation of CD4+ T cells in resting PBMC (A), Control MLR (B) and mPEG-MLR (C). Denoted in B are the proliferation (*1-4*) peaks of the alloresponsive subpopulation. Shown is the flow cytometric analysis of a representative experiment of human PBMC

The ultimate efficacy of immunocamouflage of allogeneic cells in MLRs is primarily assessed by the loss of proliferation. As shown in Figure 7, polymer grafting to either immunologically disparate population results in the loss of cell proliferation. [Wang *et al.*, 2011] Importantly, this is not due to any loss of viability of the polymer modified cells as direct mitogen stimulation yields normal nearly identical proliferation rates as unmodified cells (as measured by CFSE or ^{3}H-thymidine incorporation; not shown). The loss of proliferation is consequent to the global immunocamouflage of the receptor-ligand markers described in Table 1.

In vivo cell trafficking of allogeneic donor cells is also of importance in immunological studies. While this can be done using radiolabelled cells, it is a low resolution assay and is often quantitated as simply CPM per organ. In contrast, flow cytometry can provide significantly improved information. In murine studies it is possible to look at the proliferation of allogeneic donor cells based on flow cytometric analysis of the murine haplotype (H2). In an *in vivo* murine model of transfusion associated graft versus host disease (TA-GVHD) in which mice are transfused with allogeneic cells, significant proliferation of the donor cells is observed in lymphatic tissues such as the spleen after 28 days (Figure 8). [Chen & Scott, 2003, Chen & Scott, 2006] In contrast, if the allogeneic donor cells are PEGylated prior to their transfusion, minimal allorecognition of the foreign host tissues occurs and there is no significant proliferation of the donor splenocytes (Figure 8). While not shown, CFSE labelling can also be an important flow cytometric tool for simultaneously monitoring the trafficking and proliferation of donor cells *in vivo*. Both H2 markers and/or CSFE can be further coupled with the use of fluorescent antibodies against lymphocyte cell surface markers (*e.g.*, CD4, CD25, IL-17R, *etc.*) making it possible to follow *in vivo* lymphocyte differentiation. Due to the non-toxic nature of CFSE, labelled viable cells can be recovered via cell flow cytometric cell sorting for further *in vitro* analysis.

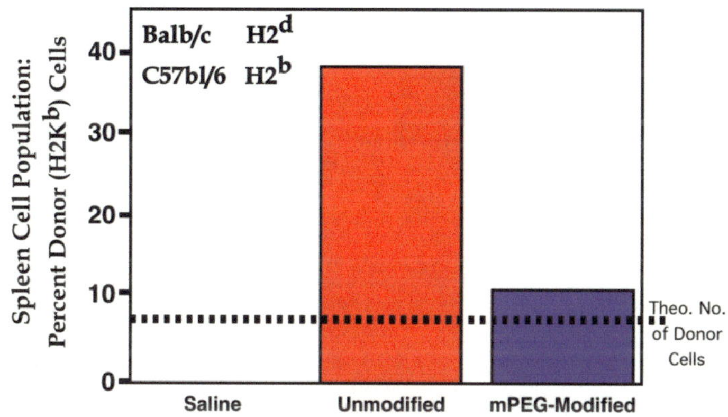

Fig. 8. Immunocompetent Balb/c mice (H2K^d) were transfused with 1.5 x 10^7 unmodified or mPEG-modified C57Bl/6 splenocytes (H2K^b) on days 0 and 14. At day 28, mice were sacrificed and the *in vivo* donor cell proliferation was assessed by flow cytometry using an anti-H2K^b monoclonal antibody. Shown are the mean precent donor cells within the spleens of the recipient animals (n=4/group)

Differentiation of naïve T cells is an important regulator of the immune response or lack of response. [Heidt *et al.*, 2010, Nistala & Wedderburn, 2009, O'Gorman *et al.*, 2009, Oukka, 2007] As our understanding of the biological functions of T cells has expanded a vast array of T cell subsets, all of which have unique immunological functions and phenotypes, have been described. Indeed, T cell differentiation is a crucial indicator of whether an inflammatory or tolerogeneic response is induced consequent to exposure to control or polymer-modified allogeneic tissue. Fortunately, flow cytometry provides a high throughput tool for the analysis of T cell differentiation.

Consequent to the immunocamouflage of the receptor-ligands involved in adhesion, allorecognition and costimulation (*see* Table 1) T cell activation and proliferation was significantly attenuated (*see* Figures 7-8). However, these findings did not elucidate if there was a differential proliferation effect between T cell subsets. Hence, flow cytometric T cell subset phenotyping was used to further investigate the effects of immunocamouflage on T cell differentiation both *in vitro* and *in vivo*. [Afzali *et al.*, 2007, Hanidziar & Koulmanda, 2010, Heidt *et al.*, 2010, Mitchell *et al.*, 2009, Weaver & Hatton, 2009] For example, as shown in Figure 9, *in vivo* challenge with unmodified allogeneic cells results in the upregulation of proinflammatory Th17 cells and a downregulation of immunosuppressive Treg cells within the spleen as determined by flow cytometry. [Wang *et al.*, 2011] In contrast, the immunocamouflage of the allogeneic cells resulted in increased Treg cells significantly above that of naïve mice and a virtually complete abrogation of the expected Th17 increase. Importantly, soluble polymer as well as unmodified or mPEG-modified syngeneic cells demonstrated no effects on the *in vivo* differentiation of Treg or Th17 cells. Similar finding in the lymph nodes and blood were observed. Indeed, as summarized in Figure 10, the immunocamouflage of allogeneic human (*in vitro*) and mouse (*in vitro* and *in vivo*) leukocytes has been experimentally shown to dramatically influence T cell differentiation resulting in the induction and persistence of a tolerogeneic/anergic state. [Chen & Scott, 2003, Chen & Scott, 2006, Wang *et al.*, 2011]

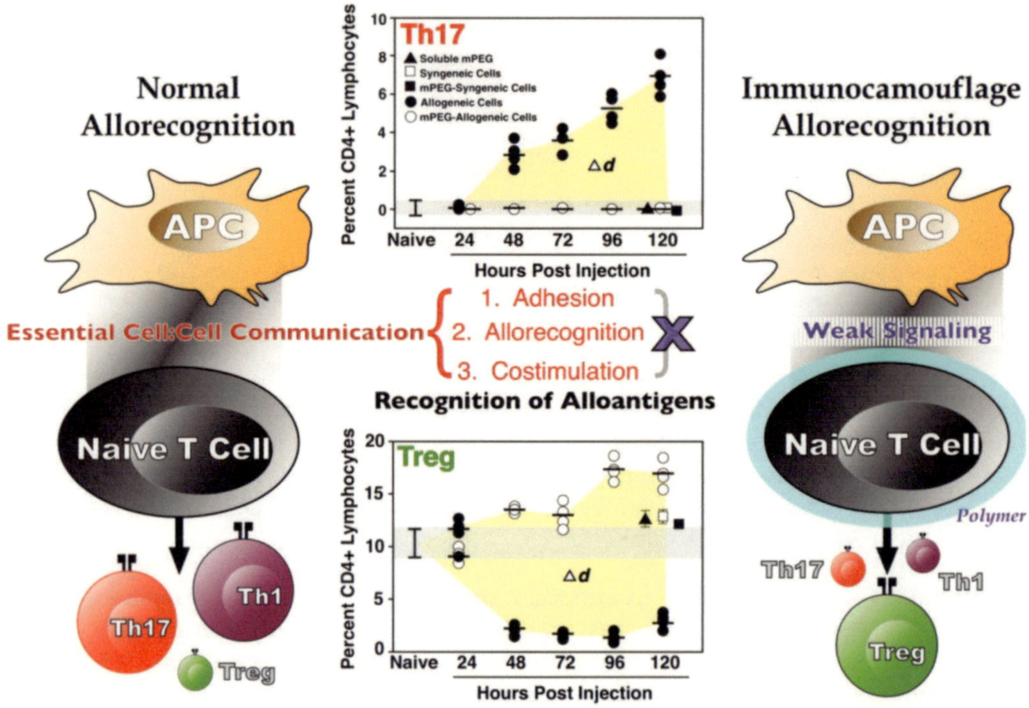

Fig. 9. Flow cytometric studies demonstrate that immunocamouflage of allogeneic murine splencoytes alters the *in vivo* systemic differentiation of Th17 and Treg lymphocytes. Shown are the percent Th17 and Treg CD4+ lymphocytes within the spleen of animals transfused with control or mPEG allogeneic splencocytes. Similar finding in the lymph nodes and blood were observed. Grey bars denote baseline levels of Th17 and Treg cells in naïve animals. The Δ*d* (yellow area) denotes the absolute difference between unmodified and mPEG-modified allogeneic splenocytes *Derived from Wang, Chen and Scott (2011)*

T cell subset differentiation is driven by variable intracellular signaling cascades triggered by the adhesion, allorecognition, costimulatory and cytokine receptor-ligand interactions occurring at the membrane of the naïve T cell. In the case of immunosuppressive Treg cells and the proinflammatory Th17 cells, the key nuclear transcription factors FoxP3+ and RORγ+, respectively, are used to detect these cell types via flow cytometry. Moreover, these markers can be combined with Phosflow™ assays to provide additional activation information. [Krutzik *et al.*, 2004] This technique combines flow cytometric analysis of phosphospecific antibodies with, for example, lymphocyte subtyping allowing for more specific identification of activated cell types. Phosphospecific antibodies are specific to tyrosine or serine phosphorylated signaling intermediates, thus antibody will only bind to a protein in its phosphorylated state. Since phosphorylation is a key mechanism of regulation in signaling pathways, this methodology enables the studies of a vast number of pathways in a variety of cells. This technology provides significantly enhanced resolution relative to western blots or ELISAs that only assess the overall activity of an entire population and that do not allow for easy isolation or phenotypic identification of the alloreactive cells involved.

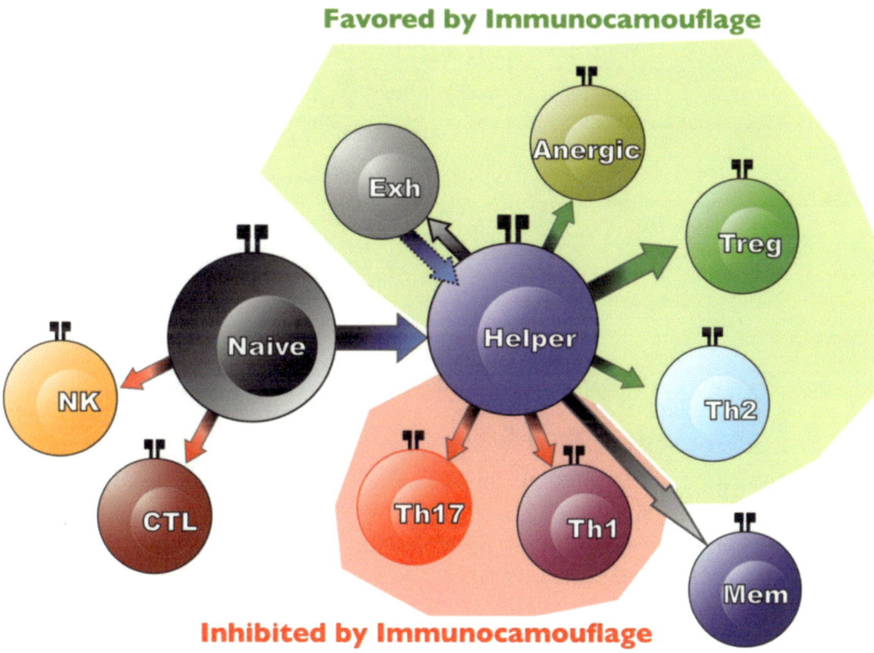

Fig. 10. Flow cytometric analysis of T cell differentiation both in vitro and in vivo demonstrates the polymer grafting to allogeneic leukocytes significantly influences the differentiation of naïve T cells. As shown diagrammatically above, immunocamouflage of allogeneic cells favors tolerogeneic/anergic T cell subsets and significantly inhibits proinflammatory T cell populations. Lymphocyte abbreviations: NK, natural killer; CTL, cytotoxic; Mem, memory; and Exh, exhausted (TCR-) T cells

For example, as illustrated in Figure 11, initiation of differentiation of the Th17 T cell lineage is controlled by the master regulatory transcription factor RORγ. This transcription factor is upregulated in response to IL-6 and TGF-β that, together with the T cell receptor (TCR) signal, initiate differentiation of Th17 from naive T cells via the Gp130-STAT3 pathways. [Kitabayashi *et al.*, 2010, Nishihara *et al.*, 2007] Il-6 acts directly to promote the development of Th17 by binding to the membrane IL-6 receptor of T cells and its signal transducer protein Gp130. Binding of the cytokine induces activation (phosphorylation) of Jaks which serve as a docking site for STAT3. STAT3 is then phosphorylated by Jak inducing its dimerization, nuclear translocation and DNA binding. To assess the activation of this pathway consequent to mitogen or allostimulation, cells can be fixed, permeabilized and stained for phosphospecific (Tyr705) STAT3 and analyzed via flow cytometry.

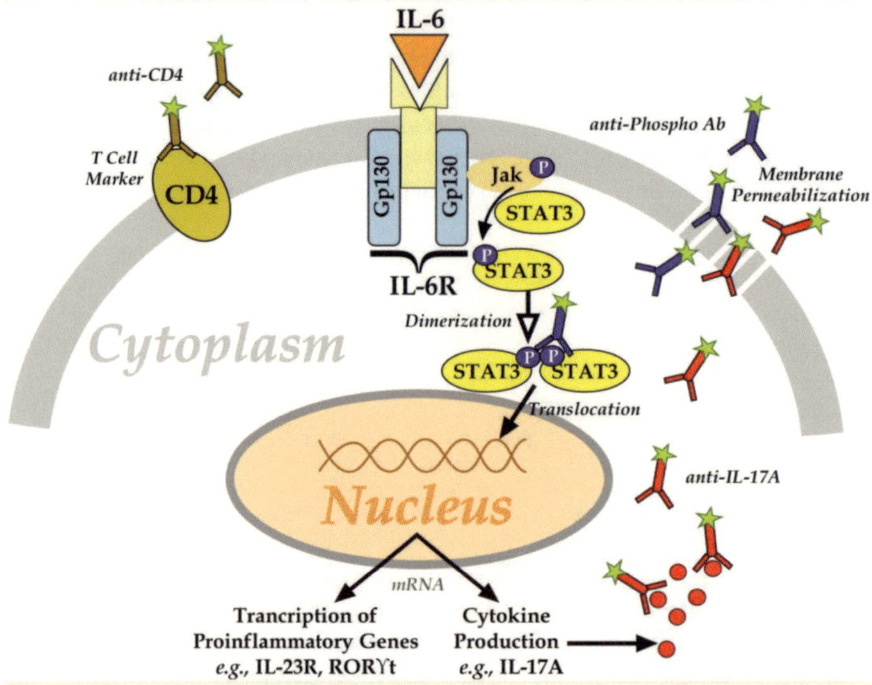

Fig. 11. Phosphospecific flow cytometry can measure the phosphorylation state of intracellular proteins at the single cell level. Many different phosphorylation states can be measured simultaneously in each cell, along with other intracellular (*e.g.*, IL-17A) and/or surface (e.*g.*, CD4) markers, enabling complex signaling networks to be resolved. Phosflow assays are performed by stimulating cells, fixing and permeabilizing before staining with phosphospecific fluorophore conjugated antibody for flow cytometric analysis

Thus, by using the wide variety of flow cytometric tools available, it is possible to detect changes within a small subpopulation of a heterogenous cell population without need to go through expensive cell sorting or purification steps. Finally, powerful analysis can be done using multiple parameter flow cytometer staining. However, timing of phosphorylation events with membrane surface phenotype expression, gene transcription and cytokine release still pose a significant challenge in the utilization of the Phosflow™ technology.

5. Conclusion

Flow cytometry has assumed an increasingly important role in the diagnosis and monitoring of disease progression or regression in modern medicine.[Chesney *et al.*, 2011, Dieterlen *et al.*, 2011, Hedley *et al.*, 2011, Hernandez-Fuentes & Salama, 2006, Mittag & Tarnok, 2011, Panzer & Jilma, 2011, Tung *et al.*, 2007, Venet *et al.*, 2011] Indeed, flow cytometry has proved to be an exceptionally powerful tool in assessing the rejection or acceptance of allogeneic tissues. Flow cytometry is essential in characterizing both *in vitro* and *in vivo* immunological response including cell proliferation (CSFE staining and murine

H2 determination), cytokine expression (cytometric bead array), intra-cellular signaling cascades, lymphocyte differentiation (*e.g.*, Tregs and Th17 cells) and *in vivo* cell trafficking (*e.g.*, thymus, spleen, lymph node and blood). Moreover, the flow cytometry tools available for immunological studies continue to expand thereby enhancing our ability to decipher the immune response to non-self antigens. By using the unique tools provided by flow cytometry, our own studies have been better able to elucidate the mechanisms by which the polymer-mediated immunocamouflage of allogeneic cells influences T cell differentiation (both *in vitro* and *in vivo*) to produce a stable tolerogeneic/anergic state. [Chen & Scott, 2003, Chen & Scott, 2006, Murad *et al.*, 1999a, Wang *et al.*, 2011]

6. Acknowledgment

This work was supported by grants from the Canadian Blood Services, Canadian Blood Services-Canadian Institutes of Health Research (CBS-CIHR) Partnership Fund and Health Canada. The views expressed herein do not necessarily represent the view of the federal government of Canada. We thank the Canada Foundation for Innovation and the Michael Smith Foundation for Health Research for infrastructure funding at the University of British Columbia Centre for Blood Research.

7. References

Abadja, F., Videcoq, C., Alamartine, E., Berthoux, F., Mariat, C. (2009) Differential effect of cyclosporine and mycophenolic acid on the human regulatory T cells and TH-17 cells balance. *Transplant Proc,* 41(8), 3367–3370.

Afzali, B., Lombardi, G., Lechler, R. I., Lord, G. M. (2007) The role of T helper 17 (Th17) and regulatory T cells (Treg) in human organ transplantation and autoimmune disease. *Clin Exp Immunol,* 148(1), 32–46.

Allison, A. C. (2000) Immunosuppressive drugs: the first 50 years and a glance forward. *Immunopharmacology,* 47(2-3), 63–83.

Battaglia, M. (2010) Potential T regulatory cell therapy in transplantation: how far have we come and how far can we go? *Transpl Int,* 23(8), 761–770.

Bonnotte, B., Pardoux, C., Bourhis, J. H., Caignard, A., Burdiles, A. M., Chehimi, J., Mami-Chouaib, F., Chouaib, S. (1996) Inhibition of the human allogeneic mixed lymphocyte response by cyclosporin A: relationship with the IL-12 pathway. *Tissue Antigens,* 48(4 Pt 1), 265–270.

Bradley, A. J., Murad, K. L., Regan, K. L., Scott, M. D. (2002) Biophysical consequences of linker chemistry and polymer size on stealth erythrocytes: size does matter. *Biochim Biophys Acta,* 1561(2), 147–158.

Bradley, A. J., Scott, M. D. (2004) Separation and purification of methoxypoly(ethylene glycol) grafted red blood cells via two-phase partitioning. *J Chromatogr B Analyt Technol Biomed Life Sci,* 807(1), 163–168.

Chen, A. M., Scott, M. D. (2001) Current and future applications of immunological attenuation via pegylation of cells and tissue. *BioDrugs,* 15(12), 833–847.

Chen, A. M., Scott, M. D. (2003) Immunocamouflage: prevention of transfusion-induced graft-versus-host disease via polymer grafting of donor cells. *J Biomed Mater Res A,* 67(2), 626–636.

Chen, A. M., Scott, M. D. (2006) Comparative analysis of polymer and linker chemistries on the efficacy of immunocamouflage of murine leukocytes. *Artif Cells Blood Substit Immobil Biotechnol,* 34(3), 305–322.

Chesney, A., Good, D., Reis, M. (2011) Clinical utility of flow cytometry in the study of erythropoiesis and nonclonal red cell disorders. *Methods Cell Biol,* 103, 311-332.

Cote, I., Rogers, N. J., Lechler, R. I. (2001) Allorecognition. *Transfus Clin Biol,* 8(3), 318–323.

Dallman, M. J. (2001) Immunobiology of graft rejection. In *Pathology and immunology of transplantation and rejection* (S. Thiru, H. Waldmann, eds.), Blackwell Science Ltd, Oxford, UK, 1-19.

Devetten, M. P., Vose, J. M. (2004) Graft-versus-host disease: how to translate new insights into new therapeutic strategies. *Biol Blood Marrow Transplant,* 10(12), 815–825.

Dieterlen, M. T., Eberhardt, K., Tarnok, A., Bittner, H. B., Barten, M. J. (2011) Flow cytometry-based pharmacodynamic monitoring after organ transplantation. *Methods Cell Biol,* 103, 267–284.

Goldstein, D. R. (2011) Inflammation and transplantation tolerance. *Semin Immunopathol,* 33(2), 111–115.

Hanidziar, D., Koulmanda, M. (2010) Inflammation and the balance of Treg and Th17 cells in transplant rejection and tolerance. *Curr Opin Organ Transplant,* 15(4), 411–415.

Hedley, D. W., Chow, S., Shankey, T. V. (2011) Cytometry of intracellular signaling: from laboratory bench to clinical application. *Methods Cell Biol,* 103, 203–220.

Heidt, S., Segundo, D. S., Chadha, R., Wood, K. J. (2010) The impact of Th17 cells on transplant rejection and the induction of tolerance. *Curr Opin Organ Transplant,* 15(4), 456–461.

Hernandez-Fuentes, M. P., Salama, A. (2006) In vitro assays for immune monitoring in transplantation. *Methods Mol Biol,* 333, 269–290.

Kitabayashi, C., Fukada, T., Kanamoto, M., Ohashi, W., Hojyo, S., Atsumi, T., Ueda, N., Azuma, I., Hirota, H., Murakami, M., Hirano, T. (2010) Zinc suppresses Th17 development via inhibition of STAT3 activation. *Int Immunol,* 22(5), 375–386.

Kleinman, S., Chan, P., Robillard, P. (2003) Risks associated with transfusion of cellular blood components in Canada. *Transfus Med Rev,* 17(2), 120–162.

Krutzik, P. O., Irish, J. M., Nolan, G. P., Perez, O. D. (2004) Analysis of protein phosphorylation and cellular signaling events by flow cytometry: techniques and clinical applications. *Clin Immunol,* 110(3), 206–221.

Le, Y., Scott, M. D. (2010) Immunocamouflage: the biophysical basis of immunoprotection by grafted methoxypoly(ethylene glycol) [mpeg]. *Acta Biomater,* 6, 2631–2641.

Li, J., Lai, X., Liao, W., He, Y., Liu, Y., Gong, J. (2011) The dynamic changes of Th17/Treg cytokines in rat liver transplant rejection and tolerance. *Int Immunopharmacol,* 11, 962–967.

McCoy, L. L., Scott, M. D. (2005) Broad spectrum antiviral prophylaxis: Inhibition of viral infection by polymer grafting with methoxypoly(ethylene glycol). In *Antiviral Drug Discovery for Emerging Diseases and Bioterrorism Threats* (T. PF, ed.), Wiley & Sons, Hoboken, NJ, *379–395.*

Mitchell, P., Afzali, B., Lombardi, G., Lechler, R. I. (2009) The T helper 17-regulatory T cell axis in transplant rejection and tolerance. *Curr Opin Organ Transplant,* 14(4), 326–331.

Mittag, A., Tarnok, A. (2011) Recent advances in cytometry applications: preclinical, clinical, and cell biology. *Methods Cell Biol,* 103, 1-20.

Muller, Y. D., Seebach, J. D., Buhler, L. H., Pascual, M., Golshayan, D. (2011) Transplantation tolerance: Clinical potential of regulatory T cells. *Self Nonself,* 2(1), 26-34.

Murad, K. L., Gosselin, E. J., Eaton, J. W., Scott, M. D. (1999a) Stealth cells: prevention of major histocompatibility complex class II-mediated T-cell activation by cell surface modification. *Blood,* 94(6), 2135-2141.

Murad, K. L., Mahany, K. L., Brugnara, C., Kuypers, F. A., Eaton, J. W., Scott, M. D. (1999b) Structural and functional consequences of antigenic modulation of red blood cells with methoxypoly(ethylene glycol). *Blood,* 93(6), 2121-2127.

Nishihara, M., Ogura, H., Ueda, N., Tsuruoka, M., Kitabayashi, C., Tsuji, F., Aono, H., Ishihara, K., Huseby, E., Betz, U. A., Murakami, M., Hirano, T. (2007) IL-6-gp130-STAT3 in T cells directs the development of IL-17+ Th with a minimum effect on that of Treg in the steady state. *Int Immunol,* 19(6), 695-702.

Nistala, K., Wedderburn, L. R. (2009) Th17 and regulatory T cells: rebalancing pro- and anti-inflammatory forces in autoimmune arthritis. *Rheumatology (Oxford),* 48(6), 602-606.

Noris, M., Casiraghi, F., Todeschini, M., Cravedi, P., Cugini, D., Monteferrante, G., Aiello, S., Cassis, L., Gotti, E., Gaspari, F., Cattaneo, D., Perico, N., Remuzzi, G. (2007) Regulatory T cells and T cell depletion: role of immunosuppressive drugs. *J Am Soc Nephrol,* 18(3), 1007-1018.

O'Gorman, W. E., Dooms, H., Thorne, S. H., Kuswanto, W. F., Simonds, E. F., Krutzik, P. O., Nolan, G. P., Abbas, A. K. (2009) The initial phase of an immune response functions to activate regulatory T cells. *J Immunol,* 183(1), 332-339.

Oukka, M. (2007) Interplay between pathogenic Th17 and regulatory T cells. *Ann Rheum Dis,* 66 Suppl 3iii87-90.

Panzer, S., Jilma, P. (2011) Methods for testing platelet function for transfusion medicine. *Vox Sang,* 101(1), 1-9.

Rossi, N. A., Constantinescu, I., Brooks, D. E., Scott, M. D., Kizhakkedathu, J. N. (2010a) Enhanced cell surface polymer grafting in concentrated and nonreactive aqueous polymer solutions. *J Am Chem Soc,* 132(10), 3423-3430.

Rossi, N. A., Constantinescu, I., Kainthan, R. K., Brooks, D. E., Scott, M. D., Kizhakkedathu, J. N. (2010b) Red blood cell membrane grafting of multi-functional hyperbranched polyglycerols. *Biomaterials,* 31(14), 4167-4178.

Scott, M. D., Bradley, A. J., Murad, K. L. (2003) Stealth erythrocytes: effects of polymer grafting on biophysical, biological and immunological parameters. *Blood Transfusion,* 1, 244-265.

Scott, M. D., Murad, K. L., Koumpouras, F., Talbot, M., Eaton, J. W. (1997) Chemical camouflage of antigenic determinants: stealth erythrocytes. *Proc Natl Acad Sci U S A,* 94(14), 7566-7571.

Suthanthiran, M., Strom, T. B. (1995) Immunobiology and Immunopharmacology of Organ Allograft Rejection. *Journal of Clinical Immunology,* 15, 161-171.

Sutton, T. C., Scott, M. D. (2010) The effect of grafted methoxypoly(ethylene glycol) chain length on the inhibition of respiratory syncytial virus (RSV) infection and proliferation. *Biomaterials,* 31(14), 4223-4230.

Tung, J. W., Heydari, K., Tirouvanziam, R., Sahaf, B., Parks, D. R., Herzenberg, L. A., Herzenberg, L. A. (2007) Modern flow cytometry: a practical approach. *Clin Lab Med,* 27(3), 453–68, v.

Venet, F., Guignant, C., Monneret, G. (2011) Flow cytometry developments and perspectives in clinical studies: examples in ICU patients. *Methods Mol Biol,* 761, 261–275.

Wang, D., Toyofuku, W. M., Chen, A. M., Scott, M. D. (2011) Induction of immunotolerance via mPEG grafting to allogeneic leukocytes. *Biomaterials,* 32, 9494–9503.

Weaver, C. T., Hatton, R. D. (2009) Interplay between the TH17 and TReg cell lineages: a (co-)evolutionary perspective. *Nat Rev Immunol,* 9(12), 883–889.

Weigt, S. S., Wallace, W. D., Derhovanessian, A., Saggar, R., Saggar, R., Lynch, J. P., Belperio, J. A. (2010) Chronic allograft rejection: epidemiology, diagnosis, pathogenesis, and treatment. *Semin Respir Crit Care Med,* 31(2), 189–207.

Weston, S. A., Parish, C. R. (1990) New fluorescent dyes for lymphocyte migration studies. Analysis by flow cytometry and fluorescence microscopy. *J Immunol Methods,* 133(1), 87–97.

8

Multiplexed Cell-Counting Methods by Using Functional Nanoparticles and Quantum Dots

Hoyoung Yun[1], Won Gu Lee[2] and Hyunwoo Bang[1]
[1]*School of Mechanical and Aerospace Engineering, Seoul National University*
[2]*Department of Mechanical Engineering, Kyung Hee University*
Republic of Korea

1. Introduction

This chapter mainly deals with investigation and development of intensity-based cell-counting methods using fluorescent silica nanoparticles (SiNPs) and quantum dots (QDs) for differential counting of leukocytes. The proposed cell-counting methods enable us to simultaneously measure multiple subsets of human blood cells using a single detector without fluorescence compensation due to an inherent signal overlap of emission spectra from multiple fluorescent labels. At the beginning of the chapter, brief history and theoretical background of multicolor flow cytometry and previous intensity-based cell-counting methods are reviewed. Subsequently, motivation and objectives of the proposed methods are introduced with current issues in this field.

Antonie van Leeuwenhoek (Holland, 1632-1723) is the first person who observed blood cells and micro-organisms in suspension using the simple microscope (~300 X). As microscopy techniques have rapidly developed, the first commercial microscope with ultraviolet (UV) was presented by Carl Zeiss (Germany) in 1904 and the phase-contrast microscope that allowed for the study of colorless and transparent biological materials were invented in 1932. Meanwhile, George Gabriel Stoke (1819–1903) first described a fluorescence difference between excitation and emission spectra known as the Stokes shift in the Mid-1800's. A fluorescent antibody technique developed by Albert Coons (1912–1978) in 1941, who labeled antibodies with fluorescein isothiocyanate (FITC), thus he gave birth to the field of immunofluorescence. From Mid-1900's, scientists began to interest in automated cell-counting techniques, not just in observation of cells. Moldovan described the first flow cytometer concept using glass capillary tubes mounted on a microscope stage (Moldavan, 1934), although this device could not measure meaningful cell-signals because of capillary blocking and interference of signals by using narrow tubes. When wider tubes were used, the device could not count cell population. In 1947, a photoelectric counter, which uses light source and photomultipliers (PMTs), was developed and this device is the first working flow cytometer (Gucker Jr et al., 1947). To test the efficiency of gas mask filters against particles, the device used filtered air to carry and constrain the sample particles. A hydrodynamic focusing concept for reproducible delivery of cells suspended in a fluid was introduced by Crossland-Taylor in 1953. Using this device, accurate counts of blood cells were obtained (Crosland-Taylor, 1953). The first impedance-based flow cytometer by using the Coulter principle was developed in 1953 (Coulter, 1953). This principle was used in the first demonstration of cell sorting in 1965 (Fulwyler, 1965). The first commercial fluorescence-based flow cytometry device (ICP 11, Partec, Germany) reached the market in 1969. Fluorescence Activated Cell Sorter (FACS) was developed by Leonard A. Herzenberg (Herzenberg et al., 1976) and firstly commercialized by Becton Dickinson (BD, USA) in 1974.

In 1977, the first multi-parametric cell counting method using monoclonal antibodies (Loken et al., 1977), which was called a two-color immunofluorescence method, was developed by Leonard A. Herzenberg and his colleagues. Subsequently, they described a three-color immunofluorescence detection system in 1984 (Parks et al., 1984) and this was beginning of the multicolor world of flow cytometry.

In 1934	Moldovan described the first flow cytometer (Moldavan, 1934)
In 1947	The photoelectric counter was developed (Gucker Jr et al., 1947) The first working flow cytometer
In 1953	Development of the concept of hydrodynamic focusing (Crosland-Taylor, 1953) The first impedance-based flow cytometry device (The coulter counter) (Coulter, 1953)
In 1965	The coulter principle was used in the first demonstration of cell sorting (Fulwyler, 1965)
In 1969	The first commercial fluorescence-based flow cytometry device was developed (ICP 11, Partec, Germany)
In 1974	The Fluorescence Activated Cell Sorter (FACS) was developed by Leonard Herzenberg and first commercialized by Becton Dickinson (BD) (Herzenberg et al., 1976)
In 1977	Two-color immunofluorescence using monoclonal antibodies and FACS was demonstrated (Loken et al., 1977) The fluorescent antibody technique (immunofluorescence) developed by Albert Coons (Coons et al., 1941), who labeled antibodies with fluorescein isothiocyanate (FITC)
In 1984	Three-color analysis: beginning the multicolor world of flow cytometry (Parks et al., 1984) Robert Murphy developed FCS 1.0 file standard (Murphy et al., 1984)

Table 1. Important developments in flow cytometry and multicolor immunofluorescence

The ability to simultaneously measure multiple parameters is the most powerful aspect of flow cytometers and enables a wide range of applications, including clinical applications and research applications. Recently, flow cytometers are the most commonly used automated cell counting and sorting devices for analyzing particles, beads or cells suspended in a fluid stream (Laerum et al., 1981, Shapiro, 1983). It has been widely applied in multi-parametric studies on the physical and/or chemical characteristics of cells, leukocyte differentiation for cell based diagnostics, and immunoreaction based on micro beads (Brando et al., 2000, HOUWEN, 2001). These applications require multi-parametric information from multiple cytometers or a single cytometer equipped with multiple photomultiplier tubes (PMTs) to simultaneously detect target samples tagged with fluorescent dyes having different emission wavelengths (Janossy et al., 2000, Glencross et al., 2002, Janossy et al., 2003). More recently, a flow cytometer equipped with multiple light sources and multiple detectors that can measure up to 16 optical parameters at the same time has been developed (Cottingham, 2005) and new methods to measure even more parameters have been suggested (Darzynkiewicz et al., 1999, Perfetto et al., 2004, Kapoor et al., 2007). Such developments can significantly enhance the reliability of cell based diagnostics and even make it possible to develop new diagnostic methods using the information given by the additionally acquired parameters.

Similarly, in parallel to developing the high performance flow cytometers requiring multi-parameter detection capabilities, portable flow cytometers have been recognized as an important tool for particular applications such as HIV/AIDS screening in developing countries and regions with limited medical facilities and resources (Cohen, 2004, Bonetta, 2005, Lee et al., 2010). Several foundations have provided support to ensure sustainable access to CD4$^+$ T-cell testing for developing countries and many researchers have made effort to develop CLIA (Clinical Laboratory Improvement Amendments)-waived flow cytometry or POC (Point-of-care) cell counting method.

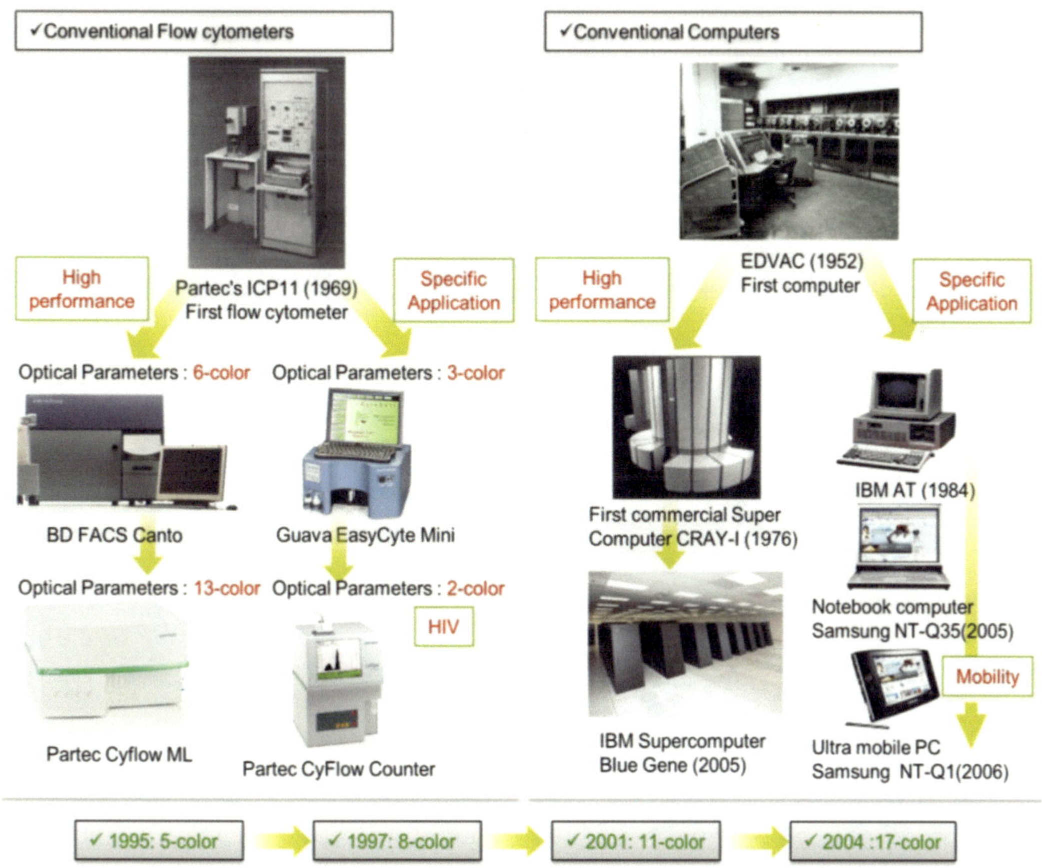

Fig. 1. The key trends of development of flow cytometers. Like computers, both of the high performance flow cytometer and the inexpensive portable flow cytometer have their own important role. (Figure sources from partec.com, bd.com, guavatechnologies.com, Samsung.com, ibm.com)

Since the invention of the first computer (EDVAC, 1952), there are two trends in history of development of computers: super computers for high performance and personal computers for mobility. In the same manner, flow cytometers will have been developing in two types: high performance flow cytometers for multi-parametric cellular analysis and inexpensive portable flow cytometers for point-of-care applications.

Multiplexed cell-counting methods in this chapter could be applied to both of high performance applications for measurement of multiple parameters on cells and point-of-care applications by using portable flow cytometers. The ability of these intensity-based cell counting methods to simultaneously measure multiple parameters by using single detector enables us to increase the number of detectable parameters per detector without fluorescence compensation. Therefore, conventional flow cytometers can detect more parameters without increase of detectors and portable flow cytometers can minimize the number of detectors.

2. Multicolor flow cytometry

2.1 One-color immunofluorescence and fluorescence dyes

An immunofluorescence staining is a technique used for analysis of biological samples. This technique allows detection of specific antigens or proteins by binding an antibody conjugated with a fluorescent dye such as fluorescein isothiocyanate (FITC) (Coons et al., 1941). For example, a CD4 antigen used for a HIV/AIDS screening is one of the most famous cell surface antigens of leukocytes. Biological samples, such as cells and tissue sections, stained by immunofluorescence can be analyze by fluorescence microscopes, confocal microscopes, or automated cell analyzers including a flow cytometer (Loken et al., 1977, Ledbetter et al., 1980).

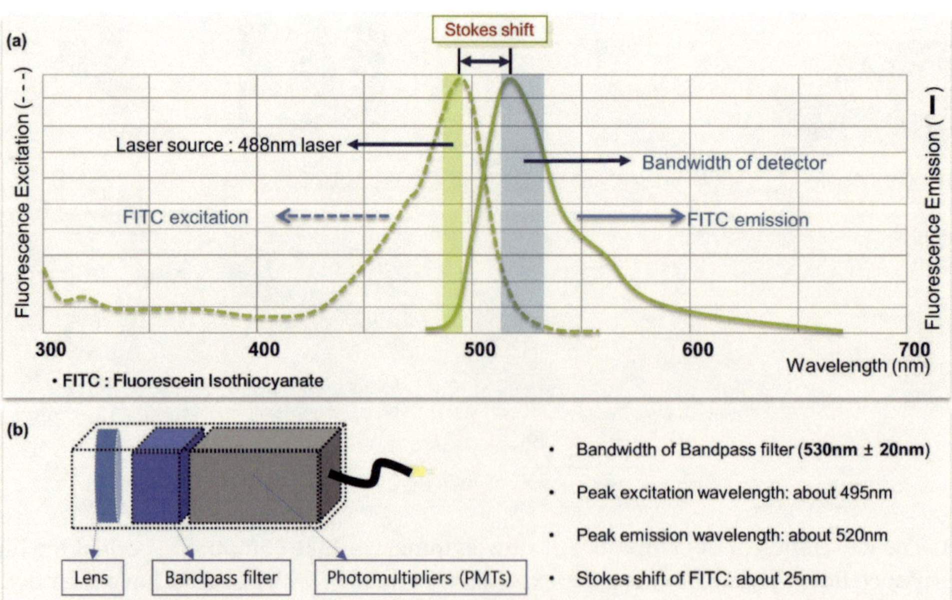

Fig. 2. Example of one-color immunofluorescence and graph of the Stokes shift of FITC

Basically, the immunofluorescence uses the Stokes shift which is a fluorescence difference between a peak excitation and emission wavelengths of the same electronic transition. As shown in Fig. 2, the peak excitation and emission wavelength of FITC is approximately 495nm and 520nm, respectively. Therefore, the Stokes shift of FITC, which is the most common used fluorescence dye in 1-color immunofluorescence, is 25nm. By using a 488nm excitation light source, an optical bandwidth filter (530nm ± 20nm), and a detector (PMTs), we can detect and count a desired marker in cells or biological samples.

Desirable fluorescence dyes for flow cytometry have several properties as follows: 1. they have biologically inertness, which means that they do not affect cells and bind directly to cellular elements; 2. are easily conjugated to monoclonal antibodies; 3. have an emission spectrum overlap as little as possible with cellular autofluorescence, which is natural fluorescence of some molecules in cells (Monici, 2005); 4. have a high cell-associated fluorescence intensity. The high fluorescence intensity enables us to distinguish positively immunofluorescence stained cells from unstained cells. The high fluorescent brightness results from fluorescence dyes with the following characteristics: 1. a high the molar absorptivity; 2. a high quantum yield; 3. the low autofluorescence; 4. a high sensitivity detector; and 5. the ability to conjugate multiple fluorescence dyes to each detecting site (Baumgarth et al., 2000).

The intensity of fluorescent dyes can be calculated by simple equations and appropriate assumptions. Fluorescent intensity could be written as (Walker, 1987)

$$I(z) = I_e(z)A\Phi L\varepsilon C \tag{1}$$

where I is the measured fluorescence intensity at time point z along the excitation beam path, Ie is the intensity of the excitation light beam at point z, A is the fraction of fluorescence light collected, Φ is the quantum efficiency, L is the length of the sampling volume along the path of the excitation beam, ε is the molar absorptivity, and C is the molar concentration of the fluorescence dye.

Fluorescent dyes	Absorbance maximum	Fluorescence emission	Molar Absorptivity $(M\text{-}cm)^{-1}$ (ε)	Quantum efficient (Φ)	Brightness (A.U.)	Brightness (*vs.* R-PE)
R-Phycoerythrin (R-PE)	490 nm 565 nm	578 nm	1,970,000	0.82	1,615,400	1
FITC	494 nm	518 nm	65,700	0.98	64,386	1/25
Propidium Iodide (PI, intercalating agent)	536 nm	716 nm	5,900	0.09	531	1/3042

Table 2. The brightness of the most common used fluorescence dyes

2.2 Two-color immunofluorescence and fluorescence dyes

Two-color immunofluorescence for two-parameter detection requires two fluorescence dyes having different emission spectra but similar excitation spectra, such as FITC and R-Phycoerythrin (R-PE). This method can be used to measure two cell populations at the same time by labeling the green florescent dye to one cell type and the red fluorescent dye to another cell type with two fluorescent detectors and a single excitation light source. To count $CD4^+$ T-cells (T-helper cells) and $CD45^+$ (leukocytes) cells which are subsets of

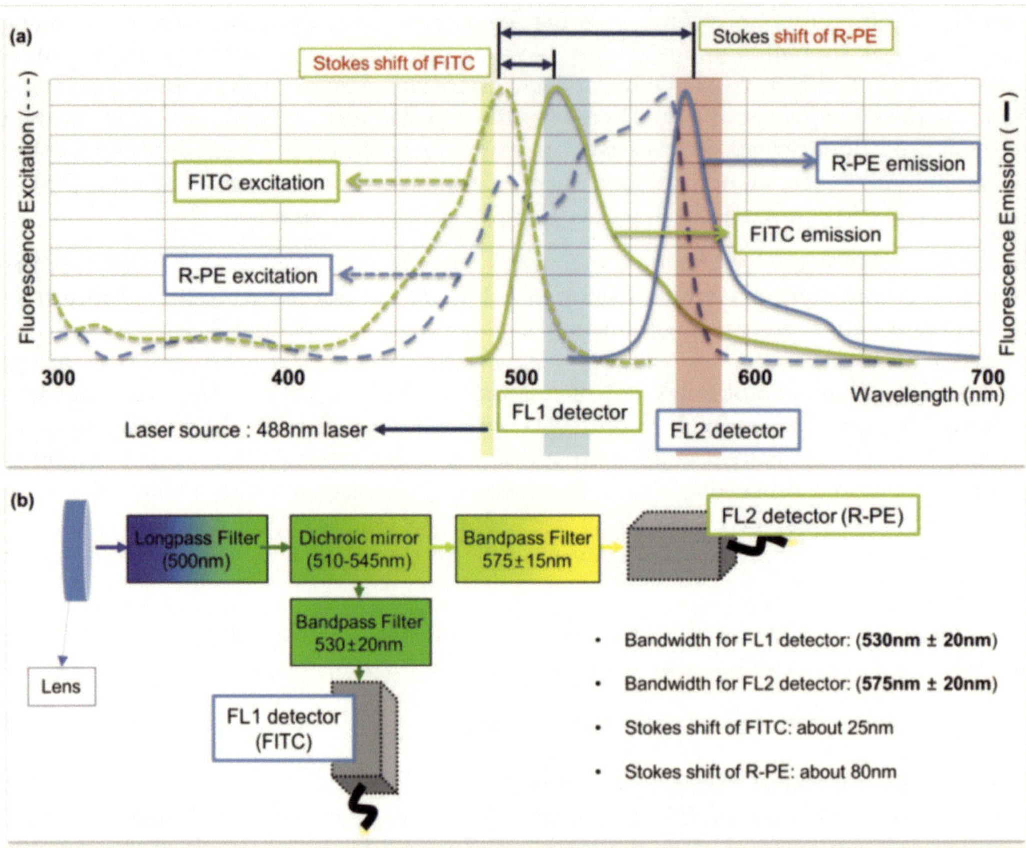

Fig. 3. (a) Excitation and emission wavelength curves of FITC and R-PE. (b) Schematic representation of an optical measurement system for two-parameter fluorescence detection. This system utilizes one laser source (488nm blue laser) and two detectors (PMTs)

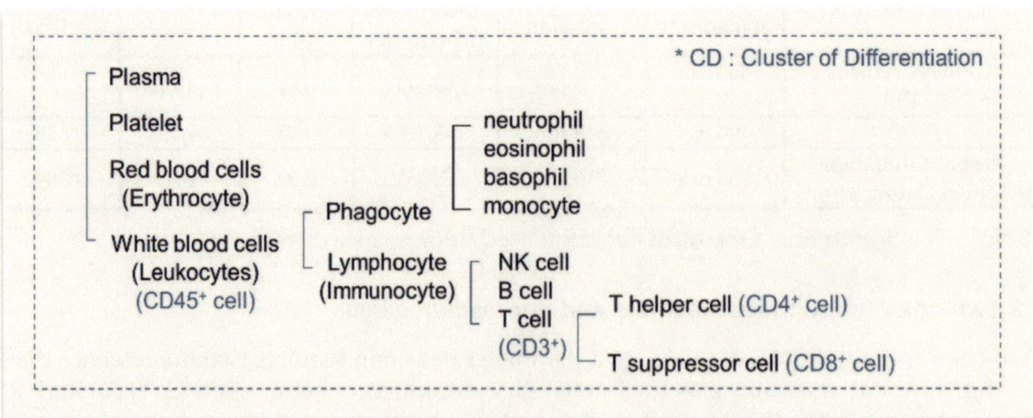

Fig. 4. A brief description of human blood subsets. T-helper cells ($CD4^+$ T-cells) are one of the most important cell types for HIV/AIDS screening because $CD4^+$ T-cells are known to be attacked by Human Immunodeficiency Virus (HIV)

leukocytes simultaneously, a mixture of FITC conjugated anti-CD45 monoclonal antibodies and R-PE conjugated anti-CD4 monoclonal antibodies are generally used. To detect additional cell types, additional fluorescence dyes with different emission wavelengths and additional detectors have to be used.

Two-color immunofluorescence utilizes a difference in the Stokes shift between two fluorescence dyes having similar excitation spectra. Therefore, we can count two different types of cells with one laser source and two PMTs. Fig. 3 shows an example of simultaneous two-parameter detection by using FITC and R-PE. The peak excitation wavelength of FITC and R-PE is 490 nm and 494 nm, respectively. 518 nm and 578 nm is the peak emission wavelength of FITC and R-PE, respectively. The optical measurement system consists of one blue laser (488 nm), one emission filter for a FITC detection (FL1, 530 ± 20 nm), and another emission filter for a R-PE detection (FL2, 575 ± 20 nm) positioned in front of each PMTs.

Fig. 5 shows an example of 2-color flow cytometry for HIV/AIDS screening. In HIV/AIDS screening, the number of $CD4^+$ T-cells in blood provides important information for antiretroviral treatment. For example, $CD4^+$ T-cell counts below 200 cells/µl require the start of antiretroviral treatment in adults (over 13 years old) (Masur et al., 2002). However, lymphocyte subsets (including $CD4^+$ T-cells) of infants and young children are higher than those of adults, therefore the ratio of $CD4^+$ T-cells to other blood cells, i.e., CD4/CD45%, CD4/CD8% or CD4/CD3%, is a more reliable indicator of HIV infection than absolute $CD4^+$ T-cell counts(Shearer et al., 2003, Organization, 2006). In general, to quantify the percentage of $CD4^+$ T-cells, two fluorescent dyes with different emission wavelengths should be assigned to each of the desired blood cell types and analyzed by a flow cytometer equipped with two PMTs. Recently, new alternative methods for affordable $CD4^+$ T-cell counting using microfluidic devices and label-free $CD4^+$ T-cell counting methods were proposed for resource-poor settings (Rodriguez et al., 2005, Cheng et al., 2007, Ateya et al., 2008).

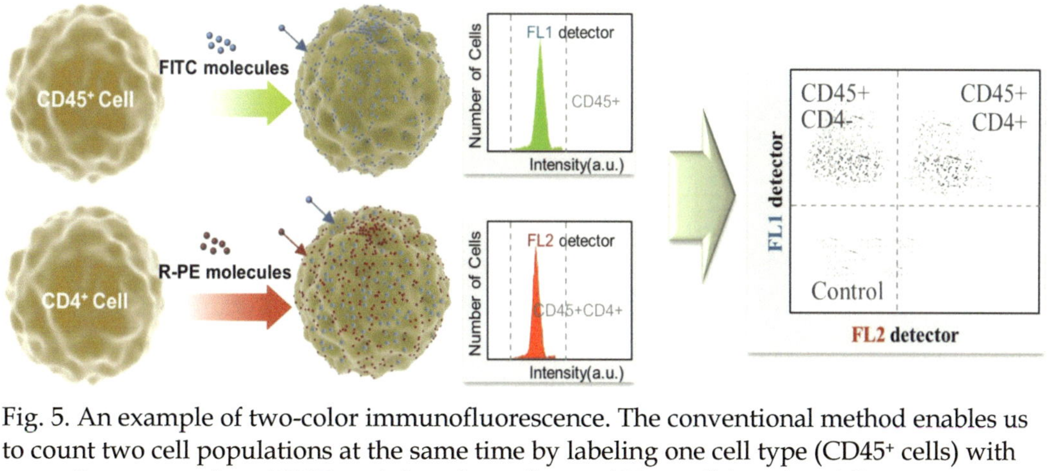

Fig. 5. An example of two-color immunofluorescence. The conventional method enables us to count two cell populations at the same time by labeling one cell type ($CD45^+$ cells) with green fluorescent dyes (FITC) and the other cell type ($CD4^+$ cells) with red fluorescent dyes (R-Phycoerythrin (R-PE)). Actually, $CD4^+$ cells are labeled with both FITC and R-PE because $CD4^+$ cells are subset of $CD45^+$ cells. HIV/AIDS screening can be performed from a simultaneous counting of $CD4^+$ T-cells and $CD45^+$ cells (Yun et al., 2010)

2.3 Multi-color immunofluorescence and fluorescence dyes

The ability to measure multi-parametric cellular information is limited by the number of fluorescence dyes that can be simultaneously measured. When designing experiments for multi-color flow cytometry that include the use of new fluorescence dye complexes, careful consideration must be given to the choice of fluorescence dyes. A desirable combination of fluorescence dyes for multi-color immunofluorescence exhibits little spectral overlap among

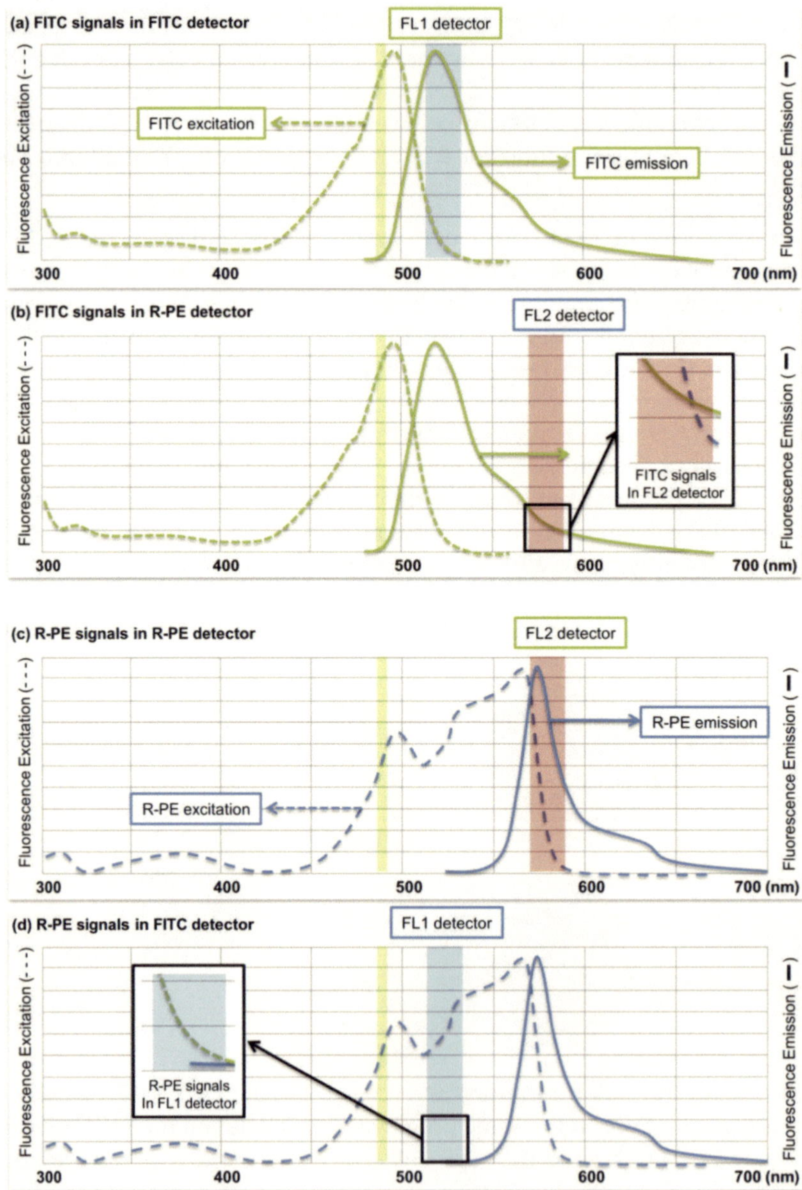

Fig. 6. The compensation problem. (a,b) FITC signals in FL1 and FL2 detectors. (c,d) R-PE signals in FL2 and FL1 detectors. FITC signals in the PE detector create most problems

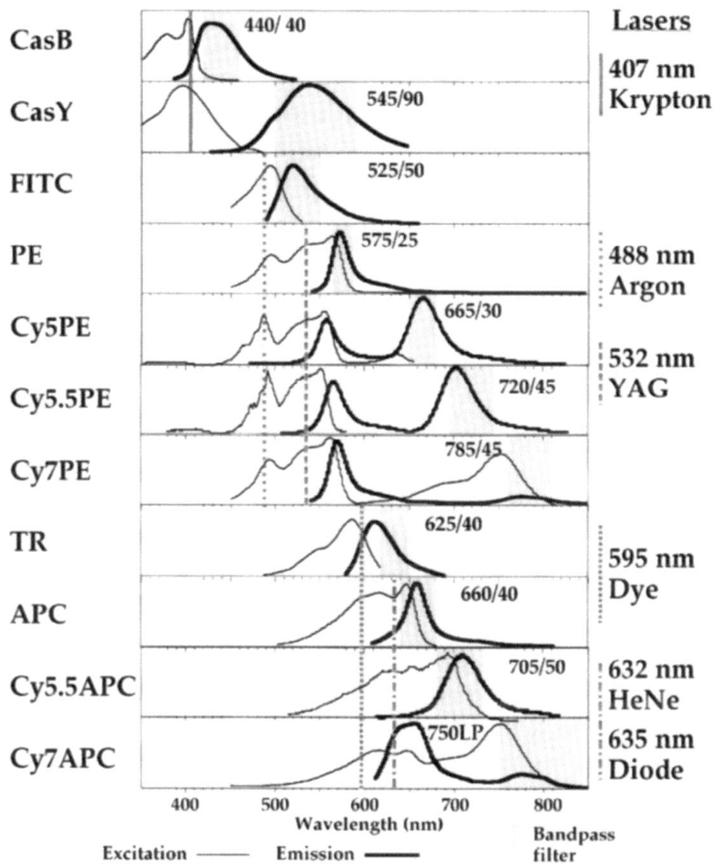

Fig. 7. An example of successful dye combination for multi-color analysis (11 colors) adapted from (Baumgarth et al., 2000). Currently, violet and green excitation light sources are provided by 405-nm violet diodes and 532-nm green solid state lasers, respectively.

each other (Baumgarth et al., 2000). The inherent overlap of emission spectra from antibody fluorescent labels makes compensation necessary. This is of particular importance when you attempt to make simultaneous immunofluorescence measurements from several cell-bound antibodies. To eliminate an error due to the overlap in the detected fluorescent signals from adjacent emission wavelengths, we should have additional compensation procedures before each flow cytometry test (Tung et al., 2004).

For flow cytometry analysis of two-parameter detection, the most common combinations of fluorescent dyes are FITC and R-PE. This is because both FITC and R-PE could be excited by a single light source such as a 488 nm blue laser but resulting in different emission spectra. However, because most fluorescent dyes do not have a sharp emission peak, the inherent overlap of emission spectra from these fluorescent labels makes compensation a necessity. In the case of FITC and R-PE in Fig. 6, spectral overlap between FITC and PE produces signals that are detected by both the FL1 and FL2 detectors. Therefore, the amount of FITC fluorescent signals being detected by the R-PE detection channel (FL2) and the amount of R-PE fluorescent signals being detected by FITC detection channel (FL1) should be compensated and eliminated. For example, to obtain pure R-PE signals, the amount of spectral overlap can be corrected by subtracting a percentage of FITC signals from the total signal generated by the R-PE detection channel. Therefore, to make simultaneous measurements of multiple immune cell subsets, this compensation procedure should be performed before testing samples. Fig. 7 shows a successful combination of fluorescence dyes for multi-color (11-color) flow cytometry excited by three different laser lines.

3. Intensity-based multiplexed cell-counting methods

3.1 Conventional intensity-based cell-counting methods

Cell counting methods by using differences in fluorescence intensities with a single detector (a single fluorescent detection channel) have been applied to some applications such as an apoptosis measurement (Darzynkiewicz et al., 1992, Schmid et al., 2007), a bead-based absolute cell counting method (Dieye et al., 2005), a cell cycle assay based on measurement of DNA contents in a cell, or counting two specific subsets of cells having same kinds of binding sites but different number of binding sites. For example, $CD4^+$ T-cells and monocytes, which are subsets of leukocytes, have same CD4 epitopes but different averages of 47,000 and 6,500 binding sites per cell, respectively. (Mandy et al., 1997, Denny et al., 1996, Bikoue et al., 1996). In 1986, Fluorescence-intensity multiplexing methods for counting different types of cell populations using dilution of fluorophores labeled reagents with unlabeled antibodies were presented (Bradford et al., 2004, Horan et al., 1986). This study has a significant impact in multi-parametric cytometry because the method can increase the number of parameter per detector without increase of additional detectors and the compensation procedure.

3.2 Multiplexed cell-counting method using silica nanoparticles

Several types of nanoparticles such as quantum dots (QDs) (Smith et al., 2006), gold nanoparticles (Daniel et al., 2004), and dye-dope SiNPs (Yan et al., 2007, Burns et al., 2006) have been demonstrated as versatile labeling reagents for bioimaging (Sharma et al., 2006) and biosensing (Yan et al., 2007). Among them, dye-doped SiNPs provide features such as high fluorescent intensity (Ow et al., 2005), excellent photostability (Santra et al., 2001, Santra et al., 2006), and ease of surface modification for bioconjugation (Qhobosheane et al., 2001). Using dye-doped SiNPs showing 10- and 100-fold increased detection sensitivity in flow cytometry analysis compared to standard methods, Tan *et al.* have suggested a flow cytometry based cancer cell detection method when the probes have relatively weak affinities or when the receptors are expressed in low concentration on the target cell surfaces (Estevez et al., 2009). The higher brightness of dye-doped SiNPs was the main reason we adopted this nanoparticle for a proposed fluorescent intensity-based multi-cell counting method. Based on an intensity difference between fluorescent dye-doped SiNPs and conventional fluorescence dyes, the multi-parameter detection method using a single detector with flow cytometry was evaluated by carrying out simultaneous counting of $CD4^+$ T-cells and $CD45^+$ cells.

Fluorescent dyes are classified by size. Among them, small molecule fluorescence dyes such as FITC, Cy5, and Alexa dyes could be doped to directly nanoparticles to obtain brighter fluorescent dyes complexes while maintaining a same excitation and emission spectra. On the other hand, fluorescent proteins such as R-PE, allophycocyanin (APC) cannot be directly

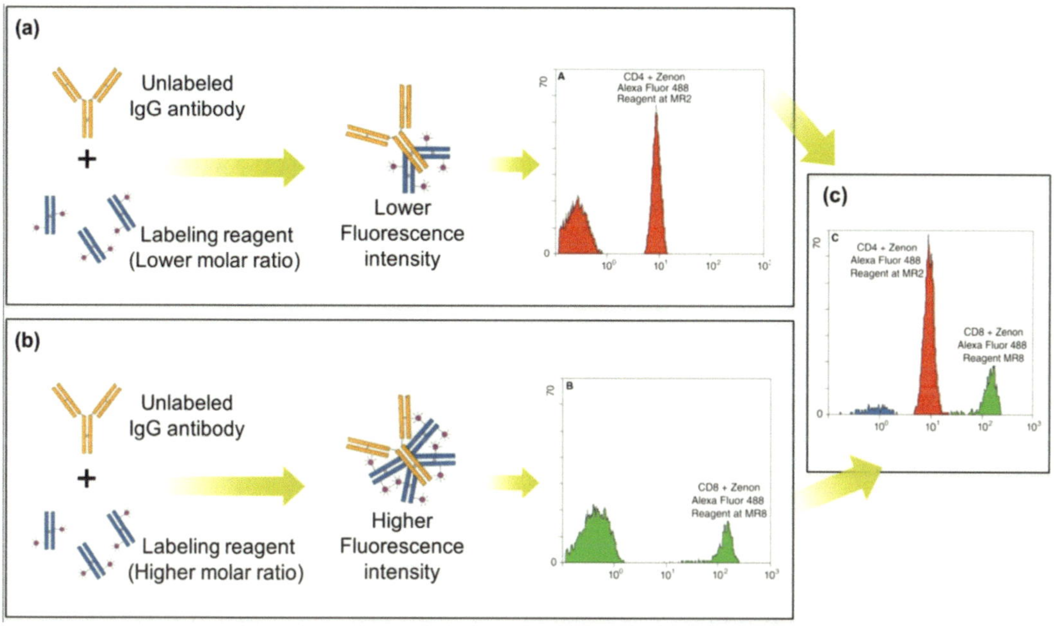

Fig. 8. Fluorescence-intensity multiplexing analysis by varying the labeling reagent (fluorescence dyes)-to antibody molar ratio (Bradford et al., 2004). This immunolabeling technology allows for multiple antigen detection per detection channel using a single fluorophore. (a) Labeling scheme for lower fluorescence intensity. Histogram shows $CD4^{+}$ T-cells labeling with a complex of CD4 antibodies and reagents having lower fluorescence intensity (a molar ratio of a labeling reagent to a primary antibody is 2). (b) Labeling scheme for higher fluorescence intensity. Histogram shows $CD8^{+}$ T-cells labeling with a complex of CD8 antibodies and fluorescence reagents having higher intensity (a molar ratio of a labeling reagent to a primary antibody is 8). (c) Histogram of simultaneous counting of $CD4^{+}$ cells and $CD8^{+}$ cells by a single detection channel

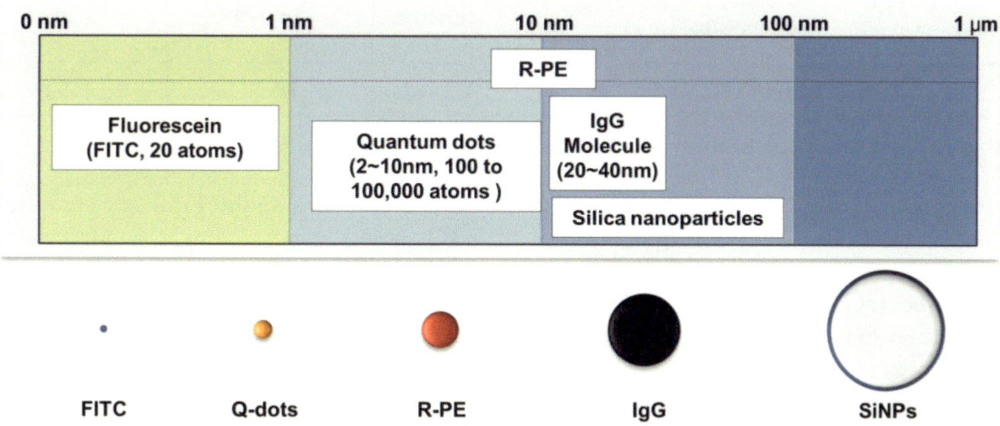

Fig. 9. The size of materials, including several types of fluorophores, immunoglobulin G (IgG), quantum dots, and silica nanoparticles

doped to nanoparticles because fluorescent proteins are much larger than small fluorophores relatively. In order to apply fluorescent proteins to intensity-based cell counting, fluorescent proteins should be used with fluorophores doped silica nanoparticles which have similar excitation and emission wavelengths with the fluorescent proteins.

The intensity of those fluorescent dye complexes can be calculated by simple equations and appropriate assumptions. From that calculation we can obtain a feasible combination of fluorophores doped nanoparticles and fluorescent proteins for intensity-based differential counting. To use fluorescent proteins in intensity based cell-counting, ideally, small molecule fluorophores having identical excitation and emission wavelengths as the fluorescent proteins itself need to be tagged to the SiNPs. Because there was no readily available combination of fluorophores and fluorescent proteins with same emission wavelengths, fluorophores which have adjacent excitation and emission wavelengths with fluorescent proteins was selected. The intensity of fluorescent dye-doped SiNPs can be calculated as following.

$$I(z) = n \times I_e(z) A \Phi L \varepsilon C \qquad (2)$$

where n is the number of fluorophores on a single silica nanoparticle. For example, the number of FITC molecules on a single nanoparticle (n) can be calculated theoretically as following Table 2. The majority of fluorescent dyes have a nonspherical shape. Fluorescein (FITC) is also a nonspherical solute with sizes of 0.47, 0.81, and 1.09 nm in different directions (Cvetkovic et al., 2005). Therefore, the size of fluorescent dye should be determined by using the appreciate method.

Method	size	The number of dyes per SiNP	Brightness (vs. FITC-IgG)
The stokes radius (Deen, 1987)	0.44 nm	40,568	5,795
The density of dyes (1kDa/1nm3)	0.9 nm	9696	1,385
The equivalent spherical diameter (Jennings et al., 1988, Cvetkovic et al., 2005)	0.7 nm	16,028	2,289
The maximum size	1.1 nm	6490	927

Table 3. Theoretical calculation of brightness of FITC-doped SiNPs

Table 3 shows the sizes (ranging from 0.44 nm to 1.1 nm) of a single FITC molecule with different methods. Therefore, the number of FITC molecule per a single nanoparticle is theoretically from 6490 to 40,568 and the relative intensity of FITC-doped SiNPs in FITC conjugated IgG is from 927 to 2,289. This theoretical value of the intensity deference is higher than experimental results from previous studies (Lian et al., 2004, Ow et al., 2005, Estevez et al., 2009, Yun et al., 2010). These results demonstrated dye-doped SiNPs is 10-100 times brighter than their constituent fluorophore. The reason for this relatively low intensity from the theoretical calculation is because fluorescent dyes were lost during the synthesis of dyes-doped SiNPs or photobleached (Santra et al., 2006). When considering these factors, the above equation of fluorescence intensity (2) is written as follows.

$$I_{SiNPs} = [n \times I_e(z) A\Phi L\varepsilon C] \times P \times L \quad (3)$$

Where P is the factor of photobleaching ranging from 0 to 1 and L is the factor of the fraction of remaining dyes ranging from 0 to 1. Accordingly, the intensity of small fluorophores doped SiNPs relative to a fluorescent protein can be defined as

$$I_{RELATIVE} = \frac{[I_e(z) A\Phi L\varepsilon C]_{PROTEIN}}{[n \times I_e(z) A\Phi L\varepsilon C \times P \times L]_{SiNPs}} \quad (4)$$

If $I_{relative} \geq 100$ or $I_{relative} \leq 0.01$, the intensity based cell-counting method using the intensity difference between small fluorophore doped SiNPs and fluorescent protein can be applied. For example, when using Propidium Iodide (PI, ε=5900/*M/Cm* and Φ=0.09) in combination with R-PE, Equation 4 could be transformed and simplified as 15,000/nPL approximately. Therefore, at conditions of no photobleaching (P=1) and no loss during the synthesis (L=1), less than 150 or more than 1,500,000 PI molecules need to dope SiNPs to analyze the two parameters using R-PE conjugated antibodies and PI-doped SiNPs.

Fig. 10 shows a concept of simultaneous counting of two subsets of leukocytes by using a combination of FITC-doped silica nanoparticles and FITC molecules. Although this study showed good correlation between the proposed method and a conventional method (R = 0.936, R^2 = 0.876), regression analysis from these results is not sufficient yet for the developed method to replace the conventional method in clinical setting. Some technical issues, such as nonspecific binding of silica nanoparticles, should be resolved.

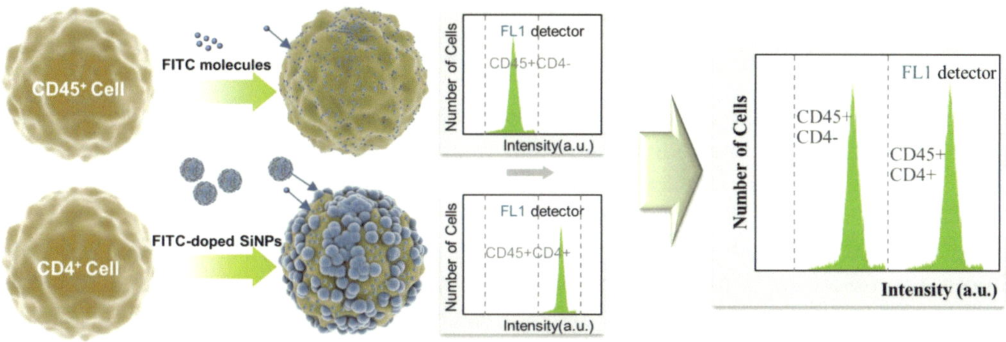

Fig. 10. An example of multiplexed cell counting using silica nanoparticles. This method utilized a dye combination of FITC and FITC-doped SiNPs instead of R-PE (Yun et al., 2010). Actually, $CD4^+$ cells are labeled with both FITC and FITC-doped SiNPs because $CD4^+$ cells are subset of $CD45^+$ cells

3.3 Multiplexed cell-counting method using quantum dots

Instead of the method by using much brighter fluorescence dyes such as FITC-doped silica nanoparticles, a method by using much darker dyes than general fluorophores can be applied to the multiplexed cell counting. Fig. 11 shows this counting concept. The proposed method also enables simultaneous counting of two subsets of leukocytes using a single detector by using quantum dots 605 (QDs 605) instead of FITC dyes in the conventional method. A combination of Q-dots 605 and R-Phycoerythrin (R-PE) can be used for making a

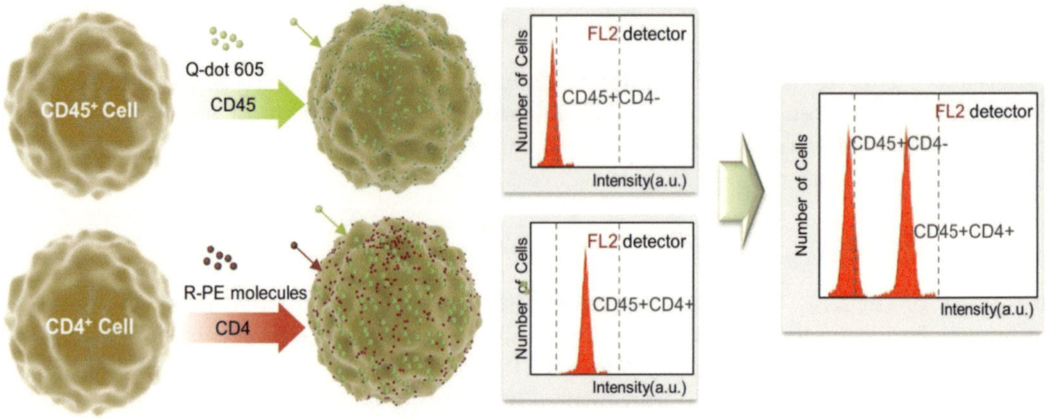

Fig. 11. An example of multiplexed cell counting using quantum dots. By using a complex of Q-dot 605 conjugated $CD45^+$ cells and R-PE conjugated CD4+ T-cells with a specific emission filter (from 564 to 606 nm), we can simultaneously count two different cell types ($CD45^+$ and CD4+ T-cells) in a single fluorescent channel. Actually, $CD4^+$ cells are labeled with both Q-dot 605 and R-PE because $CD4^+$ cells are subset of $CD45^+$ cells

similar effect in the multiplexed counting method with dye-doped silica nanoparticles. Q-dots 605 and R-PE have similar fluorescence intensity with a wide band width filter. However, by using a specific emission filter (from 564 to 606 nm), Q-dots 605 conjugated antibodies were detected as 10-100 times darker than R-PE conjugated antibodies.

4. Conclusion

Conventional flow cytometry requires multiple detectors for simultaneous identification of multiple subsets of immune cells because this method measures a single fluorescence dyes conjugated antibody per detector (PMTs). The ultimate goal of multiplexed cell-counting methods is to increase detectable parameters per fluorescence channel. These methods enable us to simultaneously measure multiple types of samples using a single detector without a troublesome fluorescence compensation procedure. In order to use the intensity-based counting in various fluorescent fields, this chapter suggests feasible combinations of fluorescence dyes and theoretical analysis to quantify an intensity difference between combinations. The combinations are classified into three groups; 1) fluorophores and fluorophore-doped silica nanoparticles which have same excitation and emission wavelengths; 2) fluorescent proteins and fluorophore-doped silica nanoparticles which have similar excitation and emission wavelengths; 3) combinations of fluorescence dyes such as quantum dots 605 and R-PE, which have different excitation and emission wavelengths. Multiplexed cell-counting methods in this chapter can be applied to both high performance flow cytometers for measurement of multiple parameters on cells and inexpensive portable flow cytometers. By using the ability of these intensity-based cell counting methods, conventional flow cytometers can detect more parameters without increase of detectors and portable flow cytometers can minimize the number of detectors. This study can be the building block for a more powerful and truly portable flow cytometer for various clinical cytometry applications.

5. Acknowledgment

This research was supported by Basic Science Research Program through the National Research Foundation of Korea (NRF) funded by the Ministry of Education, Science and Technology (2010-0005219)

6. References

Ateya, D. A., Erickson, J. S., Howell, P. B., Hilliard, L. R., Golden, J. P. & Ligler, F. S. 2008. The good, the bad, and the tiny: a review of microflow cytometry. *Analytical and Bioanalytical Chemistry,* Vol. 391, No. 5, pp. 1485-1498,

Baumgarth, N. & Roederer, M. 2000. A practical approach to multicolor flow cytometry for immunophenotyping. *Journal of immunological methods,* Vol. 243, No. 1-2, pp. 77-97,

Bikoue, A., George, F., Poncelet, P., Mutin, M., Janossy, G. & Sampol, J. 1996. Quantitative analysis of leukocyte membrane antigen expression: normal adult values. *Cytometry Part B: Clinical Cytometry,* Vol. 26, No. 2, pp. 137-147,

Bonetta, L. 2005. Flow cytometry smaller and better. *Nature Methods,* Vol. 2, No. 10, pp. 785-795, 1548-7091

Bradford, J., Buller, G., Suter, M., Ignatius, M., Beechem, J., Probes, M. & Eugene, O. 2004. Fluorescence-intensity multiplexing: simultaneous seven-marker, two-color immunophenotyping using flow cytometry. *Cytometry Part A,* Vol. 61A, No. 2, pp. 142-152,

Brando, B., Barnett, D., Janossy, G., Mandy, F., Autran, B., Rothe, G., Scarpati, B., D'avanzo, G., D'hautcourt, J.-L., Lenkei, R., Schmitz, G., Kunkl, A., Chianese, R., Papa, S. & Gratama, J. W. 2000. Cytofluorometric methods for assessing absolute numbers of cell subsets in blood. *Cytometry,* Vol. 42, No. 6, pp. 327-346, 1552-4957

Burns, A., Ow, H. & Wiesner, U. 2006. Fluorescent core-shell silica nanoparticles: towards "Lab on a Particle" architectures for nanobiotechnology. *Chemical Society Reviews,* Vol. 35, No. 11, pp. 1028-1042,

Cheng, X., Irimia, D., Dixon, M., Sekine, K., Demirci, U., Zamir, L., Tompkins, R. G., Rodriguez, W. & Toner, M. 2007. A microfluidic device for practical label-free CD4+ T cell counting of HIV-infected subjects. *Lab on a Chip,* Vol. 7, No. 2, pp. 170-178,

Cohen, J. 2004. Monitoring treatment: At what cost? *Science,* Vol. 304, No. 5679, pp. 1936-1936, 0036-8075

Coons, A. H., Creech, H. J. & Jones, R. N. 1941. Immunological properties of an antibody containing a fluorescent group. *Experimental Biology and Medicine,* Vol. 47, No. 2, pp. 200, 1535-3702

Cottingham, K. 2005. Incredible shrinking flow cytometers. *Analytical Chemistry,* Vol. 77, No. 3, pp. 73a-76a,

Coulter, W. H. 1953. *Means for counting particles suspended in a fluid.* United States patent application 2656508.

Crosland-Taylor, P. 1953. A device for counting small particles suspended in a fluid through a tube. *Nature,* Vol., No. 171, pp. 37-38,

Cvetkovic, A., Picioreanu, C., Straathof, A., Krishna, R. & Van Der Wielen, L. 2005. Relation between pore sizes of protein crystals and anisotropic solute diffusivities. *J. Am. Chem. Soc,* Vol. 127, No. 3, pp. 875-879,

Daniel, M. & Astruc, D. 2004. Gold Nanoparticles: Assembly, Supramolecular Chemistry, Quantum-Size-Related Properties, and Applications toward Biology, Catalysis, and Nanotechnology. *Chem. Rev,* Vol. 104, No. pp. 293-346,

Darzynkiewicz, Z., Bedner, E., Li, X., Gorczyca, W. & Melamed, M. R. 1999. Laser-Scanning Cytometry: A New Instrumentation with Many Applications. *Experimental Cell Research,* Vol. 249, No. 1, pp. 1-12,

Darzynkiewicz, Z., Bruno, S., Del Bino, G., Gorczyca, W., Hotz, M. A., Lassota, P. & Traganos, F. 1992. Features of apoptotic cells measured by flow cytometry. *Cytometry,* Vol. 13, No. 8, pp. 795-808,

Deen, W. 1987. Hindered transport of large molecules in liquid filled pores. *AIChE Journal,* Vol. 33, No. 9, pp. 1409-1425, 1547-5905

Denny, T., Stein, D., Mui, T., Scolpino, A., Holland, B. & Endowment, F. 1996. Quantitative determination of surface antibody binding capacities of immune subsets present in peripheral blood of healthy adult donors. *Cytometry Part B: Clinical Cytometry,* Vol. 26, No. 4, pp. 265-274,

Dieye, T. N., Vereecken, C., Diallo, A. A., Ondoa, P., Diaw, P. A., Camara, M., Karam, F., Mboup, S. & Kestens, L. 2005. Absolute CD4 T-cell counting in resource-poor settings: direct volumetric measurements versus bead-based clinical flow cytometry instruments. *JAIDS Journal of Acquired Immune Deficiency Syndromes,* Vol. 39, No. 1, pp. 32, 1525-4135

Estevez, M., O'donoghue, M., Chen, X. & Tan, W. 2009. Highly fluorescent dye-doped silica nanoparticles increase flow cytometry sensitivity for cancer cell monitoring. *Nano Research,* Vol. 2, No. 6, pp. 448-461,

Fulwyler, M. 1965. Electronic separation of biological cells by volume. *Science,* Vol. 150, No. 3698, pp. 910,

Glencross, D., Scott, L., Jani, I., Barnett, D. & Janossy, G. 2002. CD45-assisted PanLeucogating for accurate, cost-effective dual-platform CD4+ T-cell enumeration. *Cytometry Part B: Clinical Cytometry,* Vol. 50, No. 2, pp. 69-77,

Gucker Jr, F., O'konski, C., Pickard, H. & Pitts Jr, J. 1947. A Photoelectronic Counter for Colloidal Particles1. *Journal of the American Chemical Society,* Vol. 69, No. 10, pp. 2422-2431, 0002-7863

Herzenberg, L. & Sweet, R. 1976. Fluorescence-activated cell sorting. *Sci Am,* Vol. 234, No. 3, pp. 108-117,

Horan, P., Slezak, S. & Poste, G. 1986. Improved flow cytometric analysis of leukocyte subsets: simultaneous identification of five cell subsets using two-color immunofluorescence. *Proceedings of the National Academy of Sciences,* Vol. 83, No. 21, pp. 8361-8365,

Houwen, B. 2001. The Differential Cell Count. *Laboratory Hematology,* Vol. 7, No. 2, pp. 89-100,

Janossy, G., Jani, I. & Gohde, W. 2000. Affordable CD4+ T-cell counts on'single-platform'flow cytometers I. Primary CD4 gating. *British Journal of Haematology,* Vol. 111, No. 4, pp. 1198-1208,

Janossy, G., Jani, I. V. & Brando, B. 2003. New trends in affordable CD4+ T-cell enumeration by flow cytometry in HIV/AIDS. *Clinical and Applied Immunology Reviews,* Vol. 4, No. 2, pp. 91-107,

Jennings, B. & Parslow, K. 1988. Particle size measurement: the equivalent spherical diameter. *Proceedings of the Royal Society of London. A. Mathematical and Physical Sciences,* Vol. 419, No. 1856, pp. 137, 1364-5021

Kapoor, V., Subach, F. V., Kozlov, V. G., Grudinin, A., Verkhusha, V. V. & Telford, W. G. 2007. New lasers for flow cytometry: filling the gaps. *Nature Methods,* Vol. 4, No. 9, pp. 678-679,

Laerum, O. D. & Farsund, T. 1981. Clinical application of flow cytometry: a review. *Cytometry,* Vol. 2, No. 1, pp. 1-13,

Ledbetter, J. A., Rouse, R. V., Micklem, H. S. & Herzenberg, L. 1980. T cell subsets defined by expression of Lyt-1, 2, 3 and Thy-1 antigens. Two-parameter immunofluorescence and cytotoxicity analysis with monoclonal antibodies modifies current views. *The Journal of experimental medicine,* Vol. 152, No. 2, pp. 280, 0022-1007

Lee, W., Kim, Y., Chung, B., Demirci, U. & Khademhosseini, A. 2010. Nano/Microfluidics for diagnosis of infectious diseases in developing countries. *Advanced Drug Delivery Reviews,* Vol. 62, No. pp. 449-457,

Lian, W., Litherland, S., Badrane, H., Tan, W., Wu, D., Baker, H., Gulig, P., Lim, D. & Jin, S. 2004. Ultrasensitive detection of biomolecules with fluorescent dye-doped nanoparticles. *Analytical Biochemistry,* Vol. 334, No. 1, pp. 135-144,

Loken, M., Parks, D. & Herzenberg, L. 1977. Two-color immunofluorescence using a fluorescence-activated cell sorter. *J Histochem Cytochem,* Vol. 25, No. 7, pp. 899-907,

Mandy, F. F., Bergeron, M. & Minkus, T. 1997. Evolution of Leukocyte Immunophenotyping as Influenced by the HIV/AIDS Pandemic: A Short History of the Development of Gating Strategies for CD4 T-Cell Enumeration. *Cytometry (Communications in Clinical Cytometry),* Vol. 30, No. pp. 157-165,

Masur, P. H., Kaplan, J. E. & Holmes, K. K. 2002. Guidelines for Preventing Opportunistic Infections among HIV-Infected Persons-2002: Recommendations of the US Public Health Service and the Infectious Diseases Society of America*. *Annals of Internal Medicine,* Vol. 137, No. 5 Part 2, pp. 435-478,

Moldavan, A. 1934. Photo-electric technique for the counting of microscopical cells. *Science,* Vol. 80, No. pp. 188-189, 0036-8075

Monici, M. 2005. Cell and tissue autofluorescence research and diagnostic applications. *Biotechnology Annual Review,* Vol. 11, No. pp. 227-256, 1387-2656

Murphy, R. & Chused, T. 1984. A proposal for a flow cytometric data file standard. *Cytometry,* Vol. 5, No. 5, pp. 553-555, 1097-0320

Organization, W. H. 2006. HIV/AIDS Programme, Antiretroviral Therapy of HIV Infection in Infants and Children in Resource-Limited Settings: Towards Universal Access - Recommendations for a Public Health Approach. World Health Organization.

Ow, H., Larson, D. R., Srivastava, M., Baird, B. A., Webb, W. W. & Wiesner, U. 2005. Bright and stable core-shell fluorescent silica nanoparticles. *Nano Lett,* Vol. 5, No. 1, pp. 113-117,

Parks, D., Hardy, R. & Herzenberg, L. 1984. Three color immunofluorescence analysis of mouse B lymphocyte subpopulations. *Cytometry,* Vol. 5, No. 2, pp. 159-168, 1097-0320

Perfetto, S. P., Chattopadhyay, P. K. & Roederer, M. 2004. Seventeen-Colour Flow Cytometry: Unravelling The Immune System. *Nature Reviews Immunology,* Vol. 4, No. pp. 648-655,

Qhobosheane, M., Santra, S., Zhang, P. & Tan, W. 2001. Biochemically functionalized silica nanoparticles. *The Analyst,* Vol. 126, No. 8, pp. 1274-1278,

Rodriguez, W. R., Christodoulides, N., Floriano, P. N., Graham, S., Mohanty, S., Dixon, M., Hsiang, M., Peter, T., Zavahir, S. & Thior, I. 2005. A Microchip CD4 Counting Method for HIV Monitoring in Resource-Poor Settings. *PLoS Medicine,* Vol. 2, No. 7, pp. e182,

Santra, S., Liesenfeld, B., Bertolino, C., Dutta, D., Cao, Z., Tan, W., Moudgil, B. M. & Mericle, R. A. 2006. Fluorescence lifetime measurements to determine the core?shell nanostructure of FITC-doped silica nanoparticles: An optical approach to evaluate nanoparticle photostability. *Journal of Luminescence,* Vol. 117, No. 1, pp. 75-82,

Santra, S., Zhang, P., Wang, K., Tapec, R. & Tan, W. 2001. Conjugation of biomolecules with luminophore-doped silica nanoparticles for photostable biomarkers. *Analytical Chemistry,* Vol. 73, No. 20, pp. 4988-93,

Schmid, I., Uittenbogaart, C. & Jamieson, B. D. 2007. Live-cell assay for detection of apoptosis by dual-laser flow cytometry using Hoechst 33342 and 7-amino-actinomycin D. *Nature Protocols,* Vol. 2, No. 1, pp. 187-190,

Shapiro, H. M. 1983. Multistation multiparameter flow cytometry: a critical review and rationale. *Cytometry,* Vol. 3, No. 4, pp. 227-43,

Sharma, P., Brown, S., Walter, G., Santra, S. & Moudgil, B. 2006. Nanoparticles for bioimaging. *Advances in colloid and interface science,* Vol. 123, No. pp. 471-485,

Shearer, W. T., Rosenblatt, H. M., Gelman, R. S., Oyomopito, R., Plaeger, S., Stiehm, E. R., Wara, D. W., Douglas, S. D., Luzuriaga, K. & Mcfarland, E. J. 2003. Lymphocyte subsets in healthy children from birth through 18 years of age The pediatric AIDS clinical trials group P1009 study. *The Journal of Allergy and Clinical Immunology,* Vol. 112, No. 5, pp. 973-980,

Smith, A., Dave, S., Nie, S., True, L. & Gao, X. 2006. Multicolor quantum dots for molecular diagnostics of cancer. *Expert Review of Molecular Diagnostics,* Vol. 6, No. 2, pp. 231-244,

Tung, J. W., Parks, D. R., Moore, W. A. & Herzenberg, L. A. 2004. New approaches to fluorescence compensation and visualization of FACS data. *Clinical Immunology,* Vol. 110, No. 3, pp. 277-283,

Walker, D. A. 1987. A fluorescence technique for measurement of concentration in mixing liquids. *Journal of Physics E: Scientific Instruments,* Vol. 20, No. pp. 217-224,

Yan, J., Estevez, M., Smith, J., Wang, K., He, X., Wang, L. & Tan, W. 2007. Dye-doped nanoparticles for bioanalysis. *Nano Today,* Vol. 2, No. 3, pp. 44-50,

Yun, H., Bang, H., Min, J., Chung, C., Chang, J. K. & Han, D. C. 2010. Simultaneous counting of two subsets of leukocytes using fluorescent silica nanoparticles in a sheathless microchip flow cytometer. *Lab on a Chip,* Vol. 10, No. pp. 3243-3254,

9

Implementation of a Flow Cytometry Strategy to Isolate and Assess Heterogeneous Membrane Raft Domains

Morgan F. Khan, Tammy L. Unruh and Julie P. Deans
University of Calgary
Canada

1. Introduction

Flow cytometry is an analytical technique based on the detection and quantitation of scattered light from individual cells or particles. This is achieved by channelling particles single file past a light source and collecting the scattered light with detectors and filters positioned at specific angles. This has enabled the identification of unique cellular characteristics and is widely used in the field of medical science in both clinical and research labs to study biological phenomena including apoptosis, cell cycle progression, cell surface protein heterogeneity, and calcium signaling (Brown & Wittwer, 2000, Krishan, 1975, Vermes et al., 2000). Generally, flow cytometers are optimized to study cells with 1-30 μm diameters, with investigations of smaller cells and particles only recently becoming more widely applied. This coincides with the commercial availability of flow instruments capable of detecting synthetic beads as small as 200 nm in diameter.

Flow cytometry analysis of small particles can be performed on standard instrumentation. However, particles that fall at or below the wavelength (λ) of the incident light beam exhibit different scatter behaviour than the diffraction and interference typical of larger particles (Shapiro, 2003, Zwicker, 2010). As a result, an accurate, quantitative measure of particle size below the 1λ threshold is not possible. In addition, any sample that contains heterogeneous particles with a large size spread will be susceptible to different scatter characteristics making comparisons between these particles impossible. Despite these limitations, flow cytometry may be used for characterisation of sub-micron particles when a definitive size measure is not essential, provided the particles under investigation are subject to similar scatter characteristics. Biological applications where sub-micron flow cytometry analysis has been utilized successfully include the characterization of circulating microparticles (Abrams et al., 1990, Jy et al., 2010), and the characterization of bacteria and viruses in aquatic systems (Lomas et al., 2011). Another area of research that could benefit greatly from flow cytometry analysis and sorting is the study of plasma membrane microdomains called membrane rafts. These microdomains are essential mediators of plasma membrane function, yet they remain difficult to characterize by conventional techniques.

2. Visualizing protein heterogeneity within membrane vesicles

Initially described by Simons and van Meer (Simons & van Meer, 1988), membrane rafts are regions within eukaryotic plasma membranes created by preferential packing of saturated long-chain fatty acids and cholesterol, and implicated in diverse cellular functions, including signaling and membrane protein trafficking (Gupta & DeFranco, 2007). The liquid-ordered environment of raft domains attracts a subset of proteins largely distinct from those in the more fluid surrounding membrane. Additionally, membrane rafts are now known to be heterogeneous with respect to protein content. Intracellular raft heterogeneity is a useful model to explain the regulation of the many different signaling pathways orchestrated by the plasma membrane; only the specific subset of proteins required for a given biological process is recruited to a common region. Although raft protein heterogeneity is presumably essential to effect specific biochemical outcomes, the proteomic differences among distinct membrane microdomains have been difficult to characterize as a result of inadequacies associated with currently available biochemical tools.

Raft-based protein heterogeneity can currently be visualized on live cells with microscopy-based techniques such as fluorescence microscopy, single particle tracking and image correlation spectroscopy (Dietrich et al., 2002, Gupta & DeFranco, 2003, Lenne et al., 2006, Mutch et al., 2007). Protein motion and relative proximity to other molecules are tracked and the extent of co-localization between them dictates the likelihood of molecules residing in common raft domains (Gupta & DeFranco, 2003, Petrie & Deans, 2002). Microscopy has been extremely valuable in identifying intracellular raft protein heterogeneity; however, overlap of emission spectra between individual fluorophores limits the number of labels that can be simultaneously observed. In addition, microscopy can only be performed on known proteins and identification of unknown protein components within a distinct raft population requires a biochemical strategy.

Proteomic raft analysis can be achieved by extracting these domains from the plasma membrane (Foster et al., 2003, Jordan & Rodgers, 2003, Lin et al., 2010, Mannova et al., 2006, Nebl et al., 2002). Isolation of membrane rafts was traditionally performed in cold, non-ionic detergent, such as Triton X-100, in which raft proteins are largely insoluble (Brown & Rose, 1992). However, detergent extraction of model membranes was shown to artificially induce raft coalescence, therefore the use of detergent extraction for the purpose of characterizing intracellular heterogeneity is now generally avoided (Munro, 2003, Shogomori & Brown, 2003, Wilson et al., 2004). An alternative to detergent-extraction involves cell lysis by mechanical disruption, followed by density centrifugation to isolate the rafts to the buoyant fraction (Macdonald & Pike, 2005, Smart et al., 1995, Song et al., 1996). Membrane rafts extracted in the absence of detergent are thought to better reflect raft composition *in vivo*, although these isolates suffer from substantially greater contamination from non-raft proteins (Foster et al., 2003). Regardless of the isolation procedure, heterogeneous populations of membrane rafts are contained within a common sample. Consequently, differences between unique populations of rafts can only be achieved by enriching specific raft subsets from the biochemical isolate. There are currently no available purification schemes suitable for the investigation of dynamic, sub-microscopic cellular components. Thus, adapting flow cytometry detection and sorting to the analysis of membrane rafts would be a major advance in characterizing intracellular protein heterogeneity.

3. Visualizing protein heterogeneity within membrane vesicles

The extraction of membrane rafts from B lymphocytes was performed as described (Polyak et al., 2008). Briefly, cells were lysed by mechanical disruption and the lysate was mixed with an equal volume of 50% Optiprep solution (dark grey region in Figure 1a), followed by an overlay of 20% then 5% Optiprep solutions (light grey and white regions in Figure 1a, respectively). After centrifugation to equilibrium, the resulting step gradient was sampled at the two gradient interfaces where cellular material was observed; the 25%-20% interface (heavy membranes), and the 20%-5% interface (light membranes), as shown in Figure 1a. The light and heavy membrane fractions, as well as an unfractionated sample, were imaged by electron microscopy to evaluate the nature of the enriched cellular material (see Figure 1b-c). The heavy membrane fraction contains more organelles (ribosomes and mitochondria) and few vesicles, whereas the light membrane fraction contains sealed vesicles of varied size in addition to other cellular debris.

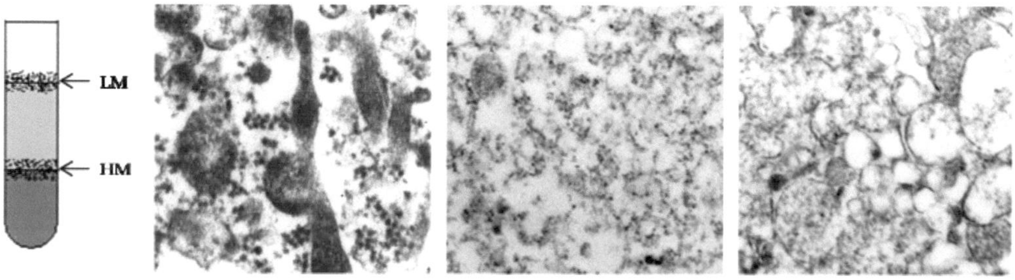

(a) (b) (c) (d)

Fig. 1. Transmission Electron Microscopy of cellular material shows enrichment of vesicles in the buoyant fraction of density gradients. BJAB B cells were mechanically lysed and subjected to gradient centrifugation. The step gradient and the location within the gradient where cellular material was confined are shown in (a). The light membrane (LM) and heavy membrane (HM) fractions were collected at the interfaces of the gradient steps. Transmission electron microscopy was performed on (b) the unfractionated material, (c) the heavy and (d) the light membrane fractions

The light membrane fraction was also observed by fluorescence and light microscopy to confirm that these vesicles are derived from the plasma membrane. BJAB B cells were labelled with the lipophilic membrane stain Vibrant-Dil. Differential Interference Contrast (DIC) and Dil-stained images from whole cells and light membranes extracted from these cells are shown in Figure 2. Imaging of whole B cells shows the successful incorporation of Dil into the plasma membrane and minimal intracellular staining. The extensive overlap between the DIC and Dil images of the light membrane fraction indicates that the majority of the vesicles are of plasma membrane origin.

To assess whether distinct membrane raft domains can be observed within the light membrane vesicles, we selected two pairs of raft-associated proteins that have been shown previously to be largely dissociated on intact cells: CD20/ surface IgM (sIgM) and CD20/linker for activation of B-cells (LAB). The degree of co-localization of sIgM and CD20 previously reported on intact BJAB cells stimulated for 1 minute was 47% (Petrie & Deans, 2002); co-localization of CD20 and LAB on intact cells was 25% (Mutch et al., 2007). BJAB

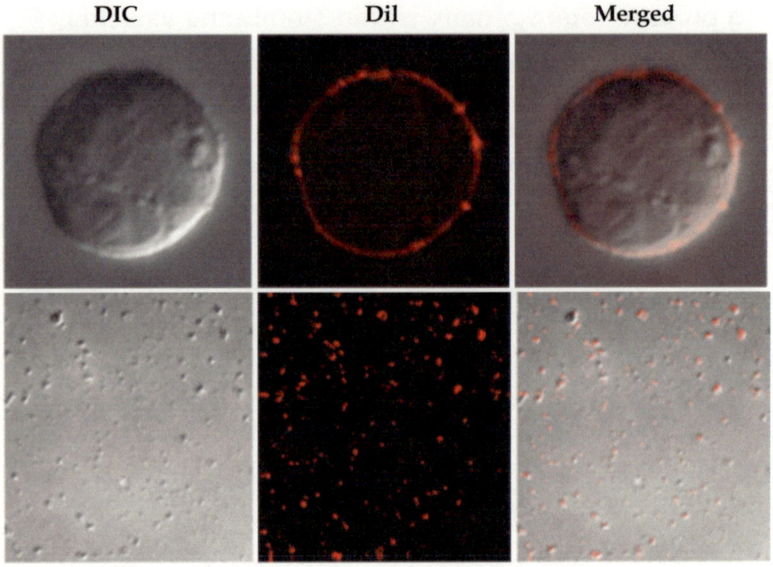

Fig. 2. Vesicles observed in the light membrane fraction originate from the plasma membrane. Whole BJAB cells were labelled with Vibrant-Dil and either imaged directly (top panels) or processed to obtain the light membrane fraction (bottom panels). The DIC images (left) and fluorescence images (centre) were merged (right)

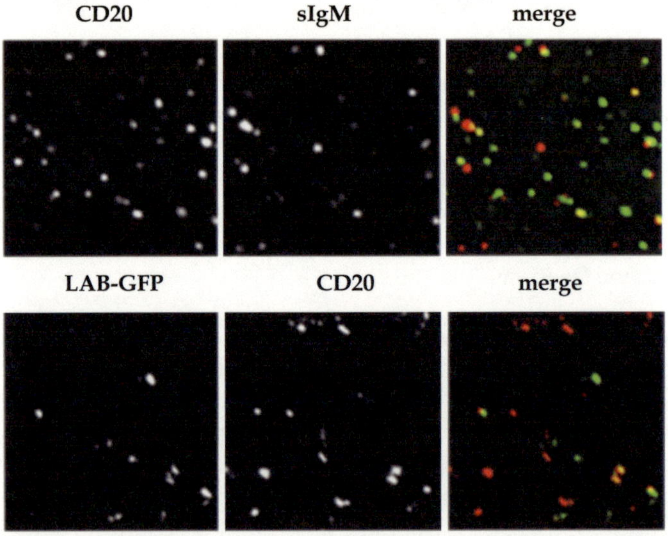

Fig. 3. Distinct membrane rafts are preserved in vesicles contained within the light membrane fraction. Membrane raft protein pairs, CD20/sIgM and LAB/CD20, were selected for analysis as these have limited co-localization in whole cells. For the CD20/sIgM analysis, BJAB cells were labelled with anti-IgM-PE and anti-CD20-AF488. For the LAB/CD20 analysis, BJAB cells that expressed LAB-GFP were labelled with anti-CD20-AF555 (bottom panel). Light membranes isolated from both sets of labelled cells were analyzed by immunofluorescence microscopy. The percentage co-localization was 49.4% for CD20/sIgM, and 30% for LAB/CD20, in agreement with values previously obtained from whole cell analysis

cells were labelled with anti-IgM-phycoerythrin (PE) and anti-CD20-Alexa Fluor 488 (AF488) for the first protein pair. The second pair utilized BJAB cells that expressed LAB tagged with green fluorescent protein (GFP) and labelled with anti-CD20-AF555. Once labelled, the light membranes were extracted and imaged by immunofluorescence microscopy (Figure 3). The percent co-localization of the sIgM/CD20 and LAB/CD20 pairings in light membrane vesicles was 49% and 30%, respectively. These values are in close agreement from conventional whole cell analysis suggesting that the vesicles in the light membrane fraction accurately represent the heterogeneity of plasma membrane rafts.

4. Single label analysis of membrane vesicles by flow cytometry

To evaluate the utility of flow cytometry for analysis of membrane raft proteins, we first wanted to determine if light membrane vesicles could be visualised by forward scatter (FSC) and side scatter (SSC) distribution on a conventional instrument (BD FACscan) in which the only modification was a reduction in the instrument threshold. Analysis in the absence of light membranes is shown in Figure 4a (left panel). This plot shows random noise generated by electronic measurements and stray light collected by the optics system, and represents a constant background present throughout the analysis of light membranes. However, when light membranes were analyzed, a clear population of vesicles could be observed beyond background noise signals (Figure 4a, middle and right panels). To estimate the size of these

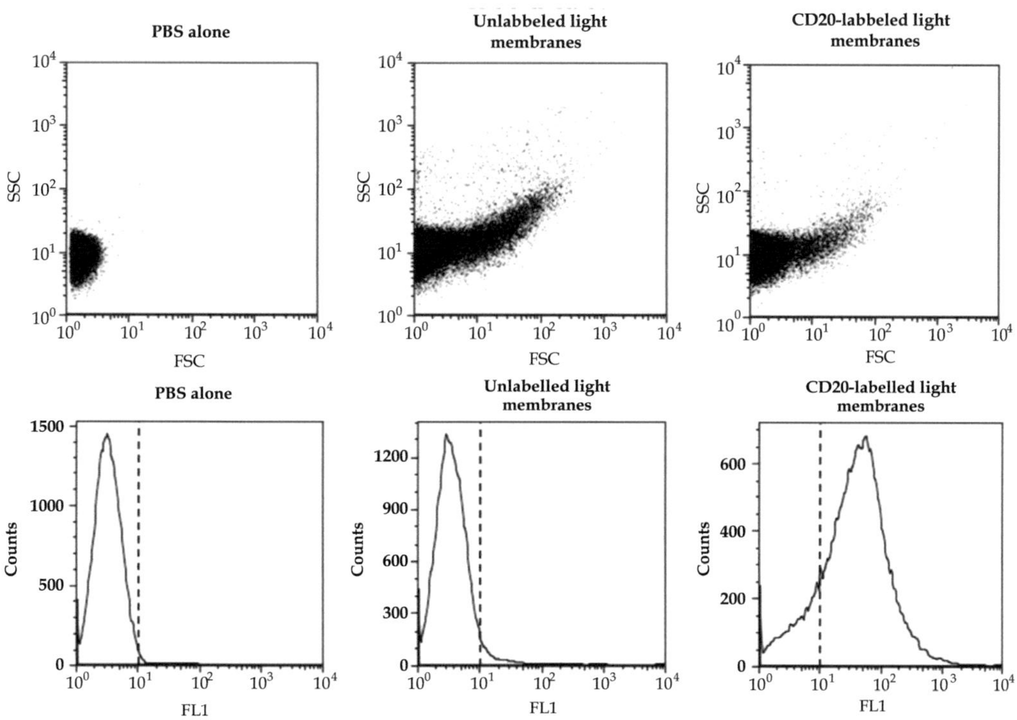

Fig. 4. Light membranes can be detected by conventional flow cytometry. Light membranes were extracted from unlabelled BJAB cells or cells labelled with anti-CD20-AF488. a) Typical FSC/SSC dot plots of the background noise (left panel) and light membranes (middle and right panels). b) Fluorescence histograms resulting from the ungated populations in (a)

vesicles, the FSC values of membrane vesicles were compared to those observed with beads of known diameter. The vesicles appeared with FSC values substantially less than the smallest bead (1 μm diameter) (data not shown), indicating that these vesicles likely measure less than the 1λ value and cannot accurately be measured.

We next evaluated the fluorescence profile of light membrane vesicles isolated from BJAB cells labelled with an anti-CD20-AF488 antibody. The ungated signals observed in the FSC/SSC plots in Figure 4(a) resulted in the corresponding fluorescence profiles shown in Figure 4b. Only samples isolated from cells that had been labelled with the fluorophore showed any fluorescence emission, indicating the specific detection of CD20-containing light membranes. To evaluate the smallest vesicles that could be detected by fluorescence, gates were placed at three different regions of the FSC/SSC plots with increasing FSC values, including a gate overlapping the background noise (gate setup shown in Figure 5a). As expected, fluorescence was observed in regions where light membranes were visible beyond the background noise (gates R2 and R3, Figure 5). The gated population that overlapped the background noise (R1) also generated a specific fluorescence signal, indicating that membrane vesicles were also present and detectable within this region (Figure 5). These data indicate that a further reduction in threshold would be beneficial as additional membrane vesicles are likely present, but excluded from analysis. One consequence of reducing the threshold is that background signals begin to dominate the FSC/SSC plot resulting in an underestimation of the event counts. However, a precise measurement of the number of events was not required for our analysis and, as the focus of subsequent experiments was the detection of fluorescence in a separate detection channel, a potentially saturated FSC channel was not problematic.

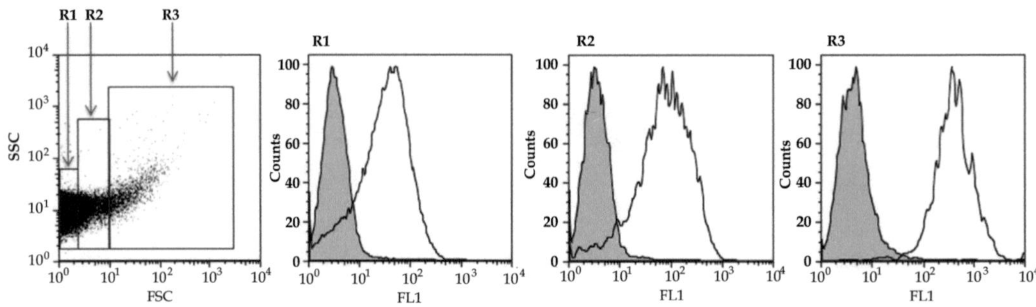

Fig. 5. Fluorescent particles can be observed in regions obscured by background noise. BJAB cells were labelled with anti-CD20-AF488. Light membranes were isolated and analyzed by flow cytometry. a) FSC/SSC plot showing gated regions R1, R2 and R3. b)-d) Fluorescence histograms of R1, R2 and R3

The fluorescence histograms shown in Figures 4 and 5 indicated that the light membranes appeared to be exclusively CD20-positive with no apparent CD20-negative population. This conflicts with microscopy data which have established that a substantial fraction of CD20 occupies separate raft domains from certain other raft proteins, such as LAB and sIgM (Mutch et al., 2007, Petrie & Deans, 2002). This suggests that a CD20-negative population of light membrane vesicles were not visualized using the current method. A dilution scheme improved the resolution of the fluorescence resulting in the observation of at least two CD20 populations (Figure 6), although a distinct CD20-negative population was still not observed.

The difficult in distinguishing distinct populations of membrane vesicles was likely the result of many membrane vesicles passing simultaneously past the light source, a consequence of the small size of membrane vesicles relative to the flow path. Dilution reduced the number of membrane vesicles detected coincidently, thus improving the resolution at the expense of acquisition time.

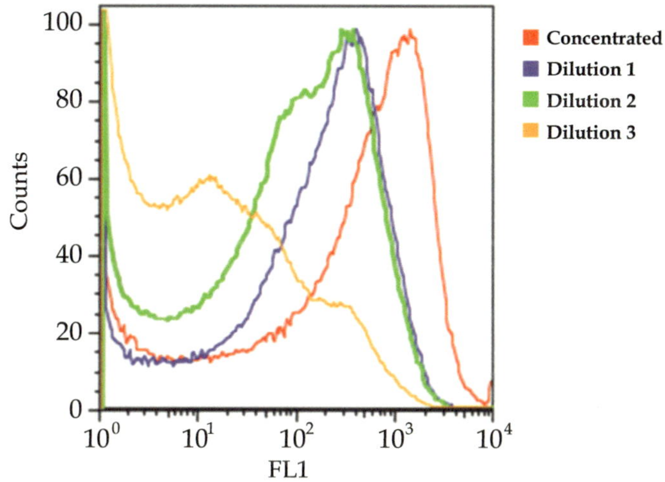

Fig. 6. CD20 heterogeneity was observed at higher sample dilutions. Light membranes obtained from anti-CD20-AF488 labelled BJAB cells were diluted 10x (dilution 1), 100x (dilution 2) and 1000x (dilution 3) from the standard volume of concentrated light membrane obtained after extraction. At greater dilutions, a bimodal distribution of CD20 fluorescence became apparent

As there was no clear CD20-negative population, we next explored the use of two fluorescence labels to determine whether flow cytometry can distinguish distinct populations of membrane raft domains.

5. Two-label analysis of membrane vesicles by flow cytometry

The B cell antigen receptor, or sIgM, translocates into rafts following antigen binding, and is found in a substantially distinct raft subset from CD20 (Figure 3). To analyse light membranes by 2-color flow cytometry, BJAB B cells were labelled with anti-CD20-AF488 and with anti-IgM-PE under activation conditions known to translocate IgM into rafts (Petrie & Deans, 2002, Polyak et al., 2008). The light membranes were extracted and analyzed on the BD FACScan flow cytometer with a reduced threshold. The fluorescence profile produced is shown in Figure 7, in which only small fractions of the total fluorescent membrane vesicles were uniquely sIgM-containing (sIgM$^+$CD20$^-$) or CD20-containing (sIgM$^-$CD20$^+$) (6% and 3%, respectively). The degree of association between sIgM and CD20 observed at 80% was substantially higher than reported by microscopy (Petrie & Deans, 2002, Polyak et al., 2008). This discrepancy between the two methods was attributed to an unknown factor specific to flow cytometry analysis. Therefore, modifications were made to the flow cytometry protocol in an attempt to increase the proportion of sIgM$^+$CD20$^-$ and IgM$^-$CD20$^+$ membrane vesicles.

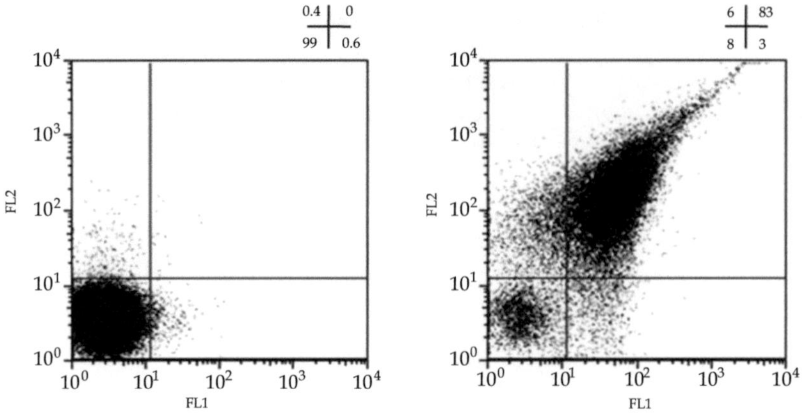

Fig. 7. Fluorescence can distinguish distinct populations of membrane raft-containing light membrane vesicles. Unlabelled BJAB B cells, or BJAB cells labelled with anti-CD20-AF488 and anti-IgM-PE were lysed and fractionated and the light membrane fractions were analysed by flow cytometry. Unlabelled light membranes showed no fluorescence (left panel) whereas fluorescence in both FL1 and FL2 channels was visible in the membranes derived from labelled cells (right panel). Populations of sIgM$^+$CD20$^-$ and IgM$^-$CD20$^+$ were present; however, the percentage of vesicles appearing as sIgM$^+$CD20$^+$ was much greater than reported by microscopy

We speculated that sIgM$^+$CD20$^-$ and IgM$^-$CD20$^+$ vesicles would be more prevalent at decreasing size. Indeed, when vesicles with progressively smaller FSC values were analyzed, the proportion of membrane vesicles exhibiting distinct fluorescence increased (Figure 8). Thus, vesicle size, as approximated by FSC, is a major factor affecting the fluorescence distribution of membrane vesicles analyzed by flow cytometry. Subsequent analyses were performed on the 20% of vesicles appearing with the lowest FSC values.

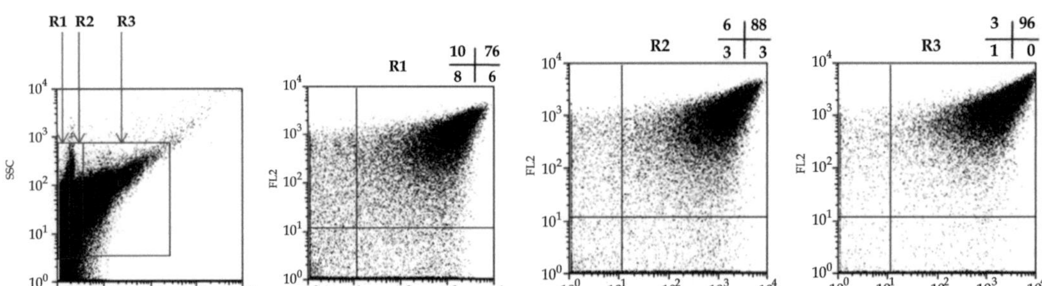

Fig. 8. Particle size influences the distribution of fluorescence. Light membranes were isolated from BJAB cells labelled with anti-CD20-AF488 and anti-IgM-PE. Gates were placed over particles with increasing FSC value (R1-R3) and the resulting fluorescence observed for the CD20$^+$sIgM$^+$ population was 76, 88 and 96%, respectively

The specificity of the association between sIgM and CD20 within the sIgM$^+$CD20$^+$ population was assessed by observing the fluorescence behaviour of light membranes isolated from cells that were separately labelled with either anti-sIgM-PE or anti-CD20-

AF488. The membrane vesicles isolated from each individually labelled cell group were mixed together in equal amounts immediately before flow cytometry analysis (Figure 9) and the fluorescence profiles then compared to light membranes isolated from cells that were labelled simultaneously (Figure 7). Flow analysis showed that even when cells were labelled separately, 62% of light membrane vesicles still exhibited positive staining for both markers, compared to 83% when rafts were isolated from cells labelled simultaneously. This suggests that when cells are labelled simultaneously, approximately 60% of the total sIgM$^+$CD20$^+$ population can be attributed to non-specific association.

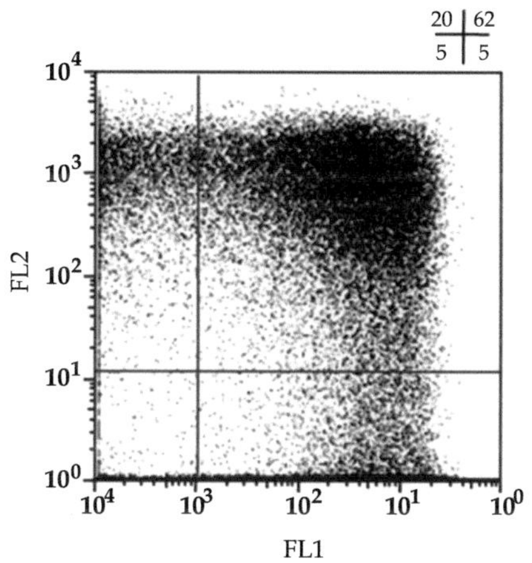

Fig. 9. Non-specific factors artifactually induce the formation of CD20$^+$sIgM$^+$ vesicles. Separate populations of BJAB cells were labelled with either anti-CD20-AF488 or anti-IgM-PE, followed by light membrane extraction. The light membranes from each population were mixed immediately before analysis by flow cytometry. The large population (62%) of CD20$^+$sIgM$^+$ vesicles must be derived from a non-specific association between single positive populations of vesicles

The residual 20% of the sIgM$^+$CD20$^+$ population approximates the reported co-localization between CD20 and sIgM in microscopy studies (Petrie & Deans, 2002). Several experiments were conducted to reduce this non-specific effect, including additional mechanical disruption of the cells, adjusting the ionic strength of the solution, and sample dilutions; however, there was no improvement in the proportion of sIgM$^+$CD20$^-$ or sIgM$^-$CD20$^+$ single fluorescence. Despite the disproportionately large sIgM$^+$CD20$^+$ population, there were still sufficient amounts of uniquely stained populations to evaluate flow cytometry sorting as a means to enrich the sIgM- and CD20- specific populations.

6. Application of flow sorting to enrich distinct sub-populations of raft containing vesicles

Flow cytometry sorting of light membranes was initially performed on BJAB cells labelled with anti-CD20-AF488. The populations selected for enrichment were the 20% most brightly labelled (CD20^{bright}) and the 20% least brightly labelled (CD20^{dim}) membrane vesicles (see Figure 10 for gate set-up). The sort was performed on a BD FACSVantage SE for approximately two hours. The resulting sorted populations were re-analyzed by flow cytometry to assess if any enrichment had taken place. The sorted, CD20^{bright} population appeared as a narrow peak (red curve shown in Figure 10). The sorted CD20^{dim} population was represented by a broad distribution (blue curve in Figure 10) that contained fewer membrane vesicles than was observed for the CD20^{bright} population. Overlaying the resulting fluorescence profiles of the sorted populations shows that the sorting did produce populations with different fluorescence intensities with only a small region of overlap between the two (Figure 10). To determine whether sufficient amounts of sorted material were present for mass spectrometry protein identification, the sorted populations were analyzed by SDS-PAGE (data not shown).

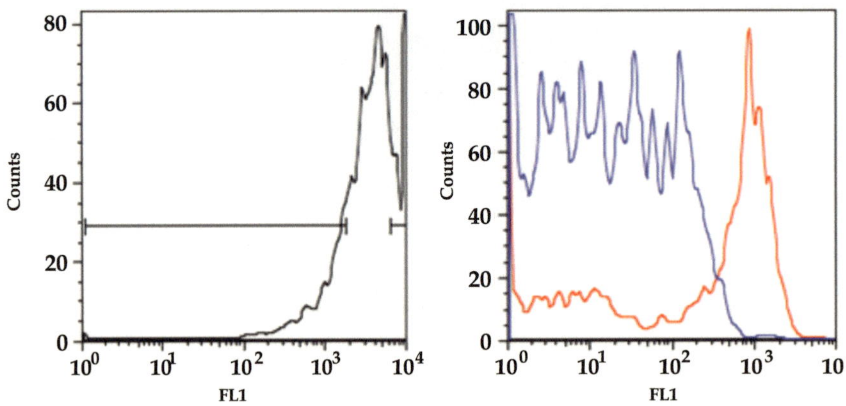

Fig. 10. Enrichment of CD20^{dim} and CD20^{bright} light membrane vesicles by flow cytometry sorting. BJAB cells were labelled with anti-CD20-AF488 followed by light membrane extraction. Light membranes were analyzed on a BD FACSVantage producing the fluorescence profile in the left panel. Sorting was performed on the 20% most dim and 20% brightest particles and the resulting purified populations were re-analyzed (right panel)

The CD20^{dim}, CD20^{bright} and a sample of unsorted material were run onto a 12.5% SDS-PAGE gel. Based on Coomassie stain intensity, the CD20^{bright} gel lane had more protein material than the CD20^{dim} population, which was in agreement with the poor population statistics observed in the flow cytometry sort. The staining pattern was similar across all three gel lanes. This was not unexpected given the limited sensitivity of regular Coomassie stains, and as a result no qualitative differences could be discerned based on SDS-PAGE analysis. Subsequently, the gel lanes corresponding to the CD20^{dim} and CD20^{bright} populations were divided into 10 gel slices, each of which was analyzed by LC-MS/MS. The number of protein identifications obtained from the CD20^{dim} population was considerably less (approximately a third) than those from the CD20^{bright} population (data not shown) confirming the protein concentration differences observed on the gel. CD20 was not identified in the CD20^{dim} population, clearly a consequence of the low protein abundance. Possibly for the same reason, no proteins were uniquely identified in this population compared to the CD20^{bright} population. Altogether, these data confirm that extracted light membranes can be sorted into distinct populations for proteomic analysis; however, greater yield from the sort is required to draw any meaningful conclusions.

Sorting of membrane vesicles isolated from BJAB cells labelled simultaneously with anti-CD20-AF488 and anti-IgM-PE, was performed on two instruments; the BD FACSVantage SE and the BD FACSAria. The compensation settings and gates on both instruments were based on vesicles with the smallest FSC value (smallest 20%), which generated the greatest proportion of $CD20^{+}IgM^{-}$ and $CD20^{-}IgM^{+}$ populations (shown in Figure 8b). During the compensation and gate setup, both instruments accommodated a reduced threshold; however, when the instruments began sorting, the noise contribution from the piezo-electric drive on the Vantage, and the additional electronic noise associated with either the Vantage or the Aria, prevented the reduction of the threshold to the optimal levels established during compensation. As a result, there was a dramatic reduction in the number of small vesicles responsible for generating the optimal fluorescence distribution. The gate was readjusted to include a greater proportion of vesicles with slightly larger FSC values. This modification resulted in only a minor proportion of vesicles appearing with a single fluorescent label (Figure 11, approximately 3% $IgM^{-}CD20^{+}$and approximately 1% $sIgM^{+}CD20^{-}$. The decrease in the proportion of distinct membrane vesicles would require an approximately 20-fold increase in sorting time to acquire quantities of sorted material similar to those obtained in the single label sort. This would have required an acquisition of approximately 30 hours and was not plausible to pursue further. Unfortunately, if reduced thresholds and low FSC gating are required for a desired experiment, sorting is not feasible with current instrumentation.

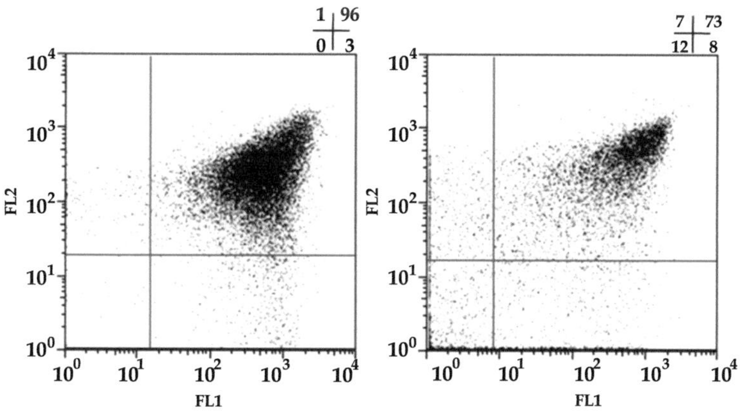

Fig. 11. Sorting particles with low FSC values results in low yields. Light membrane vesicles from BJAB cells labelled with anti-CD20-AF488 and anti-IgM-PE were analyzed on the BD FACSVantage. Initially, a low threshold setting and gate placement was possible, however when sorting was activated, the threshold increased and required gate placement on particles with higher FSC values. The result is shown in the left panel where only 3% and 1% of $CD20^{+}sIgM^{-}$ and $CD20^{-}sIgM^{+}$ was available. The same sample run on the BD FACScan in the absence of sorting resulted in the profile shown on the right panel

However, sorting light membranes is possible within specific experimental contexts. For instance, samples that do not require size gating, as observed with the single label identification of CD20 heterogeneity, can successfully be sorted with a conventional instrument. Little optimization would be required to sort sufficient $CD20^{dim}$ and $CD20^{bright}$

populations for biochemical analysis. In addition, this type of enrichment could be used for other populations of membrane raft proteins with heterogeneity observed by flow cytometry, such as GM1, as presented by Morales-Garcia et al. (Morales-Garcia et al., 2008). Even in the absence of sorting, the flow cytometry detection of membrane raft proteins could become a valuable diagnostic tool, as this method can identify heterogeneity imperceptible in conventional whole cell flow analysis.

7. Future requirements for successful flow sorting of small membrane vesicles

The threshold settings of the flow cytometer had to be reduced in order to detect smaller vesicles; however, there are still inherent limitations to using an instrument designed for cells approximately an order of magnitude larger than the membrane vesicles under investigation. The development of micro-flow cytometry systems could address many of the obstacles encountered in membrane raft analysis. The most important instrumental developments are related to the fluidics path, where poorly focused membrane vesicles will be most problematic. The use of a high flow rate (60 µl/min) was employed to minimize the central core generated by the sheath fluid. However, the substantial improvement of CD20 heterogeneity resolution at higher dilutions suggested that the diameter of the central core, even at 60 µl/min, was too large relative to the size of the vesicles. This large central core probably could not focus membrane vesicles into single file, resulting in membrane vesicles passing the laser coincidentally. The dilution of the membrane raft suspension improved the appearance of the heterogeneous populations by reducing the frequency of these coincident events at the expense of longer acquisition times. Focusing membrane vesicles into a smaller central core may not be possible using hydrodynamic focusing (Ateya et al., 2008), but recent developments in alternative focusing techniques can be applied on a scale amenable to micro-flow cytometry. The most relevant development to flow cytometry is microfluidic inertial focusing (Oakey et al., 2010). This technique exploits inertial fluidic forces within microfluidic channels to precisely position particles and has been used as a replacement for the traditional hydrodynamic focusing used in most conventional flow cytometry instruments (Oakey et al., 2010).

Another critical location of the flow path within a flow cytometer is the sorting interface. The electrostatic sorting commonly used in flow cytometry involves passing a focused cell or vesicle suspension into a vibrating nozzle. This causes the stream to break into highly uniform droplets, which are then deflected into collection tubes through the application of a voltage at precisely timed intervals. The nozzle size dictates the size of the droplet generated by this process and the recommendation for high purity sorting is that the size of the cell (or membrane vesicle in this case) should be at least 20-25% the size of the nozzle orifice (Macey, 2007). The 70 µm nozzle designed for 5-10 µm cells was the smallest available nozzle for the instruments used in this study. The membrane vesicles under observation were less than 1 µm, which would correspond to an ideal nozzle size of 5 µm. It is likely that sorting with the 70 µm nozzle would have made sorting high purity populations even more challenging, since at this size the drops formed would likely contain more than a single membrane vesicle. This is especially true since these experiments required the raft suspension to be in a small volume resulting in vesicles in close spatial proximity.

Miniaturization of the nozzle would greatly improve the effectiveness of sorting membrane vesicles by flow cytometry and is currently in development (Ateya et al., 2008). Flow cytometry sorting remains an excellent opportunity to isolate and fully characterize the protein heterogeneity in membrane raft subsets. Developments in miniaturizing flow cytometry systems are essential to sort smaller vesicles effectively.

8. Conclusion

Flow cytometry was investigated as a means to characterize proteins present in plasma membrane rafts, isolated from labelled cells as light membrane vesicles. Vesicles obtained from BJAB cells labelled with an anti-CD20 fluorescent antibody revealed heterogeneously stained populations when analysed by flow cytometry. This was used as a model system to investigate whether sorting could be employed to isolate two populations of membrane vesicles, $CD20^{dim}$ and $CD20^{bright}$. Sorting was successful, as enrichment of dim and bright fluorescence was observed on the sorted populations. Subsequent biochemical analysis was limited as the amount of protein material obtained from the sort was low. Longer sorting acquisition times would be necessary to acquire sufficient material for meaningful characterization. Flow cytometry was also used to identify membrane vesicles with distinct sIgM- and CD20-containing populations. Detection of the largest proportion of $sIgM^+CD20^-$ and $sIgM^-CD20^+$ populations required a size gate in which the smallest 20% of membrane vesicles, as determined by FSC, were selected. A reduced threshold was also required to permit the analysis of even smaller membrane vesicles. Unfortunately, enrichment of the $sIgM^+CD20^-$ and $sIgM^-CD20^+$ populations by sorting could not be performed due to the automated adjustment of instrumental threshold. This substantially reduced the proportion of membrane vesicles available for sorting and the time necessary to collect sufficient protein material for further biochemical analysis became prohibitive.

Future developments in miniaturization of flow cytometry systems (fluidics and nozzle sizes) are essential for this type of flow cytometry analysis. As the technological developments advance, it may become possible to fully characterize membrane raft domains or other cellular sub-domains that cannot be extensively studied due to limited isolation schemes.

9. Acknowledgments

The authors wish to thank Laurie Kennedy and Laurie Robertson for their assistance with sorting at the University of Calgary Flow Cytometry Core Facility. Also thanks to Wei-Xiang Dong for his assistance in collecting the TEM images at the Microscopy & Imaging Facility at the University of Calgary.

10. References

Abrams, C. S., Ellison, N., Budzynski, A. Z. & Shattil, S. J. (1990). Direct detection of activated platelets and platelet-derived microparticles in humans. *Blood,* Vol.75, No.1, (January 1990), pp. 128-138, ISSN 0006-4971

Ateya, D. A., Erickson, J. S., Howell, P. B., Jr., Hilliard, L. R., Golden, J. P. & Ligler, F. S. (2008). The good, the bad, and the tiny: a review of microflow cytometry. *Anal Bioanal Chem*, Vol.391, No.5, (July 2008), pp. 1485-1498, ISSN 1618-2650

Brown, D. A. & Rose, J. K. (1992). Sorting of GPI-anchored proteins to glycolipid-enriched membrane subdomains during transport to the apical cell surface. *Cell*, Vol.68, No.3, (February 1992), pp. 533-544, ISSN 0092-8674

Brown, M. & Wittwer, C. (2000). Flow cytometry: principles and clinical applications in hematology. *Clin Chem*, Vol.46, No.8 Pt 2, (August 2000), pp. 1221-1229, ISSN 0009-9147

Dietrich, C., Yang, B., Fujiwara, T., Kusumi, A. & Jacobson, K. (2002). Relationship of lipid rafts to transient confinement zones detected by single particle tracking. *Biophys J*, Vol.82, No.1 Pt 1, (January 2002), pp. 274-284, ISSN 0006-3495

Foster, L. J., De Hoog, C. L. & Mann, M. (2003). Unbiased quantitative proteomics of lipid rafts reveals high specificity for signaling factors. *Proc Natl Acad Sci U S A*, Vol.100, No.10, (May 2003), pp. 5813-5818, ISSN 0027-8424

Gupta, N. & DeFranco, A. L. (2003). Visualizing lipid raft dynamics and early signaling events during antigen receptor-mediated B-lymphocyte activation. *Mol Biol Cell*, Vol.14, No.2, (February 2003), pp. 432-444, ISSN 1059-1524

Gupta, N. & DeFranco, A. L. (2007). Lipid rafts and B cell signaling. *Semin Cell Dev Biol*, Vol.18, No.5, (October 2007), pp. 616-626, ISSN 1084-9521

Jordan, S. & Rodgers, W. (2003). T cell glycolipid-enriched membrane domains are constitutively assembled as membrane patches that translocate to immune synapses. *J Immunol*, Vol.171, No.1, (July 2003), pp. 78-87, ISSN 0022-1767

Jy, W., Horstman, L. L. & Ahn, Y. S. (2010). Microparticle size and its relation to composition, functional activity, and clinical significance. *Semin Thromb Hemost*, Vol.36, No.8, (November 2010), pp. 876-880, ISSN 1098-9064

Krishan, A. (1975). Rapid flow cytofluorometric analysis of mammalian cell cycle by propidium iodide staining. *J Cell Biol*, Vol.66, No.1, (July 1975), pp. 188-193, ISSN 0021-9525

Lenne, P. F., Wawrezinieck, L., Conchonaud, F., Wurtz, O., Boned, A., Guo, X. J., Rigneault, H., He, H. T. & Marguet, D. (2006). Dynamic molecular confinement in the plasma membrane by microdomains and the cytoskeleton meshwork. *EMBO J*, Vol.25, No.14, (July 2006), pp. 3245-3256, ISSN 0261-4189

Lin, S. L., Chien, C. W., Han, C. L., Chen, E. S., Kao, S. H., Chen, Y. J. & Liao, F. (2010). Temporal proteomics profiling of lipid rafts in CCR6-activated T cells reveals the integration of actin cytoskeleton dynamics. *J Proteome Res*, Vol.9, No.1, (January 2010), pp. 283-297, ISSN 1535-3907

Lomas, M. W., Bronk, D. A. & van den Engh, G. (2011). Use of flow cytometry to measure biogeochemical rates and processes in the ocean. *Ann Rev Mar Sci*, Vol.3, (January 2011), pp. 537-566, ISSN 1941-1405

Macdonald, J. L. & Pike, L. J. (2005). A simplified method for the preparation of detergent-free lipid rafts. *J Lipid Res*, Vol.46, No.5, (May 2005), pp. 1061-1067, ISSN 0022-2275

Macey, M. G., Ed. (2007). *Flow Cytometry Principles and Applications*, Humana Press Inc., ISBN 1-58829-691-1, Totowa, New Jersey.

Mannova, P., Fang, R., Wang, H., Deng, B., McIntosh, M. W., Hanash, S. M. & Beretta, L. (2006). Modification of host lipid raft proteome upon hepatitis C virus replication. *Mol Cell Proteomics*, Vol.5, No.12, (December 2006), pp. 2319-2325, ISSN 1535-9476

Morales-Garcia, M. G., Fournie, J. J., Moreno-Altamirano, M. M., Rodriguez-Luna, G., Flores, R. M. & Sanchez-Garcia, F. J. (2008). A flow-cytometry method for analyzing the composition of membrane rafts. *Cytometry A*, Vol.73, No.10, (October 2008), pp. 918-925, ISSN 1552-4930

Munro, S. (2003). Lipid rafts: elusive or illusive? *Cell*, Vol.115, No.4, (November 2003), pp. 377-388, ISSN 0092-8674

Mutch, C. M., Sanyal, R., Unruh, T. L., Grigoriou, L., Zhu, M., Zhang, W. & Deans, J. P. (2007). Activation-induced endocytosis of the raft-associated transmembrane adaptor protein LAB/NTAL in B lymphocytes: evidence for a role in internalization of the B cell receptor. *Int Immunol*, Vol.19, No.1, (January 2007), pp. 19-30, ISSN 0953-8178

Nebl, T., Pestonjamasp, K. N., Leszyk, J. D., Crowley, J. L., Oh, S. W. & Luna, E. J. (2002). Proteomic analysis of a detergent-resistant membrane skeleton from neutrophil plasma membranes. *J Biol Chem*, Vol.277, No.45, (November 2002), pp. 43399-43409, ISSN 0021-9258

Oakey, J., Applegate, R. W., Jr., Arellano, E., Di Carlo, D., Graves, S. W. & Toner, M. (2010). Particle focusing in staged inertial microfluidic devices for flow cytometry. *Anal Chem*, Vol.82, No.9, (May 2010), pp. 3862-3867, ISSN 1520-6882

Petrie, R. J. & Deans, J. P. (2002). Colocalization of the B cell receptor and CD20 followed by activation-dependent dissociation in distinct lipid rafts. *J Immunol*, Vol.169, No.6, (September 2002), pp. 2886-2891, ISSN 0022-1767

Polyak, M. J., Li, H., Shariat, N. & Deans, J. P. (2008). CD20 homo-oligomers physically associate with the B cell antigen receptor. Dissociation upon receptor engagement and recruitment of phosphoproteins and calmodulin-binding proteins. *J Biol Chem*, Vol.283, No.27, (July 2008), pp. 18545-18552, ISSN 0021-9258

Shapiro, H. M. (2003). *Practical Flow Cytometry*. Wiley-LissHoboken, New Jersey.

Shogomori, H. & Brown, D. A. (2003). Use of detergents to study membrane rafts: the good, the bad, and the ugly. *Biol Chem*, Vol.384, No.9, (September 2003), pp. 1259-1263, ISSN 1431-6730

Simons, K. & van Meer, G. (1988). Lipid sorting in epithelial cells. *Biochemistry*, Vol.27, No.17, (August 1988), pp. 6197-6202, ISSN 0006-2960

Smart, E. J., Ying, Y. S., Mineo, C. & Anderson, R. G. (1995). A detergent-free method for purifying caveolae membrane from tissue culture cells. *Proc Natl Acad Sci U S A*, Vol.92, No.22, (October 1995), pp. 10104-10108, ISSN 0027-8424

Song, K. S., Li, S., Okamoto, T., Quilliam, L. A., Sargiacomo, M. & Lisanti, M. P. (1996). Co-purification and direct interaction of Ras with caveolin, an integral membrane protein of caveolae microdomains. Detergent-free purification of caveolae microdomains. *J Biol Chem*, Vol.271, No.16, (April 1996), pp. 9690-9697, ISSN 0021-9258

Vermes, I., Haanen, C. & Reutelingsperger, C. (2000). Flow cytometry of apoptotic cell death. *J Immunol Methods*, Vol.243, No.1-2, (September 2000), pp. 167-190, ISSN 0022-1759

Wilson, B. S., Steinberg, S. L., Liederman, K., Pfeiffer, J. R., Surviladze, Z., Zhang, J., Samelson, L. E., Yang, L. H., Kotula, P. G. & Oliver, J. M. (2004). Markers for detergent-resistant lipid rafts occupy distinct and dynamic domains in native membranes. *Mol Biol Cell*, Vol.15, No.6, (June 2004), pp. 2580-2592, ISSN 1059-1524

Zwicker, J. I. (2010). Impedance-based flow cytometry for the measurement of microparticles. *Semin Thromb Hemost*, Vol.36, No.8, (November 2010), pp. 819-823, ISSN 1098-9064

10

Broad Applications of Multi-Colour Time-Resolved Flow Cytometry

Ben J. Gu and James S. Wiley
Florey Neuroscience Institutes, The University of Melbourne
Australia

1. Introduction

Flow cytometer has become an indispensable tool used in medical research. After 50 years' development, flow cytometry has been dramatically advanced in its capability and sensitivity. Different refinements of hardware and software have also been developed to accommodate the diverse applications in biomedicine, biology and chemistry. However, the basic principle is still the same: as fluorescent particles in suspension pass through one or more focused laser beams, their fluorescence emission signals are processed in real time (Sklar *et al.*, 2007). The intensity of emission signal is proportional to number of fluorescence molecules illuminated on the fluorescent particle. This feature also enables kinetic measurement of fluorescence changes over a certain period of time in a specific sub-population of particles in suspension, which is known as time-resolved flow cytometry (TR-FCM). Considering the speed and throughput of flow cytometry, TR-FCM is particular attractive in studying cellular process of molecule binding, uptake of dye and influx/efflux over a scale of seconds or minutes. Diverse applications are also applied in TR-FCM, including time-resolved fluorescence decay measurement using a pulsed laser (Condrau *et al.*, 1994a; Condrau *et al.*, 1994b), high-throughput high-content screening of air-bubble separated samples using the HyperCyt system (Edwards *et al.*, 2001b; Ramirez *et al.*, 2003), and most frequently, real-time cellular kinetics, such as Ca^{2+} influx, intracellular pH changes, cell morphology and ligand-receptor interactions. These broad applications make TR-FCM a powerful technique in discovery of cellular functions.

In this chapter, we will use studies of the P2X7 receptor as an example of the applications of TR-FCM in assessing this receptor's cellular functions in real-time. The P2X7 receptor has a ubiquitous distribution in nearly all tissues and organs of the body with the highest expression in immune cells of monocyte-macrophage origin. The receptor is present as a trimer and its activation by extracellular ATP opens a cationic channel which gradually dilates to a larger pore over tens of seconds. Activation of P2X7 is associated with massive K^+ efflux which is a cofactor for assembly of the NALP3 inflammasome and secretion of inflammatory interleukins from myeloid cells. Prolonged activation of P2X7 leads to apoptotic death of the cell. P2X7 also has a function in the absence of its ligand, namely the recognition and phagocytosis of foreign particles in the absence of opsonins (Gu *et al.*, 2010; Gu *et al.*, 2011), and these features suggest that P2X7 and its downstream signalling pathways are important in innate immunity.

1.1 Equipment required for kinetic flow cytometry

The state-of-art flow cytometry is capable of measuring up to 50,000 events per second. For kinetic flow cytometry, events are accumulated and averaged over successive time intervals, typically 1 to 10 seconds or longer. Most kinetic studies require addition of an agonist or probe either to start or during the run, which may take 2 to 5 seconds. This time limitation has prevented the use of kinetic flow cytometry in studying rapid molecular interactions occurring on a time frame of less than one second. Over the last few decades, a number of on-line injection/mixing devices have been developed to reduce the dead-time to less than one second. One of these devices is the stopped-flow and coaxial mixing (Nolan & Sklar, 1998), another commercially available device is the Time Zero system produced by Cytek (http://www.cytekdev.com/pages/Accessories.html). This device allows precise temperature control and stirring of cells suspension to which a stimulus (agonist) is delivered within one second, allowing uninterrupted measurement of cellular response.

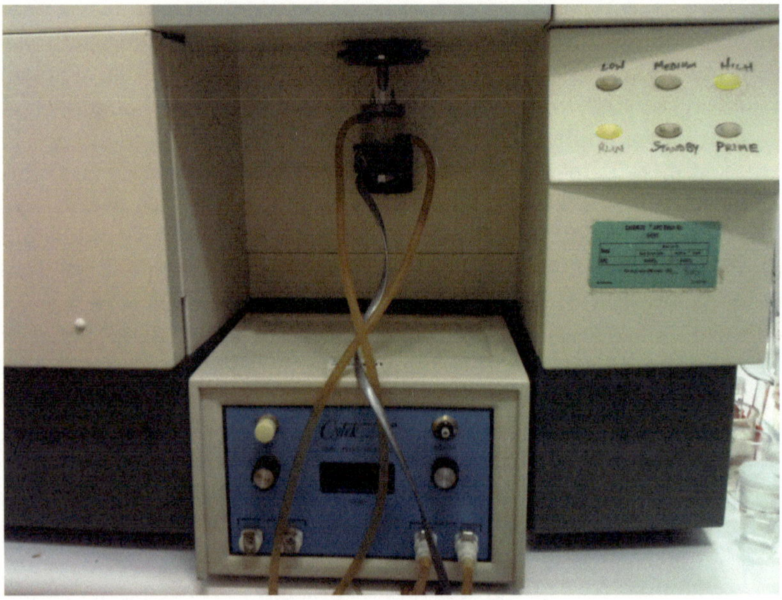

Fig. 1. A picture of Time Zero module integrated with a FACSCalibur flow cytometer

This Time Zero system is compatible with almost all the BD flow cytometers, as well as old models of Coulter flow cytometer (EPICS, Elite). It consists of two modules, the Time Zero module with water-jacket tube holder and the Air Supply module. An additional circulating water bath is also needed if temperature control is required. To install this device, the Air Supply module has to be connected to the air pressure system of the flow cytometer via a three-way valve, the sample nozzle has to be connected with a soft tubing and the short tubes (2.5 mL) have to be used instead of regular 5 mL FACS tubes. These changes may take 10-15 min to setup and another 10-15 min to clean up after each run. Since most flow cytometers are shared core facilities, other users may be affected by these changes. If subsecond cell response is not crucial for the study, an alternative way is to unscrew the sample platform (takes about 10 seconds) and fit the water-jacket tube holder on the sample bar of a BD flow cytometer (Fig. 1). The Air Supply module is therefore not needed, and regular 5 mL tubes can be used. However, the tube has to be physically removed and replaced after the addition of stimulus, which incurs a delay of 2-5 seconds before recording. In either case, a tiny stir bar (1x3 mm) has to be placed in the bottom of tube in order to mix cells. A major advantage of the Time Zero system is the device for magnetic stirring of the reaction cuvette, which maximizes the number of cell-cell interactions as well as rapidly mixing agonist or probe into the suspension. It is also a good idea to leave a small amount of water inside the water-jacket tube holder to ensure good thermal conductivity to the tube.

1.2 Quantitation of the kinetic response of cells

The two methods used to quantitate the kinetic response are either slope of a curve or area under a curve. In general, slope of a curve is more appropriate for rapid linear responses while area under a curve is more accurate for non-linear responses. Since most cellular responses are the results of multiple driving forces, and variations between each intervals are often seen in flow cytometry, area under a curve may be a better way to describe the quantitative information given by kinetic flow cytometry.

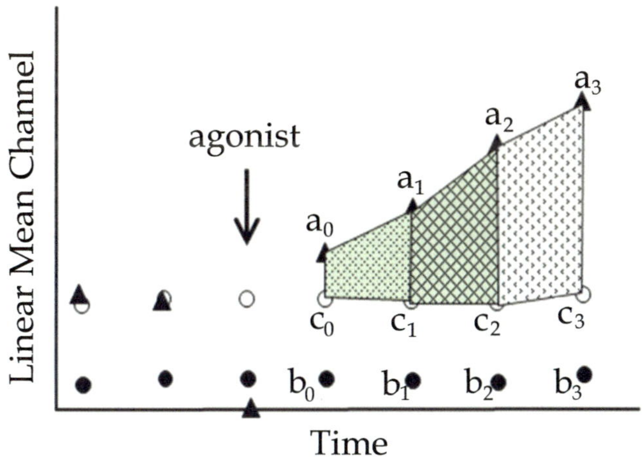

Fig. 2. A schematic illustration of area under a curve

To quantify dye uptake, arbitrary units of area under a curve in a certain time period (a number of time intervals, $n*\Delta t$) after addition of stimulus is calculated (Fig. 2). The basal line (without stimulus) has to be adjusted to the same level as the test line (with stimulus added). The area under a curve between the basal and test lines is considered as the sum of n trapezoids (Fig. 2). Therefore, the following mathematical model based on the trapezoid rule is used for the area calculation:

$a_0, a_1 \ldots a_n$ are the linear mean channel values of each interval from the ATP-induced ethidium uptake curve while $b_0, b_1 \ldots b_{60}$ are those from the basal line, and $c_0, c_1 \ldots c_{60}$ are those from the adjusted basal line. Therefore,

$\text{Area}(1) = 0.5 \times (a_0 - c_0 + a_1 - c_1) \times \Delta t$
$\text{Area}(2) = 0.5 \times (a_1 - c_1 + a_2 - c_2) \times \Delta t$
$\text{Area}(n) = 0.5 \times (a_{n-1} - c_{n-1} + a_n - c_n) \times \Delta t$

Area=0.5 x Δt x (sum(a_0,a_1,…a_{n-1})+sum(a_1,a_2,…a_n)
-sum(c_0,c_1,..c_{n-1})-sum(c_1,c_2,..c_{60}))
as c = b + Δb
$\therefore$ Area = 0.5 x Δt x (sum(a_0,a_1,…a_n)+sum(a_1,a_2,…a_n)
-(sum(b_0,b_1,..b_n)-(sum(b_1,b_2,..b_n)-2x n x Δb))

The area under a curve can then be calculated using a Microsoft Excel function.

1.3 Software for kinetic flow cytometry

Not many programs are available to process kinetic data from flow cytometry. The best freeware is WinMDI, written by Joseph Trotter of The Scripps Research Institute, La Jolla, CA 92037. The latest version of this freeware can be downloaded from http://facs.scripps.edu/software.html. WinMDI is able to calculate the mean fluorescence intensity (MFI) between defined time intervals. The data can be saved as a Tab separated text file which can then be imported by Microsoft Excel. However, WinMDI was originally written for Windows 3, and has not been updated. It can only read FCS 2.0 file, and does not recognize long file names. A brief tutorial for WinMDI by Dr Gérald Grégori can be found at http://www.cyto.purdue.edu/archive/flowcyt/labinfo/images/TutorialWinMDI.pdf. A more advanced program is FlowJo from the Tree Star Inc. Its kinetic tool can not only calculate MFI over time intervals, but also give both slope and area under the curve. The detailed instruction on the kinetic tool can be found at http://www.flowjo.com/home/tutorials/kinetics.html. Despite a number of bugs in this software, it can read FCS 3.0 file (a file format used by all latest flow cytometers) and is compatible with both Mac OS and Windows. Another software called Cyflogic (http://www.cyflogic.fi/) also includes a kinetic tool (flux trace) in its licensed version (not the free non-commercial version). Cyflogic has a similar interface as WinMDI, and can also recognize FCS 3.0 files.

In the following sections, we will use WinMDI to demonstrate how the kinetic flow cytometry analysis is performed. To use it, first choose "Display|Density Plot" on the menu, select the file, in the popup window "Format 2D Display", choose "256x256" for "Display Array Resolution" which gives a better resolution. Left click on the density plot, choose "Regions" to create a polygon gate R1 based on Forward Scatter & Side Scatter. Then choose "Display|Dot Plot" to draw a dot plot of cell marker (e.g. CD14) versus main fluorescence (e.g. Fura-red, ethidium, or YG). On "Format Dotplot" window, choose "All" for "Plot number of events". Left click on the dot plot, choose "Regions" to create a "SortRect" gate R2 based on the cell marker and main fluorescence. After the two gates are set, draw another dot plot of time versus main fluorescence. On "Format Dotplot" window, choose "All" for "Plot number of events", and check "Kinetics mode", "Overlay kinetics line" and "Draw kinetics only" to draw a kinetics line in the dot plot (KinPlot). Left click on the plot, choose "Gates", select "And" for both R1 and R2. Choose the KinPlot window, then choose "File|Save as" to save the date to a tabed text file. The file can then be imported by Microsoft Excel.

2. Ca^{2+}/Ba^{2+} influx with Fura-Red

2.1 Principles

Calcium influx/efflux is one of the most important cellular processes driven by opening of ion channels/receptors, including the P2X7 receptor. Following activation by extracellular

ATP, the P2X7 receptor opens a non-selective cation channel to allow Ca^{2+} influx and K^+ efflux. Many methods have been developed to measure P2X7 function by monitoring the cation flux through the open channel upon receptor activation. The most common ones are electrophysiological methods (patch-clamp and intracellular microelectrode), which are widely used in all receptor studies. Fluxes of divalent cations such as Ca^{2+}, Ba^{2+} as well as monovalent cations such as Rb^+, Na^+ and Li^+, have been used to study P2X7 channel function either by fluorometry with Fura-2 or with isotopes of these cations. However, interpretation of ionic flux methods requires a homogeneous cell population, while flow cytometric methods are applicable to mixed cell populations. We have developed a time-resolved flow cytometry method to monitor the influx of Ca^{2+} or Ba^{2+} into cells loaded with a fluorescent chelator, Fura-Red. Fura-Red is a fluorescent Ca^{2+} indicator which is excited by a standard argon laser (488 nm) and with emission at long wavelengths (~660 nm). This permits multi-colour analysis of Fura-Red signals in cells tagged with FITC-labelled antibodies using flow cytometry, allowing measurement of P2X7 function in specific cell types in a mixed cell population. Unlike the other fluorescent Ca^{2+} indicators, fluorescence of Fura-Red excited at 488 nm decreases once the indicator binds divalent cations such as Ca^{2+} or Ba^{2+} (Gu *et al.*, 2001; Jursik *et al.*, 2007).

2.2 Method

To study the Ba2+ influx following activation of P2X7 by ATP, mononuclear cells ($2x10^6$) are incubated in Ca^{2+} free Na medium (145 mM NaCl, 5 mM KCl, 10 mM Hepes, pH 7.5, supplemented with 0.1% BSA and 5mM glucose) with Fura-Red acetoxymethyl ester (1 µg/mL) for 30 min at 37°C. Cells are then washed twice with Na medium (with 1 mM Ca^{2+}) and labelled with FITC-conjugated cell markers for 15 min (CD14 for monocytes, CD19 for B-lymphocytes, CD3 for T-lymphocytes or CD56 for NK cells). These mononuclear cells are washed once and resuspended in K medium (150 mM KCl, 10 mM Hepes, pH 7.5, supplemented with 0.1% BSA and 5mM glucose) with 1 mM Ba^{2+} at 37°C. A small magnetic stir bar (1x3 mm) is added to the tube before it is inserted into the Time-Zero System. The FL3 voltage is adjusted to give a linear mean channel fluorescence intensity of ~700 for the gated population. No compensation is required between FL1 and FL3. ATP is added 40 sec later. Signals from mononuclear cells are acquired at about 2000 events per second on a Becton Dickinson FACSCalibur flow cytometer and the data comprising forward scatter (log mode), side scatter (log mode), FL1 (log mode), FL3 (linear mode, 1024 channels) and time (2 sec intervals) for each event are collected. Digitonin is added at the end of the run to estimate maximum values for Ca^{2+} influx. The data from each run (about 250 sec) is saved into a listmode file.

2.3 Gating and calculation

The listmode file is analysed by WinMDI. Cells are gated by forward and side scatter and by cell type specific antibodies. The linear mean channel of fluorescence intensity (1024 channels resolution) for each gated subpopulation (Fig. 4) over successive 2 sec intervals is plotted against time and saved into a text file.

The text file is then imported into *Microsoft* Excel, and the arbitrary units of area above the Ba^{2+} influx curve in 20 sec after addition of ATP is calculated using the following functions:

```
Function(C5) =AVERAGE(C$7:INDIRECT(ADDRESS(D4+5,COLUMN(),4,1),1))
```
(to calculate the average linear mean channel of basal line in the same period before ATP is added into the test tube)

```
Function(D4) =MATCH(0,D$7:D$50,0)
```
(to locate in which interval that ATP is added)

```
Function(D5) =AVERAGE(D$7:INDIRECT(ADDRESS(D4+5,COLUMN(),4,1),1))
```
(to calculate the average linear mean channel of basal line before ATP is added)

```
Function(D6) =(SUM(INDIRECT(ADDRESS(D4+10,COLUMN()-
1,4,1),1):INDIRECT(ADDRESS(D4+21,COLUMN()-1,4,1),1))+(D5-
C5)*10)+(SUM(INDIRECT(ADDRESS(D4+11,COLUMN()-
1,4,1),1):INDIRECT(ADDRESS(D4+20,COLUMN()-1,4,1),1))+(D5-C5)*8)-
SUM(INDIRECT(ADDRESS(D4+10,COLUMN(),4,1),1):INDIRECT(ADDRESS(D4+21,COLU
MN(),4,1),1))-SUM(INDIRECT(ADDRESS(D4+11,
COLUMN(),4,1),1):INDIRECT(ADDRESS(D4+20,COLUMN(),4,1),1))
```
(to calculate the first 20 sec area above Ba^{2+} influx curve after addition of ATP)

The arbitrary unit of area obtained in Function(D6) is also used to quantify the P2X7 channel function. (Excel template is available)

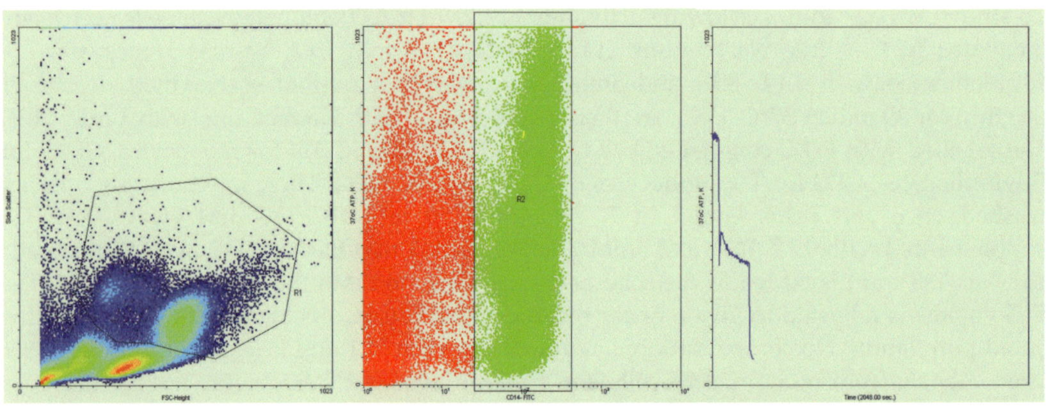

Fig. 4. Typical dotplots and gating strategy used to analyse Ba^{2+} influx by Fura-Red in CD14 positive monocytes

2.4 Notes for technique

Cation influx methods based on Fura-red fluorescence can be applied to kinetic studies in many channels/receptors which involve Ca^{2+} influx or efflux. In this study, Ba^{2+} is used as a surrogate for Ca^{2+} since cytosolic Ba^{2+} is neither pumped nor sequestered and the Ba^{2+} signal over short times represents the unidirectional influx. Most of the intracellular Ba^{2+} remains in the cytoplasmic region as mononuclear cells lack the mechanisms either to pump out intracellular Ba^{2+} or sequester this cation into intracellular organelles. Since P2X7 function is greater in Na^+ free and/or Cl^- free buffer (Humphreys & Dubyak, 1996; Wiley *et al.*, 1992), isotonic K^+ buffer is used to measure P2X7 function instead of physiological Na^+ buffer.

In measurements of Ba^{2+} influx using Fura-red, because of the long wavelength emission of Fura-Red, there is little overlap between FL1 and FL3, and the FL3-FL1 compensation setting can be ignored. This long wavelength of Fura-Red also limits the interference of yellow coloured compounds.

	A	B	C	D
1				
2		Time (min)	Basal	ATP
3				
4			2s, 20s	21
5			693.59	708.24
6				5931
7	0	0	698.8	717.8
8	1	0.033333	708.1	706.2
9	2	0.066667	696.9	715.6
10	3	0.1	689	694.9
11	4	0.133333	706.3	708.6
12	5	0.166667	690.9	715.4
13	6	0.2	687.8	702.4
14	7	0.233333	697.1	723.6
15	8	0.266667	699.7	702.3
16	9	0.3	695.1	711.3
17	10	0.333333	707.8	711.3
18	11	0.366667	692.7	711.7
19	12	0.4	686.4	716.6
20	13	0.433333	681.8	702.8
21	14	0.466667	687.1	705.4
22	15	0.5	687.2	694
23	16	0.533333	697.6	712.8
24	17	0.566667	691.3	703.5
25	18	0.6	682.5	706.6
26	19	0.633333	687.6	702
27	20	0.666667	687.5	0
28	21	0.7	702	0
29	22	0.733333	684.5	0
30	23	0.766667	690	339.7
31	24	0.8	674.2	379
32	25	0.833333	683.2	393.3

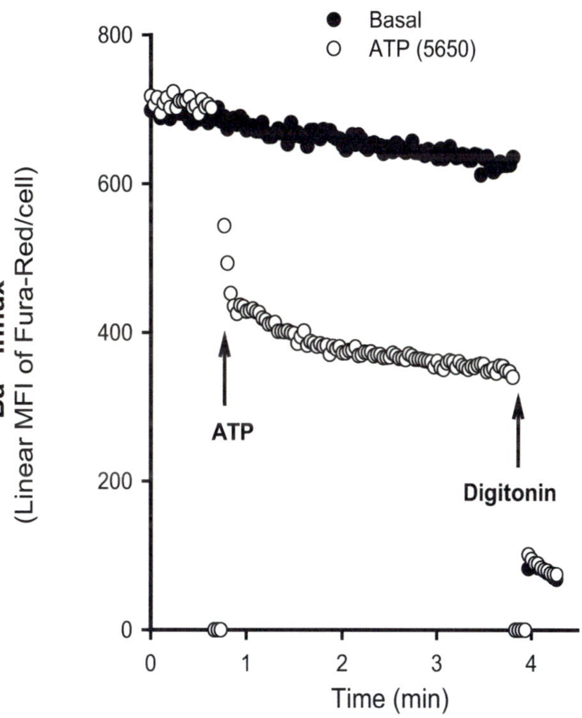

Fig. 5. An example of spreadsheet (left) and a typical curve of Ba^{2+} influx into cells (right)

3. ATP induced ethidium$^+$ uptake

3.1 Principles

A unique feature of the P2X7 receptor observed under physiological conditions is the slow further increase in permeability that develops after the initial opening of the P2X7 channel, which is readily studied by flow cytometry (Wiley *et al.*, 1998). Ethidium bromide is a phenanthridinium intercalator which binds both DNA and RNA and is generally excluded from viable cells. It has been used previously to assess cell permeabilization by ATP (Gomperts, 1983). Once bound to nucleic acids, the fluorescence is enhanced 20~30 fold. The excitation maximum is shifted to 512 nm and the emission maximum is shifted to 605 nm. This long emission wavelength allows simultaneous detection of ethidium$^+$ influx on the FL2 photomultiplier (570 to 610 nm) in the presence of FITC-labeled antibodies which are detected on the FL1 photomultiplier (525 nm). Time-resolved flow cytometry generates the mean fluorescence intensity of analysed cells over a certain time period. This technique allows a sensitive measurement of the initial rate of ethidium uptake, which is essentially unidirectional because of binding of this permeant cation to nucleic acids. By using time-resolved flow cytometry, our group has shown that there is large variation of P2X7 function among individuals (Gu *et al.*, 2000) mainly due to genetic polymorphisms which alter the function of this receptor (Gu *et al.*, 2004; Gu *et al.*, 2001; Shemon *et al.*, 2006; Skarratt *et al.*, 2005; Wiley *et al.*, 2003)

Previous methods used to measure surface P2X7 function have been semi-quantitative and unable to distinguish sub-populations within the overall cell suspension as well as being unable to distinguish live and dead cells. The two-colour time resolved flow cytometry methods described here allow quantitative assessment of the abundance of functional P2X7 receptors on the surface of different subtypes of leukocytes as well as excluding dead cells from analysis (Gu *et al.*, 2000; Jursik *et al.*, 2007).

3.2 Method

Mononuclear cells ($2x10^6$) pre-labeled with FITC-conjugated cell markers are washed once and resuspended in 100 µL Na medium with 0.1 mM Ca^{2+} at room temperature. Following the addition of 900 µL K medium, a small magnetic stir bar is added to the tube before it is inserted into the Time-Zero System which controls temperature and allows magnetic stirring. The FL2 voltage is set at around 595V with a gain of 5.0, at which the linear mean channel fluorescence intensity for Quantum PE standard beads with MESF 300747 is 48±1 (256 linear scale) and the peak channel for right reference standard PE high level beads (MESF ~560,000) is 100±1 (256 linear scale). The compensation of FL1-FL2 and FL2-FL1 is 7% and 8% respectively. Ethidium bromide (25 µM) is added, followed 40 s later by addition of 1.0 mM ATP. Mononuclear cells are acquired at approximately 1000 events per second by a Becton Dickinson FACSCalibur flow cytometer and the data comprising forward scatter (log mode), side scatter (log mode), FL1 (log mode), FL2 (linear mode, 256 channels) and time (5 sec intervals) for each event are collected. The data of each run (approximately 380 sec) is saved into a listmode file.

3.3 Gating and calculation

The listmode file is analysed by WinMDI. Cells are gated by forward and side scatter and by cell type specific antibodies (Fig. 6). Cells with maximum ethidium$^+$ uptake (254 channels or over) are considered as fully permeable necrotic cells and therefore excluded from the assay. The kinetic linear mean channel of fluorescence intensity for each gated subpopulation over successive 5 sec intervals is plotted against time and saved into a text file.

To quantify ethidium$^+$ uptake, arbitrary unit of area under the uptake curve in the first 5 min after addition of ATP is calculated. The basal line (without ATP) is firstly adjusted to the same level as the test line (with ATP added after 40 sec). The area under the ethidium uptake curve between the basal and test lines is considered as the sum of 60 trapezoids (Fig. 1a).

The text file is then imported into *Microsoft* Excel, and the area under the ethidium$^+$ uptake curve is calculated using the following functions:

Function(C5)=AVERAGE(C$7:INDIRECT(ADDRESS(D4+5,COLUMN(),4,1),1))
(to calculate the average linear mean channel of basal line in the same period before ATP is added into the test tube)

Function(D4) =MATCH(0,D$7:D$30,0)
(to locate in which interval that ATP is added)

Function(D5) =AVERAGE(D$7:INDIRECT(ADDRESS(D4+5,COLUMN(),4,1),1))
(to calculate the average linear mean channel of basal line before ATP is added)

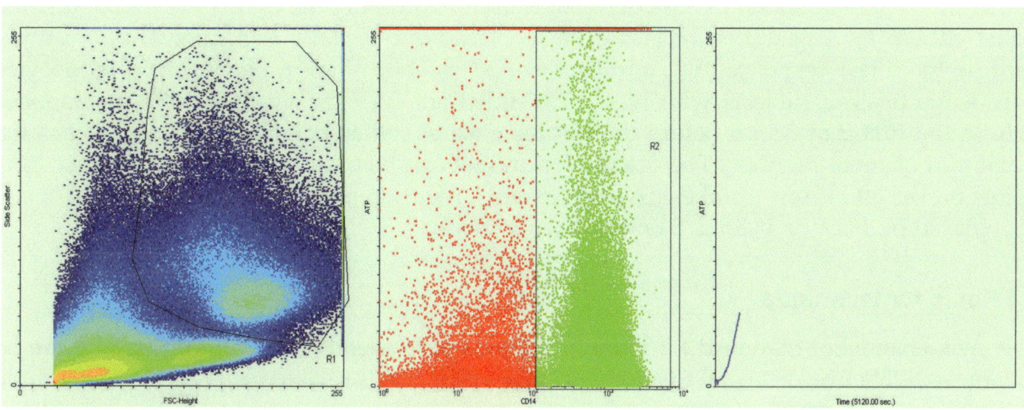

Fig. 6. Typical dotplots and gating strategy used to analyse ethidium⁺ uptake by CD14 positive monocytes

	A	B	C	D	E
1					
2					
3		Time (min)	CD14 basal	CD14 ATP	
4			5s	6	3221
5			1.74	1.66	8654
6				26278	16871
7	0	0	1.5	1.5	
8	1	0.083333	1.9	1.3	
9	2	0.166667	2.1	1.7	
10	3	0.25	2	2.2	
11	4	0.333333	1.2	1.6	
12	5	0.416667	1	0	
13	6	0.5	1.9	2	
14	7	0.583333	1.5	3.3	
15	8	0.666667	2.2	3.8	
16	9	0.75	1.8	5.8	
17	10	0.833333	2.4	7.2	
18	11	0.916667	2	9.4	
19	12	1	2.1	11	
20	13	1.083333	2.5	12.8	
21	14	1.166667	2.3	15.8	
22	15	1.25	2.5	16.6	
23	16	1.333333	2.9	18.7	

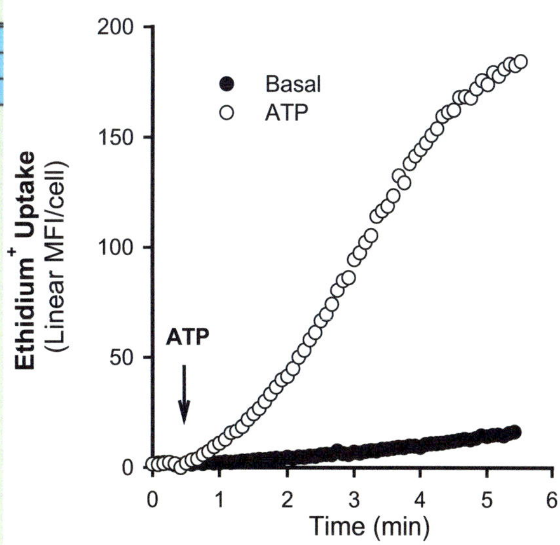

Fig. 7. An example of spreadsheet (left) and a typical curve of ethidum⁺ uptake (right)

Function(D6)
=2.5*(SUM(INDIRECT(ADDRESS(D4+8,COLUMN(),4,1),1):INDIRECT(ADDRESS(D4+5*12+8,COLUMN(),4,1),1))+SUM(INDIRECT(ADDRESS(D4+9,COLUMN(),4,1),1):INDIRECT(ADDRESS(D4+5*12+7,COLUMN(),4,1),1))-SUM(INDIRECT(ADDRESS(D4+8,COLUMN()-1,4,1),1):INDIRECT(ADDRESS(D4+5*12+8,COLUMN()-1,4,1),1))-SUM(INDIRECT(ADDRESS(E4+9,COLUMN()-1,4,1),1):INDIRECT(ADDRESS(D4+5*12+7,COLUMN()-1,4,1),1))-(D5-C5)*120)
(to calculate uptake curve in the first 5 min after area under ethidium+ uptake curve after addition of ATP)

The arbitrary unit obtained in Function(D6) is used to quantify the P2X7 pore function. Time frame chosen for calculation of ATP-induced ethidium$^+$ uptake is 5 min. This is simply because the linear response after addition of ATP is about 5 min. However, in monocytes from some healthy subjects with high P2X7 function, ATP may induce a linear response only in the first 2 or 3 min before the fluorescence of cell-associated ethidium reaches the maximum channel number. The calculation model can be readily adapted to shorter time points on the ethidium$^+$ uptake curve. To do this, the time point in above function (5*) can be replaced by 2*, 3* or 4* for 2, 3 or 4 min respectively.

3.4 Notes for technique

The peak channel of Standard PE Reference Beads measured on linear mode in FL2 can be as large as ±20% from one day to another. Therefore it is essential to calibrate the instrument daily before each set of experiments. Furthermore, ethidium$^+$ concentration, temperature and the composition of the suspending buffer are critical parameters. The area under the ethidium$^+$ uptake curve increases proportionally with the ethidium$^+$ concentration up to about 100 µM. Excess ethidium$^+$ however might bind to mitochondrial membranes and lead to inaccurate results. Moreover, P2X7 function is dependent on temperature. We have shown that P2X7 agonists fail to induce ethidium$^+$ uptake at 12°C, which is gradually restored by a temperature rise up to a physiological value of 37°C. Results are further altered by the absence or presence of Ca^{2+}, Cl^- and Na^+ ions in the acquisition medium. Small amounts of extracellular Ca^{2+} (~10 µM) in the medium are always included to maintain cell membrane integrity. However, high concentration of Ca^{2+} may reduce the ATP activity by binding to its active species, ATP^{4-} or by direct competition for permeation (Wiley *et al.*, 1996). Isotonic K^+ or sucrose media remove the inhibitory effect of Na^+ and/or Cl^- ions on P2X7 function, which facilitates the detection of differences in P2X7 function among individuals. Since multiple factors cause large alterations in the area under the ethidium uptake curve, it is essential to keep standardized assay conditions.

ATP-induced ethidium$^+$ uptake is directly proportional to the concentration of ethidium cation over the range 1 to 100 µM, consistent with permeation of ethidium$^+$ through a dilated pore. 25 µM ethidium bromide is routinely used for measurement of uptakes over a 3 to 5 minute time course. The pore formation by activated P2X7 is also sensitive to temperature. P2X7 function decreases at lower temperature while at 12°C or lower, ATP-induced ethidium$^+$ uptake is almost completely abolished. It has been reported that removal of extracellular Cl^- as well as extracellular Na^+ enhances permeability responses and stimulates the function of the P2X7 receptor (Michel *et al.*, 1999). P2X7 function measured by ATP-induced ethidium$^+$ uptake is greatest in Na^+ free, Cl^- free sucrose medium, less in KCl medium, and least in NaCl medium.

Leukocyte subtypes are identified by monoclonal antibodies and we observed that unconjugated anti-CD14, CD3, CD19 or CD16 antibody did not affect ATP-induced ethidium+ uptake. Thus, with the correct FL2-FL1 compensation, the positively gated population should give a similar value of area under ethidium+ uptake curve as the negatively gated population. While the extremely bright fluorescence of ethidium+ makes for accuracy in the uptake measurement, it does make the correct compensation between FL1 and FL2 essential. While under-compensation of FL2-FL1 leads to high basal level of ethidium+ uptake, any over-compensation of FL2-FL1 dramatically reduces the area under ethidium+ uptake curves. Meanwhile, if the FL1-FL2 compensation is too high or too low, the R2 gated population (Fig. 6) will incline towards left or right, respectively. Ethidium+ uptake can also exclude the necrotic or apoptotic cells from the live cells in the suspension, simply by excluding fluorescent events at the maximum fluorescent channel intensity at zero time which defines the fully permeabilized cells present.

4. Phagocytosis of fluorescent latex beads

4.1 Introduction

Phagocytosis is a fundamental aspect of the innate immune system which is preserved in specialized cells of all metazoans. Human monocytes suspended in saline media (without serum) rapidly phagocytose a range of foreign particles which are internalized into a phagosome via rearrangement of the actin-myosin cytoskeleton. This innate immune function requires recognition of foreign particles by one or more scavenger receptors on the monocyte surface. We have recently shown that an intact P2X7-nonmuscle myosin heavy chain IIA complex in monocyte/macrophages can regulate the phagocytosis of a range of non-opsonized particles including latex beads, and live and dead *Staphylococcus aureus* and *Escherichia coli* (Gu *et al.*, 2010).

Technical advances in the assessment of phagocytosis have allowed rapid advances in our knowledge of molecular interactions associated with engulfment of particles by phagocytes. Confocal microscopy has shown that internal membranes within the cell fuse with plasma membrane during the course of particle ingestion, and that recycling endosomes are the primary source of membrane for enlargement of phagocytic cup (Touret *et al.*, 2005). Flow cytometric assessment of particle engulfment has to some extent replaced microscopic observation (Steinkamp *et al.*, 1982) particularly as the kinetics of uptake of fluorescent targets by phagocytes can be followed by instruments capable of time-resolved measurements in a stirred cuvette at 37ºC (Gu *et al.*, 2010). These assays of phagocytosis by flow cytometry usually include measurements of fluorescence particle uptake by cells pre-incubated with cytochalasin D (CytD), an inhibitor of F-actin polymerization and phagocytic cup formation and this control condition allows the assay to distinguish engulfment of particles from adhesion. Particle size is also important in flow studies which generally employ fluorescent particles ranging from 1 to 3 μm in diameter.

Various methods have been employed in phagocytosis studies. However, no published method reflects the quantitative particle uptake in real time although this parameter is important to fully assess the engulfment ability of phagocytes. In this section, we describe a quantitative method to measure the phagocytic ability of human monocytes using time-resolved two-colour flow cytometry.

4.2 Method

Mononuclear cells (2×10^6 in 100 µL) are pre-labeled with APC conjugated-anti CD14 followed by addition of 900 µL Na medium with 0.1 mM Ca^{2+} with a small magnetic stir bar. The tube is inserted into the Time-Zero System (from Cytek Development, Fremont, CA, USA) which monitors temperature (37ºC) and allows magnetic stirring. 5 to 10 µL yellow-green carboxylated fluorescent polystyrene latex microspheres (YG bead, 1 µm, from Polyscience, Warrington, PA) are added 20 sec later. Linear MFI of YG fluorescence is collected in FL1 (voltage: 380-420, gain: 2.0). Events are acquired at about 1500 events per second by a Becton Dickinson FACSCalibur flow cytometer. The data of each run are collected for about 7 min and saved into a listmode file.

4.3 Gating and calculation

The listmode file is analysed by WinMDI. Cells are gated by forward and side scatter and by cell type specific antibodies (Fig. 8). The linear mean channel of fluorescence intensity for each gated subpopulation over successive 10 sec intervals is plotted against time to yield kinetic data which is saved into a text file.

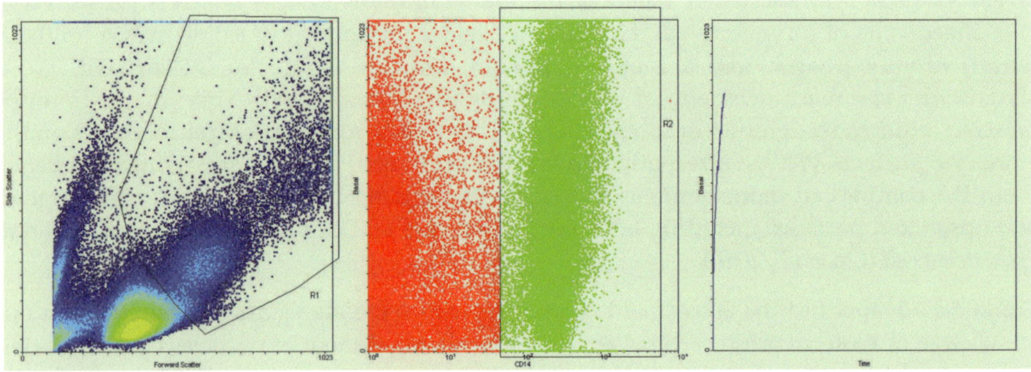

Fig. 8. Typical dotplots and gating strategy used to analyse YG bead uptake by $CD14^+$ monocytes

To quantify bead uptake, arbitrary units of area under the uptake curve in first 6.5 min after addition of beads is calculated. The area is considered as the sum of 39 trapezoids, which is calculated by the following mathematical model. The text file is then imported into *Microsoft* Excel, and mathematical calculation of the area under the bead uptake curve is programmed using the following functions:

C5, D5 and E5 are the lowest value among C6, D6 and E6, represent the threshold to exclude the background fluorescence intensity.

Function(C6)=INDIRECT(ADDRESS(MATCH(30,C$9:C$32,1)+10,COLUMN(),4,1),1)
(To calculate initial levels of fluorescence intensity)

Function(C7)=5*(C$6+2*SUM(INDIRECT(ADDRESS(MATCH(30,C$9:C$32,1)+11,COLUMN(),4,1),1):INDIRECT(ADDRESS(MATCH(30,C$9:C$32,1)+6.5*6+9,COLUMN(),4,1),1))+INDIRECT(ADDRESS(MATCH(30,C$9:C$32,1)+6.5*6+10,COLUMN(),4,1),1))-C$6*6.5*6*10
(To calculate area under YG bead uptake curve in the first 6.5 min)

The area under the YG bead uptake curve is calculated over the time frame of 6.5 min, because the uptake of beads is usually maximal at this time point. However, the calculation model can be readily adapted to different time points on the YG bead uptake curve. To do this, the time point in above function (ie 6.5) can be replaced by the desired time in minutes.

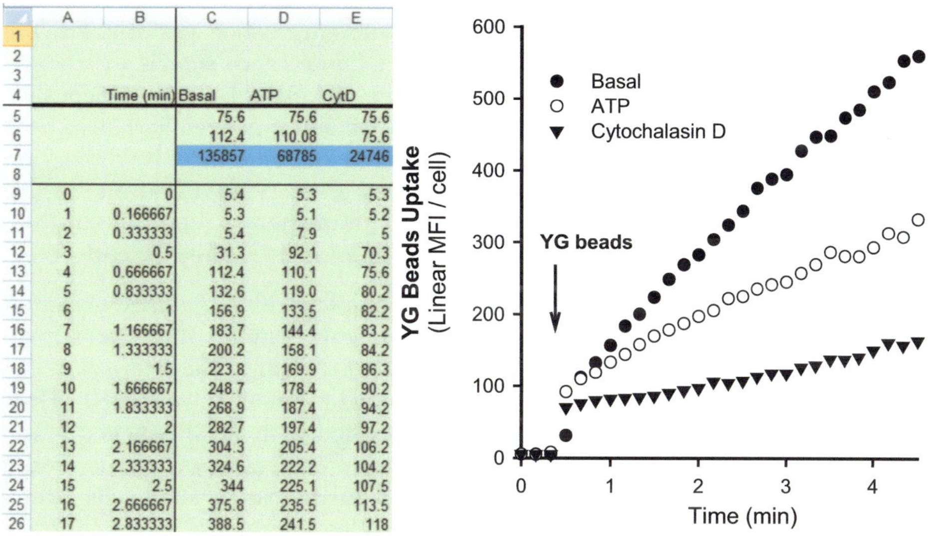

	A	B	C	D	E
1					
2					
3					
4		Time (min)	Basal	ATP	CytD
5			75.6	75.6	75.6
6			112.4	110.08	75.6
7			135857	68785	24746
8					
9	0	0	5.4	5.3	5.3
10	1	0.166667	5.3	5.1	5.2
11	2	0.333333	5.4	7.9	5
12	3	0.5	31.3	92.1	70.3
13	4	0.666667	112.4	110.1	75.6
14	5	0.833333	132.6	119.0	80.2
15	6	1	156.9	133.5	82.2
16	7	1.166667	183.7	144.4	83.2
17	8	1.333333	200.2	158.1	84.2
18	9	1.5	223.8	169.9	86.3
19	10	1.666667	248.7	178.4	90.2
20	11	1.833333	268.9	187.4	94.2
21	12	2	282.7	197.4	97.2
22	13	2.166667	304.3	205.4	106.2
23	14	2.333333	324.6	222.2	104.2
24	15	2.5	344	225.1	107.5
25	16	2.666667	375.8	235.5	113.5
26	17	2.833333	388.5	241.5	118

Fig. 9. An example of spreadsheet (left) and a typical curve of YG bead uptake (right)

4.4 Notes for technique

The time resolved flow cytometry based method described here allows real-time quantitative assessment of the phagocytic function of peripheral blood monocytes labeled with APC conjugated CD14 antibody. The excitation and emission wavelength of APC is well separated from the YG-beads containing fluorescein (APC: Ex. 633nm, Em. 660nm; YG: Ex. 441nm, Em. 486nm), thus the compensation setting of the flow cytometer can be ignored. Although lymphocytes do not phagocytose 1 µm YG bead in this setting (Gu *et al.*, 2010), the $CD14^+$ gating is necessary to exclude uptake of YG beads by the small number of neutrophils which contaminate the Ficoll separated mononuclear population.

Since the bead size is much less than cell size, multiple beads transit through the laser beam together with the cell, leading to a considerable fluorescence background. In addition, some YG beads may also adhere to cell surface non-specifically. Thus cytochalasin D (a potent phagocytosis inhibitor) is used to assess fluorescence intensity due to background resulting from above factors.

Many factors can affect this phagocytosis assay including the nature of bead surface. The total uptake of negatively charged carboxylate beads is higher than the uptake of uncharged beads suggesting the negatively charged carboxyl groups on the bead surface facilitates their uptake by monocytes. The bead size, cell:bead ratio, pH and temperature are critical parameters affecting uptake. Uptake of 1 µm beads is maximal at a pH 6.5-7.5 and 37°C in serum-free Na medium with 0.1 mM Ca^{2+}. This method can be used to compare the phagocytic ability of monocytes from different individuals, especially if a standard protocol is used and the flow cytometer is carefully calibrated from day-to-day.

5. Protein complex dissociation

5.1 Principle

Fluorescence resonance energy transfer (FRET) is one of the major techniques used for protein interaction studies. Confocal or fluorescent microscopes with photobleach or fluorescence lifetime modules are the common instruments which perform FRET based measurements. However, microscopy can only detect fluorescence signals in a single cell, and cannot measure multiple fluorescence emission wavelengths simultaneously. This limitation on confocal microscope makes flow cytometer an attractive alternative for FRET based measurement. The time-resolved fluorescence decay measurement by flow cytometry has been used to study molecule interactions (Condrau *et al.*, 1994a; Condrau *et al.*, 1994b; Deka & Steinkamp, 1996). However, this technique requires major modification to a flow cytometer since a pulsed laser has to be used in order to measure fluorescence lifetime.

The P2X7 receptor has been shown to form a protein complex with nonmuscle myosin heavy chain IIA (NMMHC-IIA) in its unactivated state, and this complex dissociates following activation of P2X7 by extracellular ATP (Gu *et al.*, 2009). To study the interaction of these two proteins in a large cohort of live cells, we developed a time-resolved FRET (TR-FRET) flow cytometry method. The HEK-293 cells are transfected with AcGFP-tagged NMMHC-IIA and DsRed-tagged P2X7. The NMMHC-P2X7 interaction is assessed by monitoring the fluorescence intensity changes of AcGFP and DsRed in double positive cells over 10-15 minutes after addition of P2X7 agonist. This method does not require any modification of the flow cytometer, and can be readily adapted to study the interaction within the intact cell of virtually any two tagged proteins expressed in a large cohort of transfected live cells.

5.2 Method

HEK-293 cells co-transfected with *pAcGFP-N1-MYH9* (the gene encoding NMMHC-IIA) and *pDsRed-monomer-N1-P2RX7* (1:4) are resuspended in Na medium with 0.1 mM $CaCl_2$ at a concentration of 2.0×10^6/mL. The cell suspension (2 mL) is stirred and temperature maintained at 37°C using a Time Zero module. ATP (1.0 mM) is added 2 min after the tube is inserted. Cells are analysed at about 1500 events/s on a FACSCalibur flow cytometer. The voltage settings and compensation are established using non-transfected cell and cells transfected with either AcGFP or DsRed. The FSC, SSC, log FL1, log FL3 and the time are collected into a FCS 2.0 file.

5.3 Gating and calculation

Fluorescent events are gated by forward and side scatter and by AcGFP and DsRed fluorescence intensity. The log mean channel of fluorescence intensity for each gated subpopulation over successive 5-s intervals is analysed by WinMDI software and saved into a text file.

To quantify levels of protein dissociation, arbitrary unit of area under/above the kinetic fluorescence curve in first 12 min after addition of ATP is calculated. The text file is then imported into *Microsoft* Excel spreadsheet, and mathematical calculation of the area under/above curve is programmed using the following functions:

Function(C4)=MATCH(0,C$7:C$40,0) ; *To calculate when ATP is added.*

Function (C5)=AVERAGE(C$7:INDIRECT(ADDRESS(C$4+5,COLUMN(),4,1),1))
To calculate the base line.

Function(C6)
=0.5*5*(INDIRECT(ADDRESS(C$4+7,COLUMN(),4,1),1)+2*SUM(INDIRECT(ADDRESS(C$4+8,COLUMN(),4,1),1):INDIRECT(ADDRESS(C$4+12*12+6,COLUMN(),4,1),1))+INDIRECT(ADDRESS(C$4+12*12+7,COLUMN(),4,1),1))-C$5*12*12*5
To calculate area above/under curve (Log mode)

Funciton(D7)=IF(C7=0,0,POWER(10,(C7+1)/256))
To transform the log MFI to artificial linear MFI. The rest data in Column D are transformed using the same function by "Ctrl-D" command.

Function(D6)
=0.5*5*(INDIRECT(ADDRESS(D$4+7,COLUMN(),4,1),1)+2*SUM(INDIRECT(ADDRESS(D$4+8,COLUMN(),4,1),1):INDIRECT(ADDRESS(D$4+12*12+6,COLUMN(),4,1),1))+INDIRECT(ADDRESS(D$4+12*12+7,COLUMN(),4,1),1))-D$5*12*12*5
To calculate area above/under curve (Linear mode)

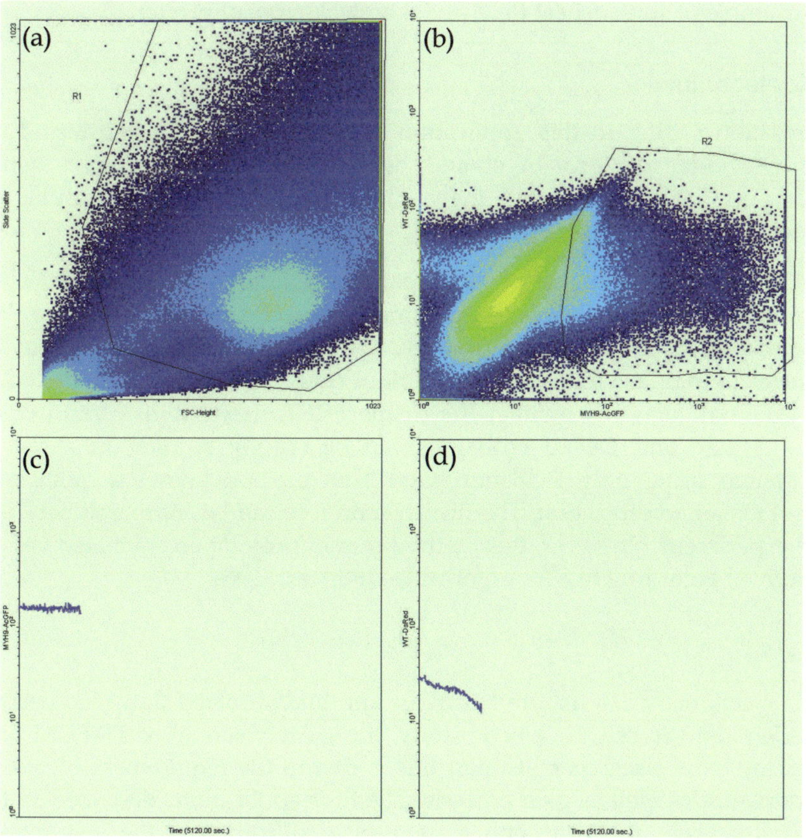

Fig. 10. Typical dotplots and gating strategy used to analyse protein-protein interaction. **a.** The FSC and SSC of HEK-293 cells gated by gate R1. **b.** The AcGFP+DsRed+ HEK-293 cells gated by R2. **c.** Changes in fluorescence of AcGFP tagged NMMHC-IIA. **d.** Kinetic P2X7 with time of DsRed tagged fluorescence

	A	B	C	D	E	F
1						
2		Time (min)	Wild Type P2X7 with BzATP			
3			AcGFP		DsRed	
4			18	18	18	18
5			605.71	234.78	400.21	36.95
6			9455	21248	-27681	-6960
7	0	0	594.8	212.4926	406	38.8905
8	1	0.083333	602.9	228.5517	407.4	39.3833
9	2	0.166667	612.7	249.6121	399.5	36.682
10	3	0.25	601.7	226.0981	400.3	36.9469
11	4	0.333333	618.7	263.453	402.9	37.8211
12	5	0.416667	606.4	235.8611	398.1	36.223
13	6	0.5	604.6	232.0732	402.3	37.6176
14	7	0.583333	599.2	221.0707	406.3	38.9956
15	8	0.666667	601.4	225.4888	400	36.8473
16	9	0.75	614.3	253.2303	403	37.8552
17	10	0.833333	605.5	233.9595	403.2	37.9233
18	11	0.916667	611.7	247.377	399.1	36.5503
19	12	1	613.7	251.8674	398	36.1904
20	13	1.083333	601.1	224.8812	398.8	36.4518
21	14	1.166667	598.7	220.0788	392.8	34.5367
22	15	1.25	606.2	235.4372	393.3	34.6924
23	16	1.333333	603.5	229.7884	392.6	34.4747
24	17	1.416667	0	0	0	0
25	18	1.5	596	214.7985	397.3	35.9633
26	19	1.583333	610.5	244.7214	392.7	34.5057
27	20	1.666667	608.7	240.7912	398	36.1904
28	21	1.75	600.2	223.0681	391.1	34.0127

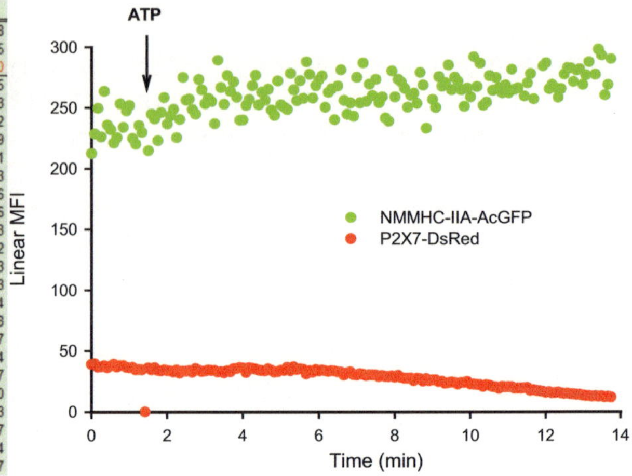

Fig. 11. An example of spreadsheet (left) and a typical curve of protein dissociation (right)

5.4 Notes for technique

The compensation setting in this application is critical. HEK-293 transfected with either AcGFP- or DsRed-tagged protein should be used to establish correct compensation. Although data on FL2 is not collected, the voltage should still be set at a similar level to FL1 to enable compensation between FL1 and FL3.

AcGFP and DsRed is a good pair of FRET partners for flow cytometry. Both AcGFP and DsRed are monomers, thus possible self-polymerization can be avoided. A regular 488 laser is optimized to excite AcGFP fluorescence signal but has gives little excitation of DsRed. The emission wavelength of AcGFP is in the optimum range for excitation of DsRed. Therefore, the DsRed emission signal is mainly due to the FRET effect. With careful compensation settings, the AcGFP and DsRed emissions can be readily studied in a real time flow cytometry system using only a 488nm laser. This method allows a quick and reliable assessment of protein dissociation. The dissociation rate can be compared between samples in the same experiment. However, this method cannot provide an estimated value for FRET efficiency derived according to Förster formulae (Förster, 1948).

6. Discussion

Although flow cytometry is a mature technique and time-resolved flow cytometry (TR-FCM) has been widely used in cellular kinetic study, the great potential of TR-FCM has not been fully realized by most researchers. In part this is due to the requirement of modification of existing instruments as well as data analysis. The four applications described in this chapter are simple and feasible, requiring only minimum modification of the flow cytometer. The Time-Zero module can be easily set up in less than 5 min. If this module is not available, a small beaker with 37°C water can substitute for temperature control. The analysis software is free and the example of MS Excel templates are available. We hope above four examples may encourage the use of TR-FCM in more cellular kinetic studies.

The new generation of flow cytometers, such as Accuri C6 from BD, MACSQuant Analyzer from Miltenyi Biotec, Cyan from Beckman Coulter, Attune Acoustic Focusing Cytometer from Invitrogen, uses "plugs" to deliver sample for analysis (Edwards *et al.*, 2001a). This analyses precise defined volume and the sample vessel need not be pressurized. However, none of these cytometers can perform TR-FCM applications described in this chapter, although all have the time parameter for acquisition. Manufacturers have not realized the importance of TR-FCM, and its marketing value. In fact, with small modification of the sample platform and the acquisition software, these new generation of flow cytometers can easily be upgraded for TR-FCM.

7. References

Condrau, M.A., Schwendener, R.A., Niederer, P. & Anliker, M. (1994a). Time-resolved flow cytometry for the measurement of lanthanide chelate fluorescence: I. Concept and theoretical evaluation. *Cytometry*,Vol. 16,No.3, pp.187-94

Condrau, M.A., Schwendener, R.A., Zimmermann, M., Muser, M.H., Graf, U., Niederer, P. & Anliker, M. (1994b). Time-resolved flow cytometry for the measurement of lanthanide chelate fluorescence: II. Instrument design and experimental results. *Cytometry*,Vol. 16,No.3, pp.195-205

Deka, C. & Steinkamp, J.A. (1996). Time-resolved fluorescence-decay measurement and analysis on single cells by flow cytometry. *Appl Opt*,Vol. 35,No.22, pp.4481-9

Edwards, B.S., Kuckuck, F.W., Prossnitz, E.R., Okun, A., Ransom, J.T. & Sklar, L.A. (2001a). Plug flow cytometry extends analytical capabilities in cell adhesion and receptor pharmacology. *Cytometry*,Vol. 43,No.3, pp.211-6

Edwards, B.S., Kuckuck, F.W., Prossnitz, E.R., Ransom, J.T. & Sklar, L.A. (2001b). HTPS flow cytometry: a novel platform for automated high throughput drug discovery and characterization. *Journal of biomolecular screening*,Vol. 6,No.2, pp.83-90

Förster, T. (1948). Intermolecular energy migration and fluorescence. *Annalen der Physik*,Vol. 437,No.2, pp.55-75

Gomperts, B.D. (1983). Involvement of guanine nucleotide-binding protein in the gating of Ca2+ by receptors. *Nature*,Vol. 306,No.5938, pp.64-6

Gu, B.J., Rathsam, C., Stokes, L., McGeachie, A.B. & Wiley, J.S. (2009). Extracellular ATP dissociates nonmuscle myosin from P2X7 complex: this dissociation regulates P2X7 pore formation. *Am J Physiol Cell Physiol*,Vol. 297,No.2, pp.C430-439

Gu, B.J., Saunders, B.M., Jursik, C. & Wiley, J.S. (2010). The P2X7-nonmuscle myosin membrane complex regulates phagocytosis of non-opsonized particles and bacteria by a pathway attenuated by extracellular ATP. *Blood*,Vol. 115,No.8, pp.1621-1631

Gu, B.J., Saunders, B.M., Petrou, S. & Wiley, J.S. (2011). P2X7 is a scavenger receptor for apoptotic cells in the absence of its ligand extracellular ATP. *Journal of Immunology*,Vol. 187,No.5, pp.2365-2375

Gu, B.J., Sluyter, R., Skarratt, K.K., Shemon, A.N., Dao-Ung, L.P., Fuller, S.J., Barden, J.A., Clarke, A.L., Petrou, S. & Wiley, J.S. (2004). An Arg307 to Gln polymorphism within the ATP-binding site causes loss of function of the human P2X7 receptor. *Journal of Biological Chemistry*,Vol. 279,No.30, pp.31287-95

Gu, B.J., Zhang, W., Worthington, R.A., Sluyter, R., Dao-Ung, P., Petrou, S., Barden, J.A. & Wiley, J.S. (2001). A Glu-496 to Ala polymorphism leads to loss of function of the human P2X7 receptor. *Journal of Biological Chemistry*,Vol. 276,No.14, pp.11135-42

Gu, B.J., Zhang, W.Y., Bendall, L.J., Chessell, I.P., Buell, G.N. & Wiley, J.S. (2000). Expression of P2X7 purinoceptors on human lymphocytes and monocytes: evidence for nonfunctional P2X7 receptors. *American Journal of Physiology - Cell Physiology*,Vol. 279,No.4, pp.C1189-97

Humphreys, B.D. & Dubyak, G.R. (1996). Induction of the P2Z/P2X7 nucleotide receptor and associated phospholipase D activity by lipopolysaccharide and IFN-gamma in the human THP-1 monocytic cell line. *Journal of Immunology*,Vol. 157,No.12, pp.5627-37

Jursik, C., Sluyter, R., Georgiou, J.G., Fuller, S.J., Wiley, J.S. & Gu, B.J. (2007). A quantitative method for routine measurement of cell surface P2X(7) receptor function in leucocyte subsets by two-colour time-resolved flow cytometry. *J Immunol Methods*,Vol. 32567-77

Michel, A.D., Chessell, I.P. & Humphrey, P.P. (1999). Ionic effects on human recombinant P2X7 receptor function. *Naunyn-Schmiedebergs Archives of Pharmacology*,Vol. 359,No.2, pp.102-9

Nolan, J.P. & Sklar, L.A. (1998). The emergence of flow cytometry for sensitive, real-time measurements of molecular interactions. *Nature Biotechnology*,Vol. 16,No.7, pp.633-8

Ramirez, S., Aiken, C.T., Andrzejewski, B., Sklar, L.A. & Edwards, B.S. (2003). High-throughput flow cytometry: validation in microvolume bioassays. *Cytometry Part A: the journal of the International Society for Analytical Cytology*,Vol. 53,No.1, pp.55-65

Shemon, A.N., Sluyter, R., Fernando, S.L., Clarke, A.L., Dao-Ung, L.P., Skarratt, K.K., Saunders, B.M., Tan, K.S., Gu, B.J., Fuller, S.J., Britton, W.J., Petrou, S. & Wiley, J.S. (2006). A Thr(357) to Ser polymorphism in homozygous and compound heterozygous subjects causes absent or reduced P2X(7) function and impairs ATP-induced mycobacterial killing by macrophages. *Journal Of Biological Chemistry*,Vol. 281,No.4, pp.2079

Skarratt, K.K., Fuller, S.J., Sluyter, R., Dao-Ung, L.P., Gu, B.J. & Wiley, J.S. (2005). A 5 ' intronic splice site polymorphism leads to a null allele of the P2X(7) gene in 1-2% of the Caucasian population. *Febs Letters*,Vol. 579,No.12, pp.2675

Sklar, L.A., Carter, M.B. & Edwards, B.S. (2007). Flow cytometry for drug discovery, receptor pharmacology and high-throughput screening. *Curr Opin Pharmacol*,Vol. 7,No.5, pp.527-34

Steinkamp, J.A., Wilson, J.S., Saunders, G.C. & Stewart, C.C. (1982). Phagocytosis: flow cytometric quantitation with fluorescent microspheres. *Science*,Vol. 215,No.4528, pp.64-6

Touret, N., Paroutis, P., Terebiznik, M., Harrison, R.E., Trombetta, S., Pypaert, M., Chow, A., Jiang, A., Shaw, J., Yip, C., Moore, H.P., van der Wel, N., Houben, D., Peters, P.J., de Chastellier, C., Mellman, I. & Grinstein, S. (2005). Quantitative and dynamic assessment of the contribution of the ER to phagosome formation. *Cell*,Vol. 123,No.1, pp.157-70

Wiley, J.S., Chen, J.R., Snook, M.S., Gargett, C.E. & Jamieson, G.P. (1996). Transduction mechanisms of P2Z purinoceptors. *Ciba Foundation Symposium*,Vol. 198149-60; discussion 160-5

Wiley, J.S., Chen, R., Wiley, M.J. & Jamieson, G.P. (1992). The ATP4- receptor-operated ion channel of human lymphocytes: inhibition of ion fluxes by amiloride analogs and by extracellular sodium ions. *Archives of Biochemistry & Biophysics*,Vol. 292,No.2, pp.411-8

Wiley, J.S., Dao-Ung, L.-P., Li, C., Shemon, A.N., Gu, B.J., Smart, M.L., Fuller, S.J., Barden, J.A., Petrou, S. & Sluyter, R. (2003). An Ile-568 to Asn Polymorphism Prevents Normal Trafficking and Function of the Human P2X7 Receptor. *Journal of Biological Chemistry*,Vol. 278,No.19, pp.17108-17113

Wiley, J.S., Gargett, C.E., Zhang, W., Snook, M.B. & Jamieson, G.A. (1998). Partial agonists and antagonists reveal a second permeability state of human lymphocyte P2Z/P2X7 channel. *American Journal of Physiology - Cell Physiology*,Vol. 44,No.5, pp.C1224-C1231

11

Application of Flow Cytometry in the Studies of Microparticles

Monika Baj-Krzyworzeka, Jarek Baran, Rafał Szatanek and Maciej Siedlar
Department of Clinical Immunology, Jagiellonian University Medical College, Cracow, Poland

1. Introduction

Many cell types including leukocytes, platelets and endothelial cells release small membrane fragments called microparticles (MP). MP are shed during cell growth, activation, proliferation, senescence and apoptosis. MP contain proteins (intracellular as well as surface markers), mRNA and miRNA of the cells they have originated from. Based on the release mechanism, size and phenotype, MP are frequently divided into two categories: exosomes and ectosomes called also microvesicles. There is no doubt that the biological significance of MP has been largely overlooked for many years, regarding them as merely cellular fragments or debris. Nowadays, MP are being recognized as an important regulator of cellular interactions under physiological and pathological conditions. MP are present in all body fluids and physiologically serve various functions like blood clotting, enhance cell adhesiveness, increase cell aggregation, etc. They mediate cell-to-cell communication by transferring cell surface receptors, mRNA, and miRNA from the cell of origin to target cells. The growing body of literature regarding the role of MP in many pathologies has recently progressed from describing the association of elevated MP number with disease stage (e.g. cancer, sepsis) through understanding how MP may contribute to thrombosis, preeclampsia and tumor progression, and finally, to using MP as a source of antigens in new forms of vaccines against infectious or malignant diseases.

Flow cytometry is a preferred method in the studies of MP because of its ability to quantitate the absolute number of particles and multicolor analysis attributes, allowing detection of several markers simultaneously. However, despite its usefulness, flow cytometry has some limitations in this field. The definition of MP using flow cytometry is still an area of great debate. In this review we propose a comprehensive summary of the possibilities, advantages and disadvantages of flow cytometry as a "gold standard" in the studies of MP.

2. Overview of different forms of microparticles

2.1 Definition of various MP – plenty is a plaque

MP are defined as a mixture of heterogeneous vesicles size-wise, and there is a number of schemes trying to classify them by considering their different characteristics (i.e. origin, size, distinct cell surface and/or internal determinant patterns, etc.), which may become confusing at times.

One of the most routinely used schemes in defining MP is their cellular origin [Heijnen et al., 1999, Hess et al., 1999, Dumaswala et al., 1984, Ginestra et al., 1998, Zitvogel et al., 1998]. This method utilizes flow cytometry to compare the cell membrane determinant composition as well as the internal cargo of MP with that of the original cell. Scientists that chose this method do not restrict themselves to just one surface/cellular determinant, but use many, in order to define the MP most precisely. It is very desirable in this case to have a unique determinant (present on/in the original cell and its MP) that would definitely establish the MP origin. Based on this classification method, scientists then use terminology that stresses out the MP origin, i.e. dendritic cell-derived microvesicles, erythrocyte-derived microvesicles, platelet-derived microvesicles, etc. [Heijnen et al., 1999, Hess et al., 1999, Dumaswala et al., 1984, Ginestra et al., 1998, Zitvogel et al., 1998].

Another way of defining MP considers two populations of MP, ectosomes and exosomes, depending on the place of origin within the same cell [Pilzer et al., 2005, Rak et al., 2010]. Thus, ectosomes are considered to be vesicles which are formed upon plasma membrane vesiculation, where as exosomes are generated within endosomal structures inside a cell [Al-Nedawi et al., 2009]. Ectosomes are relatively larger than exosomes with their size ranging from 100-1000 nm in diameter, and their outer membrane is rich in phosphatidylserine (PS) residues [Al-Nedawi et al., 2009, Del Conde et al., 2005]. Ectosomes are also associated with the formation of lipid rafts, membrane regions containing high levels of cholesterol and signaling complexes. Exosomes, on the other hand, have a lower abundance of PS residues compared to ectosomes and are usually smaller (30-100 nm) in diameter [Simpson et al., 2009]. They also seem to transport a different type of cargo than other MV originating from the same cell, showing more transporting selectivity for intracellular proteins/molecules.

Another group of MP that is often regarded as a separate population is derived from tumor cells. The most important criterion in defining TMV seems to be the assessment of their tumor origin [Yu et al., 2005, Bergmann et al., 2009, Kim et al., 2003, Huber et al., 2005]. Here, again, flow cytometry is used as the means of establishing the determinant composition (surface and/or internal) of TMV which is then compared to that of the tumor cells.

Considering the different ways of MP classification it has to be kept in mind that there is no clear, well-defined approach that could be applied for MP differentiation. Many of the methods mentioned above tend to overlap, which when used separately, could result in defining the same MP population. There is a growing need of trying to establish clear-cut guidelines that would help properly define the different types of MP. Figure 1 is a representation of the heterogeneity of MP and their different nomenclature. It also depicts some possible determinants that can be transported by particular MP population.

2.2 Isolation of MP from biological fluids or culture supernatants – The devil is in the details

There is no real consensus or a uniform protocol on MP isolation from different types of biological fluids or culture supernatants. Most of the time, people who try to isolate MP develop their own protocols which tend to incorporate their particular interests as well as the availability of equipment in their laboratory setting. The other side to this problem is sample preparation such as collecting, processing temperature, etc. as well as how the samples should be stored and prepared for future use.

The most commonly used methodology for MP isolation is differential centrifugation which employs a number of different centrifugation steps characterized by different centrifugal forces and centrifugation times. The concept behind this type of methodology is to purify the sample in such a manner as to obtain the correct MP population. Although, differences between the protocols exist, there seems to be a general agreement on the purification of the MP sample from cells and other larger cellular fragments that remain after a sample collection. This is regardless of the sample origin, whether it is culture supernatants, plasma or any other biological fluid. Thus, the initial purification step is set at a relatively low centrifugal force (around 200-500xg) for a short time period (app. 10 min.) to get rid of the larger fragments/cells from the sample [Orozco et al., 2010, Baran et al., 2010]. The next step, which centrifugal force ranges between 10,000-17,000xg and is set between 30 min. to 1 hour, is designed either to obtain the MP or to further purify the sample of unwanted cellular fragments or MP [Ayers et al., 2011, Baran et al., 2010, Gelderman & Simak, 2008]. One has to consider its interest because at this speed some of the MP can be lost which might be of significance. Thus, if platelet-derived MP (PMP), whose presence is predominant in plasma samples, is a subject of the study then the pellet obtained after this centrifugation step will mainly consist of them. At this step, one has to also consider the impact of size with regards to MP because if exosomes (part of MP population), which are considered to be smaller vesicles, are the subject of the study then they will remain in the supernatant, and the next centrifugation step/steps is/are considered to be crucial to obtain them (centrifugal force up to 150,000xg) [Grant et al., 2011, Baran et al., 2010, Al-Nedawi et al., 2008].

The adopted form of verifying the individual steps of the different centrifugation protocols employs flow cytometry. Staining the pellet or supernatant samples obtained during the different phases of the protocol with appropriate antibodies and then analyzing them using flow cytometry seems to be the method of choice by many groups. The idea behind it is to trace the MP fractions, whether present in the pellets or supernatants that come off during each step of the centrifugation protocol. Thus, for example, if platelet-free sample is required, one would stain the pellet and supernatant obtained after the initial and the 10,000-17,000xg centrifugation steps to check for platelet markers (i.e. CD41, CD61) [Baran et al., 2010]. The depletion of $CD41^{+}$ or $CD61^{+}$ entities would then signal that sample purification was successful and that further sample processing can be initiated (Fig. 2 represents an example of a marker tracing (CD61) on MP in the supernatant fractions of a plasma sample obtained during different centrifugation steps). Analogically, flow cytometry is used when the final MP population is obtained and needs verification or characterization with respect to the surface determinant profile.

Another form of centrifugation, which is also commonly used in MP isolation, involves the application of a sucrose gradient [Lamparski et al., 2002, Keller et al., 2011, Zhong et al., 2011]. In the case of the sucrose gradient filtration method, a sucrose gradient is created by gently overlaying a sucrose layer of lesser concentration on top of the layer with higher sucrose concentration in some defined concentration increments in an appropriate test tube. Next, the sample is placed on top of the sucrose density gradient and subjected to a high centrifugal force (app. 150,000xg) for an extended time period. During the centrifugation step, the sample particles move through the gradient until they reach the sucrose density that matches their own, where they stop. At the end of this step, the obtained fractions that contain MP according to their different densities, can be removed and utilized in further tests.

Another method for isolating MP which is gaining interest is referred to as microfluidic immunoaffinity method [Chen et al., 2010, Hsu et al., 2008]. The propagators of this procedure point out that this method is much faster in comparison to differential centrifugation or sucrose gradient filtration and that it yields higher MP recovery rates [Chen et al., 2010]. Another major advantage to this method seems to point out to the fact that smaller sample volumes are being used as well as the isolated MP remain relatively "untouched" (the impact of centrifugal force being excluded) thus resembling more accurately their native state i.e. shape, determinant surface profile, etc. The principle behind this method is to selectively bind MP populations to antibody-coated surfaces [Chen et al., 2010, Hsu et al., 2008, Choi et al., 2011, Cheng et al., 2007] . The method utilizes a flow channel of different dimensions, depending on the initial sample volume to be processed, which surface is chemically modified in order to later coat it with appropriate antibodies. The outcome of such modification results in the preparation of a column that is coated with an antibody that recognizes a surface determinant characteristic for particular MP population. Next, a sample is injected into the channel and the appropriate MP are immobilized on its surface. This is followed by a washing step which purpose is to elute the immobilized MP which then can be used for further tests (protein analysis, RNA isolation, etc.).

Another aspect of MP isolation that has a major impact on MP quality is sample collection, preparation and storage [Dey-Hazra et al., 2010, Trummer et al., 2009, Shah et al., 2008]. Unfortunately, here again no uniform protocols exist that would state the proper way to address these issues. As with different isolation protocols, the sample collection, preparation and/or storage depend on individual needs and settings characteristic of the study. However, there seems to be a general understanding that freshly obtained samples are the best to work with and that multiple "freezing and thawing" has a substantial impact on both the MP number as well as the surface determinant expression, which suggest that, if possible, should be avoided (see section 2.1.1) [Dey-Hazra et al., 2010, Trummer et al., 2009, Shah et al., 2008].

2.3 Sizing of MP and estimation of their absolute number by flow cytometry – Role of instrumentation

Flow cytometric analysis of MP appears to be the most favored method used for their characterization [Jy et al. 2004]. Typically, MP are identified as particles with a forward scatter smaller than an internal standard consisting of 1-1.5 μm sized latex particles [Shet et al., 2003]. Light scattering is a basic phenomenon for detecting and characterizing particles in modern flow cytometry. A light beam directed at a particle can interact with it through reflective, refractive and diffractive effects. Then, information about a particle or aggregates of particles can be derived from the changes in direction and intensity of the scattered light [Kim & Ligler 2010]. Collecting scattered light at various angles from the incident beam has been reported to provide different types of information about the particle, including both size and density [Shvalov et al., 1999]. Typically, forward scattered light (0.5-5°) can provide approximate information about the size of particle [Shapiro 2004]. It should, however, be

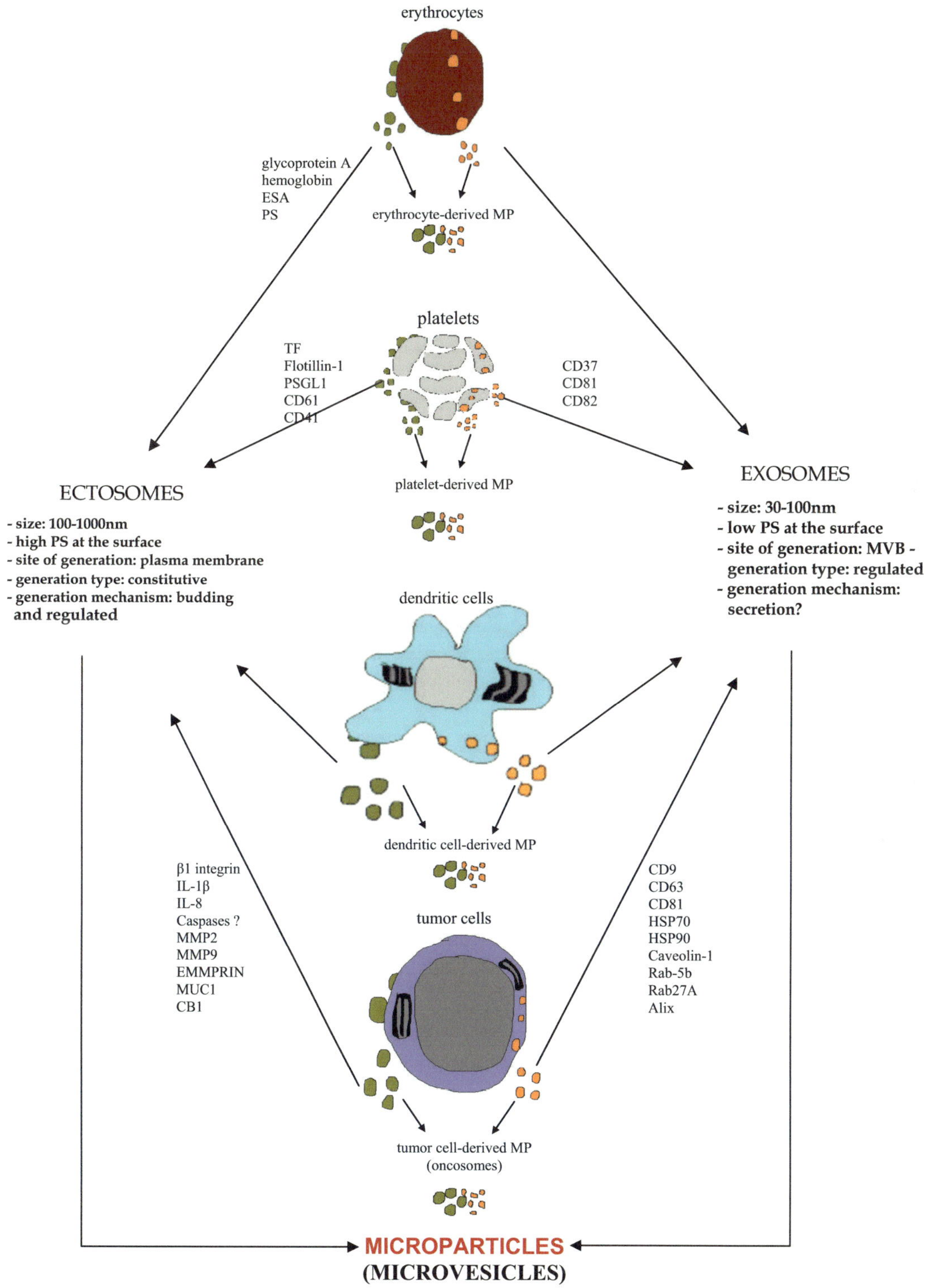

Fig. 1. Heterogeneity of microparticles

noted that the intensity of FSC is not related directly to particle size [Becker et al., 2002]. On the other hand, side-scattered light (15-150°) is often collected at 90° angle and provides information about smaller particles or granularity of internal structures. Measuring side-scattered and forward scattered light has become a standard in biomedical research, enabling cells to be distinguished by size and granularity.

A problem with MP in a standard flow cytometry is that they cannot reliably be detected when setting a forward scatter as a trigger, as they are smaller than the wavelength of a laser light used, and cannot always be discriminated from the background noise. Moreover, forward scatter is the most variable signal between instruments of different manufacturers and its proper alignment is crucial. It is affected by refractive index mismatches between sheath fluid and sample, beam geometry, polarization, beam stop position and collection angle [Nebe-von-Caron, 2009]. Unfortunately, there are a lot of data published in peer reviewed journals based on the assumption that a forward scatter signal of certain size beads represents similar size in MP. The problems with this approach have been already highlighted, and nowadays it is recommended to use log side scatter for comparative analysis of MP and beads, as all the instruments show good correlation with regards to side scatter response, being capable of reproducing the same level of sensitivity against the particular 190 nm latex particles [Nebe-von-Caron, 2009]. While the identification of MP on the basis of the light scattered parameters tests the limit of sensitivity of flow cytometry, some investigators have overcome this problem by setting the parameters of the instrument to detect fluorescence as a trigger (Horstman et al, 1994). Thus while analyzing MP one should look at log side scatter versus log fluorescence of the selected staining triggered on fluorescence and side scatter at the instrument noise level (if triggered on two channels) or either of the two, depending on the analysis needed [Nebe-von-Caron 2011].

Enumeration of MP by flow cytometry

Flow cytometry can also be used to enumerate MP (usually in the plasma) by adding, as an internal standard, a known number of fluorescent latex beads (Flow-Count Fluorospheres, Beckman-Coulter) or using tubes containing already predefined number of them (TruCount tubes, BD Biosciences). The number of MP present in the sample is derived from the following formula (1) and adjusted for the final dilution of the original sample [Baran et al, 2010]:

$$\text{MP count} = \frac{\text{No. of events in region containing MP}}{\text{No. of events in absolute count bead region}} \times \frac{\text{No. of beads per test}}{\text{Test volume [}\mu\text{l]}} \quad (1)$$

Alternatively, if the flow cytometry instrument delivers the sample to the optics by screw-driven syringe at a known rate, then the sample MP count can be calculated [Orozco & Lewis, 2010].

Role of instrumentation

Recently, a class of flow cytometers has been developed which allows the detection of particles of down to 100 nm in size. The developers of these cytometers state that the unique optical design of the apparatus eliminates the unwanted light thus giving the best signal to noise ratio. Due to these adjustments, the cytometers are supposedly representing the highest light scatter sensitivity and resolution available making it an attractive tool in MP research. Additionally, they also offer the volumetric-based absolute count ability of

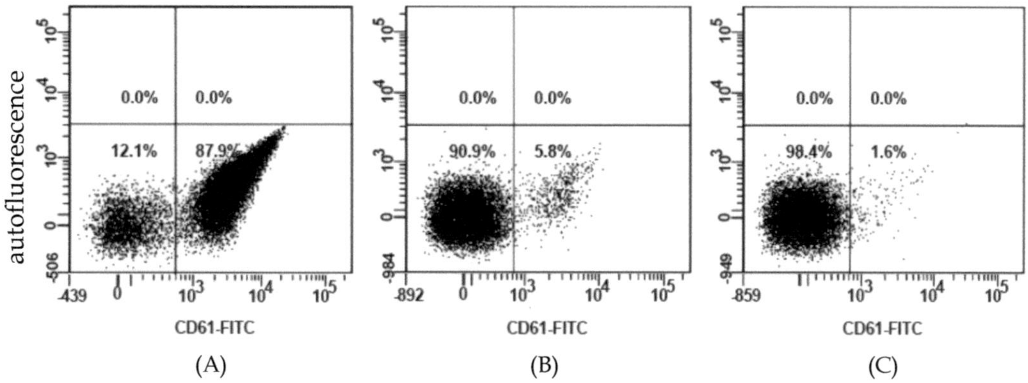

Fig. 2. Tracking of CD61 expression to follow platelets and PMP elimination in a gastric patient plasma sample subjected to differential centrifugation. A- initial plasma; B- plasma subjected to centrifugation at 15,000xg; C- plasma subjected to centrifugation at 50,000xg

samples as well as high fluorescence sensitivity making their use even more practical. One of such product is manufactured by Apogee Flow Systems and allows detection of particles less than 150 nm using 3 light scatter detectors. However, for appropriate MP detection an even lower detection limit is required as compared to microspheres [Chandler, et al. 2011]. For smaller particles, like exosomes (< 100 nm in diameter) some other approaches can be introduced to allow their analysis by flow cytometry. Caby et al. in a very elegant study have presented detection and characterization of peripheral blood exosomes by flow cytometry analysis using CD63-coated latex beads, which can be easily detected by standard instrumentation [Caby et al., 2005]. Other approaches introduce electrical detection systems to detect beads with attached MP/exosomes. Those are based on the work of Wallace Coulter, who demonstrated that electrical charge can be used to detect, size and count particles in solution. Advances in nanotechnologies have drawn many research groups to develop Coulter counters on chip-based platforms [Kim & Ligler 2010]. Holmes et al. has demonstrated a microfabricated flow cytometer for rapid analysis of microspheres using impedance for particle detection [Holmes et al., 2007]. Such cytometers could measure impedance at high (10 MHz) and low (0.5 MHz) frequencies to distinguish mixed bead populations [Kim & Ligler, 2010]. These beads may be coated with antibodies capturing MP/exosomes of different origin.

2.4 Multicolor flow cytometry analysis of MP

Multicolor flow cytometry analysis of MP, using monoclonal antibodies, opened a new way of extensive investigation and characterization of MP. Multicolor analysis is used to detect the cellular origin of MP based on their phenotype. Gelderman and Simak have developed a three-color flow cytometric assay for immunophenotyping MP that are present in plasma [Gelderman & Simak, 2008]. The assay has been used to study MP present in plasma of healthy donors and in patients with paroxysmal nocturnal hemoglobinuria, sickle cell anemia, and in patients with acute ischemic stroke [Simak et al., 2002, Simak et al., 2004, Simak et al., 2002a]. With the use of monoclonal antibodies conjugated to different fluorochromes, a combination of three or even more antigens can be analyzed on a single particle. In addition, annexin V conjugated to a fluorochrome can be used to detect PS on

MP. Some authors limit the analysis of MP to only PS positive ones, however, it has been shown that only a limited population of MP in blood binds annexin V. Although immunophenotyping of MP seems to be a straightforward procedure, here are some methodological requirements in MP staining with monoclonal antibodies. First of all, monoclonal antibodies should be directly conjugated to fluorochomes (indirect staining is not recommended), and fluorochromes used should be as bright as possible (FITC – fluorescein isothiocyanate and PerCP – peridinin-chlorophyll-protein complex conjugated antibodies are not recommended). The titration of antibodies using MP prepared from their parental cells *in vitro* as well as from plasma, should be a rule. Gelderman and Simak recommend the use of two clones against different epitopes of an antigen to confirm specificity of detection [Gelderman & Simak, 2008]. In regard to identification of cellular origin, they suggest using glycophorin A (CD235a) and the leukocyte common antigen (CD45) for detection of red blood cell and leukocyte derived MP, respectively. Platelet-derived MP are detected using monoclonal antibodies against GPIIb (CD41) or GPIIIa (CD61). Monoclonal antibodies to CD14, CD66b, CD4, CD8 and CD20 are used to detect MP from monocytes, granulocytes, T helper, T suppressor and B lymphocytes, respectively. For endothelial-derived MP the use of anti-PECAM (CD31), anti-CD34, anti-E selectin (CD62E) and anti-Endoglin (CD105) monoclonal antibodies is recommended [Gelderman & Simak 2008]. And finally, relevant isotype controls to detect the nonspecific staining should be used in parallel. It is of importance to keep in mind that the presence of specified antigen on MP does not clearly identify their cellular origin. In some cases MP may absorb a soluble antigen circulating in the plasma that is derived from another cell type. A good example is absorption of prostate antigen (PSA) by human monocytes [Faldon et al., 1996]. Thus MP derived from such monocytes might be positive for PSA.

3. Biology of platelet derived microvesicles (PMP)

PMP are the most abundant MP population in blood stream constituting approximately 70-90% of circulating MP [Horstman et al., 1999]. First demonstration of "platelet dust" was done in 1967 by Wolf [Wolf, 1967]. Nowadays, it is known that PMP may be released by activated as well as resting platelets, both in circulation and *in vitro* experiments. A body of experimental and clinical data has shown the association between PMP and diseases.

3.1 Characteristics of PMP

3.1.1 Methods of PMP generation and their phenotype analysis by flow cytometry

Blood platelets activated by a variety of stimuli undergo shape change and degranulation. During this process platelets secrete thin walled vesicles called microparticles or microvesicles (PMP) and smaller exosomes. Under physiological conditions PMP are released after activation with agonists such as epinephrine, adenosine diphosphate, thrombin or collagen [Matzdorff et al., 1998], and also by exposure to complement protein C5b-9 or high shear stress (higher than physiological), [Holme et al., 1997]. *In vitro*, PMP may be generated by stimulation of platelets with physiological factors like thrombin [George, 1982], thrombin and collagen [Baj-Krzyworzeka et al., 2002], or nonphysiological agonist like calcium ionophore [Forlow et al., 2000]. PMP shedding was also described in stored and apoptotic platelets [Jy et al., 1995].

Preanalytical stages like blood sampling site (cubital vein, central venous caterer), needle diameter, discharge of the first portion of blood, collection (Vacutainer, tube, etc), anticoagulant and transport circumstances are extremely important for PMP quality and quantity. Blood should be anticoagulated with 3.8% sodium citrate (9:1 v/v, BD Vacutainer blood collection tubes are recommended) as versenate salts lead to platelet aggregation. Changes in temperature, like overheating or cooling should be avoided. Also, shaking of blood may induce PMP release from platelets as well as other blood cells. The delay between sampling and further processing should be as short as possible (less than 1 hour), as storage results in increased number of PMP [Simak & Gelderman, 2006, Kim et al., 2002].

The protocols for obtaining PMP differ between laboratories and their standardization is a subject of debate. The first step in standardization was undertaken by the Scientific Standardization Committee of the International Society on Thrombosis and Haemostasis. The Committee recommends double centrifugation step to ensure removal of platelets from platelet poor plasma (PPP) and washing PPP samples to remove non specific particles, however these procedures may results in the loss of MP [Ayers et al., 2011]. Differential centrifugation-protocol results in isolation of PMP that in many cases contain exosomes. To avoid the exosomes contamination Grant et al. proposed filtration of PPP through a 0.1 μm pore size filter [Grant et al., 2011]. MP may be also isolated from PPP by capturing them using immobilized annexin V which binds to PS present on PMP and other MP. In this assay, MP are captured with biotinylated annexin V, then incubated with streptavidin-coated plates, and after being washed used for further experiments [Mallat et al.,1999].

Flow cytometry in PMP analysis

Flow cytometry allows the analysis of large numbers of PMP using tiny volume (about 5 μl) of plasma [Simak & Gelderman, 2006, Michelson et al., 2000]. It is of importance to use double filtered (0.2 μm) sheath fluid (e.g. phosphate buffered saline - PBS) for flow cytometry analysis of PMP. Generally, an accepted background "noise" consists of 25-50 events per second when filtered PBS is run.

Size. Standard beads of different sizes (diameter) may, to some extend, be used for PMP sizing, e.g. monodisperse fluorescent Megamix beads (BioCytex). However, one has to be aware that size related data derived from beads and that derived from biological particles are not fully comparable [Lacroix et al., 2010].

It is generally accepted that PMP are larger than 100 nm, but at the same time it should be noted that PMP are very heterogeneous size-wise. The upper limit of PMP size is about 1.5 μm. Additionally, distinguishing between PMP aggregates and platelet-PMP aggregates by flow cytometry may cause problems [Simak & Gelderman, 2006], because of their size overlap. Better results in platelet/PMP sizing can be achieved by using impedance-based flow cytometry instead of light-scatter based one. For this purpose electron microscopy or AFM analysis are highly recommended [Yuana et al., 2011].

Number. App. 75% of laboratories use flow cytometry to enumerate PMP in clinical samples [Lacroix et al., 2010]. However, a variety of preanalytic and analytic variables may lead to variations in PMP values in healthy individuals ranging from 100 to 4000 x 10^3 per μl [Robert at al., 2009]. Although, standardization in PMP count is still inadequate some steps have been already undertaken to uniform this procedure. Three Scientific and Standardization Subcommittees of the International Society on Thrombosis and Haemostasis (ISTH) have initiated a project aimed at standardizing an enumeration of cellular MP by flow cytometry. The main objective was to establish the resolution and the level of background noise of the instruments, and to define reproducibility of PMP count in plasma using flow cytometers manufactured by different vendors. The study demonstrated that different systems were heterogeneous with respect to FSC resolution and background noise. In 2010 the Scientific and Standardization Committee of the International Society on Thrombosis and Haemostasis proposed procedures to be followed for obtaining good reproducibility in PMP count by flow cytometry [Lacroix et al. 2010]. The advised strategy is based on the use of size-calibrated fluorescent beads (0.5 μm and 0.9 μm) in a fixed ratio (Megamix) to gate PMP in a defined size-restricted window [Robert et al. 2009]. However, the procedure seems to be more adequate for Beckman-Coulter instruments rather than Becton-Dickinson's, as the former measure the forward-scattered light at a relatively wide angle (1-19°) compared to the latter (1-8°) [Lacroix et al. 2010].

Phenotype. Flow cytometry is used as a method of choice for PMP phenotyping. Similarly to platelets, almost all PMP, express glycoprotein complex IIb-IIIa (CD41/CD61) [Heijnen et al., 1999, George, 1982], CD42a [Simak and Gelderman, 2006, Matsumoto et al., 2004]. Caution is recommended when staining for glycoprotein Ib (CD42b) as only 40-50% of PMP express this marker. Usually, large PMP stain better than the small ones [Zdebska et al., 1998]. Other markers were also detected on PMP, such as: CD31, PAR1, CXCR4, CD154, PF4, as well as ligands for annexin V or lactadherin [Ayers et al., 2011, Baj-Krzyworzeka et al., 2002, Fig 3.]. It has been suggested that $CD41^{+}$ and $CD42^{+}$ PMP represent two different populations, thus it is important to use both of these markers for better assessment. PMP released by activated platelets express also platelet activation markers such as CD62P and activated complex GPIIb-IIIA [Michelson, 2000]. Flaumenhaft et al. showed that cultured megakariocytes shed MP positive for CD41 and concluded that a part of blood $CD41^{+}$ MP

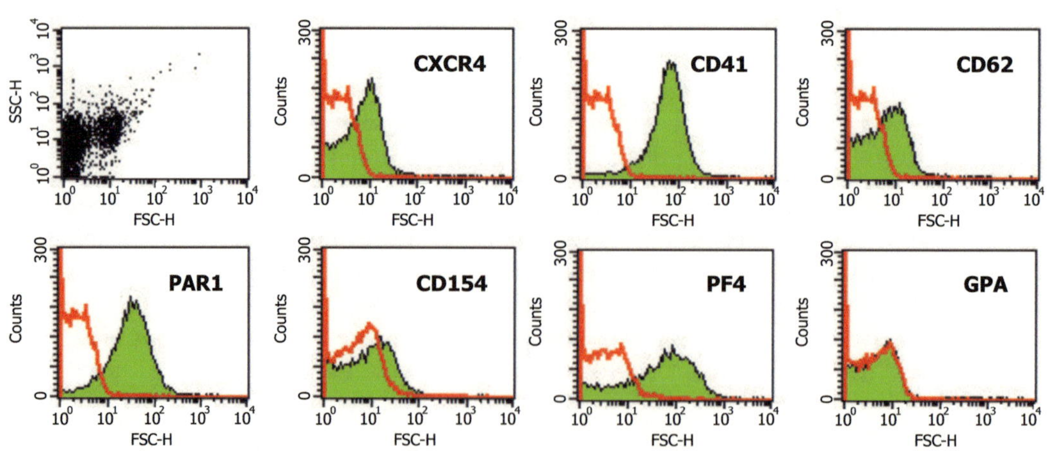

Fig. 3. Expression of selected surface proteins on PMP obtained from platelets stimulated by calcium ionophore A23187. Staining with an isotype control is shown as a red line. GPA-glycophorin A (negative marker)

are of megakaryocyte origin [Flaumenthaft et al., 2009, 2010]. They recommended multicolor flow cytometric analysis (CD41, CD62P and LAMP-1) to distinguish PMP from megacaryocyte-derived MP [Flaumenthaft et al., 2009, 2010]. Flow cytometry analysis of PMP needs standardization comprising consensual panel of antibodies (clones, concentration) and beads specification. It appears that labeling low amounts of PMP results in higher variability of MFI (Mean Fluorescence Intensity) in comparison to labeling higher amounts of PMP [Orozco & Lewis, 2010]. Moreover, it should be noted that differences in *in vitro* research protocols for PMP generation result in variable PMP subpopulations which differ in size, marker expression, protein content and thrombogenic potential [Baj-Krzyworzeka et al., 2002, Dean et al., 2009, Sandberg et al., 1985].

3.1.2 Role of PMP in modulation of biological activity of human cells

Interactions of cells with PMP may result in modulation of biological function in the following ways:

- First, PMP may provide interactions between cells without the need for direct cell-to-cell contact.
  For instance, PMP activate and stimulate neutrophils to secrete proteases, may induce the transformation of peripheral blood monocytes into endothelial progenitor cells [Prokopi et al., 2009], and may facilitate the interactions between leukocytes and endothelial cells [Forlow et al., 2000, Barry et al., 1998]. PMP may also interact with $CD34^+$ cells and increase their bone marrow homing [Janowska-Wieczorek et al., 2001].
- Second, PMP can bind to target cells and fuse with their membranes, resulting in the acquisition of new surface antigens and thus new biological properties and activities of the target cells. For example, the chemokine receptor, CXCR4 which is present on PMP, may be transferred to various cells and make them susceptible to infection by X4-HIV [Rozmysłowicz et al., 2003]. PMP may also transfer GPIIb/IIIa to neutrophils (allowing its interaction with CD18) and neutrophil activation [Salanova et al., 2007] or transfer CD40L which may activate B cells [Sprague et al., 2008].
- Third, PMP may act as "transfer vehicles" which may deliver/exchange protein, lipids, mRNA or even pathogens to target cells. For instance, PMP may change cell activity by lipid transfer [Barry et al., 1997] or may deliver CCL23, CXCL4,7, FGF and TGF [Dean et al., 2009], thus transferring chemoattractant capabilities to various cells [Baj-Krzyworzeka et al., 2002, Fig. 4.]

3.2 PMP in health and disease (counting and procoagulant activity)

Changes in circulating PMP level have been described in patient with many disease states.

Hemostasis and thrombosis

The PMP number is decreased in preterm neonates compared with adults [Rajasekhar et al., 1994]. Patients with Castaman's defect and Scott syndrome, whose platelets are defective, also have a defect in generation of PMP [Castaman et al., 1996, Weiss et al., 1994], which is associated with a bleeding tendency. On the other hand, an increased number of PMP suggests a potential prognostic marker for arherosclerotic vascular disease [Boulanger et al., 2006, Michelsen et al., 2008], transient ischemic attacks, cardiopulmonary bypass and

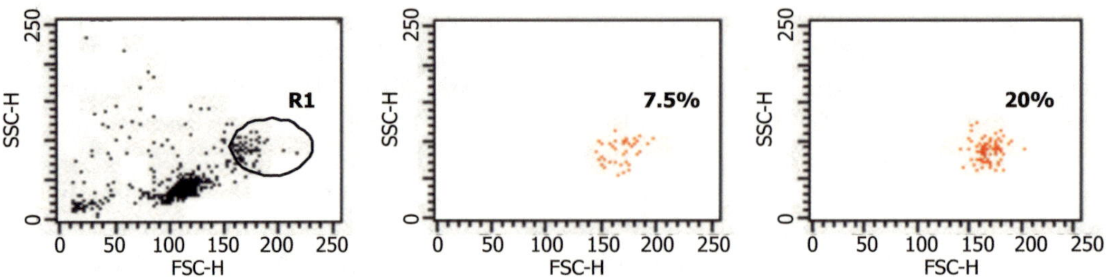

Fig. 4. Chemotactic activity of human blood monocytes to PMP analyzed by flow cytometry. The dot-plots show: monocytes defined in PBMC population by FSC and SSC parameters – region R1 (left); spontaneous chemotaxis of monocytes to culture medium without serum (middle) and chemotaxsis of monocytes to PMP (right)

thrombocytopenias (heparin-induced, thrombotic and idiopathic thrombocytopenic purpura) [Sheriadan et al., 1986, Warkentin et al., 1994]. PMP are strongly procoagulant as they contain the anionic phospholipid PS. Procoagulant PMP are present *in vivo* in blood of patients with activated coagulation and fibrinolysis including patients suffering from Disseminated Intravascular Coagulation (DIC), however, such PMP are also found in healthy donors but in low amounts only [Holme et al., 1994]. An elevated number of PMP was described in patients with diabetes mellitus, which causes the development and progression of artherosclerosis in these patients [Nomura et al., 1995].

Cancer

Although there is no set standard for monitoring PMP levels, some studies have shown that their number is elevated in the plasma of cancer patients as compared to the normal samples suggesting that the tumor itself may be responsible for stimulating their release presumably to enhance its survival. For example, elevated numbers of PMP were detected in plasma of patients with gastric cancer or in urine of patients with bladder cancer [Kim et al., 2003]. Microvesicles derived from activated platelets was also reported to induce metastasis and angiogenesis in lung cancer [Janowska-Wieczorek et al., 2005].

Inflammatory diseases

Boilard et al. demonstrated that platelets are crucial for the development of arthritis. They showed that PMP may facilitate arthritis progression [Boilard et al., 2010]. Other authors reported increased level of PMP in septic patients [Nieuwland et al., 2000, Mostefai et al., 2008]. Suprisingly, early elevated level of PMP and endothelial MP may predict a more favorable outcome in severe sepsis [Soriano et al., 2005].

4. Blood leukocyte derived MP

Major part (~80%) of MP present/detected in serum/blood is released by platelets, while the remaining ~20% constitute MP shed by erythrocytes, leukocytes and endothelial cells [Ratajczak et al., 2006].

Leukocyte-derived MP circulate in the blood stream under normal conditions and are rapidly up-regulated by inflammatory stimuli, e.g. polymorphonuclear leukocytes (PMNs) stimulated with fMLP (formyl-methionyl-leucylphenylanin), calcium ionophore, IL-8 or PMA release small vesicles very quickly (in the matter of minutes) [Hess et al., 1999, Mesri et al., 1999]. Analysis of these MP by flow cytometry showed expression of complement receptor 1 (CR1, CD35), CD66b, HLA class I, LFA-1/CD11a, Mac-1/CD11b, CD62L, CD46, CD55, CD16 and CD59 [Gasser et al., 2003]. However, PMN-MP did not express detectable amount of others PMNs markers like CD32 and CD87 [Gasser et al., 2003]. In general, PMN-MP may be distinguished from other non-PMN-MP by expression of CD66b and annexin V binding.

MP released by monocytes can be defined by CD14, CD18 and TF expression [Aharon et al., 2008]. Moreover, these microvesicles contain caspase-1 and may deliver a cell death signal to e.g. vascular smooth muscle cells [Sarkar et al., 2009]. MP generated by the human monocytic cell line U937 were positive for the co-stimulatory molecules CD80 and CD86, whereas the expression of the adhesion molecules CD11a, CD11c (the DC marker and complement receptor 4), HLA-DR and the scavenger receptor CD36 were rather low. Also, expression of HLA class II molecules such as HLA-DR, HLA-DP and HLA-DQ was lower on MdM (monocyte-derived macrophages)-derived MP than MP of mature or immature DC [Kolowos et al., 2005]. Kolowos et al observed that MP derived from LPS-stimulated MdM showed high expression of the activation marker CD71 in comparison to MP of untreated or UV-B irradiated MdM. Stimulation of another monocytic cell line (THP-1) by starvation or by endotoxin and calcium ionophore A23187 resulted in the release of MP which expressed exosomal marker Tsg 101, monocyte markers (CD18, CD14) and active tissue factor (TF) [Aharon et al., 2008]. The number of monocyte-derived MP was elevated in meningococcal sepsis and in patients with acute coronary syndromes [Nieuwland et al., 2000].

MP derived from B lymphocytes (defined by the expression of CD19) and DC have the capacity to present antigens to induce antigen-specific T-cell responses [Raposo et al., 1996, Zitvogel et al., 1998]. Dendritic cell-derived MP showed expression of HLA class I and II, as well as costimulatory molecules CD80 and CD86 [Wieckowski & Whiteside, 2006] and may present antigens to T cells [Montecalvo et al., 2008]. DC- derived exosomes were proposed to be a short range mechanism to spread alloantigen during T cell allorecognition.

Exosomes from activated T cells can mediate "activation-induced cell death" in a cell-autonomous manner, defined by the nature of the initial T cell activation events and can play central roles in both central and peripheral deletion events involved in tolerance and homeostasis [Prado et al., 2010]. On the other hand thymic cell-derived MP express several proteins that are known to be involved in leukocyte rolling on endothelial surfaces, as well as in transendothelial leukocyte migration [Turiak et al., 2011].

5. Tumor derived microvesicles – Biology and function

Tumor derived microvesicles (TMV), also called oncosomes, are released by tumor cells during their activation (Fig. 5) by different stimuli, hypoxia, irradiation, exposure to proteins from an activated complement cascade and exposure to shear stress [Ratajczak et al., 2006].

Flow cytometry is the standard method to detect and count TMV in human plasma or ascites [Baran et al., 2010]. The number of MV (mainly platelet-derived) in cancer patients is usually elevated and may correlate with distant metastasis, however, it does not correlate with the tumor size [Hejna et al., 1999, Borsig et al, 2001]. More informative is the level of MV specific for tumor cells, e.g hepatic in hepatocellular carcinoma patients which directly correlates with the tumor size [Brodsky et al., 2008]. Counting of specific TMV is possible when specific markers of tumors are known and mAb for flow cytometry are available.

TMV were reported to reprogram endothelial cells by increasing their proangiogenic activity by inducing VEGF production [Al-Nedawi K., et al., 2009; Skog J., et al. 2008]. Also, TMV containing EMMPRIN have been shown to transactivate matrix metalloproteinase (MMP) in peritumoral stromal cells thus increasing tumor spread [Siddhu et al. 2004]. It has been also suggested that polymerization of fibrin by TMV may cause an increase in the entrapment and adhesiveness of tumor cells [Castellana et al. 2010].

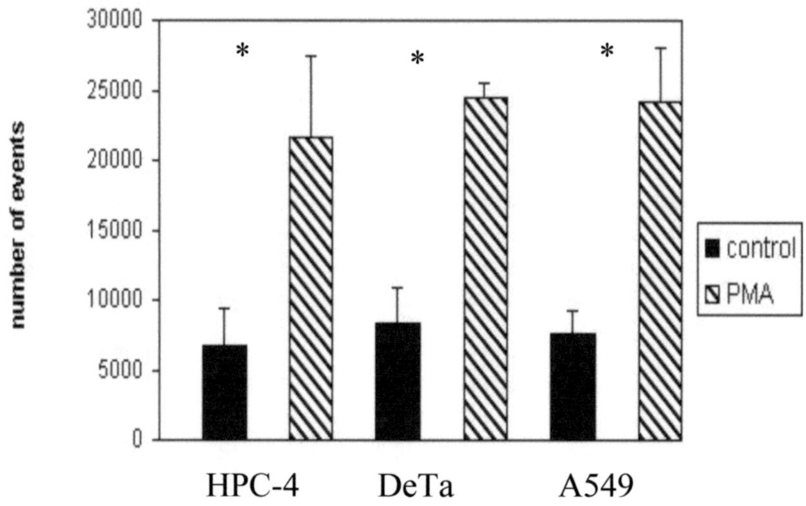

Fig. 5. Comparison of TMV number in culture supernatants from control and stimulated with PMA (100ng/ml) human cell lines: HPC-4 (pancreatic adenocarcinoma), DeTa (colorectal adenocarcinoma) and A549 (lung carcinoma). The number of events (TMV) recorded in the supernatants during 20s of acquisition using FACSCalibur. * $p<0.01$

5.1 TMV as a carrier for proteins, mRNA and miRNA (flow cytometry, Western blotting, real-time PCR)

TMV display a broad spectrum of bioactive substances and receptors on their surface. TMV from melanoma, glioma, breast, lung and pancreatic tumor cell lines express several surface molecules such as CD44, CD63, CD95L, CD147 (extracellular matrix metalloproteinase inducer, EMMPRIN), EpCAM, MUC1, oncogenic receptor EGFRvIII, integrins, chemokine receptors, TNF receptors and HLA molecules [Andreola et al., 2002, Dolo et al., 1995, Friedl et al., 1997, Fritzsching et al., 2002, Sidhu et al., 2004, Taylor and Gercel-Taylor, 2005, Al-Nedawi et al., 2008, Baj-Krzyworzeka et al., 2006]. Membrane – anchored receptors presented on tumor cell are usually present on TMV, but the level of their expression does not always correlate with that on the original cells, e.g. CD44H expression on pancreatic adenocarcinoma cells is abundant but on their TMV rather low [Baj-Krzyworzeka et al., 2006]. At the same time, TMV expressed a higher percentage of CD44 variants (v6 and v7/8) than tumor cells [Baj-Krzyworzeka et al., 2006]. Expression of tumor markers such as Her-2/neu, c-MET, EMMPRIN and MAGE-1 was confirmed by Western blotting [Baran et al., 2010].

The complete characterization of TMV protein content is possible only by mass spectrometry-based proteomic analysis. In an elegant study, Choi et al. identified in microvesicles/exosomes derived from the plasma of colorectal cancer patients 846 proteins involved in tumor progression. [Choi et al., 2011].

TMV contain mRNA for chemokines, growth factors, cytoskeleton proteins and tumor markers, as assessed by real-time PCR [Baj-Krzyworzeka et al., 2006, 2011, Ratajczak et al., 2006, Baran et al., 2010]. TMV may transfer mRNA and smaller RNA molecules, such as microRNA to responding cells [Ratajczak et al., 2006, Camussi et al., 2010]. Also, exosomes contain microRNAs and small RNA but very little mRNA [Zomer et al., 2010].

In conclusion MP can be considered as "macro messengers" as they can deliver proteins, mRNA and microRNA at the same time.

5.2 Tracking of fluorescently labeled TMV *in vitro* and *in vivo*

The phenomenon of protein/receptor transfer by MP was described for the first time by Mack et al. Transfer of CCR5 positive MP to T cells enable M- tropic HIV-1 infection [Mack et al. 2000]. Transfer of PMP increased adhesion of "painted" cells to fibrinogen [Baj-Krzyworzeka et al., 2002]. The same mechanism of receptor transfer was observed in the case of TMV. After a short incubation time transfer of TMV-related molecules CCR6, CD44v7/8 to monocyte was observed [Baj-Krzyworzeka et al., 2006]. Moreover, transferred receptors remained functional [Mack et al., 2000, Baj-Krzyworzeka et al., 2006]. To assess TMV location in monocytes confocal microscopy and flow cytometry analyses with extracellular fluorescence quenching were employed [Baj-Krzyworzeka et al., 2006]. In this study, TMV were labeled with PKH-26 red dye and were added to human monocytes followed by incubation. Crystal violet solution was used for quenching extracellular fluorescence coming only from membrane-attached TMV [Van Amersfoort & Van Strijp, 1994]. After 24h, strong red fluorescence was observed which was not quenched by crystal violet [Fig. 6]. This suggests that by that time most of TMV localized intracellularly. Thus TMV not only adhere to cell membrane (transfer of receptors) but are also effectively engulfed. By the use of other methods e.g. live-cell fluorescence microscopy, it was indicated that exosomes were internalized through endocytosis pathway, trapped in vesicles and transported to perinuclear region, but not to the nucleus. The inverted transport of lipophilic dye from perinuclear region to cell peripheries was revealed, possibly caused by recycling of the exosome lipids. The idea that TMV or other MV proteins are re-expresed (recycled) on cell membrane after engulfment is extremely attractive but still not proven [Muralidharan-Chari at al., 2010]. Outward transport of exosome lipids was presented by Tian et al. [Tian et al., 2010]. The authors suggested the separation of exosome lipids and proteins as lipids are recycled and proteins were trapped in lysosomes. They also suggested that exosomes internalization did not occur through the fusion [Tian et al. 2010].

Similar studies with the used of fluorescently labeled exosomes injected into the footpads of mice were performed by Hood et al. to follow nodal trafficking of melanoma exosomes [Hood et al., 2011]. The authors present (using fluorescent microscopy) a novel tumor exosome dependent model of lymphatic metastatic progression that supports the hypothesis that exosomes may be instrumental in melanoma cell dissemination [Hood et al. 2011].

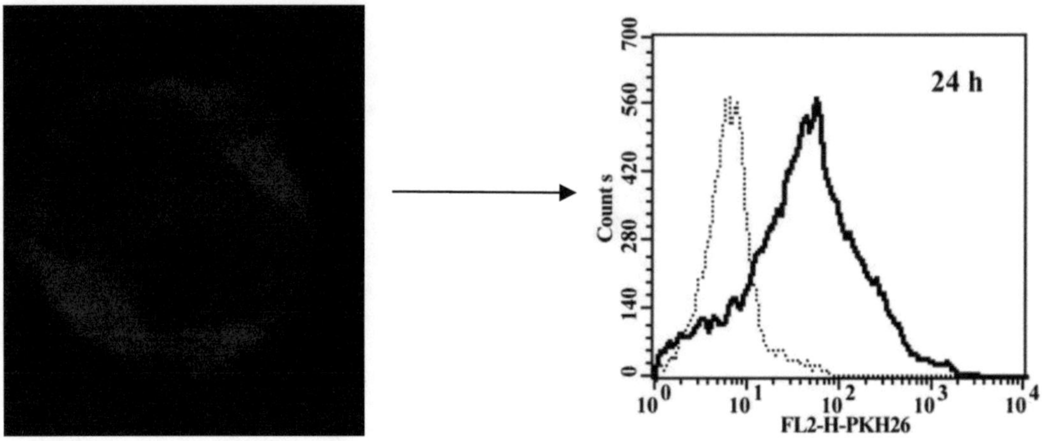

Monocytes engulfed PKH-26 labelled TMV

Crystal violet did not change strong red fluorescence of monocytes. Monocytes in medium (dotted line) or with PKH-26 labelled TMV (bold line) followed by crystal violet quenching.

Fig. 6. Tracking of fluorescently labeled TMV in human monocytes. Left panel presents confocal microscopy image after 24h incubation of PKH26 labeled-TMV with human blood monocytes; right panel presents the assessment of crystal violet quenching in these cells by flow cytometry [Baj-Krzyworzeka et al., 2006, modified)

5.3 TMV/exosomes interactions with the immune system cells (monocytes, lymphocytes, dendritic cells)

It is widely accepted that the immune system can control tumor growth especially at the early phases of its development [Dun, et al. 2004]. Based on our observations TMV may activate blood monocytes as judged by a significant increase in HLA –DR expression (higher MFI) and morphological changes [Fig. 7]. Monocytes are a heterogeneous population of blood cells. In particular, the different expression of CD14 and of CD16 is used to define the major subsets, the so called "classical' $CD14^{++}$ $CD16^{-}$ MO, typically representing up to 90-95% of all MO, and 'non-classical' $CD14^{+}CD16^{++}$. The $CD14^{++}CD16^{-}$ and $CD14^{+}CD16^{++}$ monocyte subpopulations interact with TMV with different results e.g. $CD14^{++}$CD16-engulfed more TMV than $CD14^{+}CD16^{++}$ cells [Fig. 8, Baj-Krzyworzeka et al., 2010]. However, at some point of tumor growth control process, immune surveillance of tumors fails, leading to the local or systemic progression of the tumor. The escape mechanisms adopted by the tumor cells lead to silencing of their immunogenic profile by activating immunosuppressive/ deviating pathways. The mechanisms by which cancer cells escape immune surveillance is still unknown, however, growing evidence suggests that TMV as well as MP released by the immune cells may play an important role in this phenomenon. It has been hypothesized that

TMV shedding may be a way for the tumor cells to dispose of "unwanted", immunogenic molecules from their surface. Indeed, apoptosis-inducing proteins and terminal components of complement have been shown to be shed *via* TMV in some tumors [Abid Hussein et al. 2007; van Doormaal, et al. 2009; Camussi et al. 1987; Sims et al. 1988]. Moreover TMV can modulate the function of tumor infiltrating lymphocytes *via* FasL expression which

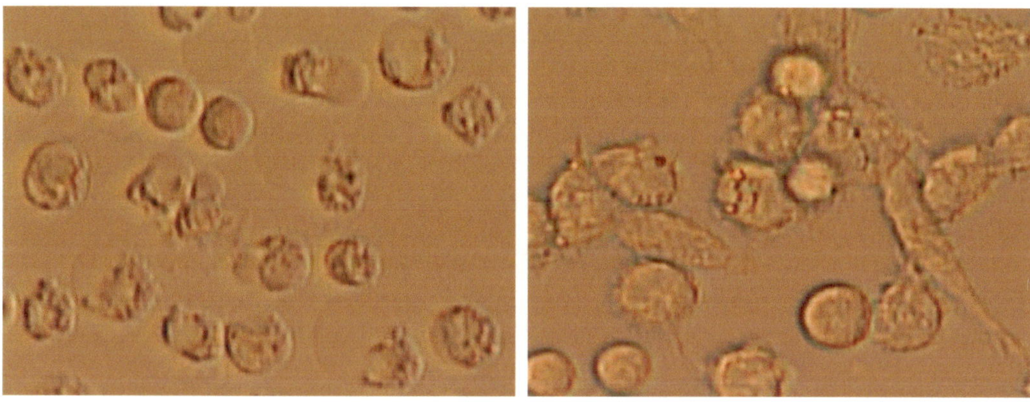

(A) (B)

Fig. 7. Light microscopy image of human monocytes cultured for 24h alone (A) or in the presence of TMV (B)

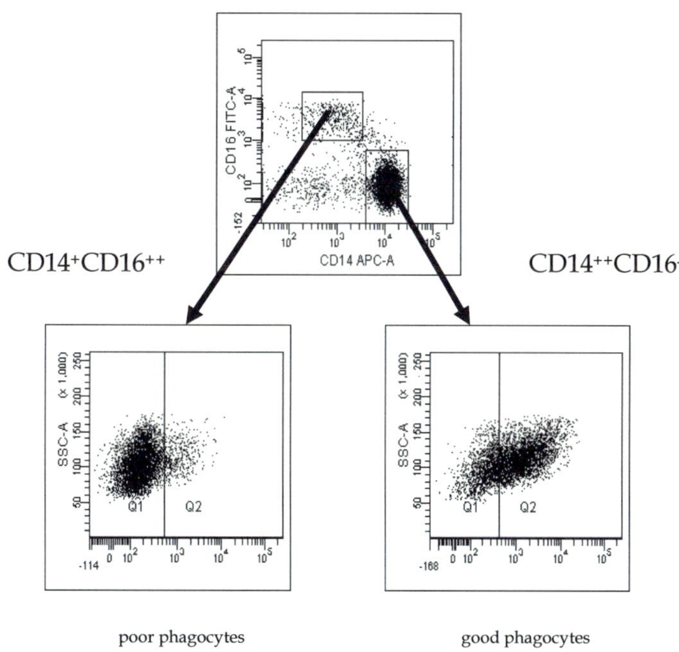

Fig. 8. Engulfment of PKH-labeled TMV by monocyte subpopulations. Flow cytometry analysis of $CD14^{++}CD16^{-}$ (right panel) and $CD14^{+}CD16^{++}$ (left panel) cells exposed to PKH26 labeled-TMV_{HPC} for 18 h followed by quenching of extracellular fluorescence with crystal violet. [Baj-Krzyworzeka et al., 2010, modified]

induce apoptosis of Fas-bearing immune cells [Whiteside, 2005, Abrahams et al., 2003, Bergmann C., et al. 2009]. Suppressive activity of TMV was also described by Szajnik et al. [Szajnik et al., 2010]. In this study, TMV induced generation of Treg and enhanced their expansion. TMV mediate the conversion of CD4+CD25neg T cells into CD4+CD25high FOXp3+ Treg as judged by flow cytometry. Tumor-derived MP derived from melanoma and colorectal carcinoma that expressed TRAIL, are responsible for apoptosis of tumor-specific T cells [Iero M. et al. 2008]. Natural killer (NK) cells upon contact with TMV lose their cytolytic potential through the downregulation of perforin expression [Liu C., et al. 2006]. Blood-derived exosomes from melanoma patients have been shown to promote the generation of myeloid-derived suppressor cells (MDSCs) from peripheral blood monocytes [Frey 2006]. MDSCs have potent immunosuppressive functions that can suppress T cell immune responses by a variety of mechanisms [Soderberg et al., 2006, Liu et al., 2010].

5.3.1 Flow cytometry detection of cytokine and chemokine secretion by monocytes stimulated with TMV

Simultaneous analysis of many parameters/factors in one sample is possible by modern bead-based immunoassays called cytometric bead array. Based on the broad range of fluorescently labeled beads coated with specific capture monoclonal antibodies, the measurement of multiple proteins from a small volume of a single sample, such as serum or culture supernatants became possible. Each bead population in the array has unique fluorescence intensity so the beads can be mixed and run together in one tube. Such systems are accessible from different manufacturers, e.g FlexSet (BD Bioscience) or xMAP (Luminex Corporation) and are compatible with different flow cytometry systems. The FlexSet beads are discriminated in FL-4 (red) and FL-5 (far red) channels, while the concentration of specified proteins, e.g. cytokines are determined by anti-cytokine PE-conjugated detection antibodies to form complexes (Fig. 9). The intensity of FL-2 (orange) fluorescence (due to anti-cytokine PE-conjugated monoclonal antibodies binding) is directly proportional to cytokine concentration in the sample which is calculated from standard curves.

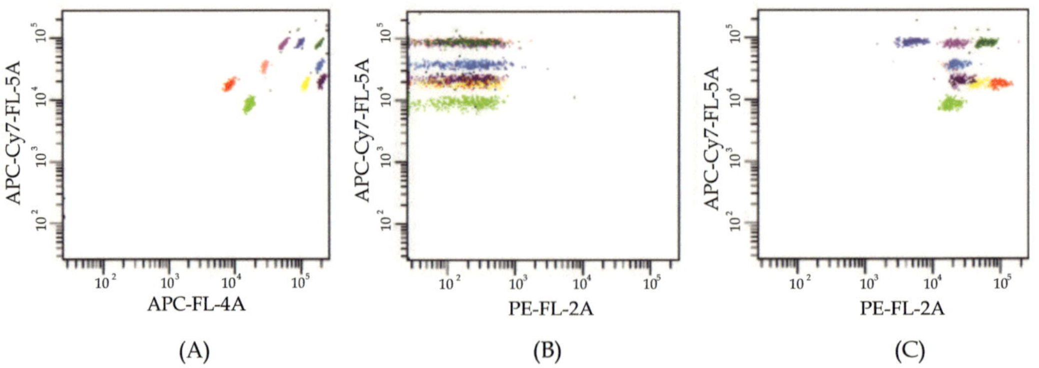

Fig. 9. Flow cytometry bead array analysis of nine different soluble factors. A – beads discrimination according to FL4 and FL5 fluorescence, B- negative control sample, C- positive sample. Analysis performed by FACSCanto flow cytometer

For our purposes we use FlexSet system followed by FACSCanto analysis of chemokine and cytokine secretion by monocytes stimulated with TMV (Fig. 10). This technique is fast and credible, but there are some limitations to this method. For instance, it is difficult to adjust the concentration of all tested parameters in one sample to be in the detection range [Baj-Krzyworzeka et al., 2011].

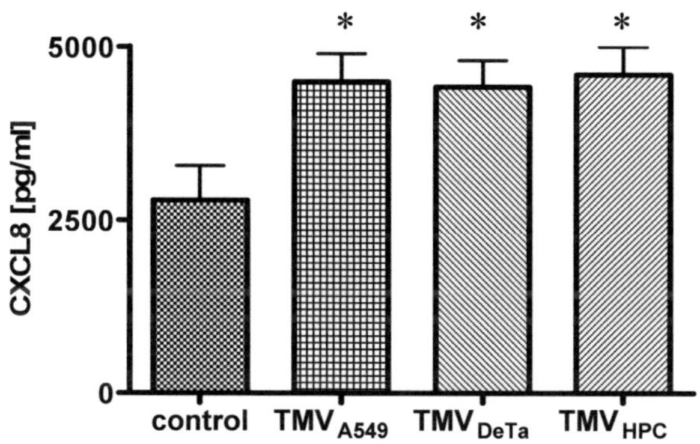

Fig. 10. The secretion of CXCL8 (IL-8) by monocytes cultured alone (control) or stimulated with TMVs after 18 h culture. The level of chemokine in the culture supernatants was determined by FlexSet method. Data (mean±SD) from four independent experiments are presented. *$p<0.05$ compared to the control [Baj-Krzyworzeka et al., 2011, modified]

5.3.2 Intracellular production of reactive oxygen (ROI) and nitrogen (RNI) intermediates measured by flow cytometry

The intracellular production of O_2^- and H_2O_2 may be easily and effectively measured by flow cytometry using oxidation-sensitive fluorescent probes, such as hydroethidine (HE, Sigma) and dihydrorhodamine 123 (DHR123, Sigma), respectively [Baj-Krzyworzeka et al., 2007]. Similarly to tumor cells, TMV induce ROI production by monocytes. Using flow cytometry we were able to establish that $CD14^{++}CD16^{-}$ cells are the major producers of ROI [Baj-Krzyworzeka et al., 2007, 2010].

Production of RNI (NO) may be also assessed by flow cytometry using intracellular staining diaminofluorescein-2 (DAF-2). A significantly higher percentage of DAF-2 positive cells was found among $CD14^{+}CD16^{++}$ cells in comparison to $CD14^{++}CD16^{-}$ cells suggesting that the former are the main producers of NO [Baj-Krzyworzeka et al., 2010].

5.3.3 Chemotactic activity of blood leukocytes induced by TMV measured by flow cytometry

TMV were described to induce chemotaxis of blood leukocytes [Baj-Krzyworzeka et al., 2011], fibroblasts and endothelial cells [Wysoczynski et al., 2009, Castellana et al., 2009]. For non-adherent cells, their chemotactic activity can be measured in Transwell 24-well plates with adequate size (e.g. 5 or 8 μm) pore filter (Costar Corning, Cambridge, MA, USA) followed by flow cytometry analysis. The cells were gated according to their FSC/SSC parameters and counted during a 20 s acquisition period at the high flow rate. Also phenotyping of migrating cells is possible. Data are expressed as the percentage of the cell input corrected by the percentage of cells which migrated spontaneously to the medium. [Baj-Krzyworzeka et al., 2011]. Chemotactic migration of granulocytes, monocytes and lymphocytes to TMVA549 assessed by flow cytometry is presented in Fig. 11.

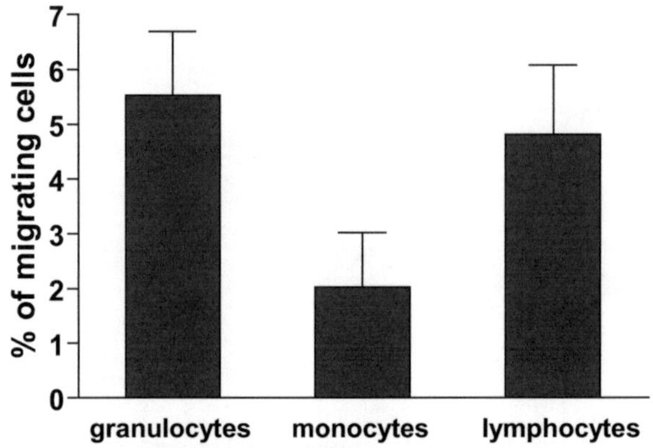

Fig. 11. Chemotaxis of human peripheral blood leukocytes to TMV_{A549} analyzed by Transwell assay followed by flow cytometry counting. Data are expressed as the percentage of the cell input number corrected by the percentage of cells, which migrated spontaneously to the medium alone. Results (mean±SD) from four independent experiments are presented. [Baj-Krzyworzeka et al., 2011 modified]

6. A new perspective in MP studies by flow cytometry

6.1 Future of instrumentation

The inability of conventional flow cytometers to measure objects smaller than 200 nm uncovers a technological gap which results in inadequate information with regards to MP data acquisition [Dragovic et al., 2011, Vasco et al., 2010]. As the MP field is becoming more attractive to the scientific community, with its wide-range applications in many types of medical fields especially, there is a growing interest of companies in the development of appropriate technology that would enable to study the whole spectrum of MP.

At the same time it must be pointed out that even with the resolution adjustments of these flow cytometers the MP fraction of 100 nm and less in size (exosomes) is still undetectable by direct measurement, which only stresses out that there is still room for improvement in this technology. An alternative way to assess MP employs the nanoparticle tracking analysis technology with the size resolution being at app. 50 nm [Dragovic et al., 2011, Vasco et al., 2010]. The principal behind it involves a finely focused laser beam that is introduced to a diluted sample through a glass prism. The laser beam then illuminates the particles in the sample and their images are transmitted through a camera mounted on a microscope onto a computer screen. The result is a short video (a compilation of frame-by-frame images), that is analyzed with appropriate computer software to first identify particles and then track their Brownian movement. The measured velocity of the particle movement is then used in calculating particle size by applying two-dimensional Stokes-Einstein equation. Additionally, this technology enables counting of particles as well as it can be equipped with modules measuring particles zeta potential and fluorescence signals when stained with appropriate antibodies conjugated with different fluorochromes.

6.2 MP as biomarkers

Monitoring of MP (PMP, TMV) level in plasma and other body fluids may be informative for effectiveness of anti-cancer treatment and for prediction of distant metastases. Also, measurement of protein composition of MP (phenotype analysis) may be useful to monitor the efficacy of anti-cancer treatment as therapeutic drugs are expulse from tumor cell *via* MP. Additionally, protein composition of MP might reflect molecular changes in tumor cells.

The whole concept behind studying MP appeared from an idea that they may represent another mode of cell-to-cell communication. The active release of MP by one cell type to another with specific surface determinant composition and internal cargo may have a profound impact on many types of normal and pathological conditions. This form of interpretation of the MP release may explain many phenomena that at present are not well-understood, i.e. angiogenesis, metastasis, M2 polarization of macrophages, etc.

Although the use of MP as biomarkers is not a gold standard, however, a number of reports shows that in certain situations they should be taken under consideration as predictors of various pathological conditions.

There is an increasing evidence that an elevated MP number is associated with certain diseases, which in itself may serve as a feasible predictor. For example, Kim et al. reported that the level of circulating platelet-derived MP is elevated in patients with gastric cancer [Kim et al., 2005]. An increase in MP number was also observed in several cardiovascular pathologies including stroke, hypertension and acute coronary syndromes [VanWijk et al., 2003]. Another group showed that an elevated MP number might be responsible in the development of atherosclerosis [Diamant et al., 2004]. Although most of the data regarding elevated MP numbers comes from platelet-derived MP, which constitute about 80% of the total blood MP population, however, MP may be also generated by other cell. An elevated MP number derived from endothelial cells was observed in arterial stiffness in hemodialysed patients [Amabile et al., 2005]. Fibroblasts were also shown to shed abundant numbers of MP in rheumatoid arthritis [Distlar et al., 2005]. Monitoring of MP levels is not restricted to blood only. Other bodily fluids may also serve as a source of information on elevated MP numbers. For instance, recent discovery of elevated MP numbers present in urine in patients developing acute kidney injury may also point to the usefulness of the MP level monitoring [Zhou et al., 2006]. Also, malignant effusions such as ascites fluids were also shown to have elevated MP numbers [Andre et al., 2002].

Besides the assessment of elevated MP numbers what seems to be even more promising with respect to biomarker monitoring is to try to establish their phenotypic/internal cargo composition and, hopefully, correlate it with appropriate pathological conditions. Tissue factor (TF) (responsible for coagulation) is overexpressed in many types of cancers, i.e. bladder, brain, colon, gastric [Patry et al., 2008, Brat & Van Meir et al., 2004, Hron et al., 2007, Yamashita et al., 2007]. TF^{+} MP were observed in blood of patients with colorectal cancer which were trapped and then fused with the membrane of activated platelets thus propagating and even initiating coagulation which in turn favored tumor cell invasiveness and metastasis [Hron et al., 2007]. Also, MP bearing CD147/extracellular metalloproteinase (MMP) inducer derived from ovarian cancer cells stimulated proangiogenic activities of human umbilical vein endothelial cells (HUVECs) [Millimaggi et al., 2007]. In inflamed and atherosclerotic endothelium, it was shown that platelet-derived MP transported and deposited substantial amounts of RANTES (CCL5) promoting monocyte recruitment [Mause et al., 2005]. Dendritic cell-derived MP (Dex) were shown to deliver peptide-loaded MHC class I/II molecules to naïve DC, which in turn were able to fully stimulate cognate T cells [Krogsgaard & Davis et al., 2005]. Circulating MP have been also reported to be responsible for an inflammatory response in sepsis. It has been shown that they may provoke endothelium inflammation by lysophosphatidic acid and thus stimulating chemotactic migration of platelets/leukocytes to the endothelium. This in turn may lead to the production of monocyte cytokines such as IL-1β, IL-8 and tumor necrosis factor-α resulting in further inflammation enhancement [Mortaza et al., 2009, Lynch & Ludlam, 2007, Gambim et al., 2007]. MV monitoring may be also beneficial in the case of venous thrombosis in cancer patients. Tumor cells (different types of tumors) often are characterized by high procoagulant potential mostly due to the overexpression of surface TF [Ran & Thorpe, 2002, Yu et al., 2005, Dvorak & Rickles, 2006]. Release of TF^{+} MV from the tumor cells into circulation may be the cause of coagulation system activation by generating thrombin which in turn results in the formation and subsequent deposition of fibrin in blood vessels thus creating a favorable niche for metastasis [Rak et al., 2006, Hron et al., 2007, Tesselaar et al., 2007]

Altogether, looking at MP as biomarkers may be useful in a proper assessment of a number of diseases and serve as a feasible explanation of certain biological processes.

7. Conclusion

Flow cytometry should be considered as a method of choice for detection and analysis of MP in biological fluids. Polychromatic flow cytometry analysis, especially, is recommended for establishing a cellular source and antigen composition of analyzed MP. However, for exosomes characterization, standard flow cytometers, due to their detection limits, are not suitable. In this case, some other approaches, such as adsorption of exosomes to anti-tetraspanin coated latex beads, may be introduced thus overcoming limits of currently available instrumentation. In addition to MP analysis, flow cytometry allows enumeration of their numbers in biological samples. This possibility seems to be of importance as absolute numbers of MP may have a clinical relevance in monitoring life threatening diseases such as cancer, sepsis and thrombosis.

8. Acknowledgment

This work was supported by the Polish National Science Centre (NCN, grant no. K/PBW/000784). We wish to thank dr. Kazimierz Weglarczyk for skilful help in preparation of flow cytometry data.

9. References

Abid Hussein, M.N.; Böing, A.N.; Sturk, A.; Hau, C.M. & Nieuwland, R. (2007). Inhibition of microparticle release triggers endothelial cell apoptosis and detachment. *Thromb Haemost*. Vol. 98, No. 5, (November 2007), pp. 1096-1107.

Abrahams, V.M.; Straszewski, S.L.; Kamsteeg, M.; Hanczaruk, B.; Schwartz, P.E.; Rutherford, T.J. & Mor, G. (2003). Epithelial ovarian cancer cells secrete functional Fas ligand. *Cancer Res*, Vol. 63, No. 17, (September 2003), pp. 5573-5581

Aharon, A.; Tamari, T.& Brenner, B. (2008). Monocyte-derived microparticles and exosomes induce procoagulant and apoptotic effects on endothelial cells. *Thromb. Haemost.* Vol. 100, No. 5, (November 2008), pp. 878-885

Al-Nedawi, K.; Meehan, B.; Micallef, J.; Lhotak, V.; May, L.; Guha, A. & Rak, J. (2008). Intercellular transfer of the oncogenic receptor EGFRvIII by microvesicles derived from tumour cells. *Nat Cell Biol*, Vol. 10, No.5, (May 2008), pp. 619-624

Al-Nedawi, K.; Meehan, B. & Rak, J. (2009). Microvesicles: messengers and mediators of tumor progression. *Cell Cycle*. Vol. 8, No. 13, (July 2009), pp. 2014-2018.

Amabile, N.; Guérin, A.P.; Leroyer, A.; Mallat, Z.; Nguyen, C.; Boddaert, .J; London, G.M.; Tedgui, A. & Boulanger. C.M. (2005). Circulating endothelial microparticles are associated with vascular dysfunction in patients with end-stage renal failure. *J Am Soc Nephrol*. Vol. 16, No. 11, (November 2005), pp. 3381-3388.

André, F.; Schartz, N.E.; Chaput, N.; Flament, C.; Raposo, G.; Amigorena, S.; Angevin, E. & Zitvogel, L. (2002). Tumor-derived exosomes: a new source of tumor rejection antigens. *Vaccine*. 2002 Dec 19Vol. 20, Suppl 4, (December 2002), pp. A28-31.

Andreola, G.; Rivoltini, L.; Castelli, C.; Huber, V.; Perego, P.; Deho, P.; Squarcina, P.; Accornero, P.; Lozupone, F.; Lugini, L.; Stringaro, A.; Molinari, A.; Arancia, G.; Gentile, M.; Parmiani, G. & Fais, S. (2002). Induction of lymphocyte apoptosis by tumor cell secretion of FasL-bearing microvesicles. *J Exp Med*, Vol. 195, No. 10, (May 2002), pp. 1303-1316

Ayers, L.; Kohler, M.; Harrison, P.; Sargent, I.; Dragovic, R.; Schaap, M.; Nieuwland, R.; Brooks, S.A. & Ferry, B. (2011). Measurement of circulating cell-derived microparticles by flow cytometry: sources of variability within the assay. *Thromb. Res*, Vol. 127, No. 4, (April 2011), pp. 370-377.

Baj-Krzyworzeka, M.; Baran, J.; Weglarczyk, K.; Szatanek, R.; Szaflarska, A.; Siedlar, M. & Zembala, M. (2010) Tumour-derived microvesicles (TMV) mimic the effect of tumour cells on monocyte subpopulations. *Anticancer Res*, Vol. 30, No. 9, (September 2010), pp. 3515-3519.

Baj-Krzyworzeka, M.; Majka, M.; Prawico, D.; Ratajczak, J.; Vilaire, G.; Kijowski, J.; Reca, R.; Janowska-Wieczorek, A. & Ratajczak,M.Z. (2002). Platelet-derived microparticles stimulate proliferation, survival, adhesion and chemotaxis of hematopoietic cells. *Exp Hematol*, Vol.30, No.5 (May 2002), pp. 450-459.

Baj-Krzyworzeka, M.; Szatanek, R.; Weglarczyk, K.; Baran, J. & Zembala, M. (2007). Tumour-derived microvesicles modulate biological activity of human monocytes. *Immunol Lett*, Vol. 113, No. 2, (November 2007), pp. 76-82

Baj-Krzyworzeka, M.; Szatanek, R.; Weglarczyk, K.; Baran, J.; Urbanowicz, B.; Brański, P.; Ratajczak, M.Z. & Zembala, M. (2006). Tumour-derived microvesicles carry several surface determinants and mRNA of tumour cells and transfer some of these determinants to monocytes. *Cancer Immunol Immunother*, Vol. 55, No. 7, (November 2005), pp. 808-818

Baj-Krzyworzeka, M.; Weglarczyk, K.; Mytar, B.; Szatanek, R.; Baran, J. & Zembala, M. (2011). Tumour-derived microvesicles contain interleukin-8 and modulate production of chemokines by human monocytes. *Anticancer Res*. Vol. 31, No. 4, (April 2011), pp. 1329-1335.

Baran, J.; Baj-Krzyworzeka, M.; Weglarczyk, K.; Szatanek, R.; Zembala, M.; Barbasz, J.; Czupryna, A.; Szczepanik, A. & Zembala, M. (2010). Circulating tumour- derived microvesicles in plasma of gastric cancer patients. *Cancer Immunol Immunother*, Vol. 59, No. 6, (June 2010), pp. 841-850

Barry, O.P.; Pratico, D.; Lawson, J.A. & FitzGerald, G.A. (1997). Transcellular activation of platelets and endothelial cells by bioactive lipids in platelet microparticles. *J Clin Invest*, Vol. 99, No. 9, (may 1997), pp. 2118-2127.

Barry, O.P.; Pratico, D.; Saavani, R.C. & FitzGerald, G.A. (1998) Modulation of monocyte-endothelial cell interactions by platelet microparticles. *J Clin Invest*, Vol. 102, No. 1, (July 1998), pp. 136-144

Becker, C.K.; Parker, J.W.; Hechinger, M.K.; Leif, R. (2002). Is forward scatter monotonic on commercial flow cytometers? Poster presented at the ISAC XXI Congress, San Diego, CA, (May 2002).

Bergmann, C.; Strauss, L.; Wieckowski, E.; Czystowska, M.; Albers, A.; Wang, Y.; Zeidler, R.; Lang, S. & Whiteside, T.L. (2009). Tumor-derived microvesicles in sera of patients with head and neck cancer and their role in tumor progression. *Head Neck*, Vol. 31, No. 3, (March 2009), pp. 371-380.

Boilard, E.; Nigrovic, P.A; Larabee, K.; Watts, G.F.; Coblyn, J.S.; Weinblatt, M.E.; Massarotti, E.M.; Remold-O'Donnell, E.; Farndale, R.W.; Ware, J. & Lee, D.M. (2010). Platelets amplify inflammation in arthritis via collagen-dependent microparticle production. *Science*, Vol. 327, No. 5965, (January 2010), pp. 580-583

Borsig, L., Wong, R., Feramisco, J., Nadeau, D.R., Varki, N.M. & Varki, A. (2001). Heparin and cancer revisited: mechanistic connections involving platelets, P-selectin, carcinoma mucins, and tumor metastasis. *Proc Natl Acad Sci U S A*. Vol. 98, No. 6, (March 2001), pp. 3352-3357.

Boulanger, C.M.; Amabile, N. & Tedgui, A.(2006). Circulating microparticles: a new potential prognostic marker for atherosclerotic vascular disease. *Hypertension*, Vol.48, No. 2, (August 2006), pp. 180-186.

Brat, D.J. & Van Meir, E.G. (2004). Vaso-occlusive and prothrombotic mechanisms associated with tumor hypoxia, necrosis, and accelerated growth in glioblastoma. *Lab Invest*. Vol. 84, No. 4, (April 2004), pp. 397-405.

Brodsky, S.V.; Facciuto, M.E.; Heydt, D.; Chen, J.; Islam, H.K.; Kajstura, M.; Ramaswamy, G. & Aguero-Rosenfeld, M. (2008). Dynamics of circulating microparticles in liver transplant patients. *J Gastrointestin Liver Dis*, Vol. 17, No. 3, (September 2008), pp. 261-268

Caby, M.P.; Lankar, D.; Vincendeau-Scherrer, C.; Raposo, G.; Bonnerot, C. (2005). Exosomal-like vesicles are present in human blood plasma. *Int Immunol*. Vol. 17, No. 7, (July 2005), pp.879-87.

Camussi, G.; Bussolino, F.; Salvidio, G. & Baglioni, C. (1987). Tumor necrosis factor/cachectin stimulates peritoneal macrophages, polymorphonuclear neutrophils, and vascular endothelial cells to synthesize and release platelet-activating factor. *J Exp Med*. Vol. 166, No. 5, (November 1987), pp. 1390-1404.

Camussi, G.; Deregibus, M.C.; Bruno, S.; Cantaluppi, V. & Biancone, L. (2010). Exosomes/microvesicles as a mechanism of cell-to-cell communication. *Kidney Int*. Vol. 78, No. 9 (November 2010), pp. 838-848.

Castaman, G.; Yu-Feng, L. & Rodeghiero, F. (1996) A bleeding disorder characterized by isolated deficiency of platelet microvesicle generation. *Lancet*, Vol. 347, No. 9002 (March 1996), pp. 700-701

Castellana, D., Zobairi, F., Martinem, M.C., Panaro, M.A., Mitolo, V., Freyssinet, J.M. & Kunzelmann, C. (2009). Membrane microvesicles as actors in the establishment of a favorable prostatic tumoral niche: a role for activated fibroblasts and CX3CL1-CX3CR1 axis. *Cancer Res.* Vol. 69, No. 3, (Februery 2009), pp.:785-793.

Chandler, W.L.; Yeung, W.; Tait, J.F. (2011). A new microparticle size calibration standard for use in measuring smaller microparticles using a new flow cytometer. *J Thromb Haemost.* Vol. 9, No. 6. (June 2011), pp.1216-24.

Chen, C.; Skog, J.; Hsu, C.H.; Lessard, R.T.; Balaj, L.; Wurdinger, T.; Carter, B.S.; Breakefield, X.O.; Toner, M. & Irimia, D. (2010). Microfluidic isolation and transcriptome analysis of serum microvesicles. *Lab Chip*. Vol. 10, No. 4, (February 2010), pp. 505-511.

Cheng, X.; Irimia, D.; Dixon, M.; Sekine, K.; Demirci, U.; Zamir, L.; Tompkins, R.G.; Rodriguez, W. & Toner, M. (2007). Microfluidic device for practical label-free CD4(+) T cell counting of HIV-infected subjects. *Lab Chip*. Vol. 7, No. 2, (February 2007), pp. 170-178.

Choi, D.S.; Park, J.O.; Jang, S.C.; Yoon, Y.J.; Jung, J.W.; Choi, D.Y.; Kim, J.W.; Kang, J.S.; Park, J.; Hwang, D.; Lee, K.H.; Park, S.H.; Kim, Y.K.; Desiderio, D.M.; Kim, K.P. & Gho, Y.S. (2011). Proteomic analysis of microvesicles derived from human colorectal cancer ascites. *Proteomics*, Vol. 11, No. 13, (July 2011), pp. 2745-2751

Choi, S.; Ku, T.; Song, S.; Choi, C. & Park, J.K. (2011). Hydrophoretic high-throughput selection of platelets in physiological shear-stress range. *Lab Chip*. Vol. 11, No. 3, (February 2011), pp. 413-418.

Dean, W.L.; Lee, M.J.; Cummins, T.D.; Schultz, D.J. & Powell, D.W. (2009). Proteomic and functional characterization of platelet microparticle size classes. *Thromb Haemost*, Vol. 102, No. 4, (October 2009), pp. 711-718

Del Conde, I.; Shrimpton, C.N.; Thiagarajan, P. & López, J.A. (2005). Tissue-factor-bearing microvesicles arise from lipid rafts and fuse with activated platelets to initiate coagulation. *Blood*. Vol. 106, No. 5, (September 2005), pp. 1604-1611.

Dey-Hazra, E.; Hertel, B.; Kirsch, T.; Woywodt, A.; Lovric, S.; Haller, H.; Haubitz, M. & Erdbruegger, U. (2010). Detection of circulating microparticles by flow cytometry: influence of centrifugation, filtration of buffer, and freezing. *Vasc Health Risk Manag*. Vol. 6, No. 6, (December 2010), pp. 1125-1133.

Diamant, M.; Tushuizen, M.E.; Sturk, A. & Nieuwland, R. (2004). Cellular microparticles: new players in the field of vascular disease? *Eur J Clin Invest*. Vol. 34, No. 6, (June 2004), pp. 392-401.

Distler, J.H.; Pisetsky, D.S.; Huber, L.C.; Kalden, J.R.; Gay, S. & Distler, O. (2005). Microparticles as regulators of inflammation: novel players of cellular crosstalk in the rheumatic diseases. *Arthritis Rheum*. Vol. 52, No. 11, (November 2005), pp. 3337-3348.

Dolo, V.; Adobati, E.; Canevari, S.; Picone, M.A. & Vittorelli, M.L. (1995). Membrane vesicles shed into the extracellular medium by human breast carcinoma cells carry tumor-associated surface antigens. *Clin Exp Metastasis*, Vol. 13, No.4 , (July 1995), pp.277-286

Dragovic, R.A.; Gardiner, C.; Brooks, A.S.; Tannetta, D.S.; Ferguson, D.J.; Hole, P.; Carr, B.; Redman, C.W.; Harris, A.L.; Dobson, P.J.; Harrison, P. & Sargent IL. (2011). Sizing and phenotyping of cellular vesicles using Nanoparticle Tracking Analysis. *Nanomedicine.* Vol. 7, No. 6, (December 2011), pp. 780-788.

Dumaswala, U.J. & Greenwalt, T.J. (1984). Human erythrocytes shed exocytic vesicles in vivo. *Transfusion.* Vol. 24, No. 6, (December 1984), pp. 490-492.

Dvorak, F.H. & Rickles, F.R. (2006). Malignancy and Hemostasis. In: Coleman RB, Marder VJ, Clowes AW, George JN, Goldhaber SZ, editors. Hemostasis and thrombosis: basic principles and clinical practice. 5th ed. Philadelphia: Lippincott CompanyWilliams & Wilkins. (2006), pp. 851–873.

Fadlon, E.J.; Rees, R.C.; McIntyre, C.; Sharrard, R.M.; Lawry, J. And Hamdy, F.C. (1996). Detection of circulating prostate-specific antigen positive cells in patients with prostate cancer by flow cytometry and reverse transcription polymerase chain reaction. *Br J Cancer.* Vol. 74, No. 3, (August 1996), pp.400-405.

Flaumenhaft, R.; Bilks, J.R.; Richardson, J.; Alden, E.; Patel-Hett, S.R.; Battinelli, E.; Klement, G.L; Sola-Visner, M. & Italiano, J.E.Jr. (2009). Megakaryocyte-derived microparticles: direct visualization and distinction from platelet-derived microparticles. *Blood* Vol. 113, No. 5, pp. 1112-1121.

Flaumenhaft, R.; Mairuhu, A.T. & Italiano, J.E.Jr. (2010). Platelet-and megakaryocyte-derived microparticles. *Semin Thromb Hemost.* Vol. 36, No. 8, pp. 881-887.

Forlow, S.B.; McEver, R.P. & Nollert, M.U. (2000) Leukocyte-leukocyte interactions mediated by platelet microparticles under flow. *Blood* Vol. 95, No.4, (February 2000), pp. 1317-1323.

Frey, A.B. (2006). Myeloid suppressor cells regulate the adaptive immune response to cancer. *J Clin Invest* Vol. 116, No. 10, (October 2006), pp. 2587–2590

Friedl, P.; Maaser, K.; Klein, C.E.; Niggemann, B.; Krohne, G. & Zänker, K.S. (1997). Migration of highly aggressive MV3 melanoma cells in 3-dimensional collagen lattices results in local matrix reorganization and shedding of alpha2 and beta1 integrins and CD44. *Cancer Res,* Vol. 57, No. 10, (May 1997), pp. 2061-2070

Fritzsching, B.; Schwer, B.; Kartenbeck, J.; Pedal, A.; Horejsi, V. & Ott, M. (2002). Release and intercellular transfer of cell surface CD81 via microparticles. *J Immunol,* Vol. 169, No. 10, (November 2002), pp. 5531-5537

Gambim, M.H.; do Carmo Ade, O.; Marti, L.; Veríssimo-Filho, S.; Lopes, L.R. & Janiszewski, M. (2007). Platelet-derived exosomes induce endothelial cell apoptosis through peroxynitrite generation: experimental evidence for a novel mechanism of septic vascular dysfunction. *Crit Care.* Vol. 11, No. 5, (September 2007), pp. R107.

Gaser, O.; Hess, C.; Miot, S.; Deon, C.; Sanchez, J.C. & Schifferli, J.A. (2003) Characterisation and properties of ectosomes released by human polymorphonclear neutrophils. *Exp Cell Res,* Vol. 285, No. 2, (May 2003), pp. 243-257.

Gelderman, M.P. & Simak, J. (2008). Flow cytometric analysis of cell membrane microparticles. *Methods Mol Biol.* Vol. 484, pp.79-93.

George, J.N.; Thoi, L.L.; McManus, L.M. & Reimann, T.A. (1982). Isolation of human platelet membrane microparticles from plasma and serum. *Blood,* Vol. 60, No. 4 (October 1982), pp. 834-840.

Ginestra, A.; La Placa, M.D.; Saladino, F.; Cassarà, D.; Nagase, H. & Vittorelli, M.L. (1998). The amount and proteolytic content of vesicles shed by human cancer cell lines correlates with their in vitro invasiveness. *Anticancer Res.* Vol. 18, No. 5A, (October 1998), pp. 3433-3437.

Grant, R.; Ansa-Addo, E.; Stratton, D.; Antwi-Baffour, S.; Jori, S.; Kholia, S.; Krige, L.; Lange, S. & Inal, J.; (2011) A filtration-based protocol to isolate human plasma membrane-derived vesicles and exosomes from blood plasma.. *J Immunol Methods,* Vol. 371, No. 1-2, (August 2011), pp. 143-151.

Heijnen, H.F.; Schiel, A.E.; Fijnheer, R.; Geuze, H.K. & Sixma, J.J. (1999). Activated platelets release two types of membrane vesicles: microvesicles by surface shedding and exosomes derived from exocytosis of multivesicular bodies and alpha-granules. *Blood,* Vol. 94, No. 11, pp.3791-3799.

Hejna, M., Raderer, M. & Zieliński, C.C. (1999) Inhibition of metastases by anticoagulants. *J Natl Cancer Inst.* Vol. 91, No 1, (January 1999), pp.22-36

Hess, C.; Sadallah, S.; Hefti,A.; Landmann,R. & Schifferli, J.A. (1999) Ectosomes released by human neutrophils are specialized functional units. *J Immunol.* Vol. 163, No. 8, (October 1999), pp. 4564-4573.

Holme, P.A.; Orvim, U.; Hamers, M.J.; Solum, N.O.; Brosstad, F.R.; Barstad, R.M. & Sakariassen, K.S. (1997). Shear-induced platelet activation and platelet microparticle formation at blood flow conditions as in arteries with a severe stenosis. *Arterioscler Thomb Vasc Biol* Vol, 17, No. 4. pp. 646-653.

Holme, P.A.; Solum, N.O.; Brosstas, F.; Roger, M. & Abdelnoor, M. (1994). Demonstration of platelet derived microvesicles in blood from patients with activated coagulation and fibrinolysis using a filtration technique and western blotting. *Thromb Haemost.,* Vol. 72, No. 5, pp. 666-671.

Holmes, D.; She, J.K.; Roach, P.L. & Morgan, H. (2007).Bead-based immunoassays using a micro-chip flow cytometer. *Lab Chip.* Vol. 7, No.8, (August 2007),pp. 1048-1056.

Holmes, D.; She, J.K.; Roach, P.L.; Morgan, H. (2007). Bead-based immunoassays using a micro-chip flow cytometer. Lab Chip. Vol. 7, No. 8, (August 2007), pp.1048-56.

Hood, J.L.; San, R.S. & Wickline, S.A.(2011). Exosomes released by melanoma cells prepare sentinel lymph nodes for tumor metastasis. *Cancer Res.* Vol. 71, No. 11 (June 2011),pp. 3792-3801

Horstman, L.L. & Ahn,Y.S. (1999). Platelet microparticles : a wide-angle perspective. *Crit Rev Oncol Hematol,* Vol 30, No. 2 (April 1999), pp. 111-142.

Horstman, L.L.; Jy, W.; Schultz, D.R.; Mao, W.W. and Ahn, Y.S. (1994). Complement-mediated fragmentation and lysis of opsonized platelets: ender differences in sensitivity. J Lab Clin Med. Vol. 123, No. 4, (April 1994), pp.515-525.

Hron, G.; Kollars, M.; Weber, H.; Sagaster, V.; Quehenberger, P.; Eichinger, S.; Kyrle, P.A. & Weltermann, A. (2007). Tissue factor-positive microparticles: cellular origin and association with coagulation activation in patients with colorectal cancer. *Thromb Haemost.* Vol. 97, No. 1, (January 2007), pp. 119-123

Hsu, C.H.; Di Carlo, D.; Chen, C.; Irimia, D. & Toner, M. (2008). Microvortex for focusing, guiding and sorting of particles. *Lab Chip.* 2008. Vol. 8, No. 12, (December 2008), pp. 2128-2134.

Huber, V.; Fais, S.; Iero, M.; Lugini, L.; Canese, P.; Squarcina, P.; Zaccheddu, A.; Colone, M.; Arancia, G.; Gentile, M.; Seregni, E.; Valenti, R.; Ballabio, G.; Belli, F.; Leo, E.; Parmiani, G. & Rivoltini, L. (2005). Human colorectal cancer cells induce T-cell death through release of proapoptotic microvesicles: role in immune escape. *Gastroenterology.* 2005 Jun;Vol. 128, No. 7, (June 2005), pp. 1796-1804.

Janowska-Wieczorek, A.; Wysoczynski, M.; Kijowski, J.; Marquez-Curtis, L.; Machalinski, B.; Ratajczak, J. & Ratajczak, M.Z. (2005). Microvesicles derived from activated platelets induce metastasis and angiogenesis in lung cancer. *Int J Cancer*, Vol. 113, No.5, (February 2005), pp. 752-760

Janowska-Wieczorek, A.; Majka, M.; Kijowski, J.; Baj-Krzyworzeka, M.; Reca, R.; Turner, A.R.; Ratajczak, J.; Emerson, S.G.; Kowalska, M.A. & Ratajczak, M.Z. (2001). Platelet-derived microparticles bind to hematopoietic stem/progenitor cells and enhance their engraftment. *Blood* Vol. 98, No.10, (November 2001), pp. 3143-3149.

Jy, W.; Horstman, L.L.; Jimenez, J.J.; Ahn, Y.S.; Biró, E.; Nieuwland, R.; Sturk, A.; Dignat-George, F.; Sabatier, F.; Camoin-Jau, L.; Sampol, J.; Hugel, B.; Zobairi, F.; Freyssinet, J.M.; Nomura, S.; Shet, A.S.; Key, N.S. and Hebbel, R.P. (2004). Measuring circulating cell-derived microparticles. J Thromb Haemost. Vol. 2, No. 10, (October 2004), pp. 1842-51.

Jy, W.; Mao, W.W.; Horstman, L.; Tao, J. & Ahn, Y.S. (1995). Platelet microparticles bind, activate and aggregate neutrophils in vitro. *Blood Cells Mol Dis*, Vol. 21, No. 3, pp. 217-231

Keller, S.; Ridinger, J.; Rupp, A.K.; Janssen, J.W. & Altevogt, P. (2011). Body fluid derived exosomes as a novel template for clinical diagnostics. *J Transl Med.* Vol. 8, No. 9, (June 2011), pp. 86.

Kim, H.K.; Song, K.S.; Park, Y.S.; Kang, Y.H.; Lee, Y.J.; Lee, K,R.; Kim, H.K.; Ryu, K.W.; Bae, J.M. & Kim, S. (2003). Elevated levels of circulating platelet microparticles, VEGF, IL-6 and RANTES in patients with gastric cancer: possible role of a metastasis predictor. *Eur J Cancer* , Vol. 39, No. 2 (January 2003), pp. 184-191

Kim, H.K.; Song, K.S.; Chung, J.H.; Lee, K.R & Lee, S.N. (2005). Platelet microparticles induce angiogenesis in vitro. *Br J Haematol*, Vol. 124, No. 3, (February 2005), pp. 752-760

Kim, H.K.; Song, K.S.; Lee, E.S.; Lee, Y.J.; Park, Y.S.; Lee, K.R. & Lee, S.N. (2002). Optimized flow cytometric assay for the measurement of platelet microparticles in plasma: pre-analytic and analytic considerations. *Blood Coagul Fibrinolysis*, Vol. 13, No. 5, pp. 393-397.

Kim, J.S. & Ligler, F.S. (2010). Utilization of microparticles in next-generation assays for microflow cytometers. *Anal Bioanal Chem.* Vol. 398, No. 6, (November 2010), pp. 2373-2382

Kolowos, W.; Gajpl, U.S.; Sheriff, A.; Voll, R.E.; Hevder, P.; Kern, P.; Kalden, J.R. & Herrmann, M. (2005). Microparticles shed from different antigen-presenting cells display an individual pattern of surface molecules and a distinct potential of allogeneic T-cell activation. *Scand J Immunol*, Vol.61, (March 2005), No.3, pp.226-233.

Krogsgaard, M & Davis, M.M. (2005). How T cells 'see' antigen. *Nat Immunol.* Vol. 6, No. 3, (March 2005), pp. 239-245.

Lacroix, R.; Robert, S.; Poncelet, P.; Kasthuri, R.S.; Key, N.S. & Dignat-George F. (2010). Standarization of platelet-derived microparticle enumeration by flow cytometry with calibrated beads: results of the International Society on Thrombosis and Haemostasis SSC Collaborative workshop. *J Thromb Haemost*, Vol. 8, No 11, (November 2010), pp. 2571-2574.

Lamparski, H.G.; Metha-Damani, A.; Yao, J.Y.; Patel, S.; Hsu, D.H.; Ruegg, C. & Le Pecq, J.B. (2002). Production and characterization of clinical grade exosomes derived from dendritic cells. *J Immunol Methods.* Vol. 270, No. 2, (December 2002), pp. 211-226.

Liu, Y.; Xiang, X.; Zhuang, X.; Zhang, S.; Liu, C.; Cheng, Z.; Michalek, S.; Grizzle, W. & Zhang, H.G. (2010). Contribution of MyD88 to the tumor exosome-mediated induction of myeloid derived suppressor cells. *Am J Pathol* Vol. 176, No.5, (May 2010), pp. 2490–2499

Lynch, S.F. & Ludlam, C.A. (2007). Plasma microparticles and vascular disorders. *Br J Haematol.* Vol. 137, No. 1, (April 2007), pp. 36-48.

Mack, M.; Kleinschmidt, A.; Brühl, H.; Klier, C.; Nelson, P.J.; Cihak, J.; Plachý, J.; Stangassinger, M.; Erfle, V. & Schlöndorff, D. (2000). Transfer of the chemokine receptor CCR5 between cells by membrane-derived microparticles: a mechanism for cellular human immunodeficiency virus 1 infection. *Nat Med*, Vol. 6, No. 7, (July 2000), pp. 769-775

Mallat, Z.: Hugel, B.; Ohan, J.; Leseche, G.; Freyssinet, J.M.& Tedgui, A. (1999). Shed membrane microparticles with procoagulant potential in human atherosclerotic plaques: a role for apoptosis in plaque thrombogenicity. *Circulation*, Vol. 99, No. 3, (January 1999), pp. 348-353.

Matsumoto, N.; Nomura, S.; Kamihata, H.; Kimura, Y. & Iwasaka, T. (2004) Increased level of oxidized LDL-dependent monocyte-derived microparticles in acute coronary syndrome. *Thromb Haemost*, Vol. 91, No. 1, (January 2004), pp. 146-154.

Matzdorff, A.C.; Kuhnel, G.; Kemkes-Matthes, B. & Pralle, H. (1998). Quantitative assessment of plateletsm platelet microparticles, and platelet aggregates with flow cytometry. *J Lab Clin Med*, Vol. 131, No. 6, pp. 507-517.

Mause, S.F.; von Hundelshausen, P.; Zernecke, A.; Koenen, R.R & Weber,C. (2005). Platelet microparticles; a transcellular delivery system for RANTES promoting monocyte recruitment on endothelium. *Arterioscler Thromb Vasc Biol*, Vol. 25, No, 7, (May 2005), pp. 1512-1518.

Mesri, M. & Altieri, D.C. (1999). Leukocyte microparticles stimulate endothelial cell cytokine release and tissue factor induction in a JNK1 signaling pathway. *J Biol Chem*, Vol. 274, No. 33 (August 1999), pp. 23111-23118.

Michelsen, A. E.; Brodin, E.; Brosstad, F. & Hansen, J.B. (2008). Increased level of platelet microparticles in survivors of myocardial infarction. *Scand J Clin Lab Invest*. Vol. 68, No. 5, pp. 386-392.

Michelson, A.D.; Barnard, M.R.; Krueger, L.A.; Frelinger, A.L. 3ed & Furman, M.I. (2000) Evaluation of platelet function by flow cytometry. *Methods*, Vol. 21, No. 3, (July 2000), pp. 259-270.

Millimaggi, D.; Mari, M.; D'Ascenzo, S.; Carosa, E.; Jannini, E.A.; Zucker, S.; Carta, G.; Pavan, A. & Dolo, V. (2007). Tumor vesicle-associated CD147 modulates the angiogenic capability of endothelial cells. *Neoplasia*. Vol. 9, No. 4, (April 2007), pp. 349-57.

Montecalvo, A.; Shufesky, W.J.; Stolz, D.B.; Sullivan, M.G.; Wang, Z.; Divito, S.J.; Papworth, G.D.; Watkins, S.C.; Robbins P.D.; Larregina, A.T. & Morelli, A.E. (2008). Exosomes as a short-range mechanism to spread alloantigen between dendritic cells during T cell allorecognition. *J Immunol* 180:3081–3090

Mortaza, S.; Martinez, M.C.; Baron-Menguy, C.; Burban, M.; de la Bourdonnaye, M.; Fizanne, L.; Pierrot, M.; Calès, P.; Henrion, D.; Andriantsitohaina, R.; Mercat, A.; Asfar, P. & Meziani, F. (2009). Detrimental hemodynamic and inflammatory effects of microparticles originating from septic rats. *Crit Care Med.* Vol. 37, No. 6, (June 2009), pp. 2045-2050.

Muralidharan-Chari, V.; Clancy, J.W.; Sedgwick, A. & D'Souza-Schorey C. (2010). Microvesicles: mediators of extracellular communication during cancer progression. *J Cell Sci*, Vol.123, No. 10, (May 2010), pp. 1603-1611

Nebe-von-Caron, G. (2011). www.cyto.purdue.edu/hmarchive, Purdue Cytometry Discussion List, (November 3rd, 2011).

Nebe-von-Caron, G. (2009). Standardization in microbial cytometry. Cytometry Part A. Vol. 75, No. 2, (February 2009), pp.86-89.

Nieuwland, R.; Berckmans, R.J.; McGregor, S.; Boing, A.N.; Romijn, F.P.; Westendrop, R.G.; Hack, C.E. & Sturk, A. (2000). Cellular origin and procoagulant properties of microparticles in meningococcal sepsis. *Blood*, Vol. 95, No. 3, (February 2000), pp. 930-935.

Nomura, S.; Suzuki, M., Katsura, K.; Xie, G.L.; Miyazaki, Y.; Kido, H.; Kagawa, H. & Fukuhara, S. (1995). Platelet-derived microparticles may influence the development of athrosclerosis in diabetes mellitus. *Athrosclerosis*, Vol. 116, No. 2, (August 1995), pp. 235-240.

Nomura, S.; Suzuki, M.; Kido, H.; Yamaguchi, K.; Fukuroi, T.; Yanabu, M.; Soga, T.; Nagata, H.; Kokawa, T. & Yasunaga, K. (1992). Differences between platelet and microparticle glycoprotein IIb/IIIa. *Cytometry*, Vol. 13, No. 6, pp.:621-629.

Orozco, A.F. & Lewis, D.E. (2010). Flow cytometric analysis of circulating microparticles in plasma. *Cytometry A*, Vol.77, No.6, (June 2010), pp. 502-514.

Patry, G.; Hovington, H.; Larue, H.; Harel, F.; Fradet, Y. & Lacombe, L. (2008). Tissue factor expression correlates with disease-specific survival in patients with node-negative muscle-invasive bladder cancer. *Int J Cancer*. Vol. 122, No. 7, (April 2008), pp. 1592-1597.

Pilzer, D.; Gasser, O.; Moskovich, O.; Schifferli, J.A. & Fishelson, Z. (2005). Emission of membrane vesicles: roles in complement resistance, immunity and cancer. *Springer Semin Immunopathol*. Vol. 27, No. 3, (November 2005), pp. 375-387.

Prado, N., Cañamero, M., Villalba, M., Rodríguez, R. & Batanero, E. (2010) Bystander suppression to unrelated allergen sensitization through intranasal administration of tolerogenic exosomes in mouse. (2010) *Mol Immunol*, Vol. 47, No. 11-12, (July 2010), pp. 2148–2151

Prokopi, M.; Pula, G.; Mayr, U.; Devue, C.; Gallagher, J.; Xiao, Q.; Boulanger, C.M.; Westwood, N.; Urbich, C.; Willeit, J.; Steiner, M.; Breuss, J.; Xu, Q.; Kiechl, S. & Mayr, M. (2009). Proteomic analysis reveals presence of platelet microparticles in endothelial progenitor cell cultures. *Blood* Vol. 114, No. 3, (April 2009), pp. 723-732

Rajasekhar, D.; Kestin, A.S.; Bednarek, F.J.; Ellis, P.A.; Barnard, M.R. & Michelson, A.D. (1994). Neonatal platelets are less reactive than adult platelets to physiological agonists in whole blood. *Thromb Haemost*.Vol. 72, No. 6, (December 1994), pp.957-963.

Rak, J. (2010). Microparticles in cancer. *Semin Thromb Hemost*. Vol. 36, No. 8, (November 2010), pp. 888-906.

Rak, J.; Yu, J.L.; Luyendyk, J. & Mackman, N. (2006) Oncogenes, Trousseau syndrome, and cancer-related changes in the coagulome of mice and humans. *Cancer Res*. Vol. 66, No. 22, (November 2006), pp. 10643–10646.

Ran, S. & Thorpe, PE. (2002). Phosphatidylserine is a marker of tumor vasculature and a potential target for cancer imaging and therapy. *Int J Radiat Oncol Biol Phys*. Vol 54, No. 5, (December 2002), pp. 1479–1484.

Raposo, G.; Nijman, H.W.; Stooryogel, W.; Liejendekker, R.; Harding, C.V.; Melief, C.J. & Geuze, H.J. (1996) B lymphocytes secrete antigen-presenting vesicles. *J Exp Med*, Vol. 183, No. 3 (March 1996), pp. 1161-1172.

Ratajczak, J.; Wysoczynski, M.; Hayek, F.; Janowska-Wieczorek, A. & Ratajczak, M.Z. (2006). Membrane-derived microvesicles: important and underappreciated mediators of cel-to-cell communication. *Leukemia*, Vol. 20, No. 9, (September 2006), pp. 1487-1495

Robert, S.; Poncelet, P.; Lacroix, R.; Arnaud, L.; Giraudo, L.; Hauchard, A.; Sampol, J. & Dignat-George, F. (2009). Standarization of platelet- derived microparticle counting using calibrated beads and a Cytomics FC500 routine flow cytometer: a first step towards multicenter studies? *J Thromb Haemost*, Vol. 7, No. 1, pp. 190-197.

Rozmysłowicz, T.; Majka, M.; Kijowski, J.; Murphy, S.L.; Conover, D.O.; Poncz, M.; Ratajczak, J.; Gaulton, G.N. & Ratajczak, M.Z. (2003). Platelet and megakaryocyte-derivedd microparticles transfer CXCR4 receptor to CXCR4-null cells and make then susceptible to infection by X4-HIV. *AIDS*, Vol. 17, No. 1 (January 2003), pp. 33-42

Salanova, B.; Choi, M.; Rolle, S.; Wellner, M.; Luft, F.C. & Kettritz, R. (2007). Beta2-integrins and acquired glycoprotein IIb/IIIa (GPIIb/IIIA) receptors cooperate in NF-kappaB activation of human neutrophils. *J Biol Chem*, Vol. 282, No.38, (September 2007), pp. 27960-27969.

Sandberg, H.; Bode, A.P.; Dombrose, F.A.; Hoechli, M. & Lentz, B.R. (1985). Expression of coagulant activity in human platelets: release of membranous vesicles providing platelet factor 1 and platelet factor 3. *Thromb Res*, Vol. 39, No. 1, (July 19850, pp. 63-79.

Sarkar, A.; Mitra, S.; Mehta,S.; Raices, R. & Wewers, M.D. (2009). Monocyte derived microvesicles deliver a cell death message via encapsulated caspase-1. *PLoS One*. Vol. 4, No. 9 (September 20090, pp. 7140.

Shah, M.D.; Bergeron, A.L.; Dong, J.F. & López, J.A. (2008). Flow cytometric measurement of microparticles: pitfalls and protocol modifications. *Platelets*. Vol. 19, No. 5, (August 2008), pp. 365-72.

Shapiro, H.M. (2003). *Practical flow cytometry*. 4th ed. New York, Wiley–Liss (2003).

Sheridan, D.; Carter, C. & Kelton, J.G. (1986). A diagnostic test for heparin-induced thrombocytopenia. *Blood*. Vol. 67, No. 1, (January 1986), pp. 27-30.

Shet, A.S.; Aras, O.; Gupta, K.; Hass, M.J.; Rausch, D.J.; Saba, N.; Koopmeiners, L.; Key, N.S. and Hebbel, R.P. (2003). Sickle blood contains tissue factor-positive microparticles derived from endothelial cells and monocytes. *Blood*. Vol. 102, No. 7, (October 2003), pp.2678-83.

Shvalov, A.N.; Surovtsev, I.V.; Chernyshev, A.V.; Soini, J.T. and Maltsev, V.P. (1999). Particle classification from lightscattering with the scanning flow cytometer. *Cytometry*. Vol. 37, No. 3, (November 1999), pp.215–220.

Sidhu, S.S.; Mengistab, A.T.; Tauscher, A.N.; LaVail, J. & Basbaum, C. (2004). The microvesicle as a vehicle for EMMPRIN in tumor-stromal interactions. *Oncogene*, Vol. 23, No. 4, (January 2004), pp. 956-963

Simak, J. & Gelderman, M.P. (2006) Cell membrane microparticles in blood and blood products: potentially pathogenic agents and diagnostic markers. *Transfus Med Rev*, Vol. 20, No. 1 (January 2006), pp. 1-26.

Simak, J.; Holada, K.; D'Agnillo, F.; Janota, J.; Vostal, J.G. (2002). Cellular prion protein is expressed on endothelial cells and is released during apoptosis on membrane microparticles found in human plasma. *Transfusion*. Vol. 42, No. 3, (March 2002), pp.334-42.

Simak, J.; Holada, K.; Risitano, A.M.; Zivny, J.H.; Young, N.S.; Vostal, J.G. (2004) Elevated circulating endothelial membrane microparticles in paroxysmal nocturnal haemoglobinuria. *Br J Haematol*. Vol. 126, No. 6, (June 2004), pp.804-13.

Simak, J.; Holada, K.; Vostal, J.G. (2002a). Release of annexin V-binding membrane microparticles from cultured human umbilical vein endothelial cells after treatment with camptothecin. *BMC Cell Biol*. Vol. 3, No. 11, (May 2002).

Simpson, R.J.; Lim, J.W.; Moritz, R.L. & Mathivanan, S. (2009). Exosomes: proteomic insights and diagnostic potential. *Expert Rev Proteomics*. Vol. 6, No. 3, (June 2009), pp. 267-283.

Sims, P.J.; Faioni, E.M.; Wiedmer, T. & Shattil, S.J. (1988). Complement proteins C5b-9 cause release of membrane vesicles from the platelet surface that are enriched in the membrane receptor for coagulation factor Va and express prothrombinase activity. *J Biol Chem*. Vol. 263, No. 34, (December 1988), pp. 18205-18212.

Skog, J.; Würdinger, T.; van Rijn, S.; Meijer, D.H.; Gainche, L.; Sena-Esteves, M.; Curry, W.T. Jr.; Carter, B.S.; Krichevsky, A.M. & Breakefield, X.O. (2008). Glioblastoma microvesicles transport RNA and proteins that promote tumour growth and provide diagnostic biomarkers. *Nat Cell Biol*. Vol. 10, No. 12, (December 2008), pp. 1470-1476.

Soderberg, A.; Barral, A.M.; Soderstrom, M.; Sander, B. & Rosen, A. (2007). Redox-signaling transmitted in trans to neighboring cells by melanoma-derived TNF-containing exosomes. *Free Radic Biol Med* Vol. 43, Vol. 1, (July 2007), pp.90–99

Soriano, A.O.; Jy, W.; Chirinos, J.A.; Valdicia, M.A.; Velasquez, H.S.; Jimenez, J.J.; Horstman, L.L.; Kett, D.H.; Schein, R.M. & Ahn, Y.S. (2005). Levels of endothelial and platelet microparticles and their interactions with leukocytes negatively correlate with organ dysfunction and predict mortality in severe sepsis. *Crit Care Med*, Vol. 33, No. 11, (November 2005), pp. 2540-2546.

Sprague, D.L.; Elzey, B.D.; Crist, S.A. Waldschmidt, T.J.; Jensen, R.J. & Ratliff, T.L. (2008). Platelet-mediated modulation of adaptive immunity: unique delivery of CD154 signal by platelet-derived membrane vesicles. *Blood* Vol. 111, No. 10, (May 2008), pp. 5028-5036.

Szajnik, M.; Czystowska, M.; Szczepanski, M.J.; Mandapathil, M. & Whiteside, T.L. (2010). Tumor-derived microvesicles induce, expand and up-regulate biological activities of human regulatory T cells (Treg). *PLoS One*, Vol. 5, No. 7, (July 2010), e11469.

Taylor, D.D. & Gercel-Taylor, C. (2005). Tumour-derived exosomes and their role in cancer-associated T-cell signalling defects. *Br J Cancer* Vol. 92, No. 2, (January 20050, pp. 305-311

Tesselaar, M.E.; Romijn, F.P.; Van Der Linden, I.; Prins, F.A.; Bertina, R.M. & Osanto, S. (2007). Microparticle-associated tissue factor activity: a link between cancer and thrombosis? *J Thromb Haemost*. Vol. 5, No. 3, (March 2007), pp. 520–527.

Trummer, A.; De Rop, C.; Tiede, A.; Ganser, A. & Eisert, R. (2009). Recovery and composition of microparticles after snap-freezing depends on thawing temperature. *Blood Coagul Fibrinolysis*. Vol. 20, No. 1, (January 2009), pp. 52-56.

Turiák, L.; Misják, P.; Szabó, T.G.; Aradi, B.; Pálóczi, K.; Ozohanics, O.; Drahos, L.; Kittel, A.; Falus, A.; Buzás, E.I. & Vékey, K.(2011). Proteomic characterization of thymocyte-derived microvesicles and apoptotic bodies in BALB/c mice. *J Proteomics*. Vol. 74, no.10,pp. 2025-33.

Van Amersfoort, E.S. & Van Strijp, J.A. (1994). Evaluation of a flow cytometric fluorescence quenching assay of phagocytosis of sensitized sheep erythrocytes by polymorphonuclear leukocytes. *Cytometry*, Vol. 17, No. 4, (December 1994), pp.294-301

van Doormaal, F.F.; Kleinjan, A.; Di Nisio, M.; Büller, H.R. & Nieuwland, R. (2009). Cell-derived microvesicles and cancer. *Neth J Med*. Vol. 67, No. 7, (July 2009), pp. 266-273.

VanWijk, M.J.; VanBavel, E.; Sturk, A. & Nieuwland, R. (2003). Microparticles in cardiovascular diseases. *Cardiovasc Res*. 2003 Aug 1Vol. 59, No. 2, (August 2003), pp. 277-287.

Vasco F.; Hawe, A. & Wim, J. (2010). Critical evaluation of nanoparticle tracking analysis (NTA) by NanoSight for the measurement of nanoparticles and protein aggregates. *Pharmaceutical Research*. Vol. 27, No. 5, (May 2010), pp. 796-810.

Warkentin, T.E.; Hayward, C.P.; Boshkov, L.K.; Santos, A.V.; Sheppard, J.A.; Bode, A.P. & Kelton, J.G. (1994). Sera from patients with heparin-induced thrombocytopenia generate platelet-derived microparticles with procoagulant activity: an explanation for the thrombotic complications of heparin-induced thrombocytopenia. *Blood*. Vol. 84, No. 11, (December 1994), pp.3691-3699.

Weiss, H.J. (1994). Scott syndrome: a disorder of platelet coagulant activity. *Semin Hematol*, Vol31, No. 4, pp. 312-314

Whiteside, T.L. (2005) Tumour-derived exosomes pr microvesicles: another mechanism of tumour escape from thte host immune system? *Br J Cancer*, Vol. 92, No. 2, (January 2005), pp. 209-211

Wieckowski, E. & Whiteside, T.L. (2006) Human tumor-deried vs dendritic cell-derived exosomes have distinct biologic roles and molecular profiles. *Immunol Res*, Vol. 36, No. 1-3, pp. 247-254.

Wolf, P. (1967). The nature and significance of platelet products in human plasma. *Br J Haematol*. Vol. 13, No. 3, pp. 269-288.

Wysoczynski, M. & Ratajczak, M.Z. (2009). Lung cancer secreted microvesicles: underappreciated modulators of microenvironment in expanding tumors. *Int J Cancer*. Vol.125, No. 7, (October 2009), pp.1595-603.

Yamashita, H.; Kitayama, J.; Ishikawa, M. & Nagawa, H. (2007). Tissue factor expression is a clinical indicator of lymphatic metastasis and poor prognosis in gastric cancer with intestinal phenotype. *J Surg Oncol*. Vol. 95, No. 4, (March 2007), pp. 324-331.

Yu, J.L.; May, L.; Lhotak, V.; Shahrzad; S,. Shirasawa, S.; Weitz, J.I.; Coomber, B.L.; Mackman, N. & Rak, J.W. (2005). Oncogenic events regulate tissue factor expression in colorectal cancer cells: implications for tumor progression and angiogenesis. *Blood*, Vol. 105, No. 4, (February 2005), pp. 1734-1741.

Yuana, Y.; Bertina, R.M. & Osanto, S. (2011). Pre-analytical and analytical issues in the analysis of blood microparticles. *Thromb Haemost*, Vol. 105, No.3 (March 2011), pp. 396-408.

Zdebska, E.; Woźniak, J.; Dzieciatkowska, A. & Koscielak, J. (1998). In comparison to progenitor platelets, microparticles are deficient in GpIb, GpIb-derived carbohydrates, glycerophospolipids, glycosphingolipids, and ceramides. *Acta Biochim Pol,* Vol 45, no. 2, pp. 417-428.

Zhong, H.; Yang, Y.; Ma, S.; Xiu, F.; Cai, Z.; Zhao, H. & Du, L. (2011). Induction of a tumour-specific CTL response by exosomes isolated from heat-treated malignant ascites of gastric cancer patients. *Int J Hyperthermia.* Vol. 27, No. 6, pp. 604-611.

Zhou, H.; Pisitkun, T.; Aponte, A.; Yuen, P.S.; Hoffert, J.D.; Yasuda, H.; Hu, X.; Chawla, L.; Shen, R.F.; Knepper, M.A. & Star, R.A. (2006). Exosomal Fetuin-A identified by proteomics: a novel urinary biomarker for detecting acute kidney injury. *Kidney Int.* Vol. 70, No. 10, (November 2006), pp. 1847-1857.

Zitvogel, L.; Regnault, A.; Lozier, A.; Wolfers, J.; Flament, C.; Tenza, D.; Ricciardi-Castagnoli, P.; Raposo, G. & Amigorena, A. (1998) Eradication ofestablished murine tumors using a novel cell-free vaccine: dendritic cell-derived exosomes. *Nat Med.* Vol. 4, No.5 (May 1998), pp. 594-600.

Zomer, A.; Vendrig, T.; Hopmans, ES.; van Eijndhoven, M.; Middeldorp, J.M. & Pegtel, D.M. (2010). Exosomes: Fit to deliver small RNA. *Commun Integr Biol.*.Vol. 3, No. 5, (September 2010), pp. 447-450.

12

Flow Cytometry-Based Analysis and Sorting of Lung Dendritic Cells

Svetlana P. Chapoval
University of Maryland
USA

1. Introduction

Dendritic cells (DC) are very specialized antigen presenting cells which play critical roles in innate and adaptive immunity and in tolerance. Their major functions are to sample antigens throughout the body and to stimulate or tolerize T cells. DC consist of several distinct subsets with different tissue distribution, surface markers, and function. This chapter discusses the lung DC subsets, their specific array of distinguishing markers, various aspects of their biology and function based on the flow cytometry-derived studies for their isolation and characterization.

2. Lung DC subpopulations

Lung DC are sentinel cells originated in the bone marrow and through the peripheral circulation are constantly recruited to the lung tissue. They sense and capture antigens, and transport processed antigens to the draining lymph nodes where they interact with T cells. However, since lung DC form a heterogeneous sentinel cell population with distinct cell subtypes having different functions in the immune response, it is important to properly define these populations in order to use/stimulate the selected one(s) for a proper immune response regulation and/or protection from the disease.

2.1 Discovery of DC

DC were co-discovered in 1973 by Ralf M. Steinman and Zanvil A. Cohn at the Rockefeller University as a population of mouse spleen cells with unusual stellate morphology (Steinman & Cohn, 1973). For this fundamental discovery Ralf M. Steinman was awarded the 2011 Nobel Prize in Physiology and Medicine. The first dendritic cell in skin with a typical dendritic morphology was described in 1868 by Paul Langerhans but, due to it morphology, was mistaken for a neuronal cell (Langerhans, 1898) and later was termed a Langerhans cell. In their seminal article defining DC as a novel cell population, Steinman and Cohn noted that DC constantly extend and retract many cell processes and have many different branches present at given time point, adhere to plastic and do not display an endocytic capacity of macrophages. The other feature that distinct these two adherent cell populations is the presence of many perinuclear acid phosphatise-positive granules in the cytoplasm of macrophages, whereas DC display only few tiny granules in this area. At that time, the scientists were able to localize DC presence only in lymphoid organs (spleen, lymph nodes, and Payer's patches) but not in other tissues studied such as thymus, liver, peritoneal cavity, intestine, and bone marrow. The presence of DC in the connective tissues of all organs including lungs was discovered a few years later (Kawanami, Basset, Ferrans, Soler, & Crystal, 1981; Spencer & Fabre, 1990; Steiniger, Klempnauer, & Wonigeit, 1984). Lung DC are critical in controlling the immune response to inhaled antigen (K. Vermaelen & Pauwels, 2005).

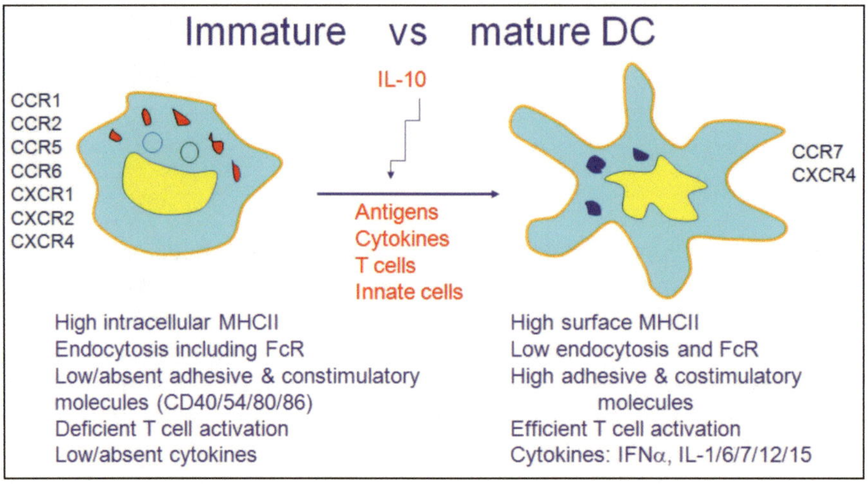

Fig. 1. Immature versus mature lung DC

Hematopoietic cell progenitor gives a rise to DC which populate the lung tissue in the immature state attracted by the specific chemokines and other mediators (K. Vermaelen & Pauwels, 2005). Immature DC display a specific set of chemokine receptors, high endocytic ability, and low T cell stimulation activity. After antigen uptake and maturation, DC upregulate adhesion and costimulatory molecule expression and cytokine production but shut down the antigen-capturing activity and limit chemokine receptor expression.

2.2 DC in the lung

DC are present in the lung tissue in an immature state (Figure 1) what means they can perform a typical function for immature DC - recognise and sample antigens but cannot stimulate T cells. The normal tissue condition without any Ag-(or other factors) induced disturbance is defined as a steady state condition. In a steady state condition, immature DC are distributed throughout the lung tissue. Depending on their lung anatomical localization site, they were originally subdivided on airway subepithelial, lung parenchymal, and visceral pleura DC (Sertl et al., 1986). However, a more common classification of lung DC in a steady state condition subdivides them on three major classes based on the cell surface marker's expression and function: conventional (c)DC, plasmacytoid (p)DC, and alveolar DC (Lambrecht & Hammad, 2009a, 2009b). DC constantly sample inhaled Ag and then mature and migrate to the T cell areas of the local lymphoid tissues, peribronchial (mediastinal) lymph nodes. Depending on many factors, including the nature and dose of Ag, the cytokine milieu at the site of Ag entry, lung DC can either stimulate a clonal expansion of Ag-specific T cells (Figure 2) or induce tolerance.

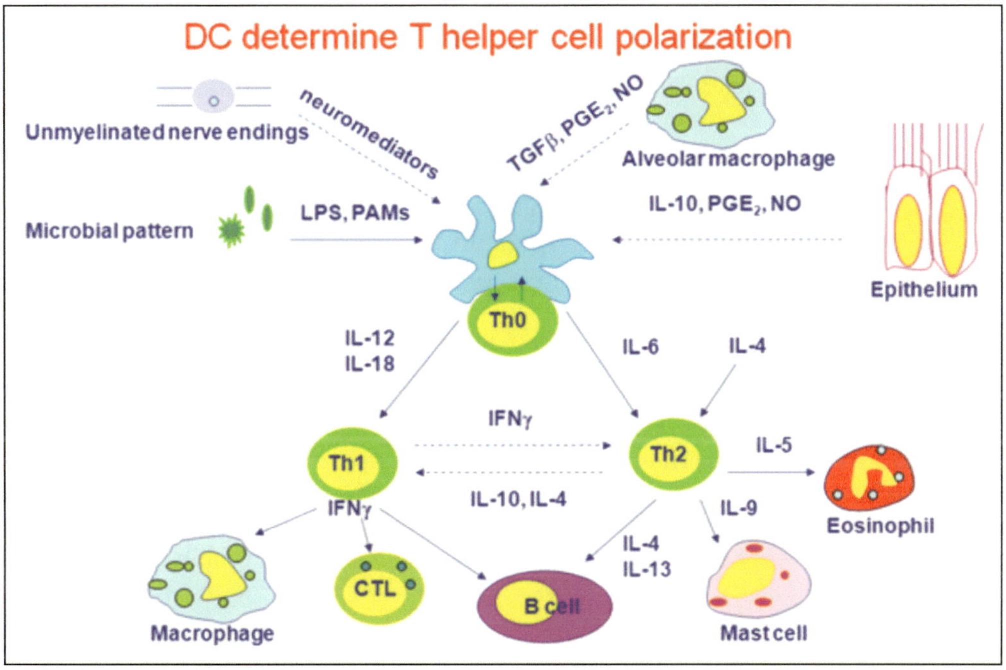

Fig. 2. DC determine Th cell polarization

DC maturation by inhaled antigen leads to their production of different cytokines which determine what type of helper T cell response will dominate, Th1 or Th2. Following DC-induced activation, generated Th cells produce a characteristic cytokine set which, in its turn, performs different functions acting on other cells involved in the response to the corresponding Ag. To avoid the potential harmful consequences of continuous lung DC activation, the cells are being kept in the immature state by different mechanisms involving products of unmyelinated nerve endings, alveolar macrophages, and airway epithelium.

The key role of DC in the interface between tolerance and immune response in the lung is a subject of many investigations (K. Vermaelen & Pauwels, 2005). Currently, two major lung DC subpopulations are defined as cDC and pDC whereas alveolar DC are not well characterized (Chapoval et al., 2009; de Heer et al., 2004; Masten et al., 2006; Ritz et al., 2004). In addition to those two well characterized DC populations, more DC subtypes can exist under inflammatory conditions (Swanson et al., 2004). As these DC differ functionally, it is important to properly subdivide and characterize them for a further definition of their role in different pathologic conditions as well as for their potential use for a DC-based therapy of different diseases. Flow cytometry provides an important, reliable, and precise tool to separate and analyse different cells based on their specific phenotypic properties. Multicolor flow cytometry allows the use of multiple parameters simultaneously which helps to clearly define DC subpopulations and status.

2.2.1 Isolation of lung cells for flow cytometric analysis

To prepare the lung cells for a flow cytometry analysis, the lungs first were perfused with 20 ml PBS via right ventricle, dissected from the thorax, and cut into small pieces using sterile surgical blades (VWR). We prepared single cell suspensions of lung cells in flow cytometry staining buffer consisting of 10% FBS supplemented PBS (free of divalent cations Ca^{2+} and Mg^{2+}) with 0.01% of sodium azide. We used two different techniques for DC isolation. In a first technique, the single cell suspensions from the mouse lungs were prepared by mincing the organs into small pieces and digesting them with type IV collagenase (Worthington Biochemical) and DNAse (Roche) for 30 min at 37^{0}C as described previously (Chapoval et al., 2009; Niu et al., 2007). For cell dissociation, digested cell suspensions were passed through a wire mesh and then through a 100 μm nylon cell strainer (BD Falcon). RBC were lyzed with Ammonium-Chloride-Potassium (K) (chloride), ACK lysis buffer (Invitrogen).

In a second technique, the digestion step was omitted and the lung single cell suspensions were freshly prepared according to a procedure reported by Piggott DA et al. (Piggott et al., 2005). Briefly, lungs were physically disrupted by pushing the tissue between two sterile glass microscope slides (Thermoscientific). Then obtained cell suspensions were passed through cell strainers to remove the tissue debris and subjected to centrifugation over the Ficoll gradient to purify a leukocyte population from the contaminating cells. RBC lysis step was excluded when using this technique as RBC (together with neutrophils and eosinophils) aggregate at the bottom of a tube whereas leukocytes remain in the cell suspension-Ficoll interface.

Similarly, human lung cells were isolated from the surgically removed lung tissues distant from a primary resected lung carcinomas by cutting tissues into pieces followed by a type IA collagenase (Sigma) enzymatic digest for 1h at 37^{0}C (Cochand, Isler, Songeon, & Nicod, 1999). The enzyme-digested tissue fragments were pushed through a stainless-steel screen and separated on a Ficoll-Paque density gradient to obtain pulmonary mononuclear cells. Cells were cultured in P10 Petri dishes in complete medium. The nonadherent cells were removed after 1 h, using three rinses of Hanks' balanced salt solution without Ca^{2+} and Mg^{2+} (HBSS). The adherent cells were incubated for an additional 16h period at 37^{0}C in complete medium. The cells released after three rinses of HBSS are referred to as loosely adherent mononuclear cell population.

DC can also be detected in the bronchoalveolar lavage (BAL) in mice (Fainaru et al., 2005; Jakubzick, Tacke, et al., 2008) and humans (van Haarst et al., 1994; Tsoumakidou et al., 2006). For BAL withdrawal in mice, airways were flushed three to four times with 1 ml of sterile endotoxin-free PBS (Chapoval et al., 1999) or 0.5 mM EDTA/HBSS (Jakubzick, Tacke, et al., 2008) using a sterile 1 ml syringe (Becton Dickinson) connected to either the blunt needle (Chapoval et al., 1999) or veterinary i.v. catheter (Chapoval et al., 2008). BAL cells were washed once with PBS or EDTA/HBSS by centrifugation. The cell pellets were resuspended in 1 mL of a corresponding buffer. Total leukocytes in BAL fluids were determined for each sample with a standard hemocytometer. For FACS analysis, BAL cells were resuspended in FACS blocking solution and stained for 30 min with appropriate conjugated Abs. BAL withdrawal in humans was performed with a flexible bronchoscope placed in the wedge position in the right middle lobe (van Haarst et al., 1994). Four aliquots of 50 ml saline were subsequently instilled and aspirated. BAL fluid was collected in siliconized bottles. BAL cells were kept at 4°C, washed twice in PBS containing 0.5% bovine serum albumin and 0.45% glucose, and subsequently filtered through a 55 μm and a 30 μm gauze. Human BAL DC selected as low autofluorescent cells were HLA-DR, L25, RFD1, and

CD68 (van Haarst et al., 1994). A portion of these cells expressed CD1a (22%) and My4 (60%). The high autofluorescent cell fraction represented alveolar macrophages which were strongly positive for APh, HLA-DR, CD68, RFD7, and RFD9.

2.2.2 Complex DC analysis using multicolor flow cytometry

Multicolor flow cytometry is a unique, useful, and powerful analytical method to identify DC subpopulations in the lung among many lung resident and inflammatory cells, to define their activation and maturation stages, to identify their surface marker expression and, therefore, to extrapolate their role in the specific lung conditions.

In our work we used the following mAbs obtained from BD Biosciences Pharmingen in multicolor flow cytometry for lung DC subpopulation detection and characterization: anti-I-A□b-biotin (AF6-120.1), anti-CD8□-PE (53-6.7), anti-CD11b- allophycocyanin-cyanin dye, APC-Cy7 (M1/70), anti-CD11c-FITC or –APC (HL3), anti-B220/CD45R-PE (RA3-6B2), anti-GR1-FITC or –APC (Ly-6G and Ly-6C). PE-Cy-5-labeled Mac1 (CD11b/CD18) Ab that were used in some experiments were obtained from Cedarlane Laboratories. DEC-205 was visualized using rat anti-mouse CD205 Ab (NLDC-145) and STAR69 (F(ab')2 goat anti-rat IgG-FITC), both from Serotec (Oxford, UK). Biotinylated rat anti-mouse F4/80 Ab (CI:A3-1; Serotec) were used in combination with SAV-FITC (BD Pharmingen) for visualization of this macrophage marker. Streptavidin-peridinin chlorophyll protein, SAV-PerCP was used as a second step reagent for biotinylated anti-I-A□^{b}. Where necessary, cells were preincubated with anti-CD16/CD32 (2.4G2) mAb for blocking cell surface FcR. Cells gated by forward- and side-scatter parameters were analyzed on either FACSCalibur or LSRII (Becton Dickinson) flow cytometer using either CELLQuest, FACSDiva, or FlowJo softwares.

2.2.3 Lung conventional DC

Proper flow cytometry-based characterization of lung DC is a complex issue as, in contrast to other organs, CD11c in the lung is expessed on DC and on a subset of lung macrophages (Jakubzick, Tacke, et al., 2008). Therefore, CD11c integrin with still undefined function (Lindquist et al., 2004; Metlay et al., 1990) can not serve as one definitive marker for lung DC. However, both cell types in the lung differ in the levels of autofluorescence (Jakubzick, Tacke, et al., 2008; Kirby, Raynes, & Kaye, 2006; K. Y. Vermaelen, Carro-Muino, Lambrecht, & Pauwels, 2001), MHC Class II expression (Jakubzick, Tacke, et al., 2008), and costimulatory molecule expression (Chelen et al., 1995).

Conventional DC are characterized as CD11c+MHCII^{low}CD11b+ cells and CD1c+CD11c+CD14-HLA-DR+ cells in mice and human, correspondingly (Chapoval et al., 2009; de Heer et al., 2004; Masten et al., 2006; Ritz et al., 2004). In mice, cDC consist more than 95% of total lung DC in a steady state condition (Maraskovsky et al., 1996; Swanson et al., 2004; K. Vermaelen & Pauwels, 2004). Lung cDC discrimination starts from elimination of autofluorescent cells based on dot plots of CD11c-empty channel (Figure 3). CD11b, an additional marker for cDC, has other alternative names: ITGAM, integrin alpha M; Mac-1, macrophage-1, consists of CD11b plus CD18; complement receptor 3, CR3 (CD11b/CD18). CD11b in complex with CD18 mediates macrophage adhesion and migration (Solovjov, Pluskota, & Plow, 2005).

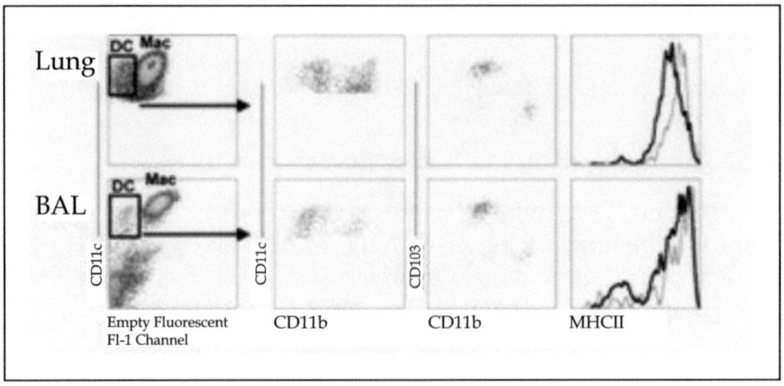

Fig. 3. Flow cytometry discrimination of lung cDC

We studied the effect of lung epithelial cell-targeted expression of vascular endothelial growth factor (VEGF) on lung DC number and activation stage. We generated these mice in order to define the role of VEGF in allergic asthma as the exaggerated levels of lung VEGF were found in asthmatic persons (Lee et al., 2004). It has been shown previously that VEGF overexpression during lung development causes a fetal death (Zheng et al., 1998). We used a dual-construct transgenic system that can be regulated externally (Ray et al., 1997). This system is based on the production of animals with two transgenic constructs. The first, CC10-rtTA construct contained the CC10 (Clara Cell 10) promoter, the rtTA (a fusion protein made up of a mutated tetracycline repressor and the herpes virus VP-16 transactivator) and human growth hormone (hGH) intronic, with its nuclear localization sequence and polyadenylation sequences. The second, tet-O-CMV-hVEGF construct contained a polymeric tetracycline operator (tet-O), minimal cytomegalovirus (CMV) promoter, human $VEGF_{165}$ cDNA, and hGH intronic and polyadenylation signals. In this system the CC10 promoter direct s the expression of rtTA to the lung. In the presence of doxycycline (Dox), rtTA is able to bind in trans to the tet-O, and the VP-16 transactivator activates VEGF gene transcription. In the absence of Dox, rtTA binding does not occur and transgene transcription is not activated.

We have found previously that lung VEGF expression induces local DC activation (Lee et al., 2004). In our research we performed the discriminatory analysis of lung cDC in WT and VEGF tg mice using different techniques (Figures 4 and 5). In Figure 4, we show that the population of cells that are considered to be macrophages with autofluorescence on empty channel (flow 6 in this study) contains both macrophages and cDC (this was supported by a Giemsa stain of sorted cytospinned cells (Chapoval et al., 2009)). Only a proper elimination of large highly autofluorescent cells on a FCS-SSC dot plot can help to distinguish these two cell populations in the whole lung cell suspension. Moreover, if lung cDC in Fig. 3 are $MHCII^{high}$, we have notices that WT mouse lung cDC are $MHCII^{low}$ (Bhandari et al., 2006; Chapoval et al., 2009; Lee et al., 2004) what makes sense considering the steady state condition of the WT mouse lung in the absence of any treatment/exposure. However, it is important to note that the procedures used for the lung DC characterization by flow cytometry (enzymatic tissue digestion, centrifugations, incubation with Ab, etc.) will all lead to the modification of the lung DC original state (K. Vermaelen & Pauwels, 2005) and, thus, different techniques, reagents used, procedure timing will impact the further cell discrimination by flow cytometry.

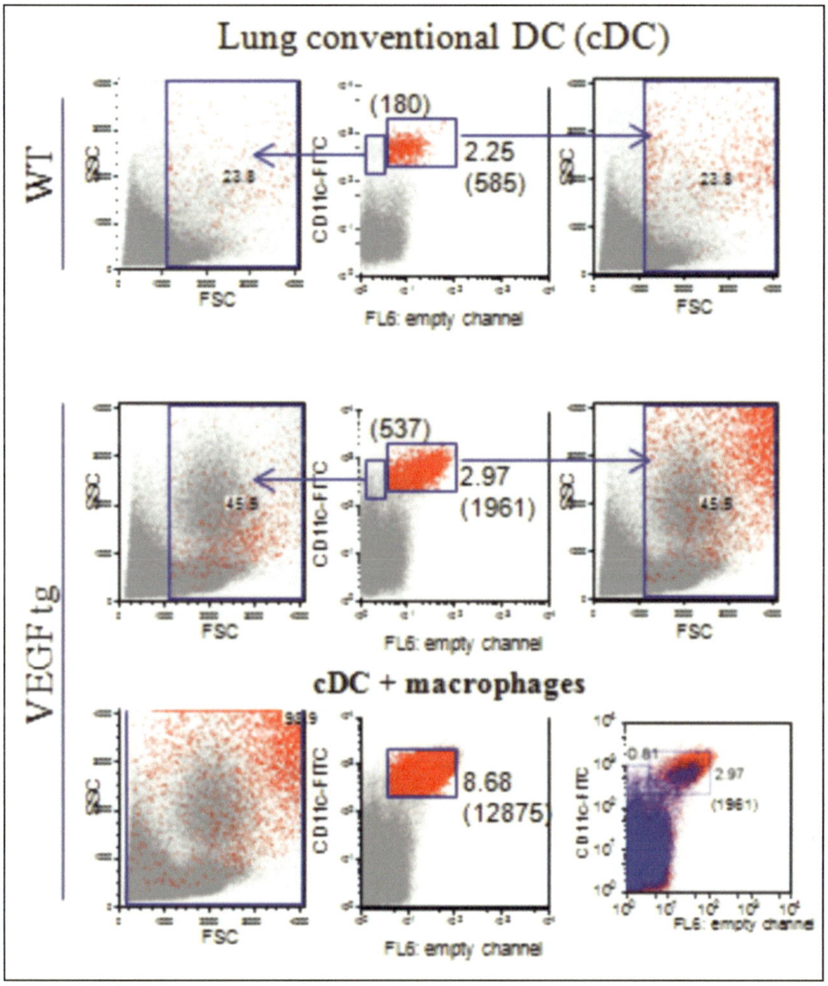

Fig. 4. Lung cDC gating strategy

The other discrimination technique was based on the assumption that CD11c+/high autofluorescent lung cells do not express MHCII and, therefore, are alveolar macrophages, whereas cDC are CD11c+MHCII+ (K. Vermaelen & Pauwels, 2004). This observation contrasts with the results obtained by us and others (Beaty, Rose, & Sung, 2007; Chapoval et al., 2009; Sung et al., 2006) (Figure 5). As it can be seen in Fig. 5, the levels of MHCII expression on macrophages and cDC are the same.

Flow cytometry of whole lung cell suspension gated on CD11c+ cells, or BAL gated on live cells, stained for CD11c vs empty FITC fluorescent channel. High autofluorescent cells are defined as macrophages (Mac), whereas low autofluorescent cells are defined as DC. The flow cytometry plots in the center show the gated DC population stained for CD11c vs CD11b or CD103 vs CD11b. On the right, the histogram plots show that both DC subsets in the lung and in BAL, CD11b^{low} DC (black line) and CD11c^{high} DC (grey line), express high levels of MHCII. Of note, this figure was provided by the Journal of Immunology as a one-time reproduction (Copyright 2008, the American Association of Immunologists, Inc.).

The other discrimination technique was based on the assumption that CD11c+/high autofluorescent lung cells do not express MHCII and, therefore, are alveolar macrophages, whereas cDC are CD11c+MHCII+ (K. Vermaelen & Pauwels, 2004). This observation contrasts with the results obtained by us and others (Beaty, Rose, & Sung, 2007; Chapoval et al., 2009; Sung et al., 2006) (Figure 5). As it can be seen in Fig. 5, the levels of MHCII expression on macrophages and cDC are the same.

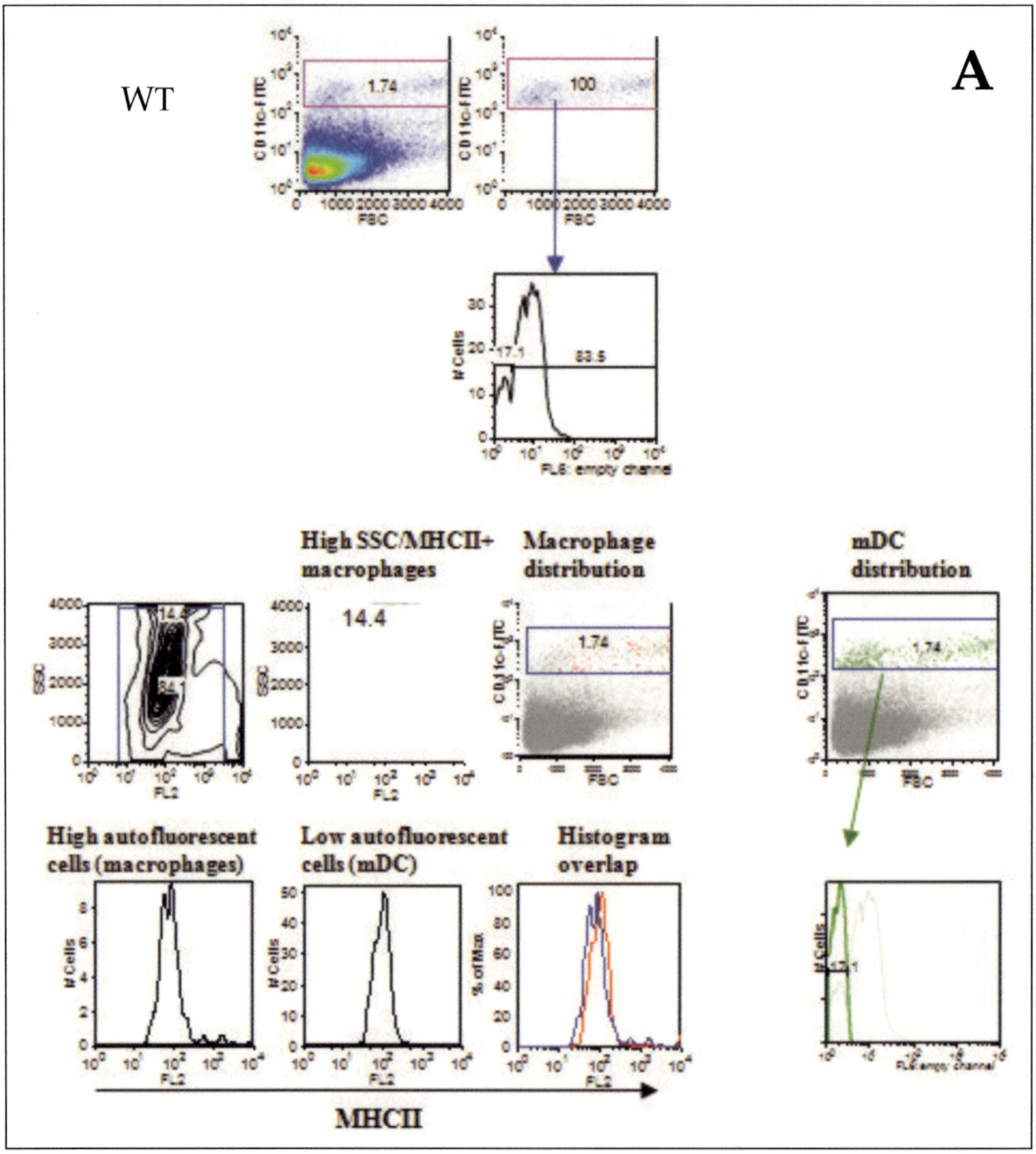

Fig. 5. (continues on next page) Application of flow cytometry gating strategies used by Vermealen K and Pauwels R (Vermaelen and Pauwels 2004) and Beaty SR and associates (Sung, Fu et al. 2006; Beaty, Rose et al. 2007) for a detailed analysis of WT (panel A) and VEGF tg (panel B) lung cDC (marked as myeloid, mDC) populations

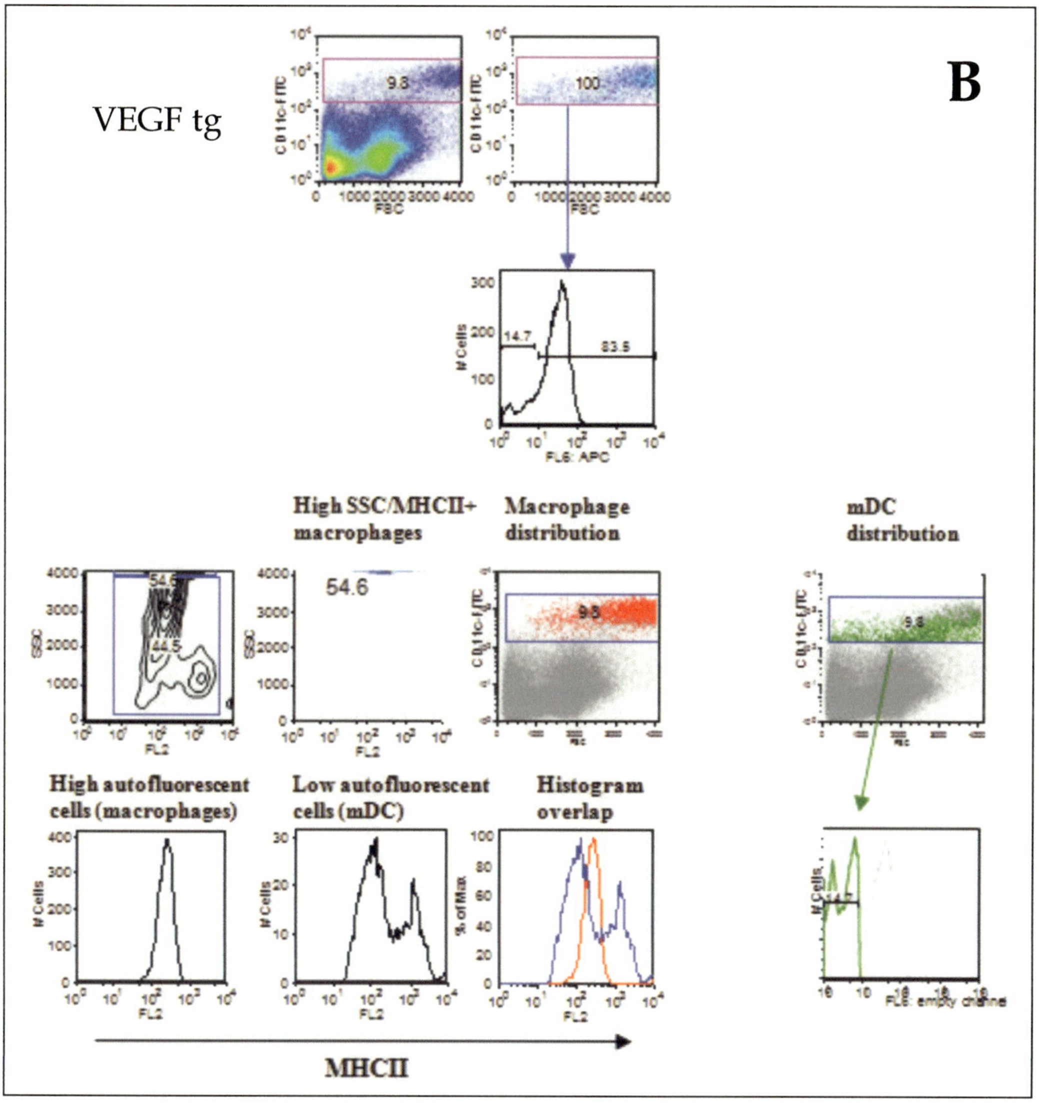

Fig. 5. Continued

We then further analyzed lung cDC using the defined above Abs to CD11c, MHCII, CD11b, DEC-205, and F4/80 cell surface markers in multicolour flow cytometry analysis using LSRII flow cytometer equipped with FACS Diva software. We identified lung cDC in WT mice as CD11c+MHCII+CD11b+F4/80^{low}DEC-205^{low} cells (Figure 6). Although it should be noted here that using anti-DEC-205 Ab for IHC of lung tissues we were able to detect an equal low number of DEC-205+ (a lectin-type receptor, (Pollard & Lipscomb, 1990) cells between WT and VEGF tg mice without DOX-containing water exposure, and, therefore, in the absence of transgene expression (Chapoval et al., 2009; Lee et al., 2004). Lung VEGF tg cDC demonstrated the increased DEC-205 and MHCII and decreased F4/80 expression. Recently, mouse lung cDC were subdivided into two subpopulations, namely CD11b+cDC and CD103+ cDC (Beaty et al., 2007; Jakubzick, Tacke, et al., 2008; Sung et al., 2006). CD103

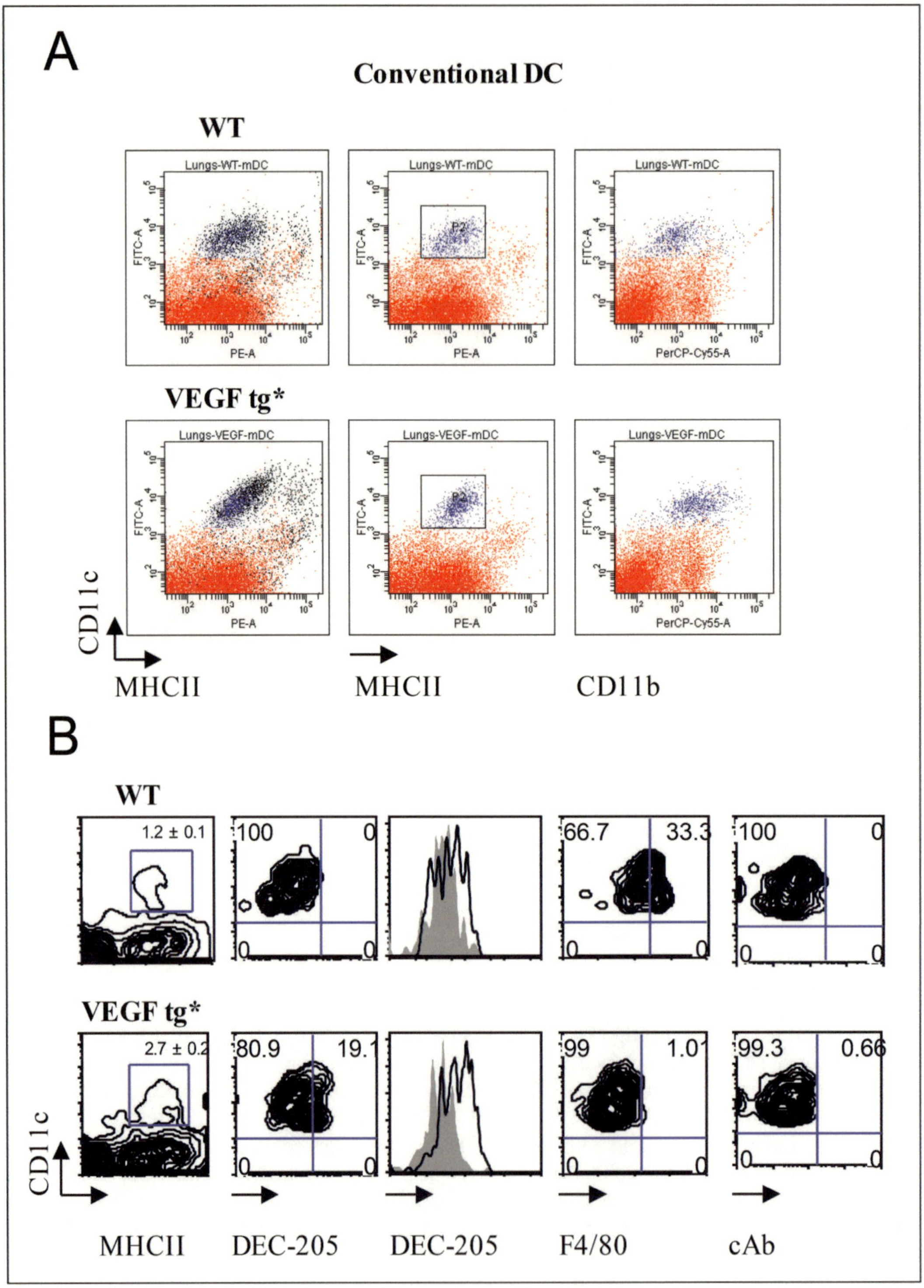

Fig. 6. Conventional DC in the lungs of WT and VEGF tg mice

is alpha E integrin which was detected on a subset of lung cDC and is also expressed on intraepithelial lymphocytes (Lehmann et al., 2002). Nevertheless, the use of this marker the helped to subdivide mouse lung tissue DC on three subclasses, pDC, CD11b+ cDC and CD103+ cDC (Beaty et al., 2007; Jakubzick, Helft, Kaplan, & Randolph, 2008; Lambrecht et al., 2000; Sung et al., 2006).

Lung cells were stained with CD11c-FITC, MHCII-PE, and CD11b-PerCP. The cells were first analyzed for forward and side scatters and gated out as shown in the blue box. Lung cDC in WT and VEGF tg mice were defined using CD11c-FITC marker and FL6 empty channel (Jakubzick, Helft, et al., 2008; Jakubzick, Tacke, et al., 2008; K. Vermaelen & Pauwels, 2004). CD11c/Fl6 dot plots of this gated population showed two CD11c^{high} WT cDC subpopulations (180 +585 cells for WT mouse lungs). Both of them were not autofluorescent in WT mice. These cells were then back-gated on the FCS and SSC dot plot. Dot plot distribution of selected cells is shown in red color. The relative and absolute numbers of the mainly macrophage-gate containing portion of WT lung cDC are equaled 2.25% / 585 cells. In contrast, the relative and absolute numbers of the portion of VEGF tg cDC were significantly higher than those found in WT mice and equaled 2.97% / 1961 cells. Population of tg lung cDC (2.25% of gated cells) showed low autofluorescence in empty FL6.

Single cell suspensions obtained from mouse lungs with omitting the enzymatic digestion step (Piggott et al., 2005) were stained with CD11c-FITC, MHCII-PE, and CD11b-PerCP. CD11c^{high} cells were gated out and analyzed for MHCII expression vs SSC. Two subpopulations of MHCII+ cells were observed in WT mouse lungs, namely SSC^{low}MHCII+ (84.1%) cells and SSC^{high}MHCII+ (14.4%) cells. The SSC^{high}MHCII+ cells composed of autofluorescent lung macrophages and they are shown in red. Most of these cells are located on the border line of SSC and where gated out in further lung cDC analysis. Lung cDC are shown in green. Lower panel for WT mice shows that both populations of autofluorescent macrophages and cDC overlap on MHCII histogram. This also applies for VEGF tg lung macrophages and cDC (two lower panels). In VEGF tg mouse lungs the number of CD11c+ SSC^{high}MHCII+ macrophages mounted to 54.6% of CD11c+ cells. Similarly to WT mice, these cells were located on the border line of SSC and where gated out from further cDC analysis.

These cells were not macrophages since macrophages were more autofluorescent and shifted more to up and right on FL6 empty channel. When macrophages were added to the dot plot, a significantly higher number of cells (8.68% / 12875 cells) in this selection box was observed. Therefore, there is a significant overlap between cDC and CD11c^{high} lung macrophages with a gating strategy based on CD11c marker and an empty channel autofluorescence.

In human, lung cDC were characterized in the enzymatically digested tissues obtained at the lung surgery (Masten et al., 2006). cDC were defined as CD1c+CD11c+CD14- HLA-DR+ cells which comprised 2% of low autofluorescent mononuclear cells in a flow cytometry analysis. The expression of CD14 together with CD11c are critical important distinguishing markers for lung cDC and macrophages, as monocytes and macrophages were CD11c-CD14+ whereas CD11c+ cDC did not express CD14. Similarly to the mouse lung DC, human lung DC in a steady state condition are in immature state as defined by the absence of expression of differentiation markers CD83 and CD1a and limited expression of costimulatory molecules (Cochand et al., 1999). In the latter study, the loosely adherent on the Petri dishes cells were further separated into DC and autofluorescent macrophages with a Coulter EPICS V based on the presence or absence of autofluorescent inclusions with a coherent INNOVA 90 light source, using a 488-nm wavelength for excitation and a 588-nm filter for emission. The gates were set to remove cell debris and to select mature alveolar macrophages and nonphagocytic DC.

2.2.4 Lung plasmacytoid DC

Plasmacytoid DC are characterized as $CD11c^{intermed}$/ B220+/GR1+ cells and CD123+CD11c-CD14-HLA-DR+ cells in mice and human, correspondingly (Chapoval et al., 2009; de Heer et al., 2004; Masten et al., 2006; Ritz et al., 2004). Plasmacytoid DC in the mouse lungs were first properly detected and functionally analyzed by Bart Lambrecht's group in 2004 (de Heer et al., 2004). This discrimination was based on CD11c and GR1 expression. The sorted cells based on this discrimination characteristic showed typical morphologies for different cell types such as eosinophils, lymphocytes, macrophages, neutrophils, and DC. pDC were targeted to the specific region based on CD11c and GR-1 expression, displayed a more immature phenotype than cDC and were $MHCII^{low}$, B220+ and CD45RB+. Confocal microscopy targeted B220+Gr1+ pDC to the lung interstitium. The elimination of these cells with the in vivo use of anti-GR1 or 120G8 depleting Abs lead to the allergic eosinophilic response in the lungs to normally inert allergen applications (Asselin-Paturel, Brizard, Pin, Briere, & Trinchieri, 2003; de Heer et al., 2004).

Lung VEGF expression increases the number of cDC in tg mouse lungs. Mouse lung tissues were obtained on day 7 of DOX water administration and processed using the enzymatic digest method. Single cell suspensions were stained with corresponding Ab and analyzed by flow cytometry. (A-B) Autofluorescent macrophages (shown in black color in panel A) were removed from the DC analysis. An upregulation of MHCII, CD11b, DEC-205 but not F4/80 expression on tg lung cDC was detected. For histograms: solid line represents isotype control rat IgG2a staining whereas transparent line shows the level of DEC-205 expression. *$p<0.0025$, WT vs tg lung mDC number (n=5/group).

We studied the effect of lung VEGF expression on local pDC number and activation employing VEGF tg mice (Chapoval et al., 2009). We have found that VEGF induced activation of lung pDC which were characterized as $CD11c^{int}$B220+GR1+ cells and upregulated MHCII, CD40, CD80, and CD86 without a substantial modulation of ICOS-L expression.

Human lung plasmacytoid DC were characterized as CD123+CD11c+CD14+HLA-DR+ cells and comprised approximately 1.0% of the low autofluorescent mononuclear cells in flow cytometry analysis of cells from the lung tissues obtained upon surgery (Masten et al., 2006). A first discrimination of DC in this study was based on CD11c and CD14 expression. Morphological examination of cytospinned cells revealed cDC enriched CD11c+CD14- cell population and pDC-enriched CD11c-CD14- cell population. These populations were further analyzed for CD3, CD19, and CD56 expression to distinguish T, B and NK cells. The elimination of these cells subsets from the analysis demonstrated that approximately 7% of CD11c-CD14-human lung cell population were pDC. A lectin type receptor BDCA-2 (Demedts, Brusselle, Vermaelen, & Pauwels, 2005) expression was present only on 9 out of

13 samples analyzed. Unexpectedly, BDCA-2 expression was also seen in the cDC subpopulation, raising concerns about the pDC specificity of this marker for lung DC. Of note, BDCA-2 is not present in mice, and Siglec-H is used to define mouse pDC (Steinman, 2010).

2.2.5 Other lung DC subtypes arising under different conditions

Maraskovsky E and associates (Maraskovsky et al., 1996) were first to demonstrate that in vivo injections of Flt3L (FMS-related tyrosine kinase 3 ligand) into the mice will lead to a dramatic increase of DC subpopulations in different organs including the lungs. Five DC subpopulations were detected in spleens of injected mice based mainly on CD8α and CD11b expression, namely

1. $CD11b^{bright}$MHCII-GR1+CD11c-,
2. $CD11b^{bright}CD11c^{dull}$MHCII+GR1+,
3. $CD11b^{bright}$CD11c+MHCII+GR1-,
4. $CD11b^{dull}$CD11c+$MHCII^{bright}$GR1-, and
5. CD11b-CD11c+$MHCII^{bright}$GR1- cells.

Populations (1-3) were also CD8α+, whereas DC in (4-5) were not expressing this lymphoid cell marker. Population (1) was highly enriched with immature granulocytes or myeloid cells as determined with Wright-Giemsa stain of sorted cell's cytospin. Last two DC subpopulations were highly enriched for veiled cells with dendritic processes. When compared for T cell stimulation activity, all 1-5 population were able to stimulate allogeneic T cells in MLR, however, DC in populations 1-2 were 30-times less efficient as compared to control freshly isolated DC. For distinguishing lung DC populations affected by Flt3L injections, the authors used DEC-205 as a selection marker considering a previously reported CD11c expression on a subset of lung macrophages. They noted a strong 8-15-times fold elevation in relative numbers of DEC-205+CD11b+ and DEC-205+CD11b- cells. A more recent publication by Masten BJ and associates (Masten, Olson, Kusewitt, & Lipscomb, 2004) focused on Flt3L injection's effect specifically on lung DC. Flt3L induced a 19-fold increase in the absolute numbers of CD11c+CD45R/B220-DC in the lungs of Flt3L-treated mice over vehicle-treated mice. Further analysis revealed a 90-fold increase in the absolute number of myeloid DC (CD11c+CD45R/B220-CD11b+ cells) and only a 3-fold increase of lymphoid DC (CD11c+CD45R/B220-CD11b- cell) from the lungs of Flt3L-treated mice over vehicle-treated mice. The authors noted 4 subpopulations of lung DC under the study conditions, namely: (1) myeloid CD11b+ CD45R/B220- DC, (2) lymphoid CD11b- CD45R/B220- DC, (3) and (4) plasmacytoid DC expressing various levels of CD11c and CD45R/B220 markers. Therefore, the use of Flt3L may be efficient in augmenting vaccine responses against different lung infectious agents and promoting anti-tumor responses. However, as for the dampening of allergic lung responses, it might not be as effective considering the fact that myeloid lung DC which are mainly upregulated by Fl3L treatment, are necessary for allergic lung response generation and sustainability (Lambrecht et al., 2000; Lambrecht, Salomon, Klatzmann, & Pauwels, 1998).

A very detailed classification of DC based on organ and tissue distribution, marker's (including chemokine receptors) expression, migration, and function was recently presented in a comprehensive review article by Alvarez, Vollmann, and von Andrian (Alvarez,

Vollmann, & von Andrian, 2008) (Table 1 shows a fraction of a table presented in this comprehensive review). As for lung DC, the authors focused only on two myeloid DC subpopulations distinguished mainly by CD103 expression, lung interstitium CD11b^{lo}CD11c+CD103+ and conducting airway CD11b^{hi}CD11c+Cd103- DC.

Dendritic cell subset	Phenotype
Precursor DC	
Hematopoietic stem and progenitor cell (HSPC)	CD45+Lin-c-Kit+Sca-1+
Macrophage DC precursor (MDP)	CD44+Lin-c-Kit^{int}CD11b-
Common dendritic projenitor (CDP)	CD44+Lin-c-Kit^{int}Flt3+
Monocyte subsets	CD115+CD11b+Ly6C $^{low/int/hi}$ F4/80^{low}CD62L+/-
Differentiated DC	
Langerhans cell	Langerin+MHCII+Dectin-1+CD1a+CD11c+CD11b+CD24a+CD205+CD45loCD8a+/-CD103-
Dermal DC (langerin+ subset)	Langerin+MHCII+CD11c^{int}CD11b^{lo}CD45^{hi}CD8a+CD103+
Dermal DC (langerin- subset)	Langerin-MHCII+CD11c+ CD24a-DEC205+
CD8a+DC	CD8a+MHCII+CD11c+CD4-CD205+SIRP-a+
CD8a-DC	CD8a-MHCII+CD11c+CD11b+CD4-SIRP-a+DCIR2+
CD8a-CD4+DC	CD8a-CD4+CD11b+MHCII+DCIR2+
Plasmacytoid DC	B220+CD11c^{lo}Ly6C+MHCII^{lo}CD4+/-CD8a+/-PDCA-1+ (human: CD123+BDCA-2+BDCA-4+)
Lung DC (2 subsets) Conducting airway DC Lung interstitium DC	 CD11b^{lo}CD11c+CD103- CD11b^{lo}CD11c+CD103+
Lamina propria DC (4 subsets)	CD11c^{hi}CD11b-CD205+CD103+ CD11c^{hi}CD11b+CD205+CD103+ CD11c^{int}CD11b^{int}CD205-CD103- CD11c^{int}CD11b+CD205-CD103-
Peyer's patch DC (3 subsets)	CD11c+CD8a+CD11b- CD11c+CD8a+CD11b+ CD11c+CD8a-CD11b-

Table 1. Phenotype of dendritic cell subsets (modified from (Alvarez, Vollmann et al. 2008)

Finally, a unifying classification of human and mouse DC subsets was recently proposed by Guilliams M and associates (Guilliams et al.) which takes into account a functional specialization and specific marker expression (Figure 7). This classification is based on the expression of CD11b, CD103, and CD207. It highlights many unanswered questions in the DC research including the proper cell determination.

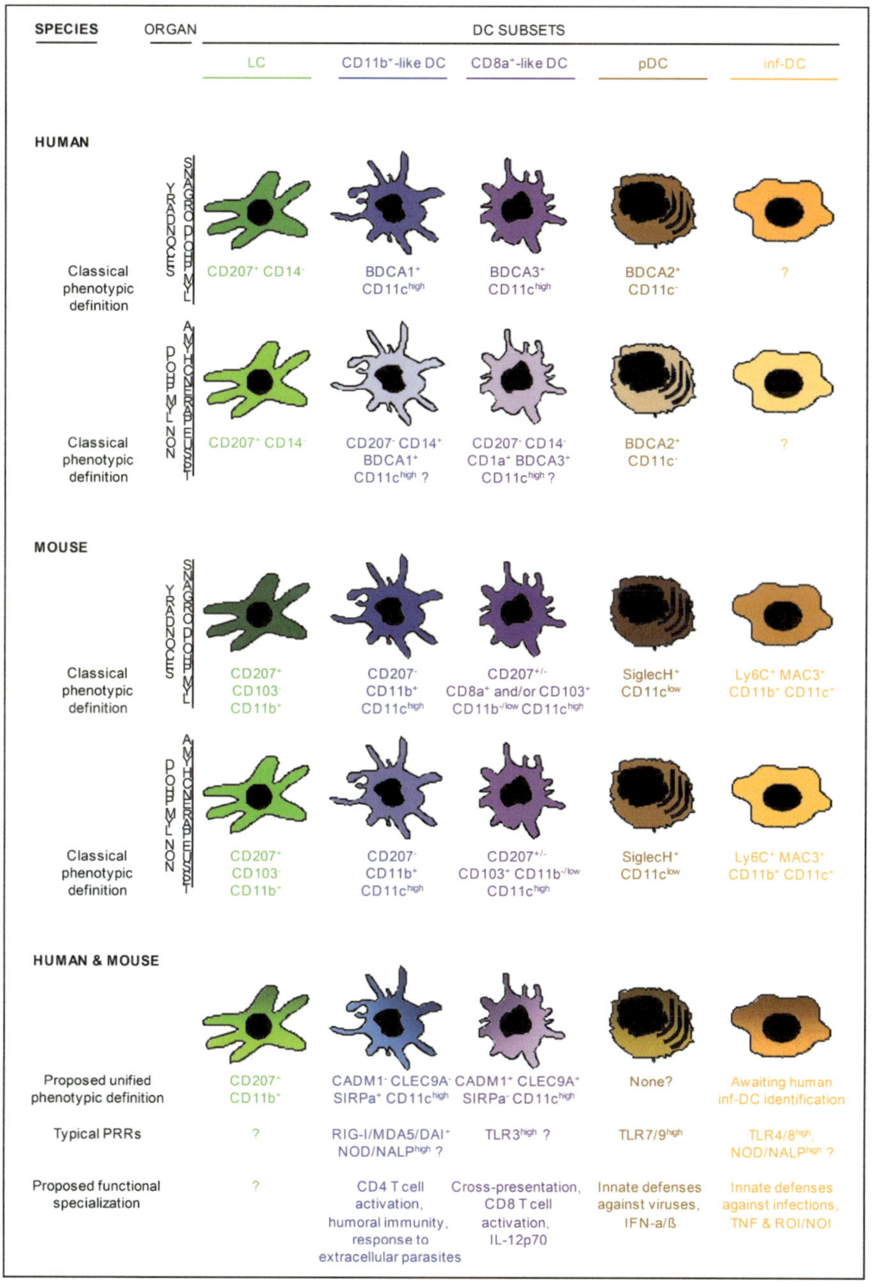

Fig. 7. A unifying model of human and mouse DC subsets (courtesy of Bernard Malissen). Human and mouse DC subsets were organized into five broad subsets irrespective of their primary location/tissue origin. These five subsets correspond to: (1) Langerhans cells (green), (2) DC-like cells (blue), (3) CD8a+ DC-like cells (violet), (4) pDC (brown), and (5) monocyte-derived inf-DC (orange). The authors suggest a general nomenclature for each DC subset (lower row, shaded colors) which is based on the unified phenotypic definition, characteristic pattern recognition receptors and functional specialization

3. Functional characteristics of lung DC

As mentioned above, the crucial functions of DC are to capture antigens throughout the body, migrate to the local lymphoid organs to deliver Ag and stimulate or tolerize T cells. The in vitro and in vivo Ag sampling by DC can be easily and specifically measured by flow cytometry (Chapoval et al., 2009; Cleret et al., 2007; Lambrecht et al., 2000; K. Y. Vermaelen et al., 2001; K. Y. Vermaelen et al., 2003). When DC acquire Ag, they become mature, upregulate their adhesion and costimulatory molecule expression, and specifically regulate chemokine receptor expression what makes them attracted to the lymphoid tissue (McColl, 2002). Ag-stimulated peripheral organ/tissue DC which downregulated inflammatory chemokine expression and upregulated CCR7 migrate to the local lymphoid tissue. These cells are called activated DC (McColl, 2002).

3.1 DC activation and maturation

As mentioned above, DC populate the lung tissue in the immature state (K. Vermaelen & Pauwels, 2005). Immature DC display high endocytic abilities and low T cell stimulation activity (Figure 1). After antigen uptake, DC undergo a complex process called maturation when they upregulate adhesion and costimulatory molecule expression and cytokine production but shut down the antigen-capturing activity. The DC conversion from immature to mature state is accompanied by a marked cellular reorganization (Shin et al., 2006) which can be detected by flow cytometry. This includes the redistribution of MHC II molecules from late endosomal and lysosomal compartments to the plasma membrane (Trombetta & Mellman, 2005; Turley et al., 2000). In addition, as mentioned above, DC downregulate their Ag uptake ability. This downregulation of some forms of endocytosis slows the clearance of MHC II from the cell surface (Sallusto, Cella, Danieli, & Lanzavecchia, 1995; Wilson, El-Sukkari, & Villadangos, 2004). Shin J-S and associates have determined the regulation of surface MHC II (Shin et al., 2006) employing bone marrow-derived DC expressing WT MHCII or mutant MHCIIβ (where single lysine of β-chain cytoplasmic domain was replaced with arginine, K>R) in flow cytometry. They have demonstrated that the MHC II β-chain cytoplasmic tail is ubiquitinated in mouse immature DC. Although only partly required for the sequestration MHC II in multivesicular bodies, this modification is essential for endocytosis. Notably, ubiquitination of MHC II was significantly downregulated with DC maturation, resulting in the cell surface accumulation of MHC II. Therefore, DC demonstrate a unique ability to regulate MHC II surface expression by selectively controlling MHC II ubiquitination.

3.2 Costimulatory molecule expression and function

In steady state conditions, lung cDC are immature and express CD11c, CD11b, low MHCII and low DEC-205 (Chapoval et al., 2009). The levels of costimulatory molecule expression on these cells vary from low to absent. To determine the effect of lung VEGF expression on local DC maturation state, we performed a flow cytometry analysis of lung digest single cell suspensions using the following marker-specific Abs for detection of costimulatory molecule expression on lung DC: anti-CD40-PE (3.23), anti-CD54-PE (3E2), anti-CD80-PE (16-10A1), anti-CD86-PE (GL1) PE-labeled, all from BD Biosciences. Anti-B7h/ICOS-L (HK5.3) Ab was obtained from eBioscience (Bhandari et al., 2006; Lee et al., 2004). PE-conjugated rat IgG2a (R35-95) and rat IgG2b (R35-38) were used as isotype controls. VEGF expression induced lung cDC activation as they upregulate MHCII, CD40, CD80, CD86, and CD54 expression on their surface (Lee et al., 2004).

3.3 In vivo antigen uptake

To track the Ag uptake by lung DC in vivo, we applied 1 μg/50 μl/mouse of OVA-FITC i.n. to WT and VEGF tg mice one time (Chapoval et al., 2009). Lung tissue and local LN digests were analyzed by flow cytometry 6h and 24h after Ag application for FITC+ cells using CD11c/MHCII/CD11b markers. We observed an increase in FITC+ DC but not Mac-1+ cell number in VEGF tg lungs by flow cytometry. Therefore, intermediately mature cDC obtained from the lung of VEGF tg mice were more efficient in Ag uptake.

Intratracheal instillations of OVA-FITC to mice with different deficiency can be used to assess the effect of such deficiency on lung DC migration. As an example, Vermaelen and associates (K. Y. Vermaelen et al., 2003) used OVA-FITC in MMP-9$^{-/-}$ mice to evaluate the effect of MMP-9 deficiency on lung DC migration. The study has shown that FITC+ cells gradually accumulate in the draining lymph nodes with a peak reaching at 24h of Ag application with no difference in lung DC migration between WT and MMP-9$^{-/-}$ mice.

4. Lung DC sorting

Highly pure isolated populations of DC are needed to evaluate their exact biological properties and function. Despite the fact that most lung DC represent rare populations among other lung cells, the high level of DC purification could be reached with either immunomagnetic (f.e. MACS technology, Milenyi Biotech) cell separation or flow cytometry-based cell sorts.

4.1 Methods of sorting

Lung conventional DC were sorted using a triple marker combination (CD11c/MHCII/CD11b) employing BD FACS Vantage or BD FACS Aria (both equipped with FACSDiva software), or Dako MoFlo (Summit software) high speed automated cell sorters (Chapoval et al., 2009) which all provide the state-of-the-art advances in the instrument set-up, cell sorting and integrated cell analysis. Autofluorescent macrophages and cell doublets are eliminated from further analysis by proper gating (Chapoval et al., 2009). The cDC sorting strategy is shown in Figure 8.

4.2 Analyses of sorted lung DC

Sorted lung DC then could be used in different in vitro assays to define the specific protein expression which could be further analyzed by flow cytometry (Beaty et al., 2007; Chapoval et al., 2009; K. Y. Vermaelen et al., 2001). The in vitro Ag uptake is an important technique to define the maturation status of DC and its functional activity. To study the in vitro Ag uptake, we subjected lung cells and sorted lung cDC to the in vitro cultures with or without increasing doses of OVA-FITC (Molecular Probes) ranging from 0.01 mg/ml to 1 mg/ml in RPMI (Life Technologies) in 24-well plates (Costar) for 30 min at 37°C. After incubation, cells were extensively washed with RPMI medium and analyzed for Ag uptake by flow cytometry. VEGF tg mDC are significantly more efficient in Ag uptake with low doses of Ag used. For example, at 10 μg of Ag only 30.2 % of WT DC were FITC+ whereas for VEGF tg

DC this number increased to 73.9%. At high dose both WT and tg cDC are equally efficient in Ag uptake.

4.3 Intracellular staining for cytokine and chemokine expression by DC

Chemokine production by lung CD11c+ cells was studied using intracellular staining (Beaty et al., 2007). Lung DC were sorted using anti-CD11c-conjugated magnetic microbeads (Miltenyi Biotec). pDC were enriched from the flow-through CD11c- cells using anti-mPDCA-1 magnetic microbeads and further sorted as PDCA-1+B220+I-A^{int} low scattered cells. CD11c+ cell fraction was further separated into subpopulations (CD103+ DC and CD11b^{hi}DC) by cell sorting on Vantage SE sorter with FACSDiva sofrware (BD Biosciences). The authors demonstrated that lung DC even without stimulation have accumulated detectable amounts of many chemokines and cytokines. Readily detectable were MIP-2, IP-10, MIP-1a, MIP-1b, RANTES, CXCL16, C10, TARC, and MDC for CD11bhi DC. Lung CD103+ DC expressed MIP-1a, CXCL16, TARC, and MDC but at much less levels. Therefore, the lung CD11bhi DC and CD103+ DC differentially express chemokines in naive mice. This difference further deepens with corresponding cell activation.

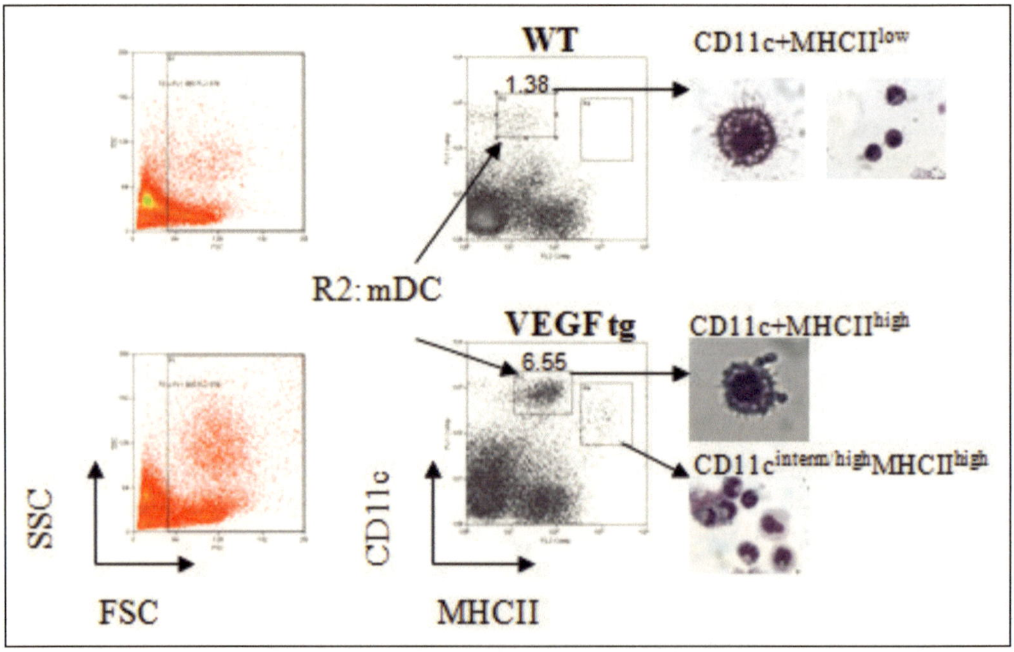

Fig. 8. Conventional lung DC acquisition and morphology. Single lung cell suspensions obtained from WT and VEGF tg mice (n=4-5 mice per experiment) were prepared with an omitting the enzymatic digestions step (Chapoval et al., 2009; Piggott et al., 2005). Cell were stained with anti-CD11c, -CD11b, and –MHCII Abs and analyzed using either FACSDiva or Summit software on cell sorters. Assigned cell populations were sorted and analyzed morphologically by Diff-Quick stain of cytospin slides prepared with 100 ml of sorted cells. The sorted cDC selected for further analysis represent CD11c+MHCIIlow population in WT mice and CD11c+MHCIIhigh population of cells in VEGF tg mice. The cells in gate 4 (CD11c$^{intermed/high}$MHCII^{high}) displayed a granulocyte-like morphology

4.4 In vivo DC migration study using sorted labeled cells

In addition to the fluorescently-labeled Ag application directly to the airways to study the lung DC migration, lung sorted or bone marrow-derived labelled DC can be introduced to the airways to track their migration with a use of flow cytometry (Lambrecht et al., 2000). This approach helps to distinguish the lymph node resident DC and DC migrated there from the lung. Bone marrow CD11c+MHCII+CD86+HSA+CD44+ICAM-1+DC were pulsed with CFSE (carboxyfluoroscein succinimidyl ester) and 1x10^6 cells were instilled intratracheally into naive mice. DC were traced in the lungs and mediastinal lymph nodes at 12h, 36h, and 120h after application. The authors have demonstrated that CFSE+ DC could be detected in BALF, digested lung tissues, and draining lymph nodes by 12h after instillation. By 36h CFSE+DC disappear from the BALF and intensively accumulate in the draining lymph nodes. A majority of injected cells had disappeared by 120h. Another study using this approach has demonstrated that by 24h approximately 2% of draining lymph node cells were CFSE+DC migrated from the lungs (Legge & Braciale, 2003). These CFSE+ DC were more mature than local DC as they showed higher levels of costimulatory molecule expression (CD40, CD80, and CD86) and upregulated MHCII expression.

Intratracheal adoptive transfer of CFSE-labeled exogenous DC has been used to study the effect of MMP-9 deficiency on DC trafficking from the lung to the mediastinal lymph nodes (K. Y. Vermaelen et al., 2003). Measuring the absolute numbers of FITC+ cells in the lymph nodes, they demonstrated no differences between MMP-9+ and MMP-9- DC reaching lymph nodes

5. Summary

In conclusion, we show and discuss in this chapter a high phenotypic and functional complexity of lung DC. None of DC subpopulation can be identified and isolated by cell sorting for further analysis based on one or two marker expression. Specific Abs at least to three-four molecules needed to be used simultaneously for a clear lung DC subpopulation differentiation. Multicolor flow cytometry measuring simultaneously 5 or more parameters has dramatically increased our ability in DC subtype biology characterization. However, the complexity of such analysis increases with the number of fluorochromes used. The use of appropriate gating strategy, inclusion of all necessary controls from the beginning of the experiment and all necessary isotype controls for the specific Abs used in the assay, proper instrument validation, correct compensation will highly contribute to obtaining relevant biological data.

6. Acknowledgment

S.P.C. is supported by NIAID R21AI076736 grant.

7. References

Alvarez, D., Vollmann, E. H., & von Andrian, U. H. (2008). Mechanisms and consequences of dendritic cell migration. *Immunity, 29*(3), 325-342.

Asselin-Paturel, C., Brizard, G., Pin, J. J., Briere, F., & Trinchieri, G. (2003). Mouse strain differences in plasmacytoid dendritic cell frequency and function revealed by a novel monoclonal antibody. [Comparative Study]. *J Immunol, 171*(12), 6466-6477.

Beaty, S. R., Rose, C. E., Jr., & Sung, S. S. (2007). Diverse and potent chemokine production by lung CD11bhigh dendritic cells in homeostasis and in allergic lung inflammation. *J Immunol, 178*(3), 1882-1895.

Bhandari, V., Choo-Wing, R., Chapoval, S. P., Lee, C. G., Tang, C., Kim, Y. K., . . . Elias, J. A. (2006). Essential role of nitric oxide in VEGF-induced, asthma-like angiogenic, inflammatory, mucus, and physiologic responses in the lung.. *Proc Natl Acad Sci U S A, 103*(29), 11021-11026.

Chapoval, S. P., Nabozny, G. H., Marietta, E. V., Raymond, E. L., Krco, C. J., Andrews, A. G., David, C. S. (1999). Short ragweed allergen induces eosinophilic lung disease in HLA-DQ transgenic mice. *J Clin Invest*, 103(12), 1707-1717.

Chapoval, S. P., Al-Garawi, A., Lora, J. M., Strickland, I., Ma, B., Lee, P. J., Homer, R. J., Ghosh, S., Coyle, A. J., Elias, J. A. (2007). Inhibition of NF-kappaB activation reduces the tissue effects of transgenic IL-13. *J Immunol*, 179(10), 7030-7041.

Chapoval, S. P., Lee, C. G., Tang, C., Keegan, A. D., Cohn, L., Bottomly, K., & Elias, J. A. (2009). Lung vascular endothelial growth factor expression induces local myeloid dendritic cell activation. *Clin Immunol, 132*(3), 371-384.

Chelen, C. J., Fang, Y., Freeman, G. J., Secrist, H., Marshall, J. D., Hwang, P. T., . . . Umetsu, D. T. (1995). Human alveolar macrophages present antigen ineffectively due to defective expression of B7 costimulatory cell surface molecules. *J Clin Invest, 95*(3), 1415-1421.

Cleret, A., Quesnel-Hellmann, A., Vallon-Eberhard, A., Verrier, B., Jung, S., Vidal, D., . . . Tournier, J. N. (2007). Lung dendritic cells rapidly mediate anthrax spore entry through the pulmonary route. *J Immunol, 178*(12), 7994-8001.

Cochand, L., Isler, P., Songeon, F., & Nicod, L. P. (1999). Human lung dendritic cells have an immature phenotype with efficient mannose receptors. *Am J Respir Cell Mol Biol, 21*(5), 547-554.

de Heer, H. J., Hammad, H., Soullie, T., Hijdra, D., Vos, N., Willart, M. A., . . . Lambrecht, B. N. (2004). Essential role of lung plasmacytoid dendritic cells in preventing asthmatic reactions to harmless inhaled antigen. *J Exp Med, 200*(1), 89-98.

Demedts, I. K., Brusselle, G. G., Vermaelen, K. Y., & Pauwels, R. A. (2005). Identification and characterization of human pulmonary dendritic cells. *Am J Respir Cell Mol Biol, 32*(3), 177-184.

Fainaru, O., Shseyov, D., Hantisteanu, S., Groner, Y. (2005). Accelerated chemokine receptor 7-mediated dendritic cell migration in Runx3 knockout mice and the spontaneous development of asthma-like disease. *Proc Natl Acad Sci U S A*, 102(30), 10598-10603.

Guilliams, M., Henri, S., Tamoutounour, S., Ardouin, L., Schwartz-Cornil, I., Dalod, M., & Malissen, B. From skin dendritic cells to a simplified classification of human and mouse dendritic cell subsets. *Eur J Immunol, 40*(8), 2089-2094.

Jakubzick, C., Helft, J., Kaplan, T. J., & Randolph, G. J. (2008). Optimization of methods to study pulmonary dendritic cell migration reveals distinct capacities of DC subsets to acquire soluble versus particulate antigen. *J Immunol Methods, 337*(2), 121-131.

Jakubzick, C., Tacke, F., Ginhoux, F., Wagers, A. J., van Rooijen, N., Mack, M., . . . Randolph, G. J. (2008). Blood monocyte subsets differentially give rise to CD103+ and CD103- pulmonary dendritic cell populations. *J Immunol, 180*(5), 3019-3027.

Kawanami, O., Basset, F., Ferrans, V. J., Soler, P., & Crystal, R. G. (1981). Pulmonary Langerhans' cells in patients with fibrotic lung disorders. *Lab Invest, 44*(3), 227-233.

Kirby, A. C., Raynes, J. G., & Kaye, P. M. (2006). CD11b regulates recruitment of alveolar macrophages but not pulmonary dendritic cells after pneumococcal challenge. *J Infect Dis, 193*(2), 205-213.

Lambrecht, B. N., De Veerman, M., Coyle, A. J., Gutierrez-Ramos, J. C., Thielemans, K., & Pauwels, R. A. (2000). Myeloid dendritic cells induce Th2 responses to inhaled antigen, leading to eosinophilic airway inflammation. *J Clin Invest, 106*(4), 551-559.

Lambrecht, B. N., & Hammad, H. (2009a). Biology of lung dendritic cells at the origin of asthma. *Immunity, 31*(3), 412-424.

Lambrecht, B. N., & Hammad, H. (2009b). Lung dendritic cells: targets for therapy in allergic disease. *Handb Exp Pharmacol*(188), 99-114.

Lambrecht, B. N., Salomon, B., Klatzmann, D., & Pauwels, R. A. (1998). Dendritic cells are required for the development of chronic eosinophilic airway inflammation in response to inhaled antigen in sensitized mice. *J Immunol, 160*(8), 4090-4097.

Lee, C. G., Link, H., Baluk, P., Homer, R. J., Chapoval, S., Bhandari, V., . . . Elias, J. A. (2004). Vascular endothelial growth factor (VEGF) induces remodeling and enhances TH2-mediated sensitization and inflammation in the lung. *Nat Med, 10*(10), 1095-1103.

Legge, K. L., & Braciale, T. J. (2003). Accelerated migration of respiratory dendritic cells to the regional lymph nodes is limited to the early phase of pulmonary infection. *Immunity, 18*(2), 265-277.

Lehmann, J., Huehn, J., de la Rosa, M., Maszyna, F., Kretschmer, U., Krenn, V., . . . Hamann, A. (2002). Expression of the integrin alpha Ebeta 7 identifies unique subsets of CD25+ as well as CD25- regulatory T cells. *Proc Natl Acad Sci U S A, 99*(20), 13031-13036.

Lindquist, R. L., Shakhar, G., Dudziak, D., Wardemann, H., Eisenreich, T., Dustin, M. L., & Nussenzweig, M. C. (2004). Visualizing dendritic cell networks in vivo. *Nat Immunol, 5*(12), 1243-1250.

Maraskovsky, E., Brasel, K., Teepe, M., Roux, E. R., Lyman, S. D., Shortman, K., & McKenna, H. J. (1996). Dramatic increase in the numbers of functionally mature dendritic cells in Flt3 ligand-treated mice: multiple dendritic cell subpopulations identified. *J Exp Med, 184*(5), 1953-1962.

Masten, B. J., Olson, G. K., Kusewitt, D. F., & Lipscomb, M. F. (2004). Flt3 ligand preferentially increases the number of functionally active myeloid dendritic cells in the lungs of mice. *J Immunol, 172*(7), 4077-4083.

Masten, B. J., Olson, G. K., Tarleton, C. A., Rund, C., Schuyler, M., Mehran, R., . . . Lipscomb, M. F. (2006). Characterization of myeloid and plasmacytoid dendritic cells in human lung. *J Immunol, 177*(11), 7784-7793.

McColl, S. R. (2002). Chemokines and dendritic cells: a crucial alliance. *Immunol Cell Biol, 80*(5), 489-496.

Metlay, J. P., Witmer-Pack, M. D., Agger, R., Crowley, M. T., Lawless, D., & Steinman, R. M. (1990). The distinct leukocyte integrins of mouse spleen dendritic cells as identified with new hamster monoclonal antibodies. *J Exp Med, 171*(5), 1753-1771.

Niu, N., Le Goff, M. K., Li, F., Rahman, M., Homer, R. J., & Cohn, L. (2007). A novel pathway that regulates inflammatory disease in the respiratory tract. *J Immunol, 178*(6), 3846-3855.

Piggott, D. A., Eisenbarth, S. C., Xu, L., Constant, S. L., Huleatt, J. W., Herrick, C. A., & Bottomly, K. (2005). MyD88-dependent induction of allergic Th2 responses to intranasal antigen. *J Clin Invest, 115*(2), 459-467.

Pollard, A. M., & Lipscomb, M. F. (1990). Characterization of murine lung dendritic cells: similarities to Langerhans cells and thymic dendritic cells. *J Exp Med, 172*(1), 159-167.

Ray, P., Tang, W., Wang, P., Homer, R., Kuhn, C., Flavell, R. A., Elias, J. A. (1997). Regulated overexpression of interleukin 11 in the lung. Use to dissociate development-dependent and -independent phenotypes. *J Clin Invest*, 100(10), 2501–2511.

Ritz, S. A., Cundall, M. J., Gajewska, B. U., Swirski, F. K., Wiley, R. E., Alvarez, D., . . . Jordana, M. (2004). The lung cytokine microenvironment influences molecular events in the lymph nodes during Th1 and Th2 respiratory mucosal sensitization to antigen in vivo. *Clin Exp Immunol, 138*(2), 213-220.

Sallusto, F., Cella, M., Danieli, C., & Lanzavecchia, A. (1995). Dendritic cells use macropinocytosis and the mannose receptor to concentrate macromolecules in the major histocompatibility complex class II compartment: downregulation by cytokines and bacterial products. *J Exp Med, 182*(2), 389-400.

Sertl, K., Takemura, T., Tschachler, E., Ferrans, V. J., Kaliner, M. A., & Shevach, E. M. (1986). Dendritic cells with antigen-presenting capability reside in airway epithelium, lung parenchyma, and visceral pleura. *J Exp Med, 163*(2), 436-451.

Shin, J. S., Ebersold, M., Pypaert, M., Delamarre, L., Hartley, A., & Mellman, I. (2006). Surface expression of MHC class II in dendritic cells is controlled by regulated ubiquitination. *Nature, 444*(7115), 115-118.

Solovjov, D. A., Pluskota, E., & Plow, E. F. (2005). Distinct roles for the alpha and beta subunits in the functions of integrin alphaMbeta2. *J Biol Chem, 280*(2), 1336-1345.

Spencer, S. C., & Fabre, J. W. (1990). Characterization of the tissue macrophage and the interstitial dendritic cell as distinct leukocytes normally resident in the connective tissue of rat heart. *J Exp Med, 171*(6), 1841-1851.

Steiniger, B., Klempnauer, J., & Wonigeit, K. (1984). Phenotype and histological distribution of interstitial dendritic cells in the rat pancreas, liver, heart, and kidney. *Transplantation, 38*(2), 169-174.

Steinman, R. M. (2010). Some active areas of DC research and their medical potential. *Eur J Immunol, 40*(8), 2085-2088.

Steinman, R. M., & Cohn, Z. A. (1973). Identification of a novel cell type in peripheral lymphoid organs of mice. I. Morphology, quantitation, tissue distribution. *J Exp Med, 137*(5), 1142-1162.

Sung, S. S., Fu, S. M., Rose, C. E., Jr., Gaskin, F., Ju, S. T., & Beaty, S. R. (2006). A major lung CD103 (alphaE)-beta7 integrin-positive epithelial dendritic cell population expressing Langerin and tight junction proteins. *J Immunol, 176*(4), 2161-2172.

Swanson, K. A., Zheng, Y., Heidler, K. M., Zhang, Z. D., Webb, T. J., & Wilkes, D. S. (2004). Flt3-ligand, IL-4, GM-CSF, and adherence-mediated isolation of murine lung dendritic cells: assessment of isolation technique on phenotype and function. *J Immunol, 173*(8), 4875-4881.

Trombetta, E. S., & Mellman, I. (2005). Cell biology of antigen processing in vitro and in vivo. *Annu Rev Immunol, 23*, 975-1028.

Tsoumakidou, M., Tzanakis, N., Papadaki, H. A., Koutala, H., Siafakas, N. M. (2006). Isolation of myeloid and plasmacytoid dendritic cells from human bronchoalveolar lavage fluid. *Immunol Cell Biol*, 84(3), 267-273.

Turley, S. J., Inaba, K., Garrett, W. S., Ebersold, M., Unternaehrer, J., Steinman, R. M., & Mellman, I. (2000). Transport of peptide-MHC class II complexes in developing dendritic cells. *Science, 288*(5465), 522-527.

van Haarst, J. M., Hoogsteden, H. C., de Wit, H. J., Verhoeven, G. T., Havenith, C. E., Drexhage, H. A. (1994). Dendritic cells and their precursors isolated from human bronchoalveolar lavage: immunocytologic and functional properties. *Am J Respir Cell Mol Biol*, 11(3), 344-350.

Vermaelen, K., & Pauwels, R. (2004). Accurate and simple discrimination of mouse pulmonary dendritic cell and macrophage populations by flow cytometry: methodology and new insights. *Cytometry A, 61*(2), 170-177.

Vermaelen, K., & Pauwels, R. (2005). Pulmonary dendritic cells. *Am J Respir Crit Care Med, 172*(5), 530-551.

Vermaelen, K. Y., Carro-Muino, I., Lambrecht, B. N., & Pauwels, R. A. (2001). Specific migratory dendritic cells rapidly transport antigen from the airways to the thoracic lymph nodes. *J Exp Med, 193*(1), 51-60.

Vermaelen, K. Y., Cataldo, D., Tournoy, K., Maes, T., Dhulst, A., Louis, R., . . . Pauwels, R. (2003). Matrix metalloproteinase-9-mediated dendritic cell recruitment into the airways is a critical step in a mouse model of asthma. *J Immunol, 171*(2), 1016-1022.

Wilson, N. S., El-Sukkari, D., & Villadangos, J. A. (2004). Dendritic cells constitutively present self antigens in their immature state in vivo and regulate antigen presentation by controlling the rates of MHC class II synthesis and endocytosis. *Blood, 103*(6), 2187-2195.

Zeng, X., Wert, S.E., Federici, R., Peters, K.G. & Whitsett, J.A. (1998). VEGF enhances pulmonary vasculogenesis and disrupts lung morphogenesis in vivo. *Dev Dyn*, 211, 215–227.

13

Stem Cell Characterization

Arash Zaminy
Department of Anatomy & Cell Biology,
Shahid Beheshti University of Medical Sciences, Tehran,
Iran

1. Introduction

One of the main problems in stem cell studies is how researchers can identify and characterize a stem cell.

Identification and characterization of stem cells is a difficult and often evolving procedure. Stem cells not only must exhibit the appropriate markers, but also a healthy and robust stem cell population must also lack specific markers. In addition to the difficulty of this area of stem cell biology markers, profiles change based on the species, site of origin and maturity (totipotent vs. multipotent) of a given population. Furthermore, stem cell populations may consist of several specific phenotypes which are often indicators of the population's general health. Flow cytometry employs instrumentation that scans single cells flowing past excitation sources in a liquid medium. It is a widely used method for characterizing and separating individual cells.

This chapter tries to explain what stem cells are, as well as to summarize current knowledge on stem cell characterization and usage of stem cells markers.

2. Stem cells

All life forms initiate with a stem cell, which is defined as a cell that has the dual capacity to self-renew and to produce progenitors and different types of specialized cells in the organism. Scientists mostly work with two kinds of stem cells from animals and humans: embryonic stem cells and non-embryonic "somatic" or "adult" stem cells.

At the beginning of human life, one fertilized egg cell – the zygote – divides into two and two becomes four (Carlson, 1996). Within 5 to 7 days, some 40 cells are produced which build up the inner cell mass encircled by an outer cell layer subsequently forming the placenta. At this phase, each of these cells in the inner cell mass has the potential to give rise to all tissue types and organs – that is, these cells are pluripotent. Finally, the cells forming the inner cell mass will give rise to the some 1013 cells that constitute a human body, organized in 200 differentiated cell types (Sadler, 2002). Many somatic, tissue-specific or adult stem cells are produced during the foetal period. These stem cells have a more limited ability than the pluripotent embryonic stem cells (ESCs) and they are multipotent – that is, they have the potential to give rise only to a limited number of cell lineages. These adult stem cells keep on in the related organs to varying degrees over the whole of a person's lifetime.

Stem cells are well-known from other cell types because of two important characteristics. First, they are unspecialized cells and the have ability to renew themselves through cell division, sometimes after long periods of inactivity. Second, under certain physiologic or experimental conditions, they can be induced to become tissue- or organ-specific cells with special abilities (Thrasher, 1966; Merok & Sherley, 2001). In some organs, such as the gut and bone marrow, stem cells divide regularly to repair and restore exhausted or damaged tissues. In other organs, however, such as the pancreas and the heart, stem cells only divide under special conditions.

3. Stem cells markers

In recent years researchers have revealed a broad range of stem cells that have unique capabilities to self-renew, grow indefinitely and differentiate or develop into multiple kinds of cells and tissues. Researchers now know that many different types of stem cells exist, but they are all found in very small populations in the human body, in some cases one stem cell in 100,000 cells in circulating blood. In addition, when scientists study these cells under a microscope, they are similar to other cells in the tissue where they are found. So, like the search for a needle in a haystack, how do scientists recognize these uncommon types of cells found in many different cells and tissues? The answer is rather simple, thanks to stem cell "markers."

What are stem cell markers? The surface of every cell in the body has specialized proteins called receptors that have the capability of selectively binding or adhering to other "signalling" molecules. There are many different types of receptors that differ in their composition and affinity for the signalling molecules. Generally, cells use these receptors and the molecules that bind to them as a way of communicating with other cells, and to perform their correct functions in the body. These cell surface receptors are commonly used as cell markers. Each cell type, for example a liver cell, has a certain combination of receptors on their surface that makes them distinguishable from other types of cells. Scientists have taken advantage of the biological exclusivity of stem cell receptors and the chemical properties of certain compounds to label or mark cells. Researchers owe much of the past success in finding and characterizing stem cells to the use of markers.

Stem cell markers are given shorthand names based on the molecules that attach to the stem cell surface receptors. For example, a cell that has the receptor stem cell antigen -1 on its surface is known as Sca-1. In many cases, a mixture of multiple markers is used to identify a particular stem cell type. So now, researchers often identify stem cells in shorthand by a combination of marker names reflecting the presence (+) or absence (-) of them. For example, a special type of haematopoietic stem cell from blood and bone marrow is described as ($CD34^{-/low}$, $c\text{-}Kit^{+}$, $Sca\text{-}1^{+}$) (Jackson et al., 2001).

Researchers employ antibody molecules that selectively bind with the receptors on the surface of the cell as a way to identify stem cells. In former years a method was developed to attach to the antibody molecule another molecule (or tag) that has the ability to fluoresce or emit light energy when triggered by an energy source such as an ultraviolet light or laser beam. Now, multiple fluorescent labels are available with emitted light that differ in colour and intensity.

Researchers exploit the combination of the chemical properties of fluorescence and unique receptor patterns on cell surfaces to identify specific numbers of stem cells. One approach for using markers is a technique known as fluorescence-activated cell sorting (FACS) (Bonner et al., 1972; Herzenberg, 2000; Julius, 1972). Researchers frequently use a FACS instrument to sort out the rare stem cells from the millions of other cells. By this method, a suspension of tagged cells (i.e. fluorescently-labelled antibodies are bound to the cell surface markers) is sent under pressure through a very fine nozzle. Upon exiting the nozzle cells pass through a light source, usually a laser, and then through an electric field. Operators apply a series of criteria. If the cell stream meets the criteria, they become negatively or positively charged. When cells are passing among an electric field, the charge difference permits the desired cells to be separated from other cells. The researchers now have a population of cells that have all of the same marker characteristics and with these cells they can conduct their research.

A second method uses stem cell markers and fluorescent antibodies to visually assess cells as they exist in tissues. Often researchers want to assess how stem cells appear in tissues and in doing so they use a microscope to evaluate them rather than the FACS instrument. In this case, a thin slice of tissue is prepared and the stem cell markers are tagged by the antibodies that have the fluorescent tag attached. The fluorescent tags are then activated either by special light energy or a chemical reaction. The stem cells will emit a fluorescent light that can easily be seen under the microscope.

4. Embryonic stem cells

An embryonic stem cell (ESC) is described by its origin. It is obtained from the blastocyst stage of the embryo. Embryonic stem cells are unique cell populations with the capability of both self-renewal and differentiation, and thus ESCs can give rise to any adult cell type. Pluripotent embryonic stem (ES) cells, like embryonal carcinoma cells, were first used as a tool to examine thoroughly early differentiation. However, the properties of ESCs identify them as being highly appropriate for making specific cell lineages in vitro. The ability of embryonic stem cells to almost limitless self-renewal and differentiation capacity has opened up the panorama of widespread applications in biomedical research and regenerative medicine.

ESCs are harvested from the inner cell mass of the pre-implantation blastocyst and have been derived from rodents (Martin, 1981; Evans & Kaufman, 1981; Doetschman et al., 1988; Graves & Moreadith, 1993), primates (Thomson et al., 1995) and humans (Thomson et al., 1998; Reubinoff et al., 2000).

4.1 Embryonic stem cell markers

Some approaches have been applied to characterize ESCs, but the most widely used approach is analysis of cell surface antigens by flow cytometry and evaluation of gene expression profile by RT-PCR or microarrays. Many cell surface antigens used to identify hESCs were first detected with antibodies prepared against pre-implantation mouse embryos and/or against mouse or human embryonal carcinoma cells (Pera et al., 2000).

Although the functions of those antigens in the continuance of undifferentiated human embryonal carcinoma cells are not necessarily clear, they may represent helpful markers for the recognition of pluripotent stem cells. These antigens include the globo-series glycolipid antigens, stage-specific embryonic antigen-3 (SSEA-3) and -4 (SSEA-4), keratan sulphate antigens TRA-1-60, TRA-1-81, GCTM2 and GCTM343, a set of various protein antigens comprising the two liver alkaline phosphatase antigens TRA-2-54 and TRA-2-49, Thy1, CD9, HLA class 1 antigens, Oct3/4, Nanog and the absence of hESC negative markers, such as SSEA-1 (Pera et al., 2000; Carpenter et al., 2003; Chambers et al., 2003; Draper et al., 2004; Heins et al., 2004; Nichols et al., 1998).

Some cell surface biomarkers are also listed in Table 1. The International Stem Cell Initiative (ISCI) established by the International Stem Cell Forum (http://www.stemcellforum.org.uk) carried out a comparative study of a large and different set of hESC lines derived from and maintained in different laboratories worldwide (Adewumi et al., 2007). Fifty-nine independent hESC lines derived from 17 laboratories in 11 countries were investigated for the expression of 17 cell surface antigens and 93 genes, which have been chosen as potential markers of undifferentiated stem cells or their differentiated derivatives (Adewumi et al., 2007). All of the independent hESC lines displayed a common expression profile for a specific set of marker antigens, despite the fact that they had different genetic backgrounds and were produced by different techniques in each laboratory. All examined cell lines expressed a comparable spectrum of cell surface marker antigens characteristic of hESCs, suggesting that there is a common set of markers that can be used to monitor, in general, the presence of pluripotent stem cells. SSEA-3 and SSEA-4 were expressed in all hESCs tests, indicating that these molecules are valuable operational markers of this cell type; however, a study revealed that they are not necessary for the pluripotency of hESCs (Brimble et al., 2007).

	Mouse ES cells	Human ES cells
SSEA-1	+	-
SSEA-3	-	+
SSEA-4	-	+
TRA-1-60	-	+
TRA-1-81	-	+
GCTM-2	-	+
Alkaline phosphatase	+	+
Oct-4	+	+
GDF-3	+	?

Table 1. Marker expression and growth properties of mouse and primate pluripotent cells

5. Haematopoietic stem cells

Blood cells are responsible for continuous preservation and immune protection of every cell type of the body. This persistent and brutal work requires blood cells, along with skin cells, to have the greatest power of self-renewal of any adult tissue. The stem cells that form blood and immune cells are known as haematopoietic stem cells (HSCs). HSCs are among the best characterized adult stem cells and the only stem cells being regularly used in clinics.

A haematopoietic stem cell is a cell isolated from the blood or bone marrow that can renew itself, can differentiate a variety of specialized cells and can mobilize out of the bone marrow into circulating blood. Since HSCs look and behave in culture like ordinary white blood cells, it has been a challenge to identify them by morphology (size and shape). Even now, scientists must rely on cell surface proteins, which generally serve as markers of white blood cells.

5.1 Haematopoietic stem cell markers

HSCs have an identity problem. First, the ones with long-term replicating ability are rare. Second, there are multiple types of stem cells. Third, the stem cells look like many other blood or bone marrow cells. So how do researchers find the desired cell populations? The most common approach is through markers that emerge on the surface of cells.

A variety of markers has been found to help distinguish and separate HSCs. Early marker efforts focused on cell size, density and recognition by lectins (carbohydrate-binding proteins derived largely from plants) (Bauman et al., 1988), but more recent attempts have focused mostly on cell surface protein markers, as defined by monoclonal antibodies. For mouse HSCs, these markers contain panels of 8 to 14 different monoclonal antibodies that recognize cell surface proteins present on differentiated haematopoietic lineages, such as the red blood cell and macrophage lineages (thus, these markers are collectively referred to as Lin) (Spangrude et al., 1988; Uchid & Weissman, 1992) as well as the proteins Sca-1 (Spangrude et al., 1988; Uchid & Weissman, 1992), CD27 (Weissman et al., 2000), CD34 (Osawa et al., 1996), CD38 (Randall et al., 1996), CD43 (Moore et al., 1994), CD90.1 (Thy-1.1) (Spangrude et al., 1988; Uchid & Weissman, 1992), CD117 (c-Kit) (Ikuta & Weissman, 1992), AA4.1 (Jordan et al., 1996) and MHC class I (Bauman et al., 1988), and CD150 (Kiel et al., 2005).

Human HSCs have been described with respect to staining for CD34 (Civin et al., 1984), CD38 (Kiel et al., 2005), CD43 (Moore et al., 1994), CD45RO (Lansdorp et al., 1990), CD45RA (Lansdorp et al., 1990), CD59 (Hill et al., 1996), CD90 (Bauman et al., 1988), CD109 (Sutherland et al., 1996), CD117 (Gunji et al., 1993), CD133 (Miraglia et al., 1997; Yin et al., 1997), CD166 (Uchida et al., 1997), HLA DR (human) (Srour et al., 1992; Tsukamoto et al., 1995) and lacking expression of lineage (Lin) markers (Baum et al., 1992). It is important to note that lineage markers are cell surface antigens that can be used for immunophenotyping cells of a particular developmental lineage. Cells that do not express these marker antigens, or express them at very low levels, are said to be lineage marker negative [lin(-)].

While none of these markers recognize functional stem cell activity, combinations (typically with 3 to 5 different markers, see examples below) led to the purification of near-homogenous populations of HSCs. The ability to obtain pure preparations of HSCs, albeit in limited numbers, has greatly facilitated the functional and biochemical characterization of these important cells. However, now there has been limited impact of these discoveries on clinical practice, as highly purified HSCs have only rarely been used to treat patients. The irrefutable advantages of using purified cells (e.g., the absence of contaminating tumour cells in autologous transplantations) have been offset by practical difficulties and increased purification costs.

HSC assays, when combined with the ability to purify HSCs, have provided increasingly detailed insight into the cells and the early steps involved in the differentiation process.

Several marker combinations have been developed that describe murine HSCs, including [CD117^{high}, CD90.1^{low}, Lin$^{neg/low}$, Sca-1^{pos}] (Morrison & Weissman, 1994), [CD90.1^{low}, Lin^{neg}, Sca-1^{pos}Rhodamine123^{low}] (Kim et al., 1998), [CD34$^{neg/low}$, CD117^{pos}, Sca-1^{pos}, Lin^{neg}] (Osawa et al., 1996), [CD150 ^{pos}, CD48^{neg}, CD244^{neg}] (Kiel et al., 2005) and side-population; cells using Hoechst-dye (Goodell et al., 1996). Each of these combinations allows purification of HSCs to near-homogeneity. Similar strategies have been widened to purify human HSCs, employing markers such as CD34, CD38, Lin, CD90, CD133 and fluorescent substrates for the enzyme, aldehyde dehydrogenase. The use of highly purified human HSCs has been mostly experimental and clinical use normally employs enrichment for one marker, usually CD34. CD34 enrichment yields a population of cells enriched for HSC and blood progenitor cells, but still contains many other cell types. However, limited trials in which highly FACS-purified CD34^{pos} CD90^{pos} HSCs were used as a source of reconstituting cells have demonstrated that rapid reconstitution of the blood system can reliably be obtained using only HSCs (Negrin et al., 2000; Vose et al., 2001).

None of the HSC markers currently used are directly linked to crucial HSC function, and consequently, even within species, markers can differ depending on genetic alleles (Spangrude & Brooks, 1992), mouse strains (Spangrude & Brooks, 1993), developmental stages (Morrison et al., 1995) and cell activation stages (Randall & Weissman, 1997; Sato et al., 1999). In spite of this, there is an obvious connection with HSC markers between divergent species such as humans and mice. However, unless the current efforts at defining the complete HSC gene expression patterns will yield usable markers that are linked to essential functions for maintaining the stemness of the cells (Ramalho et al., 2002; Ivanova et al., 2002), functional analysis will remain necessary to identify HSCs clearly (Domen et al., 1999).

Mouse	Human
CD34low/-	CD 34+
SCA-1+	CD59+
Thy1+/low	Thy1+
CD38+	CD38low/-
C-kit+	C-kit -/low

Table 2. Proposed cell surface markers of undifferentiated haematopoietic stem cells

5.2 Side population

When in adult mouse haematopoietic tissue, unpurified bone marrow cells are labelled with the membrane-permeate DNA binding dye Hoechst 33342, a very small fraction of cells extrudes this dye via a membrane pump (Goodell et al., 1996, 1997, 2001). Analysis of these cells on a flow cytometer equipped with an ultraviolet (UV) laser source allows finding of these cells; when Hoechst-labelled cells are analysed simultaneously through blue and red emission filters, the SP forms a dim tail extending from the normal G1 cell populations. These cells can reconstitute the bone marrow of lethally irradiated mice at an ED_{50} (Effective Dose 50) of fewer than 100 cells, indicating that they are highly enriched for totipotent stem cells. The SP cell subpopulation is also enriched for cells expressing the murine stem cell markers Sca-1 and c-kit, further suggesting that they contain very early haematopoietic progenitors (Goodell et al., 1996).

The SP fraction expresses an ABC transporter, Bcrp-1(ABCG2), on the cell surface and this transporter contributes to efflux of the Hoechst dye from the cells, leading to low levels of staining (Zhou et al., 2001). Interestingly, the bone marrow and peripheral immune system in ABCG2 transporter knockouts animals, is normal, suggesting that the capability to efflux Hoechst 33342 is characteristic of stem cells, but not essential for function (Uchida et al., 2002). Similar SP subpopulations have been observed in primates and humans (Kim et al., 2002; Allen et al., 2002). The SP phenotype, therefore, has become a significant marker for stem cell activity in the identification of these cells and in their physical isolation by fluorescence-activated cell sorting.

6. Mesenchymal stem cells

Stem cells from adult tissues are an interesting source for cell therapy, gene therapy and tissue engineering. These cells normally have limited lineage potential in comparison to embryonic stem cells and this can be advantageous from the viewpoint of controlling cell growth and differentiation in certain therapeutic applications (Barrilleaux et al., 2006; Barry & Murphy, 2004; Haynesworth et al., 1998).

In 1961, bone marrow was shown to have haematopoietic progenitor cells (Till & McCulloch, 1961). In the early 1970s, many investigators confirmed that bone marrow also had cells with fibroblastic morphology that could differentiate into bone, cartilage, fat and muscle (Prockop, 1997). These cells have been variously designated as marrow stromal cells or mesenchymal stem cells, and abbreviated as "MSCs." It has been demonstrated that individual cells from the bone marrow stromal population possessed multilineage potential (Pittenger et al., 1999). Since the recognition of MSCs in bone marrow, cells with the same multilineage potential have been isolated from other tissues, including trabecular bone (Noth et al., 2002; Sottile et al., 2002) , adipose tissue (Lee et al., 2004; Zuk et al., 2001) and umbilical cord (Secco, 2008). The presence of MSCs in adipose tissue has generated special interest because harvesting fat tissue is generally less invasive to the donor than harvesting bone marrow and larger quantities may be available. Adipose-derived MSCs are also called adipose-derived stem cells (ADSCs) and adipose-derived adult stromal or stem cells (ADAS cells). But in addition to ADSCs, umbilical cord is also another interesting source for MSCs and has recently gained some attention.

6.1 Mesenchymal stem cell markers

Cell surface proteins may characterize particular cell types or lineages. In some cases, the role of a specific surface protein and its role in the biology of the cell type is known. However, often the function of the protein has not been determined, but the protein has been shown to be related to a certain type of cell and can serve as a marker. Exclusive diagnostic surface markers for human MSCs have not been identified, however, several surface markers have been found to be commonly associated with hMSCs, including STRO-1, CD105 (endoglin), CD166 (activated leukocyte cell adhesion molecule, ALCAM) (Barry & Murphy, 2004; Gronthos et al., 2001) and more recently CD271 (low affinity nerve growth factor receptor, LNGFR) (Buhring et al., 2007; Quirici et al., 2002). Surface marker antigens can be used to distinguish the cells in a specific preparation and monitor their differentiation. Surface markers that are exclusively positive for a different cell type, for example, the haematopoietic surface markers CD45 and CD34, can be used to search for contamination of MSC preparations with other cell types. Surface markers have also been used for positive and negative immunoselection of MSC cell populations (Buhring et al., 2007; Simmons & Torok-Storb, 1991).

The expressed genes that appear on the hMSC surface include receptors for growth factors, matrix molecules and other cells, and point out how the hMSC will interact with its environment. The flow cytometry analysis also indicates the homogeneity of the hMSC population or whether it is a mixture of different cell types. A wide-ranging, yet incomplete, list of the surface molecules on hMSCs is provided in Table 3.

Surface antigens	
Positive	CD13, CD29, CD44, CD49b(Integrin alpha 2,5), CD54(ICAM1), cd71(Transferrin Rec), CD73(SH-3), CD105(Endoglin.SH-2), CD106(VCAM), CD166(ALCAM)
Negative	CD3, CD4, CD6, CD9, CD10, CD11a, b, CD14, CD15, CD34, CD45, D18 (Integrin beta 2), CD31 (PECAM), CD49d (Intergrin alpha 4), CD50 (ICAM3), CD62E (E-Selectin), CD117(c-kit), CD133

Table 3. Mesenchymal stem cells markers

7. Neural stem cells

Neurogenesis is defined as the procedure of generating new neurons from neural stem cells (NSCs),which consists of the proliferation and fate determination of NSCs, migration and survival of young neurons, and maturation and integration of recently matured neurons (Ming & Song, 2005).

NSCs are defined as undifferentiated cells that developmentally originate from the neuroectodermal layer during early embryogenesis. After neural tube closing, these undifferentiated precursor cells and their immediate progeny compose the neuroepithelial layer that surrounds the lateral, third and fourth ventricles in the midbrain and forebrain, and the central canal in the spinal cord. They are the main source of cells that later form all major structures of the brain and spinal cord (Maric & Barker, 2004).

NSCs have recently attracted a great deal of attention because of their inherent ability to generate all major classes of cells of the nervous system. NSCs have therefore been supposed as a useful resource for potentially repairing and restoring the physiological functions to damaged, diseased or aging neural tissues (Gang, 2000; Anderson, 2001; Temple, 2001; Vaccarino et al., 2001; Vescovi et al., 2001; Weissman et al., 2001).

However, with the accelerated interest in and growth of the NSC field, there has been growing uncertainty around the understanding of what cell phenotype actually makes up a neural stem cell. NSCs in their undifferentiated shape are characterized by a unique bipolar morphology that can help identify them from the heterogeneity associated with early culture. Derivation from human foetal material gives rise to an apparently mixed population of NSCs, exhibiting both classic bipolar NSC morphology and other cell morphologies.

7.1 Neural stem cell markers

The major research limitation is that the cellular preparations used as a source of NSCs are themselves naturally heterogeneous and consisting of both NSCs and self-renewing, but more lineage restricted, progenitors; accordingly making the retrospective studies of NSC biology skewed to an unknown degree. Adding to this is the increasing evidence that implies clear functional differences between neural stem and progenitor cells (Galli et al., 2003; Cai & Rao, 2002). Consequently, there is a critical need to use strategies to identify and isolate pure populations of NSCs and other type cells with the aim of resolving their shared or unique biological properties with respect to cell-fate determination and lineage progression.

NSCs are immunoreactive for a range of neural precursor/radial glia markers such as Nestin, Vimentin, RC2, 3CB2, Sox-2 and brain lipid-binding protein (BLBP). However, subtle differences exist between mouse and human NSCs. For example, hNS cells display moderate levels of glial fibrillary acidic protein (GFAP) expression unlike mouse NSCs (Conti et al., 2005), reflecting the differences between the species in vivo (Malatesta et al., 2000; Rakic, 2003).

So, as mentioned above, the cells which are gathered from neural tissue are heterogeneous and identifying cells is required. Therefore, some markers that are used in studies are listed below:

Neural stem cells	GFAP, Nestin, Prominin, SOX-2
Proliferating cells	Ki-67,BrdU, PCNA
Immature neurons	beta Tubulin,DCX,PSA-NCAM
Radial glia	GLAST, RC2
Mature neurons	NeuN, MAP-2, NF, BLBP
Oligodendrocyte precursors	NG2
Oligdendrocytes	O4, MBP, RIP

Table 4. Neural stem cells markers

8. Spermatogonial stem cells

Germ cells are specific cells that transfer the genetic information of an individual to the next generation. Making functional germ cells is vital for continuation of the germ line of the species. Spermatogenesis, the process of male germ cell production, takes place in the seminiferous tubules of the postnatal testis and is an extremely productive system in the body. In the mammalian testis, more than 20 million sperms per gram of tissue are created daily (Amann, 1986). The high productivity relies on spermatogonial stem cells (SSCs). Similar to other kinds of stem cells in adult tissues, SSCs are self-renewing and produce daughter cells that assign to differentiate throughout the life of the male (Meistrich & van Beek, 1993). In addition, in mammals, SSCs are unique among stem cells in the adult body, because they are the only cells that undergo self-renewal and transmit genes to subsequent generations. Furthermore, SSCs provide an excellent model to study stem cell biology due to the availability of a functional assay that clearly identifies the stem cell (Weissman et al., 2001).

Spermatogonial stem cells derive from primordial germ cells (PGCs), which in turn originate from epiblast cells (embryonal ectoderm) (Lawson KA et al., 1992). Soon after the development of the PGCs, they migrate from the base of the allantois, along the hindgut, finally reaching the genital ridges. The PGCs increase in number during migration, when these cells have reached the genital ridges; their number increases to about 10,000 per gonad (Tam and Snow, 1981). PGCs are single cells that under certain culture conditions can make colonies of cells which morphologically are similar to undifferentiated embryonic stem cells (ESCs) (Resnick JL et al., 1992).When they have arrived in the genital ridges, the PGCs are surrounded by the differentiating Sertoli cells, so seminiferous cords are formed.

The germ cells present within the seminiferous cords are different morphologically from PGCs and are called gonocytes (Clermont and Perey, 1957; Sapsford CS et al., 1962; Huckins & Clermont, 1968) or various subsequent types of pro-spermatogonia (Hilscher B et al;1974). Shortly after birth, the gonocytes restart proliferation to give rise to adult types of spermatogonia (Sapsford CS et al., 1962; Huckins & Clermont, 1968; Vergouwen RPFA et al., 1991; Novi & Saba, 1968; Bellye AR et al., 1977). This happening indicates the start of spermatogenesis.

8.1 Spermatogonial stem cell markers

Since the establishment of the transplantation technique, several new markers and characteristics of spermatogonial stem cells have been identified that can be used to isolate a population from the testis that is enriched for spermatogonial stem cells - Tables 5 and 6.

Markers for positive selection of spermatogonial stem cells	CD9 (Kanatsu-Shinohara M et al., 2004), integrin alpha 6 (Shinohara T et al., 1999), integrin beta 1 (Shinohara T et al., 1999), THY-1, CD24 (Kubota H et al., 2003)
Markers for negative selection of spermatogonial stem cells	c-kit, MHC1, Ly6A(Sca-1), CD34 (Kubota H et al., 2003)

Table 5. Overview of markers that have been successfully used to isolate spermatogonial stem cell populations from the testis by either positive or negative selection

8.2 Testicular side population

So far, four groups have separated a side population of testicular cells; meanwhile, different results were drawn as to whether these were spermatogonial stem cells. The first group reported the existence of a testicular side population. Amazingly, they did not find this population to be capable of colonizing a recipient testis after transplantation and concluded that it did not contain spermatogonial stem cells (Kubota et al., 2003).

Then, two other groups found the testicular side population to be enriched for spermatogonial stem cells (Falciatori et al., 2004; Lassalle et al., 2004). A fourth group then explained that testicular side population cells contain Leydig cell progenitors (Lo et al., 2004; de Rooij.,2004) and later failed to find spermatogonial stem cells in this population (Lo et al., 2005).

The controversial results can probably be explained by the strictness of the FACS gating and the different procedures used to separate the side population. It may be possible to isolate a very pure population of spermatogonial stem cells from the testis using the side population technique, alone or in combination with membrane markers (van Bragt et al., 2005), however, for this to be possible more research needs to be performed to determine the optimal procedures and combinations of markers.

A(s) and	GFRalpha-1(Von Schonfeldt et al., 2004, Hofmann et al, 2005) FC, MACS, IHC, ISH, WM
A(s), A (pr) and A(al)	PLZF (Buaas et al., 2004) (Costaya et al., 2004) FC, ISH, IHC, WM, Mu; OCT4 (Pesce et al., 1998) FC, ISH, IHC, WM TG; NGN3 (Yoshida et al., 2004) ISH, TG, WM, ISH; NOTCH1 (Von Schonfeldt et al., 2004) RT-PCR, IHC, SOX3 (Raverot et al., 2005) KO, IHC; c-RET (Meng et al., 2000) IHC, MACS
A spermatogonia	RBM (Jarvis et al., 2005) RT-PCR, IHC
Spermatogonia	EP-CAM (Anderson et al., 1999) FC, IHC, MACS
Premeiotic germ cells	STRA8 (Oulad Abdelghani et al., 1996) RT-PCR, ISH, IHC, WM EE2 (Koshimizu et al., 1995) WB , IHC
Cells on basal membrane and interstitium	CD9 (Kanatsu-Shinohara et al., 2004) FC, IHC, MACS
Spermatogonia, spermatocytes and round spermatids	GCNA1 (Enders & May., 1994) FC, WB, IHC
Premeiotic spermatogonia and postmeiotic spermatid	TAF4B (Falender et al., 2005) FC, KO, IHC

A(s), A-single; A (pr), pair of spermatogonia; A (al), A-aligned spermatogonia; FC, flow cytometry (including FACS); Mu, mutant mouse; TG, transgenic mouse; KO, Knockout mouse; IHC, immunohistochemistry; WM, whole mount immunostaining; WB, Western blot; ISH, in situ hybridization; RT-PCR, reverse transcriptase- PCR; MACS, magnetic-activated cell sorting

Table 6. Overview of markers used to identify spermatogonial stem cells

9. Epidermal stem cells

The skin is the body's strong outer cover that maintains the inside of the body being moist and protects the body from outside assaults by physical, environmental and biological factors. Skin and its associated hair follicles and glandular structures, sebaceous and sweat glands, are made by a stratified epithelium where the position of the cell within the tissue relates to its state of differentiation. The terminally differentiated stratum corneum, hairs and oil-filled sebocytes have a limited lifespan and are constantly shed from the body throughout the adult life. This continual shedding requires that the epithelium is replenished and restored by a stem cell population during normal maintenance of the skin and also in response to injury (Fuchs & Horsley, 2008; Watt et al., 2006). By definition, adult stem cells (ASCs) have the ability to both self-renew and make differentiated progeny (Lajitha, 1979). In healthy skin, epidermal stem cells divide uncommonly, but upon skin injury, stem cells quickly divide to repair the lesion.

There has been important progress in the recognizing of epidermal stem cells (ESCs) since the 1970s, when the idea of interfollicular epidermis was firstly suggested; later, much work was focused on the specific region of the hair follicle outer root sheath, mainly the bulge region. Hair follicle stem cells are multipotent, capable of giving rise to all cell types of the hair, the epidermis and the sebaceous gland (Morris et al., 2004).

9.1 Epidermal stem cells markers

Recognizing the ESCs is major progress in the field of skin biology which lets scientists examine their biochemical properties, lineage and their relation to other cells. There is evidence of ESCs in the bulge region of the hair follicles (Myung et al., 2009a, 2009b; Zhang et al, 2009), as well as in the interfollicular epidermis (Abbas & Mahalingam, 2009; Ambler & Maatta, 2009). When the epidermis undergoes severe damage, it may fully regenerate from the ESCs of the bulge (Watt, 2006). The ESCs present in the bulge and interfollicular epidermis are potentially interconvertible, but under normal conditions they only differentiate a more confined progeny.

ESCs can be identified in vivo by label retention or in vitro by clonogenicity, but neither of these methods allows easy isolation of stem cells for analysis. Therefore, there is a strong need for specific ESCs markers to be identified.

Identifying stem cells by their cell cycling properties has limited potential. Therefore, several research groups have undertaken wide attempts to characterize a set of stem cell specific markers. Much of this research has focused on the bulge region, as this is the most clearly defined stem cell niche in the skin (Fuchs & Horsley, 2008; Watt et al., 2006).

Many efforts have been made in recent years to recognize ESCs. The potential candidate hair follicle stem cells markers include integrin beta 1, keratin 15, keratin 19, CD71, transcription factor p63 and CD34 (Ma et al., 2004). Keratinocyte shows the characteristics of keratin intermediate filaments. In the epidermis, keratins 5 and 14 are expressed in the basal layer, while keratins 1 and 10 are found in the suprabasal layer. The hair follicle stem cells expressed the above keratins and keratins 6, 16 and 17 (Al-Refu et al., 2009; Hoang et al., 2009), and desmosomal proteins, including desmoglein, may serve as negative markers of ESCs (Wan et al., 2003).

In 2001, p63 was identified as a marker for ESCs; p63 is a transcription factor belonging to a family that contains an additional two structurally-related proteins, p53and p73 (Pellegrini et al., 2001). Although p53 fulfils an important role in tumour suppression, p63 and p73 participate in morphogenetic processes (Klein et al., 2010). Their expression is evidenced in ESCs.

CD34 is also a specific marker for bulge keratinocytes. The mouse bulge marker CD34, often used for isolating murine bulge cells, is expressed below the bulge region in human hair follicles (Ohyama et al., 2006). As mentioned before, CD34 is also a specific marker for haematopoietic stem and progenitor cells, however, much more work is needed to clarify specific markers for ESCs.

10. Conclusion

Flow cytometry is able to rapidly check thousands of cells stained with antibodies conjugated to fluorescent dyes. Each cell is individually assessed for a mixture of features such as size and biochemical and/or antigenic composition. High accuracy and sensitivity, combined with the large numbers of cells that can be examined, allows resolution of even very minor subpopulations from complex mixtures with high levels of statistical validity.

As mentioned earlier, the main problem with stem cell research is that a specific marker for each stem cell is not available for researchers and markers usually are common between some cell populations. Therefore, it is clear that we should wait to hear more from future studies to resolve this issue and introduce new and specific markers for each individual stem cell.

11. References

Abbas, O. & Mahalingam, M. (2009). Epidermal stem cells: practical perspectives and potential uses. *Br J. Dermatol.*, 161: 228-236.

Adewumi, O., Aflatoonian, B., Ahrlund-Richter, L. & Amit, M. (2007). Characterization of human embryonic stem cell lines by the International Stem Cell Initiative. International Stem Cell Initiative. *Nat. Biotechnol.*, 25, 803–816.

Allen, JD., van Loevezijn, A., Lakhai, JM., van der Valk, M., van Tellingen, O., Reid, G., Schellens, JH., Koomen, GJ. & Schinkel, AH. (2002). Potent and specific inhibition of the breast cancer resistance protein multidrug transporter in vitro and in mouse intestine by a novel analogue of fumitremorgin C. *Mol Cancer Ther.*, 1:417- 425.

Al-Refu, K., Edward, S., Ingham, E. & Goodfield, M. (2009). Expression of hair follicle stem cells detected by cytokeratin 15 stain: implications for pathogenesis of the scarring process in cutaneous lupus erythematosus. *Br J. Dermatol.*, 160: 1188-1196.

Amann, RP. (1986). Detection of alterations in testicular and epididymal function in laboratory animals. *Environ. Health Perspect.*, 70, 149–158.

Ambler, CA. & Maatta, A. (2009). Epidermal stem cells: location, potential and contribution to cancer. *J. Pathl* 217: 206-216.

Anderson, DJ. (2001). Stem cells and pattern formation in the nervous system: the possible versus the actual. *Neuron,* 30, 19–35.

Anderson, R., Schaible, K., Heasman, J. & Wylie, C. (1999). Expression of the homophilic adhesion molecule, Ep-CAM, in the mammalian germ line. *J. Reprod. Fertil.*, 116:379–84.

Barrilleaux, B., Phinney, DG., Prockop, D. J. & O'Connor, KC. (2006). Review: Ex vivo engineering of living tissues with adult stem cells. *Tissue Eng.*, 12, 3007–3019.

Barry, FP. & Murphy, JM. (2004). Mesenchymal stem cells: clinical applications and biological characterization. *Int. J. Biochem. Cell Biol.*, 36, 568–584.

Baum, CM., Weissman, IL., Tsukamoto, AS., Buckle, AM. & Peault, B. (1992). Isolation of a candidate human hematopoietic stem-cell population. *Proc Natl Acad Sci USA*, Vol 89,2804–2808.

Bauman, JG., de Vries, P., Pronk, B. & Visser, JW. (1988). Purification of murine hemopoietic stem cells and committed progenitors by fluorescence activated cell sorting using wheat germ agglutinin and monoclonal antibodies. *Acta Histochem Suppl.*, Vol 36,241–253.

Bellve, AR., Cavicchia, JC., Millette, CF., O'Brien, DA., Bhatnagar, YM. & Dym,M. (1977). Spermatogenic cells of the prepuberal mouse. Isolation and morphological characterization. *J. Cell Biol.*, 74:68- 85.

Bonner, WA., Hulett, HR., Sweet, RG. & Herzenberg, LA. (1972). Fluorescence activated cell sorting. *Rev. Sci. Instrum.*, 1972:43, 404–409.

Brimble, SN., Sherrer, ES., Uhl, EW. & Wang, E. (2007). The cell surface glycosphingolipids SSEA-3 and SSEA-4 are not essential for human ESC pluripotency. *Stem Cells*, 25, 54–62.

Buaas, FW., Kirsh, AL., Sharma, M., McLean, DJ., Morris, JL. & Griswold, MD. (2004). Plzf is required in adult male germ cells for stem cell self-renewal. *Nat Genet.*, 36:647–52.

Buhring, H-J., Battula, V L., Treml, S., Schewe, B., Kanz, L. & Vogel, W. (2007). Novel markers for the prospective isolation of human MSC. *Ann. N. Y. Acad. Sci.*, 1106, 262–271.

Cai, J. & Rao, MS. (2002) Stem cell and precursor cell therapy. *Neuromolecular Med.* 2, 233–249.

Carlson, BM. (1996). *Patten's Foundations of Embryology.* 6th edn. New York, McGraw-Hill.

Carpenter, MK., Rosler, E. & Rao, MS. (2003).Characterization and differentiation of human embryonic stem cells.*Cloning Stem Cells*,5(1):79–88.

Chambers, I., Colby, D., Robertson, M., Nichols, J., Lee, S. & Tweedie, S. (2003). Functional expression cloning of Nanog, a pluripotency sustaining factor in embryonic stem cells. *Cell*, 113(5):643–655.

Civin, CI., Strauss, LC., Brovall, C., Fackler, MJ., Schwartz, JF. & Shaper, JH. (1984). Antigenic analysis of hematopoiesis. III. A hematopoietic progenitor cell surface antigen defined by a monoclonal antibody raised against KG- 1a cells. *J. Immunol.*, Vol 133,157–165.

Clermont, Y. & Perey, B. (1957). Quantitative study of the cell population of the seminiferous tubules of immature rats. *Am J. Anat*, 100:241–68.

Conti, L., Pollard, SM., Gorba,T., Reitano, E., Toselli, M., Biella, G., Sun, Y., Sanzone, S., Ying Q-L, Cattaneo E. & Smith, A. (2005). Niche-independent symmetrical self-renewal of a mammalian tissue stem cell. *PLoS Biol*, 3:e283.

Costoya, JA., Hobbs, RM., Barna, M., Cattoretti, G., Manova, K. & Sukhwani M. (2004). Essential role of Plzf in maintenance of spermatogonial stem cells. *Nat Genet*, 36:653–9.

de Rooij, DG. & Van Bragt, MP. (2004). Leydig cells: testicular side population harbors transplantable leydig stem cells. *Endocrinology*, 2004, 145:4009–10.

Doetschman, T., Williams, P., Maeda, N. (1988). Establishment of hamster blastocyst-derived embryonic stem cells. *Dev. Biol*, 127: 224–227.

Domen, J. & Weissman, IL. (1999). Self-renewal, differentiation or death: regulation and manipulation of hematopoietic stem cell fate. *Mol Med Today.* Vol 5,201–208.

Draper, JS., Pigott, C., Thomson, JA & Andrews, PW. (2002). Surface antigens of human embryonic stem cells: changes upon differentiation in culture. *J. Anat*, 200(Part 3):249–258.

Eiges, R., Schuldiner, M., Drukker, M., Yanuka, O., Itskovitz-Eldor, J. & Benvenisty, N. (2001). Establishment of human embryonic stem cell-transduced clones carrying a marker of undifferentiated cells. *Curr. Biol.* 11, 514–518.

Ellis, P., Fagan, B. M., Magness, S. T., Hutton, S., Taranova, O., Hayashi, S., McMahon, A., Rao, M. & Pevny, L. (2004). SOX2, a persistent marker for multipotential neural stem cells derived from embryonic stem cells, the embryo or the adult. *Dev. Neurosci* 26,148-65.

Enders, GC, May JJ, 2nd. Developmentally regulated expression of a mouse germ cell nuclear antigen examined from embryonic day 11 to adult in male and female mice. *Dev. Biol.*,1994, 163:331–40.

Evans, MJ., Kaufman, MH. (1981). Establishment in culture of pluripotential stem cells from mouse embryos. *Nature*, 291:154–156.

Falciatori, I., Borsellino, G., Haliassos, N., Boitani, C., Corallini, S. & Battistini, L. (2004). Identification and enrichment of spermatogonial stem cells displaying side-population phenotype in immature mouse testis. *Faseb J*,18:376–8.

Falender, AE., Freiman, RN., Geles, KG., Lo, KC., Hwang, K. & Lamb, DJ. (2005). Maintenance of spermatogenesis requires TAF4b, a gonad-specific subunit of TFIID. *Genes Dev*,19:794–803.

Fuchs, E. & Horsley, V. (2008). More than one way to skin. *Genes Dev*, 22(8):976–985.

Gage, F.H. (2000) Mammalian neural stem cells. *Science* 287, 1433–1438.

Galli R., Gritti A., Bonfanti L., & Vescovi A.L. (2003). Neural stem cells: an overview. *Circ. Res.*92, 598–608.

Goodell, MA., Brose, K., Paradis, G., Conner, AS. & Mulligan, RC. (1996). Isolation and functional properties of murine hematopoietic stem cells that are replicating in vivo. *J. Exp Med*. Vol 183,1797–1806.

Goodell, MA, Rosenzweig M, Kim H, Marks DF, De Maria M, Paradis G, Grupp S, Seiff CA, Mulligan RC, Johnson RP. (1997). Dye efflux studies suggest that hematopoietic stem cells expressing low or undetectable levels of CD34 antigen exist in multiple species. *Nat Med*, 3:1337–1345.

Goodell, MA. (2001). Stem cell identification and sorting using the Hoeschst 33342 side population (SP). In: Robinson JP, Darzynkiewicz Z, Dean PN, Hibbs AR, Orfao A, Rabinovitch PS, Wheeless LL, editors. *Current protocols in cytometry*. New York: John Wiley & Sons; P 9.18.1–9.18 –21.

Graves, KH., Moreadith, RW. (1993). Derivation and characterization of putative pluripotential embryonic stem cells from preimplantation rabbit embryos. *Mol Reprod Devel*, 36:424–433.

Gronthos, S., Franklin, DM., Leddy, HA., Robey, PG., Storms, RW. & Gimble, JM. (2001). Surface protein characterization of human adipose tissue-derived stromal cells. *J. Cell. Physiol.* 189, 54–63.

Gunji, Y., Nakamura, M. & Osawa, H. (1993). Human primitive hematopoietic progenitor cells are more enriched in KITlow cells than in KIThigh cells. *Blood,* Vol 82,3283–3289.

Haynesworth, S. E., Reuben, D. & Caplan, A. I. (1998). Cell-based tissue engineering therapies: the influence of whole body physiology. *Adv. Drug Deliv. Rev.* 33, 3–14.

Heins, N., Englund, MC., Sjöblom, C., Dahl, U., Tonning, A., Bergh, C & Lindah, L. (2004). Derivation, characterization and differentiation of human embryonic stem cells. *Stem Cells*, 22(3):367–376.

Herzenberg, LA. & De Rosa, SC. (2000). Monoclonal antibodies and the FACS: complementary tools for immunobiology and medicine. *Immunol. Today*. 21, 383–390.

Hill, B., Rozler, E. & Travis, M. (1996). High-level expression of a novel epitope of CD59 identifies a subset of CD34& bone marrow cells highly enriched for pluripotent stem cells. *Exp Hematol.* Vol 24,936–943.

Hilscher, B., Hilscher, W., Bulthoff-Ohnolz, B., Kramer, U., Birke, A. & Pelzer, H. (1974). Kinetics of gametogenesis. I. Comparative histological and autoradiographic studies of oocytes and transitional prospermatogonia during oogenesis and prespermatogenesis. *Cell Tissue Res* ,154: 443–70.

Hoang, MP., Keady, M. & Mahalingam, M. (2009).Stem cell markers (cytokeratin 15, CD34 and nestin) in primary scarring and nonscarring alopecia. *Br J. Dermatol* 160: 609-615.

Hofmann, MC., Braydich-Stolle, L. & Dym, M. (2005). Isolation of male germ-line stem cells, influence of GDNF. *Dev. Biol*, 279:114–24.

Huckins, C. & Clermont, Y. (1968). Evolution of gonocytes in the rat testis during late embryonic and early post-natal life. *Arch Anat Histol Embryol*, 51:341–54.

Ikuta, K. & Weissman, IL. (1992) Evidence that hematopoietic stem cells express mouse c-kit but do not depend on steel factor for their generation. *Proc Natl Acad Sci USA.* Vol 89,1502–1506.

Ivanova, NB., Dimos, JT., Schaniel, C., Hackney, JA., Moore, KA. & Lemischka, IR. (2002). A stem cell molecular signature. *Science,* Vol 298,601–604.

Jackson, K., Majka, SM., Wang, H., Pocius, J., Hartley, CJ., Majesky, MW., Entman, ML., Michael, LH., Hirschi, KK. & Goodell, MA. (2001). Regeneration of ischemic cardiac muscle and vascular endothelium by adult stem cells. *J. Clin. Invest.* 107(11), 1395–1402.

Jarvis, S., Elliott, DJ., Morgan, D., Winston, R. & Readhead, C. (2005). Molecular markers for the assessment of postnatal male germ cell development in the mouse. *Hum Reprod* 2005,20:108–16.

Jorda, CT., McKearn, JP. & Lemischka, IR. (1990). Cellular and developmental properties of fetal hematopoietic stem cells. *Cell*, Vol 61,953–963.

Julius, MH., Masuda, T. & Herzenberg, LA. (1972). Demonstration that antigen-binding cells are precursors of antibody-producing cells after purification with a fluorescence-activated cell sorter. *Proc. Natl. Acad. Sci. U. S. A.* 69, 1934–1938.

Kanatsu-Shinohara, M., Toyokuni, S. & Shinohara, T. (2004). CD9 is a surface marker on mouse and rat male germline stem cells. *Biol. Reprod*, 70:70–5.

Kempermann, G., Jessberger, S., Steiner, B. & Kronenberg, G. (2004) Milestones of neuronal development in the adult hippocampus. *Trends Neurosci* 27, 447–52.

Kiel, MJ., Yilmaz, OH., Iwashita, T.,Terhorst , C. & Morrison, SJ. (2005) SLAM family receptors distinguish hematopioetic stem and progenitor cells and reveal enothelial niches for stem cells. *Cell*, 121:1109–1121.

Kim, M., Cooper, DD., Hayes, SF. & Spangrude, GJ. (1998). Rhodamine123 staining in hematopoietic stem cells of young mice indicates mitochondrial activation rather than dye efflux. *Blood,* Vol 91,4106–4117.

Kim, M., Turnquist, H., Jackson, J., Sgagias, M., Yan,Y., Gong, M., Dean, M., Sharp, JG. & Cowan, K. (2002). The multidrug resistance transporter ABCG2 (breast cancer resistance protein 1) effluxes Hoechst 33342 and is over expressed in hematopoietic stem cells. *Clin Cancer Res*, 8:22–28.

Klein, AM., Brash, DE., Jones, PH. & Simons, BD. (2010). Stochastic fate of p53-mutant epidermal progenitor cells is tilted toward proliferation by UVB during preneoplasia. *Proc Natl Acad Sci USA* 107: 270-275.

Koshimizu, U., Nishioka, H., Watanabe, D., Dohmae, K. & Nishimune, Y. (1995). Characterization of a novel spermatogenic cell antigen specific for early stages of germ cells in mouse testis. *Mol Reprod Dev*, 40:221–7.

Kubota, H., Avarbock, MR. & Brinster, RL. (2003). Spermatogonial stem cells share some, but not all, phenotypic and functional characteristics with other stem cells. *Proc Natl Acad Sci U S A* ,100:6487–92.

Lajtha, LG. (1979). Stem cell concepts. *Differentiation*, 14(1–2):23–34.

Lansdorp, PM., Sutherland, HJ. & Eaves, CJ. (1990). Selective expression of CD45 isoforms on functional subpopulations of CD34& hemopoietic cells from human bone marrow. *J. Exp Med.*. Vol 172,363–366.

Lassalle, B., Bastos, H., Louis, JP., Riou, L., Testart, J. & Dutrillaux, B. (2004). 'Side Population' cells in adult mouse testis express Bcrp1 gene and are enriched in spermatogonia and germinal stem cells. *Development*, 131:479–87.

Lawson, KA. & Pederson, RA. (1992). Clonal analysis of cell fate during gastrulation and early neurulation in the mouse. In: Ciba Foundation Symposium 165. Post implantation development in the mouse. New York: John Wiley & Sons, 3–26.

Lee, RH., Kim, B., Choi, I., Kim, H., Choi, HS., Suh, K., Bae, Y. C. & Jung, J. S. (2004). Characterization and expression analysis of mesenchymal stem cells from human bone marrow and adipose tissue. *Cell Physiol. Biochem.* 14, 311-324.

Lo, KC., Brugh,VM., Parker, M. & Lamb, DJ. (2005). Isolation and enrichment of murine spermatogonial stem cells using rhodamine 123 mitochondrial dye. *Biol. Reprod.*, 72:767–71.

Lo, KC., Lei, Z., Rao, Ch, V., Beck, J. & Lamb, DJ. (2004). De novo testosterone production in luteinizing hormone receptor knockout mice after transplantation of Leydig stem cells. *Endocrinology*, 145:4011–5.

Ma, DR., Yang , EN. & Lee, ST. (2004). A Review: The Location, Molecular Characterisation and Multipotency of Hair Follicle Epidermal Stem Cells. *Ann Acad Med Singapore*, 33:784-8

Malatesta, P., Hartfuss, E. & Gotz, M. (2000) Isolation of radial glial cells by fluorescent-activated cell sorting reveals a neuronal lineage. *Development*, 127: 5253–5263.

Maric, D. & Barker, J. L. (2004). Neural Stem Cells Redefined A FACS Perspective. *Molecular Neurobiology*: 04:30(1): 49–76.

Martin, G. Isolation of a pluripotent cell line from early mouse embryos cultured in medium conditioned by teratocarcinoma cells. *Proc Natl Acad Sci U S A* 1981, 78: 7634–7638.

Meistrich, M. L. & van Beek, M. E. A. B. (1993). Spermatogonial stem cells. In *Cell and Molecular Biology of the Testis* (C. Desjardins, and LL. Ewing, eds.), pp. 266–295. Oxford University Press, New York.

Meng, X., Lindahl, M., Hyvonen, ME., Parvinen, M., de Rooij, DG. & Hess, MW. (2000). Regulation of cell fate decision of undifferentiated spermatogonia by GDNF. *Science* ,287:1489–93.

Merok, J. R & Sherley, JL. (2001). Breaching the kinetic barrier to in vitro somatic stem cell propagation. *J. Biomed. Biotech.* 1:25–27.

Ming, G. L. & Song, H. (2005) Adult neurogenesis in the mammalian central nervous system. *Annu Rev Neurosci.,* 28, 223–50.

Minguell, JJ., Erices, A. & Conget, P. (2001). Mesenchymal stem cells. *Exp. Biol. Med.,* 226:506–520.

Miraglia, S., Godfrey, W. & Yin, AH. (1997). A novel five-transmembrane hematopoietic stem cell antigen: isolation, characterization, and molecular cloning. *Blood,* Vol 90,5013–5021.

Moore, T., Huang, S., Terstappen, LW., Bennett, M. & Kumar, V. (1994). Expression of CD43 on murine and human pluripotent hematopoietic stem cells. *J. Immunol.* Vol 153,4978–4987.

Morris, RJ., Liu, Y., Marles, L., Yang, Z., Trempus, C. & Li, S. (2004). Capturing and profiling adult hair follicle stem cells. *Nat Biotech,* 22:411-7.

Morrison, SJ. & Weissman, IL. (1994). The long-term repopulating subset of hematopoietic stem cells is deterministic and isolatable by phenotype. *Immunity,* 1:661–673.

Morrison, SJ., Hemmati, HD., Wandycz, AM. & Weissman, IL. (1995). The purification and characterization of fetal liver hematopoietic stem cells. *Proc Natl Acad Sci USA.* Vol 92,10302–10306.

Myung, P., Andl T & Ito, M. (2009b). Defining the hair follicle stem cell (Part II). *J. Cutan Pathol.,* 36: 1134-1137.

Myung, P., Andl T. & Ito, M. (2009a). Defining the hair follicle stem cell (Part I). *J. Cutan Pathol.,* 36: 1031-1034.

Negrin, RS., Atkinson, K. & Leemhuis T. (2000). Transplantation of highly purified CD34&Thy-1& hematopoietic stem cells in patients with metastatic breast cancer. *Biol. Blood Marrow Transplant,* Vol 6,262–271.

Nichols, J., Zevnik, B., Anastassiadis, K., Niwa, H., Klewe-Nebenius, D & Chambers, I. (1998). Formation of pluripotent stem cells in the mammalian embryo depends on the POU transcription factor Oct 4. *Cell,* 95(3):379–391.

Noth, U., Osyczka, AM., Tuli, R., Hickok, NJ., Danielson, KG. &Tuan, RS. (2002). Multilineage mesenchymal differentiation potential of human trabecular bone-derived cells. *J. Orthop. Res.,* 20, 1060–1069.

Novi, AM., & Saba, P. (1968). An electron microscopic study of the development of rat testis in the first 10 postnatal days. *Z Zellforsch Mikrosk Anat* , 86:313–26.

Ohyama, M., Terunuma, A., Tock, CL., Radonovich, MF., Pise- Masison, CA. & Hopping, SB. (2006). Characterization and isolation of stem cell-enriched human hair follicle bulge cells. *J. Clin Invest,* 116(1):249–260.

Osawa M., Hanada, K., Hamada, H., Nakauchi, H. (1996). Long-term lymphohematopoietic reconstitution by a single CD34low/negative hematopoietic stem cell. *Science,* Vol 273,242–245.

Oulad Abdelghani, M., Bouillet, P., Decimo, D., Gansmuller, A., Heyberger, S. & Dolle, P. (1996). Characterization of a premeiotic germ cell-specific cytoplasmic protein encoded by Stra8, a novel retinoic acid-responsive gene. *J. Cell Biol,* 135: 469–77.

Pellegrini, G., Dellambra, E., Golisano, O., Martinelli, E., Fantozzi, I., Bondanza, S., Ponzin, D., McKeon, F. & De Luca, M. (2001). P63 identifies keratinocyte stem cells. *Proc Natl Acad Sci USA* 98: 3156-3161.

Pera, M. F., Reubinoff, B. & Trounson, A. (2000). Human embryonic stem cells. *J. Cell Sci.*, 113, 5–10.

Pesce, M., Wang, X., Wolgemuth, DJ. & Scholer, H. (1998). Differential expression of the Oct-4 transcription factor during mouse germ cell differentiation. *Mech Dev*, 71:89–98.

Pittenger, MF., Mackay, AM., Beck, SC., Jaiswal, RK., Douglas, R., Mosca, JD., Moorman, MA., Simonetti, DW., Craig, S. & Marshak, DR. (1999). Multilineage potential of adult human mesenchymal stem cells. *Science*, 284, 143–147.

Prockop, DJ. (1997). Marrowstromal cells as stemcells for nonhematopoietic tissues. *Science*, 276, 71–74.

Quirici, N., Soligo, D., Bossolasco, P., Servida, F., Lumini, C. & Deliliers, GL. (2002). Isolation of bone marrow mesenchymal stem cells by anti-nerve growth factor receptor antibodies. *Exp. Hematol.*, 30, 783–791.

Rakic, P. (2003) Elusive radial glia cells: historical and evolutionary perspective. *Glia* 43: 19–32.

Ramalho-Santos, M., Yoon, S., Matsuzaki, Y., Mulligan, RC. & Melton, DA. (2002). Stemness:transcriptional profiling of embryonic and adult stem cells. *Science*, Vol 298,597–600.

Randall, TD., Lund, FE., Howard, MC. & Weissman, IL. (1996). Expression of murine CD38 defines a population of long-term reconstituting hematopoietic stem cells. *Blood*, Vol 87,4057–4067.

Randall, TD. & Weissman, IL. (1997). Phenotypic and functional changes induced at the clonal level in hematopoietic stem cells after 5-fluorouracil treatment. *Blood*, Vol 89,3596–3606.

Raverot, G., Weiss, J., Park, SY., Hurley, L. & Jameson, JL. (2005). Sox3 expression in undifferentiated spermatogonia is required for the progression of spermatogenesis. *Dev. Biol.*, 283:215–25.

Resnick, JL., Bixler, LS., Cheng, L. & Donovan, PJ. (1992). Long-term proliferation of mouse primordial germ cells in culture. *Nature*, 359:550–1.

Reubinoff, BE., Pera, MF., Fong, CY., Trouson, A., Bongso, A. (2000). Embryonic stem cell lines from human blastocysts: somatic differentiation in vitro. *Nature Biotechnol.*, 18: 399–404

Sadler, TW. (2002). *Langman's Medical Embryology*, 8th edn. Philadelphia, Lippincott Williams and Wilkins.

Sapsford, CS. (1962). Changes in the cells of the sex cords and the seminiferous tubules during development of the testis of the rat and the mouse. *Austr J. Zool*,10:178–92.

Sato, T., Laver, JH., & Ogawa, M. (1999). Reversible Expression of CD34 by Murine Hematopoietic Stem Cells. *Blood*, Vol 94,2548–2554.

Secco, M., Zucconi, E., Vieira, NM., Fogaça, LL., Cerqueira, A.,Carvalho, MD., Jazedje, T., Okamoto, OK., Muotri, AR. & Zatz, M. (2008). Multipotent stem cells from umbilical cord: cord is richer than blood! *Stem Cells*, 26: 146-150.

Shibata, T., Yamada, K., Watanabe, M., Ikenaka, K., Wada, K., Tanaka, K. & Inoue, Y. (1997) Glutamate transporter GLAST is expressed in the radial glia-astrocyte lineage of developing mouse spinal cord. *J. Neurosci.*, 17, 9212–9.

Shinohara, T., Avarbock, MR. & Brinster, RL. (1999). Beta(1)- and alpha(6)-integrin are surface markers on mouse spermatogonial stem cells. *Proc Natl Acad Sci U S A,* 1999, 96:5504–9.

Shinohara, T., Orwig, KE., Avarbock, MR. & Brinster, RL. (2000). Spermatogonial stem cell enrichment by multiparameter selection of mouse testis cells. *Proc Natl Acad Sci U S A,* 97:8346–51.

Simmons, P. J. & Torok-Storb, B. (1991). Identification of stromal cell precursors in human bone marrow by a novel monoclonal antibody, STRO-1. *Blood,* 78, 55–62.

Sottile, V., Halleux, C., Bassilana, F., Keller, H., & Seuwen, K. (2002). Stem cell characteristics of human trabecular bone-derived cells. *Bone* 30, 699–704.

Spangrude, GJ. & Brooks, DM. (1993). Mouse strain variability in the expression of the hematopoietic stem cell antigen Ly-6A/E by bone marrow cells. *Blood,* Vol 82,3327–3332.

Spangrude, GJ., Heimfeld, S. & Weissman, IL. (1988). Purification and characterization of mouse hematopoietic stem cells. *Science,* Vol 241,58–62.

Spangrude, G. & Brooks, DM. (1992). Phenotypic analysis of mouse hematopoietic stem cells shows a Thy-1- negative subset. *Blood,* Vol 80,1957–1964.

Srour, EF., Brandt, JE., Leemhuis, T., Ballas, CB. & Hoffman, R. (1992). Relationship between cytokine-dependent cell cycle progression and MHC class II antigen expression by human CD34& HLA-DR- bone marrow cells. J. *Immunol.* Vol 148,815–820.

Sutherland, DR., Yeo, EL. & Stewart, AK. (1996). Identification of CD34& subsets after glycoprotease selection: engraftment of CD34&Thy-1&Lin– stem cells in fetal sheep. *Exp Hematol.* Vol 24,795–806.

Tam, PP. & Snow, MH. (1981).Proliferation and migration of primordial germ cells during compensatory growth in mouse embryos. *J. Embryol Exp Morphol* 64:133–47.

Temple, S. (2001) Stem cell plasticity—building the brain of our dreams. *Nat. Rev. Neurosci.* 2, 513–520.

Terstappen, LW., Huang, S., Safford, M., Lansdorp, PM. & Loken, MR. (1991).Sequential generations of hematopoietic colonies derived from single nonlineage-committed CD34&CD38– progenitor cells. *Blood,* Vol 77,1218–1227.

Thomson, JA., Itskovitz-Eldor, J., Shapiro SS, et al. (1998). Embryonic stem cell lines derived from human blastocysts. *Science,* 282: 1145–1147.

Thomson, JA., Kalishman, J., Golos, TG., et al. (1995). Isolation of a primate embryonic stem cell line. *Proc Natl Acad Sci U S A,*92: 7844–7848

Thrasher, J. D. (1966) Analysis of renewing epithelial cell populations. In: *Methods in Cell Physiology,* vol. 2 (Prescott, D. M., ed.), Academic, New York, pp. 323–357.

Till, J. E. & McCulloch, C. E. (1961). A direct measurement of the radiation sensitivity of normal mouse bone marrow cells. *Radiat. Res.* 14, 213–222.

Toresson, H., Mata de Urquiza, A., Fagerstrom, C., Perlmann, T. & Campbell, K. (1999). Retinoids are produced by glia in the lateral ganglionic eminence and regulate striatal neuron differentiation. *Development,* 126, 1317–26.

Tsukamoto, A., Weissman, I. & Chen, B. (1995). Phenotypic and functional analysis of hematopoietic stem cells in mouse and man. In: Mertelsman La, ed. *Hematopoietic Stem Cells, Biology and Therapeutic Applications: Phenotypic and functional analysis of hematopoietic stem cells in mouse and man.*

Uchida, N., Leung, FY. & Eaves, CJ. (2002). Liver and marrow of adult mdr-1a/ 1b (-/-) mice show normal generation, function, and multi-tissue trafficking of primitive hematopoietic cells. *Exp Hematol.*, 30:862- 869.

Uchida, N. & Weissman, IL. (1992). Searching for hematopoietic stem cells: evidence that Thy-1.1lo Lin- Sca-1& cells are the only stem cells in C57BL/Ka-Thy-1.1 bone marrow. *J. Exp Med.*, Vol 175,175–184.

Uchida, N., Yang, Z. & Combs, J. (1997). The characterization, molecular cloning, and expression of a novel hematopoietic cell antigen from CD34& human bone marrow cells. *Blood,* Vol 89,2706–2716.

Vaccarino, FM., Ganat, Y., Zhang, Y., & Zheng W. (2001) Stem cells in neurodevelopment and plasticity. *Neuropsychopharmacology,* 25, 805–815.

van Bragt, MP., Ciliberti, N., Stanford, WL., de Rooij, DG. & van Pelt, AM. (2005). LY6A/E (SCA-1) expression in the mouse testis. *Biol. Reprod.*, 2005, 73:634–8. Epub,Jun 1.

Vergouwen, RPFA., Jacobs, SG., Huiskamp, R., Davids, JAG. & de Rooij, DG. (1991). Proliferative activity of gonocytes, Sertoli cells and interstitial cells during testicular development in mice. *J. Reprod. Fertil.*, 93:233–43.

Vescovi, A.L., Galli R., & Gritti A. (2001) The neural stem cells and their transdifferentiation capacity. *Biomed. Pharmacother.*, 55, 201–205.

von Schonfeldt, V., Wistuba, J. & Schlatt, S. (2004). Notch-1, c-kit and GFRalpha-1 are developmentally regulated markers for premeiotic germ cells. *Cytogenet Genome Res,* 105:235–9.

Vose, JM., Bierman, PJ. & Lynch, JC. (2001). Transplantation of highly purified CD34&Thy-1& hematopoietic stem cells in patients with recurrent indolent non-Hodgkin's lymphoma. *Biol. Blood Marrow Transplant,* Vol 7,680–687.

Wan, H., Stone, M., Simpson, C., Reynols, L., Marshall, J., Hart, I., Dilke, K. & Eady, R. (2003). Desmosomal proteins, including desmoglein 3, serve as novel negative markers for epidermal stem cell-containing population of keratinocytes. *J. Cell Sci.,* 116: 4239-4248.

Watt, FM., Lo Celso, C. & Silva-Vargas, V. (2006). Epidermal stem cells: an update. *Curr Opin Genet Dev.,* 16(5):518–524.

Weissman, IL., Anderson, DJ, & Gage, F. (2001) Stem and progenitor cells: origins, phenotypes, lineage commitments, and transdifferentiations. *Annu. Rev. Cell. Dev. Biol.,* 17, 387–403.

Wiesmann, A., Phillips, RL. & Mojica, M. (2000). Expression of CD27 on murine hematopoietic stem and progenitor cells. *Immunity,* Vol 12,193–199.

Yin, AH., Miraglia, S. & Zanjani, ED. (1997). AC133, a novel marker for human hematopoietic stem and progenitor cells. *Blood,* Vol 90,5002–5012.

Yoshida, S., Takakura, A., Ohbo, K., Abe, K., Wakabayashi, J. & Yamamoto, M. (2004). Neurogenin3 delineates the earliest stages of spermatogenesis in the mouse testis. *Dev. Biol.,* 269:447–58.

Zhang, YV., Cheong, J., Ciapurin, N., McDermitt, DJ. & Tumbar, T. (2009). Distinct self-renewal and differentiation phases in the niche of infrequently dividing hair follicle stem cells. *Cell Stem Cell,* 5: 267-278.

Zhao, X., Ueba, T., Christie, BR., Barkho, B., McConnell, MJ., Nakashima, K., Lein, ES., Eadie, BD., Willhoite, AR., Muotri, AR., Summers, RG., Chun, J., Lee, KF. & Gage,

FH. (2003) Mice lacking methyl-CpG binding protein 1 have deficits in adult Neurogenesis and hippocampal function. *Proc Natl Acad Sci U S A,* 100, 6777–82.

Zhou, S., Schuetz JD., Bunting KD., Colapietro AM., Sampath J., Morris JJ., Lagutina I., Grosveld GC., Osawa M., Nakauchi H., Sorrentino BP. (2001). The ABC transporter Bcrp1/ABCG2 is expressed in a wide variety of stem cells and is a molecular determinant of the side-population phenotype. *Nat Med.*, 7:1028 –1034.

Zuk, PA., Zhu, M., Mizuno, H., Huang, J., Futrell, JW., Katz, AJ., Benhaim, P., Lorenz, HP., & Hedrick, MH. (2001). Multilineage cells from human adipose tissue: implications for cell-based therapies. *Tissue Eng.*, 7, 211–228.

14

Flow Cytometric Sorting of Cells from Solid Tissue – Reagent Development and Application

P. S. Canaday and C. Dorrell
Oregon Health & Science University
USA

1. Introduction

The isolation and study of cells from solid tissues is one of the great current challenges for flow cytometry. The vast majority of mammalian cells reside within solid organs, but the application of flow cytometric techniques to such cells remains limited. The study of hematopoietic biology has been revolutionized by the development of standardized monoclonal antibodies recognizing defined antigens that permit flow cytometric isolation, definition, and characterization of blood cell types (Bendall et al., 2011; Fleming et al., 1993; Hoffman et al., 1980; Nakeff et al., 1979). Antibodies have been used to better identify and understand the role different blood cells play in the immune system (Springer et al., 1979). They have also been used to help zero in on the stem cell populations and to learn more about the processes of hematopoietic differentiation (Ikuta et al., 1992; Spangrude et al., 1988). Their use has impacted virtually every facet of hematopoietic study.

This same approach is likely to bring similar benefits to the study of solid tissue. Unfortunately, the reagents and techniques needed for studying cells from solid tissues are woefully limited. Most available surface-reactive antibodies have been defined by their activity against hematopoietic antigens. The lack of understanding about the surfaces of tissue-resident cells is one of the reasons why the isolation of adult stem cells and culture of primary cells from solid tissue remains problematic. In order to advance the study and characterization of these cells, new reagents and techniques must be developed. The development of monoclonal antibodies against solid-tissue specific antigens will help researchers sort and study subsets of cells from other organs. It will allow for comparison between subsets of cells from the same tissue and similar subsets from different tissues. It is likely that, as with the hematopoietic field, new subsets and classes of cells will be discovered. Hopefully, the development of more monoclonal antibodies will not only move research forward but will also aid in the development of therapeutic technologies.

This chapter will include information about the history of monoclonal antibodies with a focus on how they impacted the field of flow cytometry. The development of novel monoclonal antibodies and examples of their successful application to the field of solid tissue biology will be described, and suggestions will be offered for the advancement of flow cytometric research beyond the hematopoietic field.

2. A brief overview of the history of hematopoietic antibody production

In order to better understand how antibodies will benefit the study of solid tissues, it is helpful to examine how they have benefited the study of hematopoietic tissue. The study of hematopoietic tissue has been immensely successful and there is much benefit to be gained by understanding and learning from what has been done before.

2.1 Hybridomas

The advent of monoclonal antibody-producing hybridomas revolutionized the field of cytometry. Kohler and Milstein originally described the creation of immortal cells that produced monoclonal antibodies against a predefined target (Kohler and Milstein, 1975). They did this by fusing cells from a plasmacytoma line with splenocytes from a mouse that had been immunized with sheep erythrocytes. The resulting clonal cell line possessed the useful attributes of each parent; they could be cultured indefinitely and also continued to produce the desired immunoglobulin.

Prior to the development of hybridomas, polyclonal serum was used for cell or protein recognition. While there are applications where the use of polyclonal serum is advantageous, it has the disadvantages of being a finite resource and that the antigens are not fully characterized.

The innovation of monoclonal antibodies revolutionized cell analysis by allowing precise and accurate reproducibility both between experiments and between researchers. In the beginning of the prolific development of monoclonal antibodies, individual labs would make their own antibody clones (Lemke et al., 1978; Solter and Knowles, 1978). Very quickly, it became clear that a more standardized approach would be useful; it was not always clear, for example, whether antibodies that appeared to label the same cells were binding to the same antigens. During the first HLDA (Human Leucocyte Differentiation Antigens) workshop in 1992, 15 antibodies with known targets were standardized as CD (cluster of differentiation) markers (Zola and Swart, 2005). As was reflected in the name, the HLDA was concerned primarily with blood cells, which were readily accessible and a logical place to start.

2.1.1 Uses

Flow cytometry is not the only use for monoclonal antibodies; their application in biomedical and basic research is extensive. Although immunoassays were in use prior to the development of monoclonal antibodies, the increased availability and consistency of this new reagent dramatically increased the number of potential applications. Radioimmunotherapy would not be possible without the superb specificity of monoclonal antibodies. Pathogen classification used to require hours, or even days; there are now many cases where it can be done in a matter of minutes. Microscopy has taken advantage of monoclonal antibodies to produce exquisite images and reveal the internal structure of cells in ways not previously imagined. Many other examples exist, but a comprehensive list of monoclonal antibody applications is beyond the scope of this chapter.

2.2 Use of antibodies for flow cytometry

Even before Kohler and Milstein devised monoclonal-producing hybridomas, antibodies were being used for flow cytometry. The Herzenberg group, in 1971, became the first to employ antibody labeling as a cell identification tool in flow cytometry (Herzenberg, 1971). Polyclonal anti-sera were employed in subsequent studies, such as Epstein's work on lymphocyte biology (Epstein et al., 1974). In 1977, the first paper using fluorescently-labeled monoclonal antibodies was published, and the field has never looked back (Williams et al., 1977). Since then, thousands of publications have included the use of monoclonal antibodies in flow cytometry. They have become an indispensible tool for biomedical research.

2.3 Advances in flow cytometry

Advancements in the technical aspects of flow cytometry were driven largely by the rapid generation and characterization of new monoclonal antibodies. The demand for more fluorophores, more detectors, and more lasers in order to assess multiple properties on the same cell was the impetus for significant advancements in the field. Multicolored flow cytometry allowed for the discovery of multiple subsets of cells. Three color detection using a dual laser system was developed by 1983 (Parks et al., 1984). In 1985, BD utilized microcomputing in the new FACScan, increasing cell throughput and simplifying all aspects of the cell isolation process. By the turn of the millennium, eight simultaneous 'colors' (fluorochromes) were used in flow cytometry experiments (Roederer et al., 1997). Any time a new instrument becomes available, researchers immediately begin pushing the limits of the new technology. Advances in photomultiplier tube technology and the development of better dichroic filters also helped in the development of bigger and better flow cytometers.

The rise in technology necessitated new standardized ways of analyzing the data. The FCS (Flow Cytometry Standard) was proposed in 1984 by Murphy and Chused and was summarily adopted by the scientific community at large (Murphy and Chused, 1984). This facilitated data sharing between labs.

3. Antibody production targeting cells from solid tissue

The rapid development of antibodies and cell sorting technology to meet the needs of the hematopoietic research community has laid much of the ground work required for studies of other cell types. There is an ever-growing need to be able to identify subpopulations of cells from solid tissues. Diseases such as diabetes, liver disease, and a variety of cancers have benefited, and will continue to benefit from, an expanding pool of monoclonal antibodies that can be used to further investigate them (Jarpe et al., 1990; Larsen et al., 1986; Muraro et al., 1989). Using the same approach pioneered by Milstein and Kohler, research into all systems of the body has begun to follow in the footsteps of the hematopoietic field. While there are other ways of making hybridomas, the immunization of a rat or mouse with whole cells continues to be valuable because antigens are presented in their native configuration. Thus, the resulting antibodies are likely to recognize the epitopes available in a live, intact cell. In order to use these antibodies to identify and isolate cells for growth and/or functional studies, this is an essential property.

3.1 Immunization

Modern monoclonal antibody production uses a procedure that has changed little from the methods of Köhler and Milstein (Kohler and Milstein, 1975). In brief, the mouse or rat is immunized on multiple occasions using cells obtained from the tissue of interest. Four days after the final immunization the animal is sacrificed and the spleen harvested. Splenocytes are fused with myeloma cells using polyethylene glycol and cultured on semi-solid HAT (hypoxanthine/aminopterin/thymidine) media to prevent the growth of un-fused myeloma cells. Hybridoma clones are isolated and grown individually to produce antibody for testing, and interesting clones are expanded to larger cultures and cryopreserved for further study. Of these steps, the selection of the immunogen and the treatments used to isolate it from solid tissue prior to immunization are the most critical to the success of the procedure. One can immunize with partially dissociated tissue, fully dispersed cells in suspension or a FACS-purified cell subpopulation. Each of these has advantages and disadvantages.

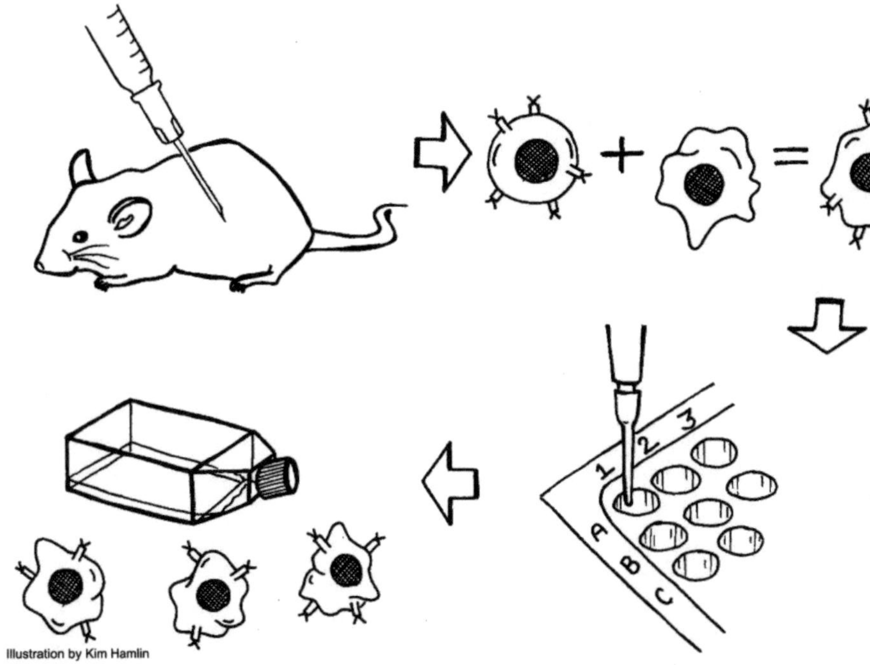

Fig. 1. Making Hybridomas. A mouse is injected with an immunogen, antibody producing splenocytes are fused with myeloma cells to produce hybridoma lines, clones are grown in 96-well plates using drug selection to exclude un-fused myeloma cells and selected clones are scaled up

Immunization using minimally-dispersed fragments of tissue is simple, quick and requires limited (if any) proteolytic enzyme treatment. Thus, this approach is most likely to preserve sensitive antigens. Because it does not exclude indigestible material (which can include important tissue substructures), this method also offers the most complete representation of all antigens in the tissue. The disadvantage is that this method includes antigenic material that gives rise to immune responses against unwanted antigens that are present in debris.

If tissue is instead enzymatically dissociated to a single-cell suspension, much of the intercellular debris can be eliminated and the cell-surface antigens are more available. Although native epitopes might be altered by proteolysis, it is important to consider that this same process will be required to recover cells for future analysis; raising antibodies against a proteolysis-sensitive antigen is of limited utility. Unfortunately, it is not always clear what the optimal digestion protocol will turn out to be for a given tissue type. If it is possible to perfuse the organ with a collagenase, this can be a very productive approach (Klaunig et al., 1981). Regardless of whether perfusion is performed, dispersal to a single-cell state usually requires three elements: Mechanical dissociation (by mincing and/or passage through a narrow aperture such as a needle), collagenase treatment (to digest extracellular matrix) and a broad-specificity protease (e.g. trypsin) to disperse tightly-associated cells. Specific protocols successfully used for tissues such as mouse liver (Dorrell et al., 2008b), and human pancreas (Dorrell et al., 2008a) are described in the next section.

Immunization with a subset of a single-cell suspension allows for the generation of antibodies targeted against a subset of cells. At a minimum, it should be possible to exclude defined "contaminating" populations such as blood and endothelium. The cell subset may be isolated using flow sorting, immunomagnetic separation, or physical properties such as density or size. This approach has the same downside as tissue digestion because the researcher must know how to digest the tissue in order to liberate the cells of interest without damaging them. In addition, the number of recovered cells tends to be smaller, meaning that the immunization might be less efficient.

A useful method for increasing the likelihood of obtaining antibodies targeted to a particular cell type is subtractive immunization (Williams et al., 1992). In this method, the first immunization uses tissue, cells and/or debris containing antigens which are irrelevant or undesirable. Subsequent treatment with cyclophosphamide kills the lymphocytes which have responded to any of these antigens, so that after subsequent immunizations with the tissue/cells of interest, only the new and relevant antigens cause an immune response. This approach was used successfully to raise antibodies against human pancreatic islet cells after pre-immunization with trypsin and calf serum, which might otherwise have been confounding antigens required for islet dispersal and cell storage (Dorrell et al., 2008a). Subtractive immunization is compatible with any of the immunogen sources described above.

3.1.1 Proven immunization strategies for mouse liver and human islets

This chapter will focus on two different tissue preparations from two dissimilar tissues. Understanding why they would be treated differently will help the researcher determine the best course of action for future tissue digestion.

Preparing single-cell solution from a mouse liver requires several stages. The first is a two-step portal vein perfusion with calcium and magnesium-free Hanks salt solution followed by a solution containing collagenase. After about twenty minutes, when the liver is visibly degraded it is removed, placed in a dish with media, and teased apart with forceps to release as many cells as possible. The resulting slurry should be allowed to flow through a 40 μm strainer. The filtered cells can be spun for two minutes at 50g in order to pellet the hepatocytes; other cell types will remain in suspension after this treatment. Tissue that does not pass through the filter should be subjected to an ex vivo digest of about 20 minutes in 2.5 mg/mL collagenase D at 37°C before collection through a 40 μm strainer. Any remaining solid tissue is then digested with 0.05% trypsin and mechanically dissociated with a pipetter. Following all of these treatments little or no undigested material should remain. At each stage, it is important to collect dissociated cells by passing them through a 40μm strainer and to store them on ice without further exposure to enzyme (Dorrell et al., 2008b; Klaunig et al., 1981).

We receive intact human islets from the Islet Cell Resource Center network. They are essentially small aggregates of cells obtained as the end product of a whole-organ perfusion protocol, and therefore require only a simple enzymatic digest to reduce to a single cell suspension. Islets are washed with calcium- and magnesium-free DPBS (Dulbecco's Phosphate-Buffered Saline) and then incubated in 0.05% trypsin at 37°C. Gentle pipetting is done every three minutes in order to aid the dissociation until the islets are visibly dispersed into a single-cell state.

3.2 Hybridoma screening

Regardless of the immunization strategy and target cell population, most of the resulting hybridomas will not produce desirable antibodies. It is therefore essential to have a strategy for evaluating many hybridomas to obtain as many useful ones as possible. Labeling of tissue sections with hybridoma supernatants followed by microscopic evaluation can be labor-intensive, but it provides invaluable information regarding cell type-specificity. A detailed anatomical knowledge of the target tissue is not generally required by the screener; the important requirement at this stage is the identification of clones that selectively label populations of cells found in common structures (e.g. ducts, blood vessels, islets, etc.).

For the screening of large numbers of hybridomas for reactivity, cryosections of OCT (Optimal Cutting Temperature) cryomatrix-embedded tissue is recommended. To save time, hybridoma supernatants can be pooled and evaluated in batches. Batches exhibiting a promising tissue labeling pattern are then reevaluated, clone-by-clone. Figure 2 illustrates immunofluorescent labeling using an antibody with an interesting labeling pattern that emerged after an immunization series using human islet cells; this one made the cut. "HIC1-8G12" labels both the ducts (as shown by co-labeling with KRT19) and a subset of cells within the islet.

Further examination revealed that these islet cells were alpha cells (as shown by co-labeling with transthyretin [TTR], which is strongly expressed in this population (Dorrell et al., 2011b)). Using "interesting labeling pattern" as a criterion for antibody selection is subjective, of course, but the study of markers like HIC1-8G12 can lead to the identification of previously unexpected relationships between cell types. Flow cytometric screening of this antibody (described in the next section) showed that this particular antibody recognizes a cell surface antigen and can be used for live cell flow cytometry studies.

4. Flow cytometry

Protocols describing analysis and sorting by flow cytometry have been developed with primary blood cells and/or transformed cell lines in mind. For solid-tissue derived cells, some modifications and special considerations are needed.

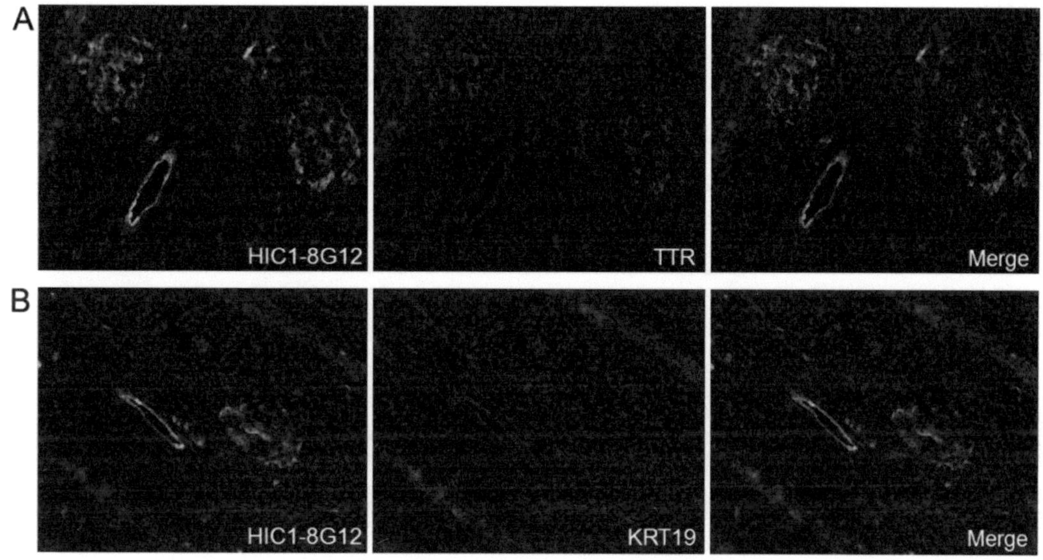

Fig. 2. Human pancreatic tissue labeling by HIC1-8G12. Co-labeling with TTR (A) or KRT19 (B) shows that this antibody binds an antigen that is present on both ducts and alpha cells

4.1 Selecting antibodies of interest by flow cytometric screening

After the initial screening on slides, it is important to determine which antibodies have cell surface reactivity. Flow cytometry is ideal for this purpose. Because the goal is to create antibodies against surface molecules, if an antibody with an interesting tissue labeling pattern does not label live cells with sufficient intensity and specificity to be distinguished by flow cytometry, it is not worth pursuing.

As discussed previously, there are many ways of getting cells into a single-cell suspension. It is recommended that if an enzymatic dispersal was used for immunization then the same method should be used to prepare cells for flow cytometry. If no enzymatic dispersal was used, it is worth taking the time to do the screening using a variety of digestion methods.

Many people worry that the dispersal method will influence the preservation of epitopes. They are right to worry. Some methods will alter or remove antigens of interest rendering them unrecognizable. We have found, for example, that the antigen recognized by one of our in-house favorite antibodies (MIC1-1C3) is unusually sensitive to digestion with Pronase, a mixture of strong proteases (Dorrell et al., 2011a). It is very important to try to optimize your digestion protocol but bear in mind that, at the end of the day, if you can't get the cells into single-cell suspension then they can't be sorted and studied in isolation.

With precious human samples, it can be much more difficult to do the experiments and learn which digestion method will work best but it is worth optimizing in the beginning for higher reproducibility later on.

As with screening on tissue sections, hybridoma supernatants can be pooled for screening by flow cytometry. This may not be necessary if the tissue section screen reduced the candidate list to a reasonable number, but will be necessary if tissue section screening was not performed or if few cells are available. During screening by flow cytometry, the antibody isotype can also be conveniently determined. Cells incubated in the supernatant from a single clone are detected using a combination of isotype-specific secondary antibodies selective for mouse or rat IgG or IgM. Figure 3 is a dot plot showing cells labeled with a mixture of primary antibodies, some IgG and some IgM. Because these were detected with both PE-conjugated anti-mouse IgM and APC-conjugated anti-mouse IgG, primary antibodies of these two isotypes can be used together.

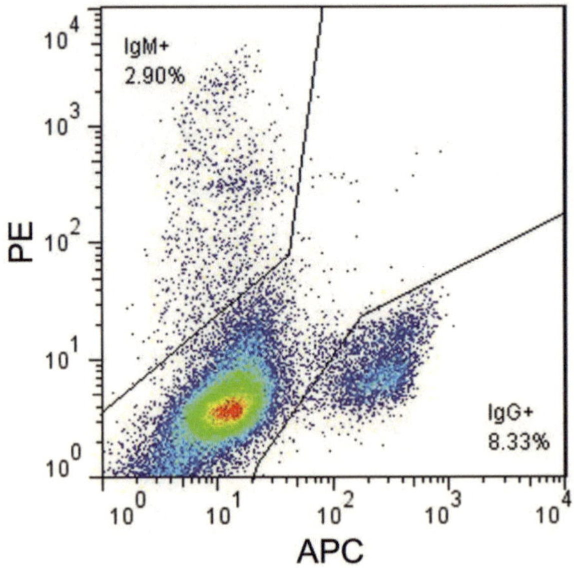

Fig. 3. Isotype specific secondary antibodies permit simultaneous detection of IgG and IgM-labeled cells

4.2 Multi-step antibody labeling to isolate populations of interest

Using unconjugated monoclonal antibodies has advantages and disadvantages. On one hand, it takes longer to label the cells because a secondary antibody is required for detection, necessitating additional steps. On the other hand, the researcher is not limited by pre-conjugated fluorochromes and can change "colors" to suit the experiment or instrument. Although pre-conjugated monoclonal antibodies marking known lineages can be an important tool in the study of solid tissue cells, such reagents are limited and most experiments will require the use of novel, unconjugated antibodies as well. Thus, despite its added complexity, a multi-step labeling protocol incorporating both fluorochrome-conjugated and unconjugated antibodies is ideal.

Generally speaking, monoclonal antibodies made against mouse antigens are made in rats and monoclonal antibodies targeting human antigens are made in mice. It is possible to do combination labeling using both conjugated and unconjugated antibodies raised in the same host species, but special care is required; a detailed protocol is provided later in this section. Polyclonal antibodies are produced by immunization of a variety of species, and are often easy to combine with monoclonal antibodies for co-detection. It is vital to know the host species of each antibody, its isotype and whether or not each secondary antibody is adsorbed to prevent cross-reactivity against immunoglobulins from another species.

Once an antibody has been found with reactivity against a cell population of interest, it is important to do a simple titration in order to ensure that the optimal concentration is being utilized. This helps to optimize the intensity of labeling by minimizing non-specific "background" labeling and also avoids waste. A proper titration involves labeling a fixed number of cells with antibody a range of different concentrations. When the antibody concentration is unknown (which is often the case for hybridoma supernatants), it is convenient to test a series of dilutions (e.g. undiluted, 1:10, 1:100, 1:500:, 1:1000). We prefer to use the highest concentration that does not result in a detectable elevation in non-specific labeling of "negative"cells. It is important to have an excess of antibody to ensure that all target antigens are saturated. The staining will be much easier to reproduce if the researcher takes the time to do one titration experiment at the beginning.

Once the sample is dissociated into single cells, it can be resuspended in holding buffer at a concentration of between $1X10^6$ and $1X10^7$ per ml. This has proven to be a good working concentration for the labeling of solid-tissue derived cells. A recommended general-purpose holding buffer is DMEM with 1% FBS and 0.1 mg/ml DNase I; this mixture provides nutrients, "blocks" cells against non-specific antibody binding by exposure to bovine immunoglobulins and reduces cell aggregation by digesting nuclear material released by dead cells.

It can be advantageous to use a combination of newly developed and commercially available antibodies. This allows for the exclusion (by electronic gating) of unwanted cell types. If multiple antibody-defined cell types are undesirable, the experiment can be simplified by using a common fluorochrome to label them for combined exclusion. This is sometimes referred to as a "dump channel". For example, if both blood and endothelium are unwanted, anti-CD45-FITC and anti-CD31-FITC can be employed together.

We have found it useful to employ a labeling technique incorporating two different unconjugated primary antibodies and three conjugated antibodies in a five color sort. This allowed us to learn whether the new antibodies were reactive against blood or endothelium in addition to epithelial subpopulations.

A sample labeling protocol follows:

Step 1. Using 5ml round-bottom tubes (polystyrene or polypropylene, of the specific type required by the instrument), incubate the appropriate samples with unconjugated primary antibodies on ice for 20 minutes. Primary antibodies that can be distinguished by isotype or host species can be combined at this stage. If the cells are prone to settling, resuspend them periodically by vortexing.

Step 2. Wash by increasing the volume and centrifuging at the speed appropriate for your cells. Aspirate all but about 50 µl of supernatant.

Step 3. Resuspend the pellet in the small volume that remains by gently flicking the tube until there is no longer a visible pellet. Do this before adding appropriate volume of holding buffer. (Failure to do this may result in clumping)

Step 4. Add all secondary antibodies and incubate for 20 minutes on ice.

Step 5. Wash as described above and resuspend in blocking buffer. This solution is holding buffer supplemented with serum/sera of the species in which the conjugated antibodies to be used in Step 6 were raised. The immunoglobulins present in such sera will block unoccupied sites on the divalent secondary antibodies added in Step 4. Allow 20 minutes for blocking to proceed, on ice.

Step 6. Add conjugated primary antibodies and incubate for 20 minutes on ice.

Step 7. Wash and resuspend in holding buffer containing a dead cell-marking agent such as propidium iodide. The optimal concentration for sorting tends to be between $1X10^6$ and $1X10^7$ depending on the amount of debris present after cell isolation. At this point, it is important to visually inspect each tube for the presence of cell clumps. If these cannot be dispersed by vortexing they must be excluded by cell straining to avoid clogging the sorter's nozzle. BD makes tubes with strainer caps that allow convenient filtration of samples immediately prior to sorting.

4.3 Sorting

There are several instrument-related considerations for sorting tissue-derived cells. The selection of optimal nozzle diameter, fluidic pressure, forward and side scatter voltage settings are all vital and will be different depending on the organ and tissue type. Furthermore, because tissue-derived cells are being stored in an unnatural environment - a single cell suspension - care must be taken to avoid cell aggregation and to minimize ongoing cell death. These are issues that seldom arise in the world of hematopoietic sorting.

Cells from solid tissues tend to be larger than hematopoietic cells so it is often necessary to use a larger nozzle in order to avoid damaging the cells or clogging the nozzle. Cells from solid tissues are also often more fragile and are potentially more likely to be damaged by the shear forces when they pass through a smaller nozzle. The correct nozzle diameter must be determined empirically, but when in doubt one should err towards using a larger nozzle and accepting reduced cell throughput.

For sorting cells from human pancreatic islets or nonparenchymal cells isolated from a mouse liver, we use a 100 µm nozzle at a pressure of 15 PSI. Under these conditions, cells were sorted at between 2,000 and 4,000 events per second with over 98% purity (Dorrell et al., 2008b). When sorting mouse hepatocytes, which are large and fragile, the optimal nozzle for highest post-sort viability is the 150 µm nozzle at 4.5 PSI (Duncan et al., 2010).

There are a few tricks to keeping cells in a single cell suspension. If a visible pellet of settled cells is observed in the source tube, the sorter's tube vortexer or manual flicking/vortexing should be employed. As discussed previously, minimizing the amount of calcium can reduce cell aggregation; a low [Ca^{2+}] holding buffer may be helpful. Keeping the sample cold using a chilling apparatus will also inhibit clumping.

Size-standard beads (e.g. 10 µm diameter) should be used to establish consistent forward and side scatter voltages. This facilitates the direct comparison of the size and granularity of cell samples collected on different days and even on different instruments. Sample-to-sample variability of solid tissue derived cells can be much greater than that of hematopoietic cells, so this sort of calibration is very important.

It is common practice when using flow cytometry with hematopoietic cells to set the voltages for the fluorescent detectors so that negative population falls below 10^1. This approach is not recommended for the more heterogeneous populations found in isolated tissue-derived cells, however. It is important to set the voltage on the PMTs so that very few cells are against the axis; if this means that some of the "negative" cells exhibit a significant degree of non-specific labeling, so be it. Note that this will be less of an issue when using software that permits visualization using a logical scale. Figure 5 illustrates how it becomes very difficult to identify distinct populations when detector voltages are set so that not all cells are on scale.

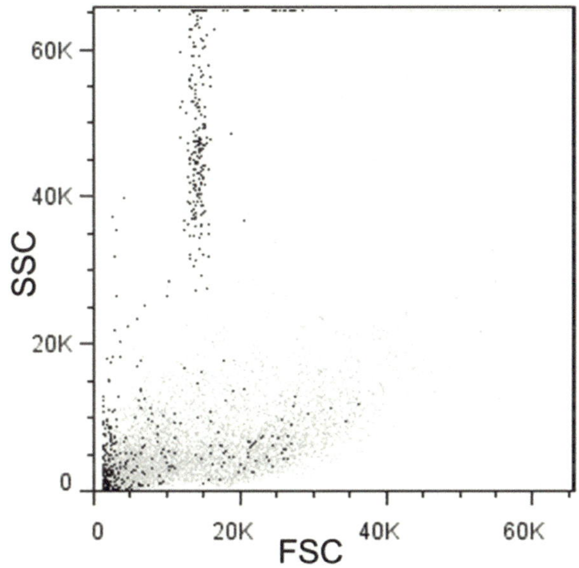

Fig. 4. 10 micron diameter beads and cells both on scale

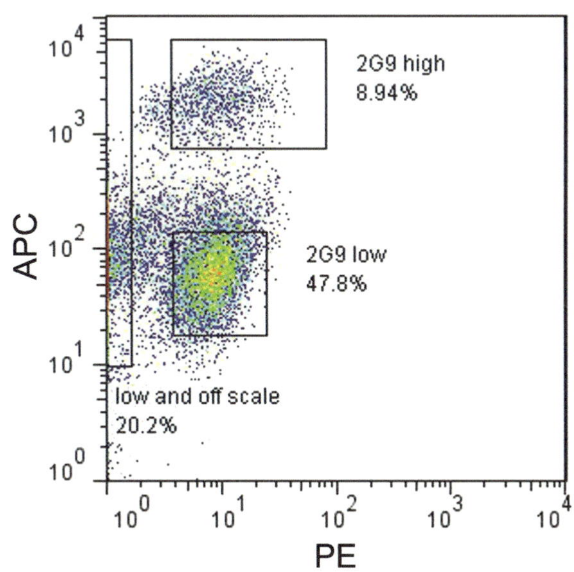

Fig. 5. Some cells are "off-scale low"

The use of "back-scattering" to evaluate the size/granularity of antibody-defined cell subpopulations requires the ability to gate on distinct populations. Since these properties are hard to predict on solid tissue-derived cells, back-scattering can reveal where the cells appear on a FSC/SSC plot and thus insure that both the optimal voltages and gating are employed.

5. Post-sort analysis

While flow cytometry data is valuable, it is the ability to isolate cell populations and do follow-up experiments that it such an overwhelmingly powerful tool. Cell populations can be analyzed for RNA content, they can be cultured, reprogrammed, transplanted, or even simply cytospun and stained for other markers.

5.1 Microarray and RT-PCR

Microarray and QRTPCR are arguably two of the most powerful tools for more comprehensive understanding of each cell type. When post-sort RNA analysis is the goal, there are a few things to keep in mind in order to acquire the highest quality RNA.

A very high purity sorted sample will result in less contamination of RNA from other cell types. A typical sort will result in a purity of 95% or higher. Unless the available cell numbers are very limited, a higher purity level is probably desirable. Re-sorting can be advantageous because it can allow you to make the initial sort faster, not aborting any events.

There are, of course, advantages and disadvantages of sorting and then resorting. The obvious advantage is that the resorted sample is very close to 100% pure; there are very few contaminating cells that might negatively affect results. A potential disadvantage is that the cells are being put through the sorter again. This increases the likelihood of them being damaged. The question of whether the RNA expression might change as the cells are subject to shear forces multiple times is a valid but hypothetical concern.

5.2 Cell culture

Culturing cells that have never been isolated before poses exciting challenges. How does one optimize culture conditions for cells that have not been thoroughly characterized? It requires trial and experimentation but at least if the cells can be analyzed first to see what genes they are expressing, the researcher has information that will aid with making educated guesses.

5.2.1 Stem cell assays

If the goal of sorting is to isolate stem/progenitor cells, there are a number of things that can be done in order to determine whether the cells of interest can be accurately described as stem cells.

One good example of this is the work done by Sato and colleagues, where LGR5 positive cells were isolated from the mouse intestine and used to initiate three dimensional cultures in Matrigel (Sato et al., 2009). In this case, previously gained knowledge, about what the stem cells were expressing and what the requirements were to maintain them, were used in order to cultivate the intestinal stem cell and maintain them indefinitely.

The most rigorous stem cell assay is transplantation. If the unique population is sorted and found to be able to engraft a recipient animal and give rise to multiple types of daughter cells it is a strong indicator that the population contains a stem cell. It is fortunate that many human stem cells are transplantable into immune-deficient mice and give rise to cells that can replace the equivalent mouse cell (Grompe, 2001; Kamel-Reid and Dick, 1988; Wang et al., 2001).

5.2.2 Cell reprogramming

There are several ways that new antibodies might contribute to the success of cell reprogramming. First, if tissue-resident progenitors can be identified and isolated, their inherent plasticity would make them obvious targets for reprogramming. Additionally, if antibodies are created against cells in various stages of development, it will aid in the understanding of cell expression and signaling during development, and the replication of these events in adult cells. Knowing what cells express at various stages of development also allows for quick assays to determine whether the researcher is on the right path.

5.2.3 Culture for research and for transplant

Currently, it is very difficult to get cells for experimentation from cadaveric human donors. Researchers need sources of tissue and unfortunately the cell lines that are available are almost always tumor-derived. This limits their utility with regard to learning about the normal biology of certain cell types. Great strides have already been made in the field of solid tissue culture with the goal of future transplantation. Tissue culture has been shown to be remarkably successful at producing skin (Ueda, 2011). There has also been some success culturing hepatocytes with the hope of creating an external liver support device (Niu et al., 2009). As our understanding becomes more comprehensive, so too will our ability to maintain these cells in culture. Eventually, tissue banks might augment or even supplant the need for cadaveric organ donation.

6. Conclusion

The more tools we have to work with, the more quickly and thoroughly we can address issues of disease and expand our understanding of healthy tissue. Being able to physically isolate different cell subtypes is crucial to that understanding if we want to utilize powerful tools, such as microarray and RNA sequencing, which require large numbers of highly purified populations of cells. Experiments using up to 17 fluorochromes and 31 metal-conjugated antibodies are already being performed on blood and bone marrow cells (Bendall et al., 2011; Perfetto et al., 2004). In our lab, we have produced a number of antibodies against solid tissue and used these to isolate and analyze defined subpopulations that were not previously accessible by flow cytometry (Dorrell et al., 2011b; Dorrell et al., 2011c). As the need for these antibodies continues, it is hoped that more researchers will contribute to the array of tools that can be used in solid-tissue research.

The HLDA has expanded their mission to include characterization of surface epitopes found on all tissues relevant to the immune system. This expansion was reinforced with a name change; they are now the HCDM (Human Cell Differentiation Molecules) (Zola et al., 2007) Unfortunately there is not the same sort of all-inclusive drive toward a comprehensive characterization and evaluation of antibodies against tissue-bound cells. We feel that a comparable initiative directed towards solid organs, using the strategies and techniques described in this document, would yield many additional tools and reagents for the study of normal and pathological tissues.

7. Acknowledgements

The authors would like to thank Kim Hamlin for illustrating figure 1.

8. References

Bendall, S.C., Simonds, E.F., Qiu, P., Amir el, A.D., Krutzik, P.O., Finck, R., Bruggner, R.V., Melamed, R., Trejo, A., Ornatsky, O.I., *et al.* (2011). Single-cell mass cytometry of differential immune and drug responses across a human hematopoietic continuum. Science *332*, 687-696.

Dorrell, C., Abraham, S.L., Lanxon-Cookson, K.M., Canaday, P.S., Streeter, P.R., and Grompe, M. (2008a). Isolation of major pancreatic cell types and long-term culture-initiating cells using novel human surface markers. Stem Cell Res *1*, 183-194.

Dorrell, C., Erker, L., Lanxon-Cookson, K.M., Abraham, S.L., Victoroff, T., Ro, S., Canaday, P.S., Streeter, P.R., and Grompe, M. (2008b). Surface markers for the murine oval cell response. Hepatology *48*, 1282-1291.

Dorrell, C., Erker, L., Schug, J., Kopp, J.L., Canaday, P.S., Fox, A.J., Smirnova, O., Duncan, A.W., Finegold, M.J., Sander, M., *et al.* (2011a). Prospective isolation of a bipotential clonogenic liver progenitor cell in adult mice. Genes Dev *25*, 1193-1203.

Dorrell, C., Grompe, M.T., Pan, F.C., Zhong, Y., Canaday, P.S., Shultz, L.D., Greiner, D.L., Wright, C.V., Streeter, P.R., and Grompe, M. (2011b). Isolation of mouse pancreatic alpha, beta, duct and acinar populations with cell surface markers. Mol Cell Endocrinol *339*, 144-150.

Dorrell, C., Schug, J., Lin, C.F., Canaday, P.S., Fox, A.J., Smirnova, O., Bonnah, R., Streeter, P.R., Stoeckert, C.J., Jr., Kaestner, K.H., *et al.* (2011c). Transcriptomes of the major human pancreatic cell types. Diabetologia *54*, 2832-2844.

Duncan, A.W., Taylor, M.H., Hickey, R.D., Hanlon Newell, A.E., Lenzi, M.L., Olson, S.B., Finegold, M.J., and Grompe, M. (2010). The ploidy conveyor of mature hepatocytes as a source of genetic variation. Nature *467*, 707-710.

Epstein, L.B., Kreth, H.W., and Herzenberg, L.A. (1974). Fluorescence-activated cell sorting of human T and B lymphocytes. II. Identification of the cell type responsible for interferon production and cell proliferation in response to mitogens. Cell Immunol *12*, 407-421.

Fleming, W.H., Alpern, E.J., Uchida, N., Ikuta, K., and Weissman, I.L. (1993). Steel factor influences the distribution and activity of murine hematopoietic stem cells in vivo. Proc Natl Acad Sci U S A *90*, 3760-3764.

Grompe, M. (2001). Mouse liver goes human: a new tool in experimental hepatology. Hepatology *33*, 1005-1006.

Herzenberg, L.A. (1971). II Selective depletion of lymphocytes. In Immunologic Intervention (Academic Press), pp. 96-104, 145-148, 281, 289.

Hoffman, R.A., Kung, P.C., Hansen, W.P., and Goldstein, G. (1980). Simple and rapid measurement of human T lymphocytes and their subclasses in peripheral blood. Proc Natl Acad Sci U S A *77*, 4914-4917.

Ikuta, K., Uchida, N., Friedman, J., and Weissman, I.L. (1992). Lymphocyte development from stem cells. Annu Rev Immunol *10*, 759-783.

Jarpe, A.J., Hickman, M.R., Anderson, J.T., Winter, W.E., and Peck, A.B. (1990). Flow cytometric enumeration of mononuclear cell populations infiltrating the islets of Langerhans in prediabetic NOD mice: development of a model of autoimmune insulitis for type I diabetes. Reg Immunol *3*, 305-317.

Kamel-Reid, S., and Dick, J.E. (1988). Engraftment of immune-deficient mice with human hematopoietic stem cells. Science *242*, 1706-1709.

Klaunig, J.E., Goldblatt, P.J., Hinton, D.E., Lipsky, M.M., Chacko, J., and Trump, B.F. (1981). Mouse liver cell culture. I. Hepatocyte isolation. In Vitro *17*, 913-925.

Kohler, G., and Milstein, C. (1975). Continuous cultures of fused cells secreting antibody of predefined specificity. Nature *256*, 495-497.

Larsen, J.K., Munch-Petersen, B., Christiansen, J., and Jorgensen, K. (1986). Flow cytometric discrimination of mitotic cells: resolution of M, as well as G1, S, and G2 phase nuclei with mithramycin, propidium iodide, and ethidium bromide after fixation with formaldehyde. Cytometry *7*, 54-63.

Lemke, H., Hammerling, G.J., Hohmann, C., and Rajewsky, K. (1978). Hybrid cell lines secreting monoclonal antibody specific for major histocompatibility antigens of the mouse. Nature *271*, 249-251.

Muraro, R., Nuti, M., Natali, P.G., Bigotti, A., Simpson, J.F., Primus, F.J., Colcher, D., Greiner, J.W., and Schlom, J. (1989). A monoclonal antibody (D612) with selective reactivity for malignant and normal gastro-intestinal epithelium. Int J Cancer *43*, 598-607.

Murphy, R.F., and Chused, T.M. (1984). A proposal for a flow cytometric data file standard. Cytometry *5*, 553-555.

Nakeff, A., Valeriote, F., Gray, J.W., and Grabske, R.J. (1979). Application of flow cytometry and cell sorting to megakaryocytopoiesis. Blood *53*, 732-745.

Niu, M., Hammond, P., 2nd, and Coger, R.N. (2009). The effectiveness of a novel cartridge-based bioreactor design in supporting liver cells. Tissue Eng Part A *15*, 2903-2916.

Parks, D.R., Hardy, R.R., and Herzenberg, L.A. (1984). Three-color immunofluorescence analysis of mouse B-lymphocyte subpopulations. Cytometry *5*, 159-168.

Perfetto, S.P., Chattopadhyay, P.K., and Roederer, M. (2004). Seventeen-colour flow cytometry: unravelling the immune system. Nat Rev Immunol *4*, 648-655.

Roederer, M., De Rosa, S., Gerstein, R., Anderson, M., Bigos, M., Stovel, R., Nozaki, T., Parks, D., and Herzenberg, L. (1997). 8 color, 10-parameter flow cytometry to elucidate complex leukocyte heterogeneity. Cytometry *29*, 328-339.

Sato, T., Vries, R.G., Snippert, H.J., van de Wetering, M., Barker, N., Stange, D.E., van Es, J.H., Abo, A., Kujala, P., Peters, P.J., *et al.* (2009). Single Lgr5 stem cells build crypt-villus structures in vitro without a mesenchymal niche. Nature *459*, 262-265.

Solter, D., and Knowles, B.B. (1978). Monoclonal antibody defining a stage-specific mouse embryonic antigen (SSEA-1). Proc Natl Acad Sci U S A *75*, 5565-5569.

Spangrude, G.J., Muller-Sieburg, C.E., Heimfeld, S., and Weissman, I.L. (1988). Two rare populations of mouse Thy-1lo bone marrow cells repopulate the thymus. J Exp Med *167*, 1671-1683.

Springer, T., Galfre, G., Secher, D.S., and Milstein, C. (1979). Mac-1: a macrophage differentiation antigen identified by monoclonal antibody. Eur J Immunol *9*, 301-306.

Ueda, M. (2011). Skin, Applied Tissue Engineering (InTech).

Wang, X., Al-Dhalimy, M., Lagasse, E., Finegold, M., and Grompe, M. (2001). Liver repopulation and correction of metabolic liver disease by transplanted adult mouse pancreatic cells. Am J Pathol *158*, 571-579.

Williams, A.F., Galfre, G., and Milstein, C. (1977). Analysis of cell surfaces by xenogeneic myeloma-hybrid antibodies: differentiation antigens of rat lymphocytes. Cell *12*, 663-673.

Williams, C.V., Stechmann, C.L., and McLoon, S.C. (1992). Subtractive immunization techniques for the production of monoclonal antibodies to rare antigens. Biotechniques *12*, 842-847.

Zola, H., and Swart, B. (2005). The human leucocyte differentiation antigens (HLDA) workshops: the evolving role of antibodies in research, diagnosis and therapy. Cell Res *15*, 691-694.

Zola, H., Swart, B., Banham, A., Barry, S., Beare, A., Bensussan, A., Boumsell, L., C, D.B., Buhring, H.J., Clark, G., *et al.* (2007). CD molecules 2006--human cell differentiation molecules. J Immunol Methods *319*, 1-5.

15

Experimental Conditions and Mathematical Analysis of Kinetic Measurements Using Flow Cytometry – The FacsKin Method

Ambrus Kaposi[1], Gergely Toldi[1], Gergő Mészáros[1],
Balázs Szalay[2], Gábor Veress[3] and Barna Vásárhelyi[2,4]
[1]*First Department of Pediatrics, Semmelweis University*
[2]*Department of Laboratory Medicine, Semmelweis University*
[3]*Analytix Ltd.*
[4]*Research Group of Pediatrics and Nephrology, Hungarian Academy of Sciences*
Hungary

1. Introduction

Flow cytometry is in use for the assessment of different cell subsets' prevalence for decades. However, the development of specific dyes sensitive for the quickly changing intracellular analytes provided an opportunity for the real-time monitoring of intracellular processes with flow cytometry. In these kinetic measurements additionally to cell prevalence values the time as a novel variable is introduced. This enables researchers to gather data on cellular functionality from a new perspective, as the recording of a kinetic parameter with flow cytometry provides information on intracellular processes in several cell subtypes in a simultaneous manner, where physiological cell-cell interactions (such as cytokines) are still present. This approach may be a useful tool in many different areas of immune research. However, the mathematical formulae to characterize the several millions of data recorded during one measurement are still missing.

During past year our team made efforts to develop algorithms to extract the biologically relevant information from these measurements.

2. Possible ways of analysis of kinetic data obtained with flow cytometry

We define here the term 'kinetic measurement' as when the distribution of a parameter measured varies over time (Figure 1). For commonly used parameters (like FSC, SSC and most fluorescent parameters) this does not apply in general and just simply observing the distribution of these parameters regardless of the time parameter is suitable for statistical comparisons of different measurements. For the description and comparison of kinetic measurements however approaches different from the standard ones should be taken. Table 1 shows a review of the analytical methods already reported in papers on kinetic flow cytometric measurements.

2.1 Dot plot

The simplest way of presenting kinetic information is using a scatter plot (or dot plot) with time parameter and measured analyte on axis x and y, respectively, when each dot represents an individual cell. This approach and variants such as density plot (Figure 1, left), contour plot or 3D densitiy plot (June et al., 1986) are widely used (Table 1). The careful selection of cutoff values enables users to compare measurements qualitatively. The use of this technique is limited by its subjective nature. It does not provide data about the magnitude or shape of the kinetic process either.

2.2 Smoothing method

A more complex approach is to average the kinetic parameter at given small time intervals and to replace the dots in the scatter plot with these averaged values (red or green curves on Figure 1, left). This approach replaces the distribution of the kinetic parameter at each different time interval with one average value calculated from that distribution (red or green lines on Figure 1, right). Another way of explaining this method is that it is essentially a smoothing of the spiked curve that goes through all the dots in the scatter plot. There are several averaging methods that could be used: mean (used in Omann et al., 1990; Lund-Johansen et al., 1992; Rijkers et al., 1993; do Céu Monteiro et al., 1999; Jakubczak et al., 2006; Schepers et al., 2009), geometric mean (Bailey et al., 2006), median (Szalay et al., 2012). The mean is sensitive to outliers and is suitable for the characterization of a normal distribution. The median separates the lower and upper 50% range of the data.

There are also different approaches to define time intervals where the averaging takes place. These include partitioning the whole time-frame into intervals of the same length (used in the method described in Section 3); partitioning the whole time-frame into intervals all containing the same number of cells; having a fixed-length time-frame and shifting it through the whole measurement and calculating the average in these (overlapping) intervals (moving average, used in Rijkers et al., 1993, Bailey et al., 2006); using local regression (lowess method, published in (Cleveland, 1979), used in (Szalay et al., 2012)); using cubic splines etc.

The result of a smoothing method is a curve describing the measurement. If one has more measurements from the same type these curves can be averaged. A curve is an easy way to understand the graphical representation of a measurement and it shows information on how a hypothetical "average" cell behaves during the measurement. When using median as averaging method 50% of the cells showed a kinetic reaction that was higher than that of the "average" cell and 50% of the cells showed a lower reaction[1].

Furthermore, different parameters with possible biological meaning can be calculated (or simply read) from the curve such as maximum (highest value), time to reach maximum, maximal slope, value at given time points, slope at given time points, AUC (area under curve) etc. Note that these calculated parameters differ from the parameters that would be recorded during the measurement for each cell: from a single measurement one can only derive a single value for each such calculated parameter. It is possible to compare the

[1] The precise mathematical formulation of "higher" and "lower" in this sense is not within the scope of this chapter.

reference	investigated cell types	dyes used	software used	graphical presentation of kinetic data	standardization against	averaging method	parameters calculated	statistical comparison
June et al., 1986	lymphocytes	Indo-1		3D intensity against time density plot mean instensity in 100 equal-length time intervals % of responding cells in 100 equal-length time intervals	first part	Mean	time to 50% maximal response % of responding cells	-
Omann et al., 1990	leukocytes	Fluo-3	BD Chronys	mean intensity of 2 s intervals with 8 s gaps against time	previous calibration of $[Ca^{2+}]$	Mean	intensity 10 s after stimulation	-
Lund-Johansen et al., 1992	monocytes, leukocytes	Fura-Red	Cyclops (Cytomation Inc)	intensity against time scatter plot	first 40 s	Mean	intensity at a given time point	t-test
1990, Norgauer et al., 1993	neutrophils	Fluo-3, Indo-1		histogram of intensity values before and 10 s after stimulation smoothed $[Ca^{2+}]$ against time averaged $[Ca^{2+}]$ at 10 s time points	previous calibration of $[Ca^{2+}]$	mean (?)	intensity 10 s after stimulation maximal intensity	-
Rijkers et al., 1993	lymphocytes	Fluo-3, SNARF-1 (Ca^{2+}), Mag-indo-1 (Mg^{2+})		intensity against time scatter plot moving mean of instensity against time	?	mean	maximal intensity	-
do Céu Monteiro et al., 1999	platelets	Fluo-3	EPICS XL-MCL, System II software	intensity against time scatter plot mean intensity every 25 s	first 20 s	mean	maximal intensity	?

Table 1. (continues on next page) Analysis methods used in a selection of articles publishing results of kinetic flow cytometric measurements. *Intensity* refers to the fluorescent intensity value of the measured kinetic parameter. These values are usually given relative to the begininng values so as to show the fold increase of intensity. We call the the method of transforming raw values into fold-increase values (or sometimes actual concentration values) *standardization*

reference	investigated cell types	dyes used	software used	graphical presentation of kinetic data	standardization against	averaging method	parameters calculated	statistical comparison
Jakubczak et al., 2006	Neutrophils	Fluo-3, Fura-Red	Statistica 6.0	mean intensity every 60 s	first 40 s	mean	slope at given time points intensity at given time points	Mann-Whitney U test
Bailey et al., 2006	PBMC, Jurkat	Fluo-3, Fura-Red, Indo-1	FCSPress 1.3	moving geometric mean intensity against time	first part	geometric mean	maximum	-
Stork et al., 2007	B lymphocytes	Indo-1	FlowJo	moving median (?) intensity against time	none	?	-	-
Demkow et al., 2009	Neutrophils	Fluo-3, Fura-Red	Statistica 6.0	-	first 40 s	mean (?)	intensity after 60s	Mann-Whitney U test
Schepers et al., 2009	granulocytes, monocytes, lymphocytes	Fluo-3		intensity against time scatter plot mean intensity every 30 s	first 30 s	mean	intensity at every 30 s	paired Wilcoxon-test
Szalay et al., 2012	T cells	Fluo3AM (cytoplasmic Ca^{2+}), Rhod2-AM (mitochondrial Ca2+ levels), Dihydroethidium (superoxide), DAF-FM diacetate (NO)	R, Statistica 7	moving median intensity against time in representative measurements	first 5 s	median	AUC maximum time to reach maximum	paired Wilcoxon-test, Mann-Whitney U test

Table 1. (continued) Analysis methods used in a selection of articles publishing results of kinetic flow cytometric measurements. *Intensity* refers to the fluorescent intensity value of the measured kinetic parameter. These values are usually given relative to the begininng values so as to show the fold increase of intensity. We call the the method of transforming raw values into fold-increase values (or sometimes actual concentration values) *standardization*

corresponding parameters of different groups of measurements with regular statistical methods, eg. Mann-Whitney U test for 2 groups (used in Jakubczak et al.; 2006, Demkow et al.; 2009, Toldi et al.; 2010b, Szalay et al., 2012), t-test (used in Lund-Johansen et al., 1992), paired Wilcoxon-test (used in Schepers et al., 2009; Toldi et al., 2010a, Szalay et al., 2012).

The fitting of these curves should be standardized as they usually should start at value 1.0. Hence the values represent relative parameter values (rpv). This can be done by dividing the

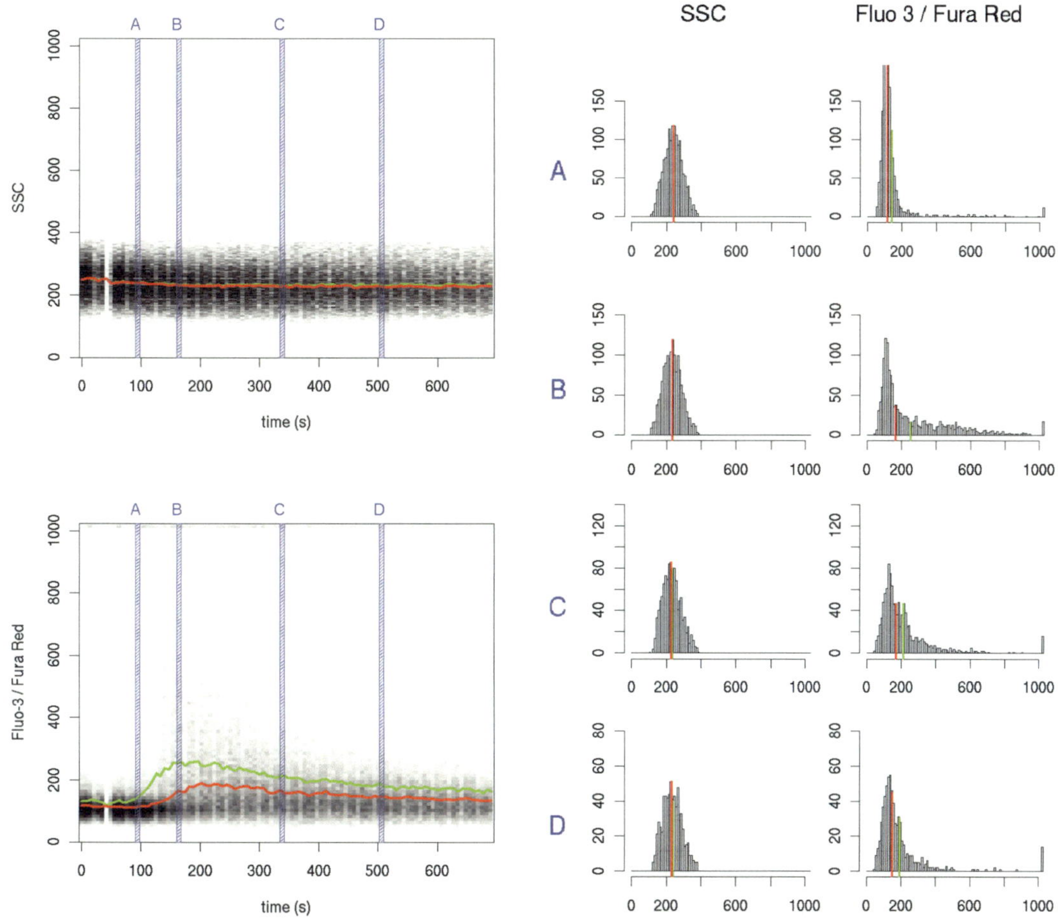

Fig. 1. Left side: 2D density plots of SSC over time and Fluo 3 / Fura Red over time in a representative Ca^{2+}-flux measurement (human CD4+ lymphocytes stimulated with PHA). Black areas represent the highest density while white areas represent zero density. The measurement interval was splitted up to 100 time intervals of equal length and medians (red curve) and means (green curve) in each interval were calculated. Right side: histograms of SSC and Fluo 3 / Fura Red parameters at 4 representative time intervals named A, B, C and D. The red line shows the place of the median and the green line that of the mean. Note that the distribution of SSC is constant over time while that of Fluo 3 / Fura Red changes: there is a sudden shift towards higher values at approx. 110 s and a slow continuous shift towards lower values afterwards

values at each time point by the value at the beginning of the experiment. This changes the values of those calculated parameters that depend on axis y (i.e. the maximum, slope parameters) but not those dependent only on axis x (i.e. time to reach maximum). Sometimes a calibration is made and the measured kinetic parameter value is converted into real biochemical/biophysical units (as in Omann et al., 1990, Norgauer et al., 1993). Another kind of standardization can be done by shifting the whole measurement by subtracting or adding a time value from/to all time points. This is useful when the exact beginning of the kinetic reaction is not known and the goal is to calculate distances from the maximal value or some well-defined time point inside the measured time-frame.

However, the value of curve parameters derived by smoothing method depends very much on the exact method used and the adjustments that are made. Adjustments have to be done for each measurement manually. Moreover, these methods are very sensitive to experimental conditions and provide no qualitative feedback on the shape of the smoothed curve. Smoothing methods are well-established for presenting but not for analyzing the data (Motulsky et al., 1987).

2.3 Fitting a model to the smoothed values

By selecting a mathematical model the assumptions that one would make about a kinetic process are made explicit (Motulsky et al., 2004). By fitting the model to the smoothed values one can test whether the measured values really follow the selected model; if so, the parameters that describe the model can be calculated. The model can be empirically determined or mechanistic. The former describes the general shape of the data and its parameters do not necessarily correspond to a biological process, while the latter is specifically formulated to describe a biological process with parameters such as dissociation constants, catalytic velocities etc. In our case the model can be formulated by a function that takes a time value and some other parameters describing the exact shape of the function and returns a numeric value that estimates the smoothed kinetic parameter value (an example of an empirically determined function is shown in Figure 2). The parameters describing the exact shape correspond to those calculated from the smoothed curve in 2.2. A series of empirical models is described in (Kaposi et al., 2008, Mészáros et al., 2011). We will describe a version improved further in Section 3. Some applications of this method are described in Section 5 (Toldi et al., 2010a-b-c, 2011a-b). Mechanistic models for calcium flux kinetics are also available (Tang et al., 1996; Politi et al., 2006). Fitting a function to the smoothed kinetic parameter values could be done by non-linear least-squares regression (Bates et al., 1988) or by one of the several robust regression methods (Motulsky et al., 2004). A robust way of testing whether the model fits the dataset is cross-validation (Picard et al., 1984).

2.4 Fitting to quantiles

An extension of the smoothing method using median averaging (method 2.2) which is orthogonal to method 2.3 comes from the idea of quantile regression (Koenker et al., 2001). One limitation of methods 2.2 and 2.3 is that they replace the distributions of the kinetic parameter at each time interval with one single value forgetting about the deviation around this average value. Replacing such a distribution with eg. 100 percentile values preserves the shape of the distribution. Afterwards, one could fit models to values corresponding to the same percentile just as in method 2.3. This is the essence of our method "FacsKin" described precisely in Section 3.

$$\text{logist+}(t;\, y0,\, y2,\, x1,\, m1) = \frac{y0 + (y2 - y0)}{1 + e^{\frac{4*m1*(-t-m1)}{y2-y0}}} \quad (y0,\, y2,\, x1,\, m \geq 0 \text{ and } y0 < y2)$$

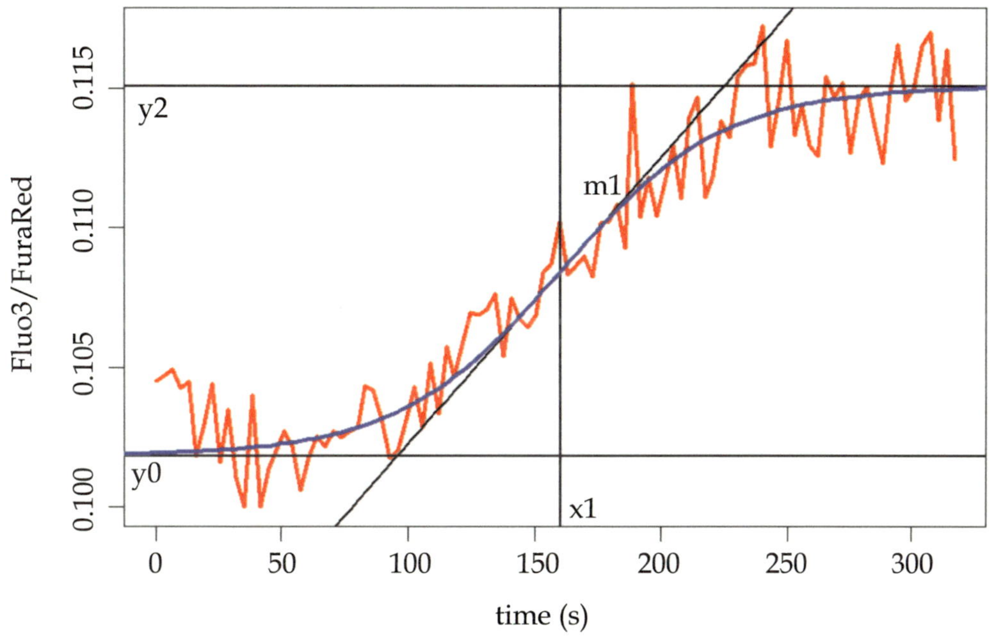

Fig. 2. A kinetic model describing kinetic reactions following an increasing sigmoid shape curve. The corresponding mathematical function is called *logist+* function and has 4 parameters that fully describe the shape of a particular logistic function (*y0, y2, x1* and *m1*, black lines with captions). The time parameter is denoted *t*. The 320 s long kinetic flow cytometric measurement time-frame was divided into 100 time intervals of equal length and the median of the kinetic parameter was calculated in each interval (red curve). The *logist+* function was fitted (blue curve) to these median values with Nelder-Mead optimization method minimizing the sum of absolute deviances (Nelder et al., 1965). The result of the current fit was: *y0=0.1018, y2=0.1151, x1=160.29, m1=0.0001026*

2.5 Fitting to the whole measurement at the same time

Replacing a distribution with percentile (or more generally, quantile) values is unnecessary if the type of the probability distribution is known. In this case fitting the parameters of the probability distribution is a more robust method than fitting functions separately to quantiles. It also helps to avoid overfitting (Hawkins, 2004). Then, it is necessary to describe the change of the parameters of the probability distribution over time by fitting a function to this change as well, one function per parameter for the probability distribution. Having a probability distribution with 2 parameters and two functions each having 8 parameters to describe their changes would result in a model containing *2*8=16* parameters (compare it with the *8*100* parameters for the functions for all 100 percentiles). The same result could be achieved by creating a mechanistic model based on the biological characteristics of the kinetic process but with parameters having exact biological meaning like dissociation constants, enzyme activities, cell types etc. However, this is a great challenge due to the large variety of cells and measurement conditions. The computational capacity required for this approach could be reduced by replacing the whole measurement with percentiles at each time interval.

2.6 Fitting to different measurements at the same time

To statistically compare different (groups of) measurements one can take the (empirical or estimated) distributions of parameters derived from fitting models separately to these measurements and compare them with statistical methods such as Kruskall-Wallis test. In this case, p values should be adjusted for multiple comparisons because each parameter has to be compared separately. A more robust method would be to define a common model for several measurements selecting parameters that are common in different measurements according to the null hypothesis and other parameters that are tested for differences.

3. Description of the FacsKin method

We developed a method for describing and comparing kinetic flow cytometry measurements using method 2.4 described in the previous section. Our aim was to provide a readily usable standard way of analyzing and comparing kinetic measurements. Previous versions of the method were published in (Kaposi et al., 2008) and (Mészáros et al., 2011). A computer program that implements the method is available at the website http://www.facskin.com. The implementation was done in Java (Oracle Inc., Redwood Shores, USA.) and R (R Development Core Team, 2006). This section describes the technical details of the method. A more user-oriented description and tutorial is the User's Guide on the website: http://www.facskin.com/node/3.

3.1 Input data

The input of the method are the time (seconds) and kinetic parameter value (raw measured intensity value or calculated ratio in case of eg. Fluo 3 / Fura Red fluorescent dyes) for each cell in the gated cell population that the user is interested in.

We divide the whole measurement into 100 equal-length time intervals. Sometimes the resolution of the time parameter isn't high enough and the cells are not evenly distributed in the time intervals. To prevent this, we recalculate time values so as to make time points evenly distributed:

$$(t'_i, t'_{i+1}, t'_{i+2}, t'_{i+3}, \ldots t'_{j-1}) := (t_i, t_i+d, t_i+2*d, t_i+3*d, \ldots, t_i+(j-i-1)*d),$$

where t_k is the old time value of the kth cell, t'_k is the new time value of the kth cell, $t_{i-1} \neq t_i = t_{i+1} = \ldots = t_{j-1} \neq t_j$, $d = (t_j - t_i) / (j - i)$. In the special case when t_{j-1} is the time value of the last cell, $t_j = t_i + (t_i - t_{i-1})$.

In each time interval we calculate the following 201 quantiles distributed equally: $1/402$, $1/402 + 1/201$, $1/402 + 2/201$, $1/402 + 3/201$, ... $1/402 + 200/201$. We use 201 quantiles so that the quartiles (0.25, 0.5, 0.75 corresponding to 51th, 101th, 151th quantile) can be obtained directly. From now on, we will use these 201 quantiles in each time interval instead of the original measurement data (we replace the original measurement data with 201*100 + 100 = 20,200 values (quantiles + time values)).

3.2 Kinetic models

We defined 5 kinetic models (Figure 3) each for different kind of kinetic measurement:

1. **constant:** the value of the kinetic parameter is constant during the measurement timeframe
2. **logist+:** the kinetic parameter starts at a given value, increases during the measurement timeframe and reaches a given value
3. **logist-:** same as *logist+*, but instead of increasing the kinetic parameter value decreases during the measurement timeframe
4. **dlogist+:** the kinetic parameter starts at a given value, increases, reaches a maximum value and then decreases and reaches a given value during the measurement timeframe
5. **dlogist-:** same as *dlogist+*, but instead of increasing and then decreasing the kinetic parameter value first decreases, reaches a minimum and then increases

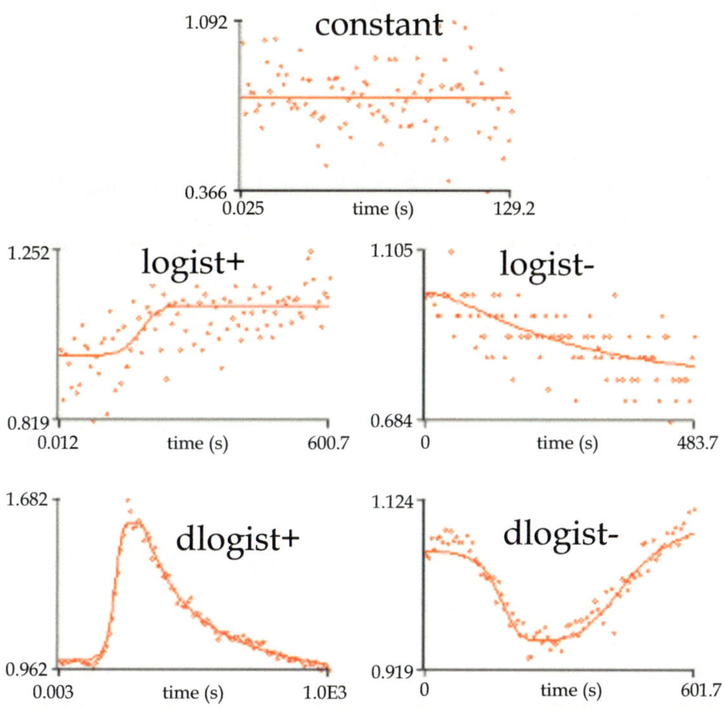

Fig. 3. Representative plots of the 5 kinetic models fitted to kinetic flow cytometric measurements (calcium flux). The dots represent the median values (quantile 0.5) at each of the 100 time intervals, the curves the functions fitted on these dots

Each model corresponds to a function. Here follows the formula and parameters for each function. Most of the parameters are constrained which means that the domain of the function is restricted to such values. *Logist+* and *logist-* differ only in their constraints and the meaning of their parameters, this is true for *dlogist+* and *dlogist-* as well. The reason for separating these functions is that we would like to avoid fitting increasing functions to some quantiles while decreasing functions to other quantiles of the same measurement.

1. **constant:** The function is a horizontal line having the same value (y) all the time. Formula:

$$constant\ (t;\ y) = y$$

Constraints: $y \geq 0$.
Parameter: y: constant value

2. **logist+:** an S-shape function that starts at a given value ($y0$) increases and reaches a higher given value ($y2$). Formula:

$$\text{logist}+(t;\ y0,\ y2,\ x1,\ m1) = y0 + \frac{y2 - y0}{1 + e^{\frac{(-t+x1)*4*m}{y2-y0}}}$$

Constraints: $y0 \geq 0$, $y2 \geq 0$, $x1 \geq 0$, $m1 \geq 0$, $y0 < y2$.
Parameters (see also Figure 2):
- $y0$: starting value. The limit of the function at $-\infty$ (minus infinity). It is not necessarily the value at time point 0. If the function begins with a steep, the starting value is lower than the value at time point 0.
- $y2$: ending value. The limit of the function at $+\infty$ (positive infinity). Not necessarily the value of the function at the end of the measurement.
- $x1$: time to reach 50% value. The time point when the function reaches the 50% value. The 50% value is the mean of the starting value and the ending value (unit: s).
- $m1$: slope at 50% value. The slope of the function at the 50% value (unit: int/s where int is the unit of the vertical axis).

3. **logist-:** an S-shape function that starts at a given value ($y0$) decreases and reaches a lower given value ($y2$). Formula:

$$\text{logist}-(t;\ y0,\ y2,\ x1,\ m1) = y0 + \frac{y2 - y0}{1 + e^{\frac{(-t+x1)*4*m}{y2-y0}}}$$

Constraints: $y0 \geq 0$, $y2 \geq 0$, $x1 \geq 0$, $m1 \geq 0$, $y0 < y2$.
Parameters:
- $y0$: starting value. The limit of the function at $-\infty$ (minus infinity). It is not necessarily the value at time point 0. If the function begins with a steep, the starting value is higher than the value at time point 0.
- $y2$: ending value. The limit of the function at $+\infty$ (positive infinity). Not necessarily the value of the function at the end of the measurement.
- $x1$: time to reach 50% value. The time point when the function reaches the 50% value. The 50% value is the mean of the starting value and the ending value (unit: s).
- $m1$: slope at 50% value. The slope of the function at the 50% value (unit: int/s where int is the unit of the vertical axis.).

4. **dlogist+:** a function that starts at a given value ($y0$), has an increasing phase, reaches a maximum ($y1$), has a decreasing phase and reaches a given ending value ($y2$). Formula:

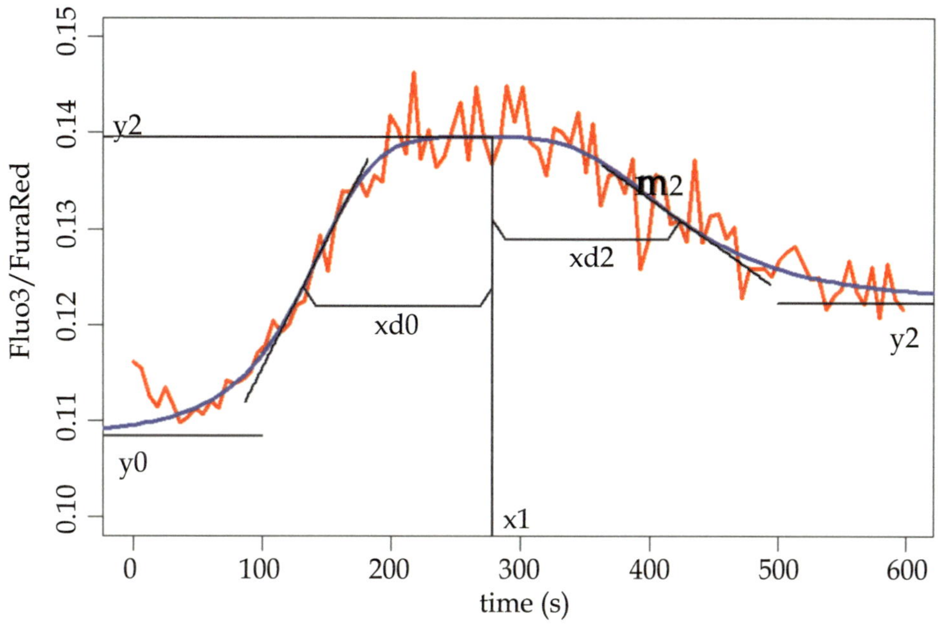

Fig. 4. Parameters of the *dlogist+* function (the formula is given in 3.2.5). The 600 s long kinetic flow cytometric measurement time-frame was divided into 100 time intervals of equal length and the median of the kinetic parameter was calculated in each interval (red curve). The d*logist+* function was fitted (blue curve) to these median values with Nelder-Mead optimization method minimizing the sum of absolute deviances (Nelder et al., 1965). The result of the current fit was: y0=0.*1083, y1=0.1395, y2=0.1222, x1=278.4, xd0=146.7, xd2=145.0, m0=2.657*10*$^{-4}$, *m2=-9.519*10*$^{-5}$

$$\text{dlogist}+(t;\, y0,\, y1,\, y2,\, x1,\, xd0,\, xd2,\, m0\; m2) = \begin{cases} y0 + \dfrac{y1-y0}{1+\left(\dfrac{x1-t}{xd0}\right)^{\frac{4*xd0*m0}{y1-y0}}}, & \text{t<x1} \\[2ex] y2 + \dfrac{y1-y2}{1+\left(\dfrac{t-x1}{xd2}\right)^{\frac{4*xd2*m2}{y2-y1}}}, & \text{t} \geq \text{x1} \end{cases}$$

Constraints: y0 ≥ 0, y1 ≥ 0, y2 ≥ 0, m0 ≥ 0, x1 ≥ 0, xd0 ≥ 0, xd2 ≥ 0, m2 ≤ 0, xd0 ≤ x1, y1 > y0, y1 > y2.

Parameters (see also Figure 4):

- y0: starting value. The limit of the function at -∞ (minus infinity). It is not necessarily the value at time point 0. If the function begins with a steep, the starting value is lower than the value at time point 0.
- y1: maximum value. The maximum of the function. It is possible that the maximum point is not in the measurement timeframe (usually meaning that the measurement does not follow this kinetic model).
- y2: ending value. The limit of the function at +∞ (positive infinity). Not necessarily the value of the function at the end of the measurement.

- x1: time to reach maximum value. The time point when the function reaches the maximum value (unit: s).
- xd0: time from the first 50% value to maximum. The distance between the time point where the function reaches the first 50% value and where the function reaches the maximum. The first 50% value is the mean of the starting value and the maximum (unit: s).
- m0: slope at first 50% value. The slope of the function at the first 50% value (unit: int/s where int is the unit of the vertical axis).
- xd2: time from maximum to the second 50% value: the distance between the time point where the function reaches the maximum and where the function reaches the second 50% value. The second 50% value is the mean of the maximum and the ending value (unit: s)
- m2: slope at second 50% value: the slope of the function at the second 50% value (unit: int/s where int is the unit of the vertical axis).

5. **dlogist-:** a function that starts at a given value (*y0*), has a decreasing phase, reaches a minimum (*y1*), has an increasing phase and reaches a given ending value (*y2*). Formula:

$$\text{dlogist}-x(t;\ y0,\ y1,\ y2,\ x1,\ xd0,\ xd2,\ m0\ m2) = \begin{cases} y0 + \dfrac{y1-y0}{1+\left(\dfrac{x1-t}{xd0}\right)^{\frac{4*xd0*m0}{y1-y0}}}, & t<x1 \\ y2 + \dfrac{y1-y2}{1+\left(\dfrac{t-x1}{xd2}\right)^{\frac{4*xd2*m2}{y2-y1}}}, & t\geq x1 \end{cases}$$

Constraints: $y0 \geq 0$, $y1 \geq 0$, $y2 \geq 0$, $m2 \geq 0$, $x1 \geq 0$, $xd0 \geq 0$, $xd2 \geq 0$, $m0 \leq 0$, $xd0 \leq x1$, $y1 < y0$, $y1 < y2$.
Parameters:

- *y0*: starting value. The limit of the function at -∞ (minus infinity). It is not necessarily the value at time point 0. If the function begins with a steep, the starting value is higher than the value at time point 0.
- *y1*: minimum value. The minimum of the function. It is possible that the minimum point is not in the measurement timeframe (usually meaning that the measurement does not follow this kinetic model).
- *y2*: ending value. The limit of the function at +∞ (positive infinity). Not necessarily the value of the function at the end of the measurement
- *x1*: time to reach minimum value. The time point when the function reaches the minimum value (unit: s).
- *xd0*: time from the first 50% value to minimum. The distance between the time point where the function reaches the first 50% value and where the function reaches the minimum. The first 50% value is the mean of the starting value and the minimum (unit: s).
- *m0*: slope at first 50% value: the slope of the function at the first 50% value (unit: int/s where int is the unit of the vertical axis).
- *xd2*: time from maximum to the second 50% value. The distance between the time point where the function reaches the minimum and where the function reaches the

second 50% value. The second 50% value is the mean of the minimum and the ending value (unit: s).

- *m2*: slope at second 50% value. The slope of the function at the second 50% value (unit: int/s where int is the unit of the vertical axis).

The parameters dependent on axis y (*y0, y1, y2, m0, m1, m2*) can be standardized by dividing each value by the *y0* parameter of the same function so that the functions start at value 1.0 and the *y0, y1* and *y2* parameters become relative parameter values (rpv) while *m0, m1* and *m2* parameters become values of rpv/s units. The standardization of the parameters dependent only on axis x in case of *dlogist+* and *dlogist-* functions is done by having *xd0* and *xd2* parameters which are measured as a distance from the maximum, not as the time to reach the 50% values.

3.3 Function fitting

Before fitting a function, we estimate the parameters by applying the lowess smoothing method (Cleveland, 1979) several times with different smoother spans. We fit models with the Nelder-Mead optimisation method (Nelder et al., 1965) to quantile values starting from the estimated parameters minimizing the sum of absolute deviances.

For all 5 functions we do the following:

1. First we use 10-fold cross validation on the three quartiles separately to get an estimation of how well the function fits the measurement data. We summate the sum of absolute distances between the function fitted to the training set and the test set (Picard et al., 1984). The test set is one tenth of the whole dataset (which is 100 time and 100 intensity values for each quartile).
2. Then we fit the function to the 201 quantiles mentioned earlier.

The result of fitting the functions is 201*(1 + 4 + 4 + 8 + 8) = 5025 parameters and the 10-fold cross validation values for the 5 functions.

3.4 Comparison

To describe a measurement, we select the best function (by looking at how well the median function fits the median (0.5 quantile) values and looking for low 10-fold cross validation values) and we create distributions of the parameters by using the corresponding parameters of the 201 functions, hence each parameter will be represented by a distribution of 201 values. For example, in case of the *dlogist+* function we can talk about the distribution of the maximum value (Figure 5). The distributions can be summarized by giving median [range] or median [quartiles] values or visually by drawing a histogram or box plot.

To compare different (groups of) measurements we select a common function that describes every measurement well. Then, we summate the distributions of each parameter by group so that each group will have one single distribution for every parameter containing (measurement count in group)*201 values. We can compare distributions of parameters between different groups by probability binning method (Roederer et al., 2001) or by calculating the overlap of the middle 50% of the distributions. The T value given by probability binning and the overlap percentage give a measure of difference between the distributions and the former method also gives a p-value (corresponding to the null hypothesis that the two distributions are equal). There is the possibility of extracting only 1 value for each parameter from one measurement, ie. the parameters of the median function (which was fitted to the 0.5 quantile values) and in this case usual nonparametric statistical methods like Mann-Whitney U test (or Kruskall-Wallis test, for more than 2 groups) can be used to compare parameters between different groups.

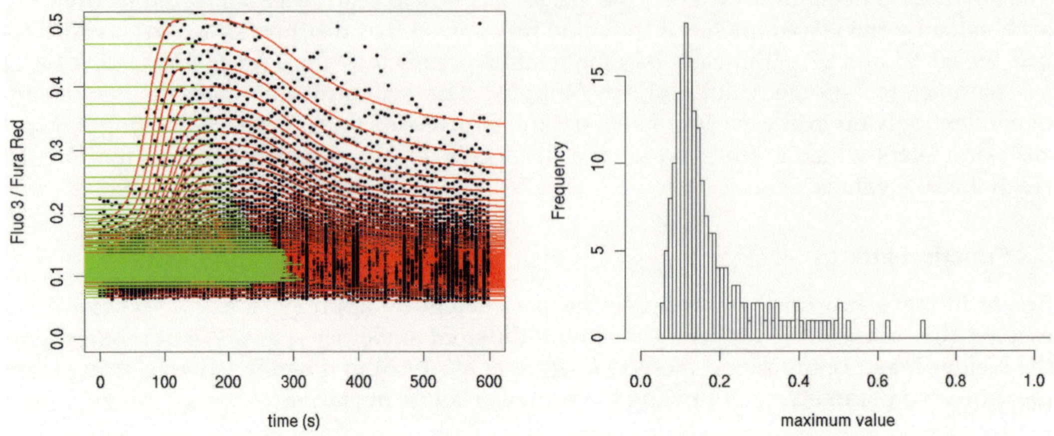

Fig. 5. Derivation of the distribution of parameter *y1* (maximum value) of the *dlogist+* function. The 600 s long kinetic flow cytometric measurement time-frame was divided into 100 time intervals of equal length and 201 quantiles were calculated in each interval (black dots). *Dlogist+* function was fitted to each quantile (red curves). The maximum parameters (green lines) of each were collected and form a distribution (histogram on the right)

4. Experimental settings

Additionally to cytoplasmic Ca^{2+} signal (June et al., 1990) the development of a number of fluorescent probes (Johnson, 2001) provided an opportunity to measure the kinetics of other intracellular parameters such as membrane potential, mitochondrial Ca^{2+} levels and superoxide generation (Mészáros et al., 2011).

The authors of this chapter are mainly interested in investigating the activation process of T-lymphocytes. The experimental procedures described below are useful when examining the first short period of T-lymphocyte activation. We optimized incubation times, temperature and dye concentrations for Jurkat cells. The precise experimental settings can be found in (Mészáros et al., 2011). It should be emphasized that these experimental conditions may be different for other cell types.

4.1 Variables to be standardized during the measurements

Cells: although human peripheral blood samples are probably the most common specimen submitted to flow cytometry laboratory, to optimize an assay for experimental purposes, the most adequate way is to use different cell lines.

How specimens are obtained, handled, and stored is intimately related to the reason for obtaining them (for example, to analyse human peripherial blood lymphocytes, samples should be taken in a heparinized tubes and stored at room temperature). In most instances it is also crucial to assess the viability of separated cells. There are several methods available for this purpose (Stoddart, 2011). Additionally, viability should be determined prior to separation procedures.

The number of cells required per assay depends on the number of experiments planned and on the expected proportion of responding cells. Experiments with cells having a homogeneous response need ~106 cells per 10-min assay to quantify the response of a major population.

Solvents: the choice of cell culture medium can be influenced by two requirements: i) the metabolic requirements of the cells and ii) the solving properties of the fluorescent dyes used. For example cyanine and oxonol dyes are hydrophobic and will tend to plate out of aqueous solutions onto the surfaces of glass and plastic test tubes and onto the tubing in flow cytometers. Most of these compounds are highly soluble in DMSO (dimethylsulfoxide) and DMF (dimethyl formamide), which, because it does not readily evaporate, is a convenient vehicle for preparation of stock and working solutions.

In our protocols given below, and generally as well, the amount of DMSO added to cell suspensions is sufficiently small to keep the overall concentration at under 1% (v/v) (Brayton, 1986).

Dyes: evaluation of live cells using flow cytometry presents some difficult challenges. One of these is the need for maintaining the stability of cells. Therefore fluourescent dyes should not be toxic. During the staining procedure the cells and the reagents must be kept at appropriate temperature and should be carefully checked for pH (7.4), since the cells and some dyes are very sensitive to temperature and pH. The staining procedure should be performed under dimmed light and incubation should be in the dark, because of the light sensitivity of fluorochroms.

Dyes and ionophores for intracellular measurements may stick to cytometer tubing. Therefore, before measurement it is important to preequilibrate the tubing to prevent baseline shift. Likewise, tubing should be thoroughly cleaned after use by flushing the instrument with bleach. In case this is not done, residual dye may migrate from the tubing into cell samples that are introduced later into the instrument, and this may produce the appearance of immunofluorescent staining in unlabeled cells. In some cases ionophore in the sample may stick to the cytometer tubing and subsequently bind to cells in a later sample, producing a real change in the signal. When there is a possibility that this could happen, it may be prudent to flush with bleach between samples.

One has to be aware of a specific problem that may occur when several dyes are used in combination, i.e., their fluorescence emission spectra may overlap. In case quantitative information is required (i.e., the amount of fluorescence has to reflect a biochemical quantity), samples stained with a single dye should be included for use in setting fluorescence compensation (Roederer, 2002).

In the last years we established some flow cytometry methods that enable the users to monitor intracellular processes (membrane potential, mitochondrial Ca^{2+} levels and superoxide generation). We optimized incubation times, temperature and dye concentrations for T-lymphocytes. The dyes used are listed in Table 2. For more cellular function probes see (Johnson, 2001).

4.2 Considerations on timing

For many kinetic experiments with flow cytometry, the cell suspensions are analyzed for a period of 5-20 min. Timing is particularly critical when the change of the intracellular parameter to be observed lasts for a few minutes or less, in which case kinetic measurements incorporating time as a measurement parameter represent the only realistic approach to obtain consistent data. Even when stimuli produce effects lasting longer, it is important to maintain a relatively constant duration of cell incubation with dyes and stimuli from sample to sample.

4.3 Control measurements

Every experiment should include a baseline measurement which runs for 1-2 minutes with no additions to the sample. This provides a view of the degree of homogenity of individual cells in the population. Ideally the population distribution is very tight, but in case of presence of different cell types in the sample, the detected fluorescent signal intensity could be very diverse. In many cases, there is marked heterogenity in the changes that occur, sometimes even in populations of cells that were previously thought to be homogeneous. A limitation of flow cytometry, however, is that it does not permit kinetic resolution of certain complex kinetic responses such as cellular oscillatory responses. This requires video microscopy with digital image analysis, a technique that is complementary to flow cytometry for the study of various parameters of cell activation (Botvinick et al., 2007).

Name of the dye	Excitation max, (nm)	Emission max, (nm)	Excitation laser line (nm)	Use
Calcium sensitive ratiometric dyes				
Fluo-3-AM	506	526	488	**Cytomplasma Ca^{2+}-level**
Fura Red	436	655	488	
Indo-1	330-361	405-475	365	
Membrane potential sensitive dyes				
DiBAC4(3)	494	516	488	**Membrane potential**
DiBAC4(5)	590	616	488	
Mitochondrial probes				
JC-1	520	530, 590	488	**Mitochondrial potential**
TMRM	543	567	488	
Rhod-2/AM	552	581	488	**Mitochondrial Ca^{2+} level**
ROS sensitive dyes				
DAF-FM diacetate	495	515	488	**NO measurement**
HE	518	605	488	**O_2^- generation measurement**

Table 2. Fluorescent probes for kinetic measurements

"Pseudo mixing test" is an important control in kinetic flow cytometry measurements. It determines whether the cell population is susceptible to mechanical shear forces like mixing and sample pressurization. These effects can activate pressure sensitive ion flux mechanisms present in some cell lines and can result in changes of the signal detection.

The fact that some of the fluorescent probes can be compartmentalized in cells forces us to use different control experiments. In order to test the validity of assay systems the use of specific activators and/or inhibitors is mandatory. At the end of the measurements to test whether the cells were properly loaded with reporter dye and whether the flow cytometry system was set up properly, the addition of positive or negative control chemicals is needed.

5. Applications of the FacsKin method

FacsKin provides a tool for the evaluation of kinetic flow cytometry data. This section presents some experiments that benefited from opportunities provided by FacsKin.

5.1 The investigation of calcium influx kinetics in Th1 and Th2 cells

Upon antigen presentation, a signal transduction pathway leads to a transient, biphasic elevation of $[Ca^{2+}]_{cyt}$ in lymphocytes (Figure 6). The first phase of the biphasic calcium signal is directly linked to the generation of IP_3, and calcium release from the endoplasmic reticulum (ER) upon the binding of IP_3 to its designated receptor (Lewis, 2001). The second phase is due to the activation of calcium release activated calcium (CRAC) channels in the cell membrane. The calcium signal converges to the activation of transcription factors leading to cytokine production and further factors needed for the development of an adequate lymphocyte response. The actual distribution of $[Ca^{2+}]_{cyt}$ depends on finely tuned interactions of mechanisms responsible for its elevation and decrease. Besides ER calcium release and calcium entry through the CRAC channels, mitochondria also contribute to the elevation of $[Ca^{2+}]_{cyt}$ via the regulation of CRAC channel functionality. However, in a later phase of lymphocyte activation, they may also take up and store large amounts of calcium via the mitochondrial calcium uniporter (MCU) and, therefore, decrease $[Ca2+]_{cyt}$ (Duchen, 2000). Other mechanisms that specifically contribute to the clearance of elevated $[Ca2+]_{cyt}$ in lymphocytes are the sarco/endoplasmic reticulum calcium ATPase (SERCA) (Feske, 2007) and the plasma membrane calcium ATPase (PMCA) (Di Leva et al., 2008).

The steps of activation begin with identical stimuli in the two major arms of T helper lymphocytes, Th1 and Th2 cells. However, they produce a different set of cytokines, and exert distinct effects on the inflammatory balance. While Th1 cells account for the development of a pro-inflammatory response, Th2 cells produce anti-inflammatory cytokines. Since the expression of cytokine genes is influenced by the characteristics of calcium influx kinetics, the differences in calcium handling of the Th1 and Th2 subset may remarkably contribute to variations in cytokine production (Dolmetsch et al., 1998). Therefore, we investigated the differences of calcium handling between Th1 and Th2 lymphocytes. We tested the contribution of the ER calcium release, the CRAC channel, the MCU, the SERCA pump and the PMCA pump to the regulation of $[Ca^{2+}]_{cyt}$ during the early period of T lymphocyte activation.

First, we compared the kinetics of calcium response in the Th1 and Th2 lymphocyte subsets following lymphocyte activation (Toldi et al., 2011a). AUC, Slope and Max values were lower in the Th2 subset. However, the t_{max} value did not significantly differ in the two subsets. The higher activity of the SERCA pump, along with the lower activity of mitochondrial calcium reuptake, and therefore of the CRAC channels account for the notion that Th2 cells go through a lower level of lymphocyte activation compared with Th1 cells upon identical activating stimuli.

In contrast to the SERCA pump, which functions from the beginning of calcium influx, the PMCA pump in Th1 cells has a role in the shaping of $[Ca^{2+}]_{cyt}$ kinetics from a stage when $[Ca^{2+}]_{cyt}$ is already elevated, thus ensuring the reconstitution of the original $[Ca^{2+}]_{cyt}$ level. This is represented in our results by the fact that the inhibition of this mechanism affects the Max values but not the Slope value in Th1 cells. The main regulator of the PMCA pump is the elevated level of $[Ca^{2+}]_{cyt}$ (Di Leva et al., 2008). Therefore, the initial calcium uptake of the ER has an important regulatory effect on the function of the PMCA pump. Since calcium reuptake by ER is more active in Th2 cells, $[Ca^{2+}]_{cyt}$ will not increase to the extent observed in Th1 cells. Therefore, it seems that $[Ca^{2+}]_{cyt}$ will not be elevated sufficiently in the Th2 subset to activate the PMCA pump during the initial phase of activation. In contrast, in Th1 cells, due to the lower extent of ER reuptake, $[Ca^{2+}]_{cyt}$ will increase sufficiently to activate the PMCA pump. Differential calcium signaling and distinct kinetics of the alterations of $[Ca^{2+}]_{cyt}$ may have an important contributing role to the production of dissimilar cytokines by Th1 and Th2 cells.

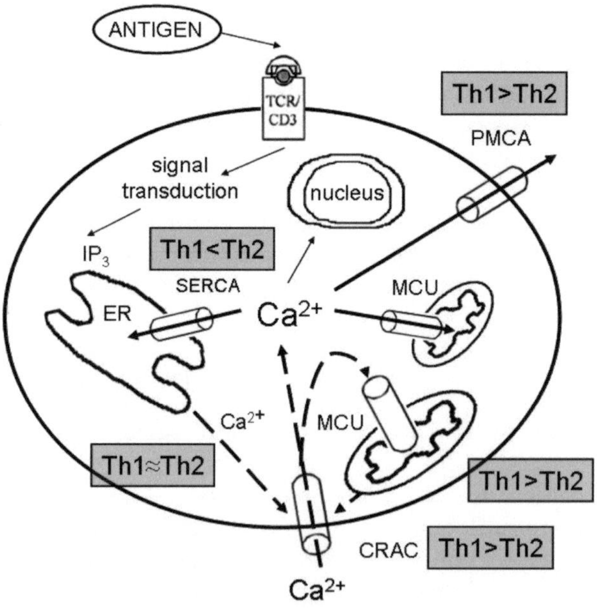

Fig. 6. The regulation of cytoplasmic free calcium level in lymphocytes. Interrupted arrows represent mechanisms responsible for the elevation, whereas bold arrows represent those responsible for the decrease of the cytoplasmic free calcium level. The differential activity of these mechanisms in Th1 and Th2 cells is marked in the gray boxes. TCR: T cell receptor, IP_3: inositol trisphosphate, ER: endoplasmic reticulum, CRAC: calcium release activated calcium channel, MCU: mitochondrial calcium uniporter, SERCA: sarco/endoplasmic reticulum calcium ATPase, PMCA: plasma membrane calcium ATPase

5.2 The role of lymphocyte potassium channels in the regulation of calcium influx

In order to maintain the electrochemical driving force for calcium entry from the extracellular space, depolarizing calcium influx needs to be counterbalanced by the efflux of cations, predominantly potassium. Therefore, lymphocyte activation is closely linked to and regulated by the function of lymphocyte potassium channels. There are two major types of potassium channels in T lymphocytes: the voltage-gated Kv1.3 and the calcium-activated IKCa1 channels. In our investigations, we studied the role of the Kv1.3 and IKCa1 channels in the process of lymphocyte activation not only in healthy individuals, but also in neonates, pregnancy and immune-mediated disorders, such as preeclampsia, multiple sclerosis and type 1 diabetes.

In healthy individuals, a triarylmethane compound (TRAM), the specific inhibitor of the IKCa1 channel decreased calcium influx in Th2 cells to a lower extent than in Th1 cells (Toldi et al., 2011b). This finding supports previous data from Fanger et al. (2000) obtained by patch clamp, showing that IKCa1 currents are smaller in Th2 cells when compared with the Th1 subset. A possible contributing element to this phenomenon might be that $[Ca^{2+}]_{cyt}$, which needs to reach a threshold to activate the IKCa1 channels, increases more rapidly in Th1 than in Th2 cells, due to the distinct function of the SERCA pump, as detailed above.

In contrast with IKCa1, the inhibition of Kv1.3 channels by a specific blocker, margatoxin (MGTX) results in a somewhat larger decrease of calcium in Th2 than in Th1 cells. Calcium influx in Th1 cells is less sensitive to the inhibition of the Kv1.3 channel. All in all, a larger amount of compensatory potassium leaves the cells through the Kv1.3 and IKCa1 channels upon lymphocyte activation in the Th1 subset, enabling a larger amount of calcium to enter from the extracellular space compared with the Th2 subset.

In healthy individuals, CD8 cells were more sensitive to the inhibition of the IKCa1 channels than the CD4 subset, responding with a higher level of decrease of the AUC value upon the application of TRAM. However, almost no difference was observed between the sensitivity of CD4 and CD8 cells to the inhibition of the Kv1.3 channel.

5.3 Lymphocyte activation and potassium channels in healthy pregnancy and preeclampsia

Both in pregnancy and in the neonatal period, the immune response and the kinetics of lymphocyte activation are altered compared with the adult, non-pregnant state. Healthy pregnancy is characterized by the development of an immune tolerance specific for the antigens presented by the developing fetus. The impairment of this tolerance and the development of an abnormal immune response play a major role in adverse pregnancy outcomes, including preeclampsia (Saito et al., 2007). This disorder is characterized by hypertension, proteinuria, edema and endothelial dysfunction usually evolving in the third trimester of pregnancy. The development of a maternal systemic inflammatory response has also been described in PE (Saito et al., 2007). An important feature of this disorder is the absence of Th2 skewness and thus the predominance of pro-inflammatory cytokines, as shown by a number of investigations (Darmochwal-Kolarz et al., 2002; Rein et al., 2002; Saito et al., 1999).

Our results indicate marked differences of calcium influx kinetics and sensitivity to Kv1.3 and IKCa1 channel inhibition (by margatoxin (MGTX) and a triarylmethane compound

(TRAM), respectively) in major lymphocyte subsets (i.e. Th1, Th2, CD4 and CD8 cells) between non-pregnant, healthy pregnant and preeclamptic lymphocytes (Toldi et al., 2010a). These properties in preeclampsia are more comparable to the non-pregnant state than to healthy pregnancy, suggesting that there is a characteristic pattern of calcium influx in healthy pregnant women that is missing in preeclamptic patients. This raises the notion that lymphocyte calcium handling upon activation may have a role in the characteristic immune status of healthy pregnancy.

AUC values of the calcium response are lower in healthy pregnancy in the Th1, CD4 and CD8 lymphocyte subsets. On contrary to Th1 cells, the activation induced calcium response of the Th2 subset is not decreased compared with the non-pregnant state. The decreased activation of the Th1 subset and the lack of decrease in Th2 cells may partly be responsible for the well established Th2 skewness in healthy pregnancy (Darmochwal-Kolarz et al., 2002; Rein et al., 2002; Saito et al., 1999). Unlike in healthy pregnancy, we could not detect a difference in the AUC values of calcium influx of Th1 and CD8 cells in preeclampsia compared to non-pregnant women. The maintained activation properties of Th1 lymphocytes in preeclamptic patients may contribute to the lack of Th2 dominance associated with normal pregnancy. It is of particular interest that calcium influx of Th2 lymphocytes in healthy pregnancy was insensitive to potassium channel inhibition, while calcium influx decreased significantly in non-pregnant samples upon treatment with the specific channel blockers. Of note, Th2 lymphocytes in preeclampsia presented with non-pregnant-like characteristics, and were also sensitive to MGTX and TRAM treatment. Since the regulatory function of Kv1.3 and IKCa1 channels on calcium influx appears to be limited in healthy pregnant samples, this may be an element contributing to the Th2 shift present in healthy pregnancy, but absent in preeclampsia. While calcium influx in CD8 and Th1 lymphocytes was resistant to potassium channel inhibition in preeclamptic, that of healthy pregnant lymphocytes was sensitive. Similarly to Th2 cells, while it is unclear whether the resistance of Th1 lymphocytes to potassium channel inhibition is reflected in their function, the insensitivity of the Th1 subset to the inhibition of regulatory lymphocyte potassium channels in preeclampsia may be linked to the Th1 skewness.

5.4 Lymphocyte activation and potassium channels in the newborn

Decreased functionality of neonatal T cells is a widely recognized experimental and clinical phenomenon. Reduced functioning is well characterized by a lower level of cytokine production compared to adult T cells (Cohen et al., 1999; García Vela et al., 2000). Several factors might be responsible for the decreased cytokine expression compared to adult lymphocytes. We hypothesized that short-term T lymphocyte activation properties are different in neonates compared to adults. We aimed to characterize the calcium influx kinetics upon activation in major T lymphocyte subsets (i.e. Th1, Th2, CD4 and CD8 cells) in the neonate, and its sensitivity to the specific inhibition of Kv1.3 and IKCa1 lymphocyte potassium channels (Toldi et al., 2010b).

Lower AUC and Max values in most of the investigated subsets suggest that short-term activation and associated calcium influx are decreased in neonatal lymphocytes, in line with the fact that newborns mount lower immune responses to distinct stimuli. Upon treatment of lymphocytes with selective inhibitors of the Kv1.3 and IKCa1 channels (MGTX and TRAM, respectively), calcium influx decreases in most investigated lymphocyte subsets isolated from adults. However, with the exception of the CD8 subset, such a reduction was not demonstrated in neonatal lymphocytes. These findings may partly explain why neonatal lymphocytes are less responsive to activating stimuli and, hence, exert a lower intensity of immune response. Our results improve the understanding of the mechanisms that prevent neonatal T cells from adequate activation upon activating stimuli, and partially elucidate previous experimental data indicating that a greater amount of stimulation is needed in neonatal lymphocytes compared with adults to achieve a similar immune response (Adkins, 1999; Cohen et al., 1999). The functional impairment of lymphocyte potassium channels may be of importance in those mechanisms.

5.5 Lymphocyte activation and potassium channels in multiple sclerosis

We also investigated calcium influx kinetics in multiple sclerosis (MS) patients without and with interferon (IFN) beta treatment compared to healthy individuals (Toldi et al., 2011b). We aimed to describe the effects of Kv1.3 and IKCa1 channel inhibitors on calcium influx, and to assess whether these inhibitors could potentially contribute to the treatment of MS via the selective reduction of lymphocyte activation as suggested before (Wulff et al., 2003). We demonstrated that the reactivity of lymphocytes isolated from MS patients receiving no IFN beta treatment is increased compared to healthy individuals, reflected by lower t_{max} and elevated Slope values in the CD4, Th1 and Th2 subsets (i.e. the peak of the calcium influx is reached more rapidly). Interestingly, these alterations were not present in the CD8 subset. Of note, while the kinetics of calcium influx is altered, comparable AUC and Max values indicate that the amount of calcium entering the lymphocytes in MS is not different from that in healthy individuals.

In healthy individuals, we found prominent differences between Th1 and Th2 cells with regard to their sensitivity to IKCa1 channel inhibition, as described above. In contrast with healthy subjects, the investigated lymphocyte subsets show altered sensitivity to the inhibition of the Kv1.3 and IKCa1 channels in MS patients without IFN beta. In this group, the inhibition of the IKCa1 channel results in a similar decrease of calcium influx in all investigated subsets. However, MGTX, the specific blocker of the Kv1.3 channel decreased the AUC value to a higher extent in CD8 cells than in CD4 cells. Therefore, the contribution of Kv1.3 channels to the activation of CD8 lymphocytes is increased in MS patients receiving no IFN beta. However, the specificity of Kv1.3 inhibition is limited to CD8 cells since other cell types, including Th1 and Th2 cells, behave in a similar manner in MS patients without IFN beta upon Kv1.3 channel inhibition. Therefore, on contrary to previous suggestions (Wulff et al., 2003), the inhibition of this channel does not seem to be specific enough, since it also affects anti-inflammatory cytokine producing Th2 cells. This would probably result in a setback of therapeutic efforts in MS. Therefore, the effects of administration of Kv1.3 channel inhibitors need to be further investigated and characterized in MS.

IFN beta therapy induces compensatory changes in calcium influx kinetics and lymphocyte potassium channel function in MS, shaping these properties more similar to those of healthy individuals. However, the suppressive effect of IFN beta treatment on lymphocyte activation is seen in Th1 cells selectively, while Th2 function is less affected. These observations might indicate a novel mechanism through which IFN beta exerts beneficial therapeutic effects on immune functionality in MS.

5.6 Lymphocyte activation and potassium channels in type 1 diabetes

In samples taken from type 1 diabetes mellitus (T1DM) patients, the activation characteristics of lymphocytes show an evident alteration compared to healthy samples (Toldi et al., 2010c). First, we noticed that the peak of calcium influx in the overall lymphocyte population and the Th1 subset is reached more rapidly in T1DM (i.e. t_{max} values were decreased), while AUC and Max values were comparable. Similarly to MS, this finding raised the notion of an increased reactivity of lymphocytes in T1DM.

In lymphocytes of healthy subjects both Kv1.3 and IKCa1 channels contribute to the maintenance of calcium influx upon activation. On the contrary, the sensitivity of T1DM lymphocytes to the inhibition of Kv1.3 channels is increased, probably due to the increased expression of Kv1.3 channels (Toldi et al., 2010c). The altered activation kinetics of T1DM lymphocytes may at least partly be attributed to the increased significance of Kv1.3 channels.

Based on promising animal data, the specific inhibition of Kv1.3 channels is under extensive investigation as a possible measure to prevent the development of the autoimmune response against pancreatic beta cells (Chandy et al., 2004). Our data indicate that by specific inhibition of Kv1.3 channels, lymphocyte activation can be modulated in T1DM. However, our findings provide clear evidence for Kv1.3 channels to have an important role in each lymphocyte subset in T1DM, including Th2 lymphocytes acting as counterbalancing factors in the development of T1DM through the production of anti-inflammatory cytokines (Yoon and Jun, 2001). Therefore, administration of Kv1.3 channel inhibitors would not have an exclusive effect on cells responsible for the autoimmune response in T1DM, but may have an impact on the activation characteristics of immune cells in general. The finding that increased significance of Kv1.3 channels in lymphocyte activation is not exclusive for a specific subset, but is characteristic for most of major lymphocyte subsets in T1DM, alerts us that the overall immunomodulatory effect upon inhibition of Kv1.3 channels in T1DM needs to be further characterized.

6. References

Adkins, B. (1999). T-cell function in newborn mice and humans. *Immunol Today*, Vol.20, No.7, (July 1999), pp. 330-335

Bailey, S., Macardle, P.J. (2006). A flow cytometric comparison of Indo-1 to fluo-3 and Fura Red excited with low power lasers for detecting Ca(2+) flux. *J Immunol Methods*, Vol.311, No.1-2, (April 2006), pp. 220-225

Bates, D.M., Watts, D.G. (1988). Nonlinear Regression Analysis and its Applications. Wiley Book, New York. ISBN 0471-816434

Botvinick, E.L. Shah, J.V. (2007). Laser-based measurements in cell biology. *Methods Cell Biol*, Vol.82, Part I, (2007), pp. 81-109.

Brayton, C.F. (1986). Dimethyl sulfoxide (DMSO): a review. *Cornell Vet*, Vol.76, No.1, (January 1986), pp. 61-90.

Chandy, K.G., Wulff, H., Beeton, C., Pennington, M., Gutman, G.A., Cahalan, M.D. (2004). K+ channels as targets for specific immunomodulation. *Trends Pharmacol Sci*, Vol.25, No.5, (May 2004), pp. 280–289

Cleveland, W.S. (1979). Robust Locally Weighed Regression and Smoothing Scatterplots. *Journal of the American Statistical Association*, Vol.74, No.368 (December 1979), pp. 829-836

Cohen, S.B., Perez-Cruz, I., Fallen, P., Gluckman, E., Madrigal, J.A. (1999). Analysis of the cytokine production by cord and adult blood. *Hum Immunol*, Vol.60, No.4, (April 1999), pp. 331-336

Darmochwal-Kolarz, D., Rolinski, J., Leszczynska-Goarzelak, B., Oleszczuk, J. (2002). The expressions of intracellular cytokines in the lymphocytes of preeclamptic patients. *Am J Reprod Immunol*, Vol.48, No.6, (December 2002), pp. 381-386

Demkow, U., Winklewski, P., Potapinska, O., Popko, K., Lipinska, A., Wasik, M. (2009). Kinetics of calcium ion concentration accompanying transduction of signals into neutrophils from diabetic patients and its modification by insulin. *J Physiol Pharmacol*, Vol.60, No.5, (November 2009), pp. 37-40

Di Leva, F., Domi, T., Fedrizzi, L., Lim, D., Carafoli, E. (2008). The plasma membrane Ca2+ ATPase of animal cells: structure, function and regulation. *Arch Biochem Biophys*, Vol.476, No.1, (August 2008), pp. 65–74

do Céu Monteiro, M., Sansonetty, F., Gonçalves, M.J., O'Connor, J.E.. (1999). Flow cytometric kinetic assay of calcium mobilization in whole blood platelets using Fluo-3 and CD41. *Cytometry*, Vol.35, No.4, (April 1999), pp. 302-310

Dolmetsch, R.E., Xu, K., Lewis, R.S. (1998). Calcium oscillations increase the efficiency and specificity of gene expression. *Nature*, Vol.392, No.6679, (April 1998), pp. 933–936

Duchen, M.R. (2000). Mitochondria and calcium: from cell signalling to cell death. *J Physiol*, Vol.529, Pt.1, (November 2000), pp. 57–68

Fanger, C.M., Neben, A.L., Cahalan, M.D. (2000). Differential Ca2+ influx, KCa channel activity, and Ca2+ clearance distinguish Th1 and Th2 lymphocytes. *J Immunol*, Vol.164, No.3, (February 2000), pp. 1153–1160

Feske, S. (2007). Calcium signalling in lymphocyte activation and disease. *Nat Rev Immunol*, Vol.7, No.9, (September 2007), pp. 690–702

García Vela, J.A., Delgado, I., Bornstein, R., Alvarez, B., Auray, M.C., Martin, I., Oña F., Gilsanz F. (2000). Comparative intracellular cytokine production by in vitro stimulated T lymphocytes from human umbilical cord blood (HUCB) and adult peripheral blood (APB). *Anal Cell Pathol*, Vol.20, No.2-3, (2000), pp. 93-98

Hawkins, D.M. (2004). The Problem of Overfitting. *J Chem Inf Comput Sci*, Vol.44, No.1 (January 2004), pp 1–12

Jakubczak, B., Wasik, M., Popko, K., Demkow, U. (2006). Kinetics of calcium ion concentration accompanying signal transduction in neutrophils from children with increased susceptibility to infections. *J Physiol Pharmacol*, Vol.57, No.4, (September 2006), pp. 131-137

Johnson, D.I. (2001). Cellular function probes. *Current Protocols in Cytometry*, Chapter4, Unit4.4, (May 2001).

June, C.H., Ledbetter, J.A., Rabinovitch, P.S., Martin, P.J., Beatty, P.G., Hansen, J.A. (1986). Distinct patterns of transmembrane calcium flux and intracellular calcium mobilization after differentiation antigen cluster 2 (E rosette receptor) or 3 (T3) stimulation of human lymphocytes. *J Clin Invest*, Vol.77, No.4, (April 1986), pp. 1224-1232

June, C.H., Rabinovitch, P.S. (1990). Flow cytometric measurement of intracellular ionized calcium in single cells with indo-1 and fluo-3. *Methods Cell Biol*, Vol.33, Chapter5, (1990), pp.37-58.

Kaposi, A.S., Veress, G., Vásárhelyi, B., Macardle, P., Bailey, S., Tulassay, T., Treszl, A. (2008). Cytometry-acquired calcium-flux data analysis in activated lymphocytes. *Cytometry A*, Vol.73, No.3, (March 2008), pp. 246-253

Koenker, R., Hallock, K.F. (2001). Quantile Regression. *Journal of Economic Perspectives*, Vol.15, No.4 (Fall 2001), pp. 143-156

Lewis, RS. (2001). Calcium signaling mechanisms in T lymphocytes. *Annu Rev Immunol*, Vol.19, (April 2001), pp. 497-521

Lund-Johansen, F, Olweus, J. (1992). Signal transduction in monocytes and granulocytes measured by multiparameter flow cytometry. *Cytometry*, Vol.13, No.7, (September 1992), pp. 693-702

Mészáros, G., Szalay, B., Toldi, G., Kaposi, A., Vásárhelyi, B., Treszl, A. (2011). Kinetic measurements using flow cytometry: new methods for monitoring intracellular processes. *Assay Drug Dev Technol*, [Epub ahead of print], (September 2011).

Motulsky, H.J., Ransnas, L.A. (1987). Fitting curves to data using nonlinear regression: a practical and nonmathematical review. *FASEB J*, Vol.1, No.5, (November 1987), pp. 365-374

Motulsky, H., Christopoulos, A. (2004). Fitting models to biological data using linear and nonlinear regression: a practical guide to curve fitting. Oxford University Press, USA

Nelder, J.A., Mead, R. (1965). A Simplex Method for Function Minimization. *Computer Journal*, Vol.7, No.4, (January 1965), pp. 308-313

Norgauer, J., Dobos, G., Kownatzki, E., Dahinden, C., Burger, R., Kupper, R., Gierschik, P. (1993). Complement fragment C3a stimulates Ca2+ influx in neutrophils via a pertussis-toxin-sensitive G protein. *Eur J Biochem*, Vol.217, No.1, (October 1993), pp. 289-94.

Omann, G.M., Harter, J.M. (1991). Pertussis toxin effects on chemoattractant-induced response heterogeneity in human PMNs utilizing Fluo-3 and flow cytometry. *Cytometry*, Vol.12, No.3, (March 1991), pp. 252-259

Picard R.R., Cook, R.D. (1984). Cross-Validation of Regression Models. *Journal of the American Statistical Association*, Vol.79, No.387 (September 1984), pp. 575-583

Politi, A., Gaspers, L.D., Thomas, A.P., Höfer, T. (2006). Models of IP3 and Ca2+ oscillations: frequency encoding and identification of underlying feedbacks. *Biophys J*, Vol.90, No.9, (May 2006), pp. 3120-3133

R Development Core Team. (2006). R: A Language and Environment for Statistical Computing. Vienna, Austria: R Foundation for Statistical Computing. ISBN 3-900051-07-0

Rein, D.T., Schondorf, T., Gohring, U.J., Kurbacher, C.M., Pinto, I., Breidenbach, M., Mallmann, P., Kolhagen, H., Engel, H. (2002). Cytokine expression in peripheral blood lymphocytes indicates a switch to T(HELPER) cells in patients with preeclampsia. *J Reprod Immunol*, Vol.54, No.1-2, (March 2002), pp. 133-142

Rijkers, G.T., Griffioen, A.W. (1993). Changes in free cytoplasmic magnesium following activation of human lymphocytes. *Biochem J*, Vol.289, No.2, (January 1993), pp. 373-377

Roederer, M., Treister, A., Moore, W., Herzenberg, L.A. (2001). Probability binning comparison: a metric for quantitating univariate distribution differences. *Cytometry*, Vol.45, No.1, (September 2001), pp. 37-46

Roederer, M. (2002). Compensation in flow cytometry. *Current Protocols in Cytometry*, Chapter 1, Unit 1.14, (December 2002).

Saito, S., Umekage, H., Sakamoto, Y., Sakai, M., Tanebe, K., Sasaki, Y., Morikawa, H. Increased T-helper-1-type immunity and decreased T-helper-2-type immunity in patients with preeclampsia. *Am J Reprod Immunol*, Vol.41, No.5, (May 1999), pp. 297-306

Saito, S., Shiozaki, A., Nakashima, A., Sakai, M., Sasaki, Y. (2007). The role of the immune system in preeclampsia. Mol. Aspects Med., Vol.28, No.2, (April 2007), pp. 192-209

Schepers, E., Glorieux, G., Dhondt, A., Leybaert, L., Vanholder, R. (2009). Flow cytometric calcium flux assay: evaluation of cytoplasmic calcium kinetics in whole blood leukocytes. *J Immunol Methods*, Vol.348, No.1-2, (August 2009), pp. 74-82

Stoddart, M.J. (2011). Cell viability assays: introduction. *Methods Mol Biol*, Vol.740, Mammalian Cell Viability, (2011), pp.1-6.

Stork, B., Neumann, K., Goldbeck, I., Alers, S., Kähne, T., Naumann, M., Engelke, M., Wienands, J. (2007). Subcellular localization of Grb2 by the adaptor protein Dok-3 restricts the intensity of Ca2+ signaling in B cells. *EMBO J*, Vol.26, No.4, (February 2007), pp. 1140-1149

Szalay, B., Mészáros, G., Cseh, A., Acs, L., Deák, M., Kovács, L., Vásárhelyi, B., Balog, A. (2012). Adaptive Immunity in Ankylosing Spondylitis: Phenotype and Functional Alterations of T-Cells before and during Infliximab Therapy. *Clin Dev Immunol*, Vol.2012, (Epub September 2011), 808724

Tang, Y., Stephenson, J.L., Othmer, H.G. (1996). Simplification and analysis of models of calcium dynamics based on IP3-sensitive calcium channel kinetics. *Biophys J*. Vol.70, No.1, (January 1996), pp. 246-263

Toldi, G., Stenczer, B., Treszl, A., Kollar, S., Molvarec, A., Tulassay, T., Rigo, J.Jr, Vasarhelyi, B. (2010a). Lymphocyte calcium influx characteristics and their modulation by Kv1.3 and IKCa1 channel inhibitors in healthy pregnancy and preeclampsia. *Am J Reprod Immunol*. Vol.65, No.2, (February 2011), pp. 154-163

Toldi, G., Treszl, A., Pongor, V., Gyarmati, B., Tulassay, T., Vasarhelyi, B. (2010b). T-lymphocyte calcium influx characteristics and their modulation by Kv1.3 and IKCa1 channel inhibitors in the neonate. *Int Immunol*, Vol.22, No.9, (September 2010), pp. 769-774

Toldi, G., Vasarhelyi, B., Kaposi, A.S., Meszaros, G., Panczel, P., Hosszufalusi, N., Tulassay, T., Treszl, A. (2010c). Lymphocyte activation in type 1 diabetes mellitus: the increased significance of Kv1.3 potassium channels. Immunol Lett. Vol.133, No.1, (September 2010), pp. 35-41

Toldi, G., Kaposi, A., Zsembery, Á., Treszl, A., Tulassay, T., Vásárhelyi, B. (2011a). Human Th1 and Th2 lymphocytes are distinguished by calcium flux regulation during the first ten minutes of lymphocyte activation. *Immunobiology*, [Epub ahead of print], (August 2011)

Toldi, G., Folyovich, A., Simon, Z., Zsiga, K., Kaposi, A., Mészáros, G., Tulassay, T., Vasarhelyi, B. (2011b). Lymphocyte calcium influx kinetics in multiple sclerosis treated without or with interferon beta. *J Neuroimmunol*, Vol.237, No.1-2, (August 2011), pp. 80-86

Wulff, H., Calabresi, P.A., Allie, R., Yun, S., Pennington, M., Beeton, C., Chandy, K.G. (2003). The voltage-gated Kv1.3 K+channel in effector memory T cells as new target for MS. *J Clin Invest*. Vol.111, No.11, (June 2003), pp. 1703–1713

Yoon, J.W., Jun, H.S. (2001). Cellular and molecular pathogenic mechanisms of insulin-dependent diabetes mellitus. *Ann N Y Acad Sci*, Vol.928, (April 2001), pp. 200–211

16

Analysis of Cellular Signaling Events by Flow Cytometry

Jacques A. Nunès, Guylène Firaguay and Emilie Coppin
Institut National de la Santé et de la Recherche Médicale, Unité 1068,
Centre de Recherche en Cancérologie de Marseille, Institut Paoli-Calmettes,
Aix-Marseille Univ., Marseille,
France

1. Introduction

All the cells are engaged on a cell communication by sending and receiving signals. Cells having the correct receptors on their surfaces will encode the plasma membrane signal recognition to intracellular signals corresponding to cellular signaling events. This process corresponds to a huge intracellular network of protein-protein or lipid-protein interactions. To avoid to be lost in this kind of maze, some general signaling pathways are most of the time present in many cell systems such as MAP kinases or PI-3 kinases pathways. These signaling pathways induce some protein phosphorylation events that can be identified by specific antibodies directed against these phosphosites (anti-phospho antibodies). Thus, these crossroads can be determined by using antibodies. A widely used method to identify these signaling events is the Western blotting or protein immunoblotting from cell extracts. However, several research groups are now developing new analytical techniques based also on the use of anti-phospho antibodies, but allowing them to detect signaling events at the single cell level. These experimental approaches are using the principles of the flow cytometry (FCM). Phosphoflow technology will provide rapid, quantitative and also multi-parameter analyses on single cells.

2. Cell signaling

In biology, cell signaling corresponds to the mechanisms of communication at the cellular level (Gomperts et al., 2009). The molecules involved in these exchanges provide three functions: transport of information via chemical signals, decoding the messages carried by these signals through receptors (intercellular communication itself), and finally transfer the orders contained in these messages to the intracellular machinery (intracellular communication).

Cellular communication may be endocrine (exchange of information remotely using hormones), paracrine (local exchanges between adjacent cells, such as neurotransmission) or autocrine (messages sent and received by the same cell to self-regulate). The molecules that carry information (hormones, mediators) can be compared with "keys" (called ligands) adapted to the "locks" represented by the receivers. In this metaphor, the intracellular signaling is comparable to a "bolt" activated by movement of the key in the lock. Despite their diversity, the signaling mechanisms are guided by common characteristics.

2.1 General laws involved in cell signaling

All the reactions based on a system [key-lock] and downstream events follow the law of mass action where molecules are engaged each other and then disengaged. These states are corresponding respectively to the reactions of association or dissociation. The affinity of one molecule for another one is defined by the ratio between association and dissociation constants. Thus, the affinity is high when the time of association is longer than the time of dissociation. These parameters are dependent of the conformational changes of the molecules. These alterations open some sites at the surface of the molecule that can be accessible, for instance, to enzymes such as the protein kinases. Thus, these opened sites become substrates for the kinases and a phosphate ion (PO_4^{3-}) is transferred. Thus, cell signaling is in part a large equilibrium between phosphorylation and dephosphorylation states for proteins and but also lipids. Edmond H. Fischer and Edwin G. Krebs were able to show that reversible protein phosphorylation affects the structure, shape, function and activity of proteins that are responsible for the regulation of nearly all aspects of cellular life (Krebs & Fischer, 1989). Fischer and Krebs received the Nobel Prize in Physiology or Medicine in 1992 for the discovery of reversible protein phosphorylation and its importance as a biological regulatory mechanism.

2.2 Intercellular signaling

Intercellular signaling is governed by ligand-receptor interactions. The families of ligands or signals often differ only by tiny molecular substitutions. The addition of a radical hydroxyl (-OH) or methyl (-CH3) is sufficient to differentiate the action of soluble mediators such as dopamine, norepinephrine and epinephrine. In the family of morphine (short sequences of amino acids called peptides and acting in a manner similar to morphine, especially by intervening in the modulation of pain), the substitution of one amino acid can alter the recognition by its ligand receiver called receptor. The study of immunological recognition provides many opportunities to demonstrate that the replacement of a few amino acids in a protein could markedly change binding properties. The antigen receptors such as the T-cell receptors (TCRs) adjust to different agonist, partial agonist and antagonist peptides by subtle conformational changes in their complementarity-determining regions (CDRs), in induced-fit mechanisms of antibody/antigen recognition (Rudolph & Wilson, 2002). This knowledge has been largely improved by high resolution of ligand-receptor co-crystal structures. Thus, various receptors recognize their ligands with different affinities. These differences are important because they help to refine considerably the transmission of information: each peptide acts optimally on its specific receptor, but is also able to affect other receptor family with a lower affinity. This heterogeneity of recognition generates an affinity gradient into the ligand-receptor interactions that in part, will explain selectivity in the intracellular encoding of the signals delivered by the receptors.

2.3 Intracellular signaling

The receptors are made up of successive sequences with the recognition motif of ligand (exposed to the outside of the cell), a transmembrane segment that provides the binding of the receptor to the plasma membrane, and finally a sequence on intracellular enzyme activity. They fall into three groups that differ in the mode of intracellular as a result of the binding of the signal. In the simplest family (insulin receptor, for example), both ends of the same molecule provide signal reception and the enzyme activation. In the two other groups, receptor and enzyme activation functions are not contained in the same protein sequence such as i) a receptor directly associated with an independent cytoplasmic enzyme (for example, the CD4 molecule associated with the Src protein tyrosine kinase family member, Lck), ii) or a receptor linked to an independent cytoplasmic enzyme by a third partner named an adaptor protein (for example, the G protein-coupled receptor (GPCR) β adrenergic receptor coupled to the adenylate cyclase via heterotrimeric G proteins).

Activation of the receptor is itself relayed by families of specialized molecules that provide signal transduction, that is to say their relays, the membrane to all intracellular processes (Fig. 1). Some of them, such as JAK (activating protein kinases called Janus, by reference to the Latin god of thresholds and crossings, to the extent that they "open" signaling downstream of receptors) (Li et al., 2008) or MAPK (mitogen-activated protein kinases) (Mendoza et al., 2011), integrate information from different receptors expressed at the cell membrane. The cell can respond appropriately, for example by phosphorylating its own receptors and thereby adjusting at all times the sensitivity of the cell to signals from its environment (the process of sensitization and desensitization). Several other main signaling pathways have been described such as the phosphatidylinositol 3-kinase-mammalian target of rapamycin (PI3K-mTOR) pathway. The signaling pathways are the major routes to control, for instance, cell differentiation, proliferation in response to extracellular stimuli. Moreover, the major pathways are playing as a concert where these pathways have common regulators and might intersect each other to co-regulate downstream events (Mendoza et al., 2011).

Figure 1 illustrates a simplest view of the major signaling pathways as vertical boxes where always lipid or protein kinase activities are involved. Upon extracellular signals induced by ligand-receptor interactions, these different boxes are turned-on by some adaptor molecules that are connecting receptors to the first steps of these signaling cascades.

Several websites are dedicated to describe these signaling pathways (for example, the Database of Cell Signaling from Science Signaling, a journal published by the American Association for the Advancement of Science (http://stke.sciencemag.org/) or the UCSD Signaling Gateway, a comprehensive resource in signal transduction (http://www.signaling-gateway.org/)). Some nuclear factor involved in gene transcription can be involved very rapidly in these signaling cascades and located transiently at the inner face of the plasma membrane such as the Nuclear Factor of kappa light chain gene enhancer in B cells (NFκB) or the Signal Transducers and Activators of Transcription (STATs). As already mentioned (Mendoza et al., 2011), the signaling pathways are inter-connected. For instance, the phosphoinositide-specific phospholipase C (PI-PLC) clives the phosphatidylinositol-4,5-bisphosphate to generate inositol-1,4,5-trisphosphate (IP3, involved in ionized Ca^{2+}) and diacylglycerol (DAG). This increase of DAG will participate to i) the activation of some serine/threonine protein kinase C (PKC) isoforms that are able to activate NFκB signaling by phosphorylating a repressor of these transcription factors (first box in Figure 1) and ii) the activation of the RAS / Extracellular signal-regulated kinases 1 & 2 (ERK-1/2) pathway via the involvement of a DAG-dependent RAS guanyl releasing protein (RasGRP) (third box in Figure 1).

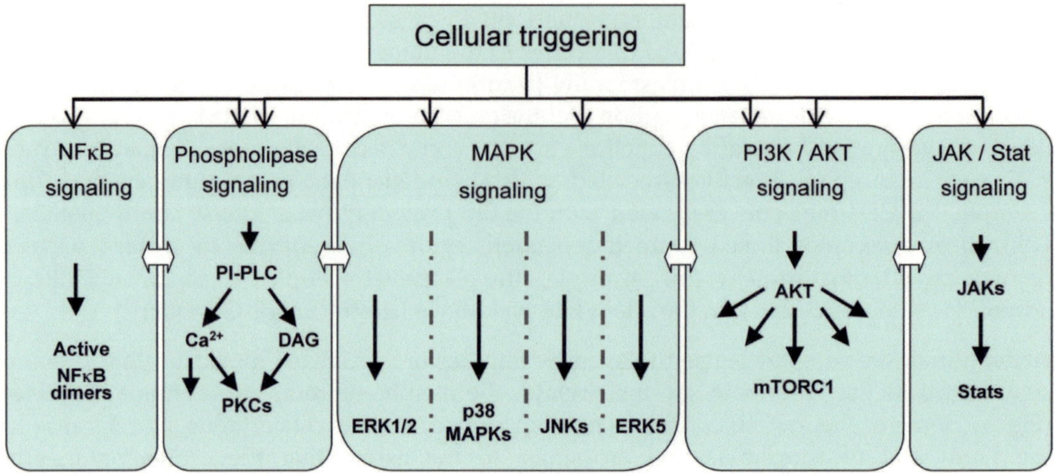

Fig. 1. Some major intracellular signaling pathways activated under an exogenous triggering are here illustrated such as Nuclear Factor of kappa light chain gene enhancer in B cells (NFκB), phosphoinositide-specific phospholipase C (PI-PLC), mitogen-activated protein kinases (MAPK), phosphatidylinositol 3-kinase (PI3K)/Akt and Janus kinase (JAK)/ Signal Transducers and Activators of Transcription (STATs). These pathways are regulated by phosphorylation steps and inter-connected (see text). These signaling cascades are activating transcription factors involved in gene expression

Thus, the intracellular signaling acts as a primary target for control of the expression of specific genes in the cell based on varying combinations of signals it receives. The intracellular signaling mechanisms involved in initiating motor responses (in muscle) or secretory (in the exocrine glands or the brain), but their main role is to control gene expression. They are thus responsible for the process of cell differentiation and a referral to a cell cycle proliferation or, conversely, apoptosis (programmed cell death, which led to the elimination of atypical cells); hence their importance in the process of tumor formation. The majority of cancers results from a dysfunction of intracellular signaling molecules, which in turn causes an imbalance between uncontrolled proliferation and loss of the ability of tumor cells to be self-destructed by apoptosis.

3. Methods for the detection of signaling events

There are several methods involving chemistry, biochemistry, microscopy and physics that are used to detect and analyze intracellular signals. Here, we briefly describe a general method used by who is interested on signal transduction as the Western blot and then we develop the experimental approaches using flow cytometers.

3.1 Western blot (also called protein immunoblot): An universal method for the detection of signaling events

The method is based on the use of electrophoresis to transfer proteins from a gel to a membrane (Towbin et al., 1979). The aim of SDS-PAGE (PolyAcrylamide Gel Electrophoresis) is to separate proteins according to their size, and no other physical feature. Western blots allow investigators to determine the molecular weight of a protein and to measure relative amounts of the protein present in different samples. Prior to SDS-PAGE, the proteins should be extracted from isolated cells or tissues. The proteins are then transferred to a membrane (for example, nitrocellulose), where they are probed using specific antibodies.

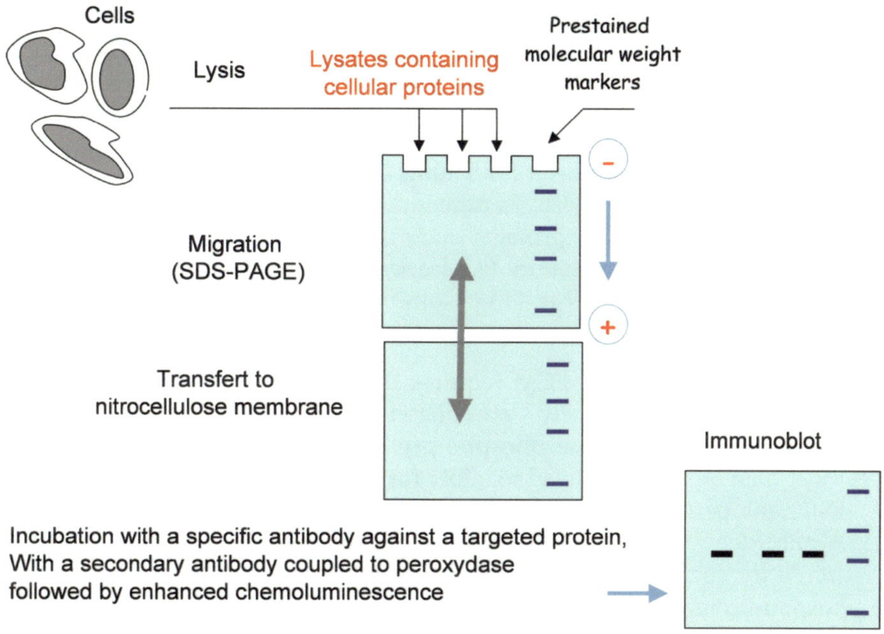

Fig. 2. Western blot method needs to extract the proteins from a reasonable number of cells (but not from a single cell)

The signaling events are governed by phosphorylation/dephosphorylation steps. When a protein is phosphorylated, its apparent molecular weight will be higher (for instance, the molecular weight of the protein Ser/Thr kinase ERK-2 will shift from 42 to 44 kDa upon phosphorylation). The ERK-2 molecular weight mobility shift detected by Western blot correlates with an increase of ERK-2 Ser/Thr kinase activity detected by *in vitro* kinase assays (Nunès et al., 1994). However, the detection of kinase activity based on slower mobility of activated kinases upon SDS-PAGE is not always validated because it does always correlate with the real enzymatic activity (Yao et al, 2000). Thus, some specific antibodies have been developed against the phosphorylated peptide sequences of activated kinases (Yung et al., 1997). Now, many anti-phosphosite antibodies against many phosphorylated proteins such as protein kinases or protein kinase substrates are commercially available. Furthermore, the quality of these antibodies employed is of great importance for the success of the detection of a specific phosphorylation step. The validation of these antibodies will be discussed later on in the text.

The conventional Western blot results are semi-quantitative and require a large number of cells (between 10^2 to 10^6 cells per point). New approaches using similar immuno-detection as Western blot, have been developed to reduce the number of cells per point. High-resolution capillary isoelectric focusing (IEF) allows isoforms and individual phosphorylated forms to be resolved using around 25 cells per point (O'Neill et al., 2006). This capillary-based nano-immunoassay is able evaluate the different ratio of unphosphorylated to mono or bi-phosphorylated ERK1/2 using anti-ERK1/2 antibodies as a probe. This system is now commercialized as the NanoPro 1000 system (ProteinSimple, Santa Clara, CA, USA). Despite all efforts in this field of the Western blot, it is virtually impossible to reach the detection of signaling events at the single cell level. By definition, the flow cytometry is able to detect events at the single cell level using specific antibodies, which is essential in a heterogeneous cell population.

3.2 Phosphoflow analysis

Flow cytometry (FCM) has been used for a long time to detect specific markers at the cell surface using antibodies labeled with fluorescent dyes. Then, similar approaches have been performed to detect intracellular proteins such as cytokine production in hematopoietic cells. Intracellular cytokine detection by FCM opens the door to analyze other intracellular proteins such as phosphorylated signaling molecules (Chow et al., 2001; Krutzik & Nolan, 2003).

Detection of phospho-proteins by FCM requires that the protein is stable and accessible to the antibody. Cells are usually stimulated and fixed with formaldehyde or paraformaldehyde to cross-link the phospho-proteins and stabilize them for analysis. The fixed cells must then be permeabilized to allow for entry of phospho-specific antibodies into the cells. Different permeabilization techniques are often useful for various subcellular locations. A mild detergent will allow for detection of cytoplasmic proteins, while alcohol may be required for antibody access to nuclear proteins. Alcohol permeabilization may also enhance phospho-protein detection using peptide specific antibodies due to the denaturing property of alcohol (Krutzik et al., 2004). This approach has been improved to visualize many parameters at the single cell level (multidimensional molecular profiles of signaling) to define cell network phenotypes in many cell types (Irish et al., 2004; Irish et al., 2006).

The consideration of signaling networks as dynamic systems is crucial for a full understanding, and this requires methods applicable to analyze individual living cells (Johnson & Hunter, 2005). A protocol has been developed to determine by FCM in a dynamic system and in single-cell, the phospho-protein activation status (Firaguay & Nunès, 2009). For this approach, a pleitropic activator of the signaling pathway such as pervanadate, has been used. In this protocol, the phospho-protein staining corresponds to a sandwich labelling to increase the brightness (for instance, a rabbit monoclonal antibody against anti-phosphoSer473 AKT followed by biotinylated anti-rabbit immunoglobulins (Ig) and then streptavidin conjuguated with the Phycoerythrin (PE).

All the specific antibodies used for phosphoflow analysis should be well optimized for this technology. For instance, it will be easier to use monoclonal antibodies than polyclonal antibodies. These antibodies should be validated in Western blot by showing that they are able to detect the targeted phospho-protein at the right molecular weight (without detecting other protein, meaning other bands on the immunoblot). Then for a proper validation in FCM, the phospho-protein staining should be sensitive to the cell treatment with some specific inhibitors of signaling pathways (for anti-phosphoSer473 AKT staining in activated cells should be decreased by a cell treatment with a PI3K inhibitor). Finally, the phospho-protein staining should be decreased or abolished in cells derived from mice invalidated for the gene encoding the targeted protein (KO mice) or in cellular models using a RNA interference.

Using validated anti-phospho-protein antibodies, this phosphoflow analysis is able to define signaling events upon receptor triggering (multi intracellular phospho-protein staining) at the single cell level (multi extracellular surface marker staining). This purpose is illustrated in Figure 3.

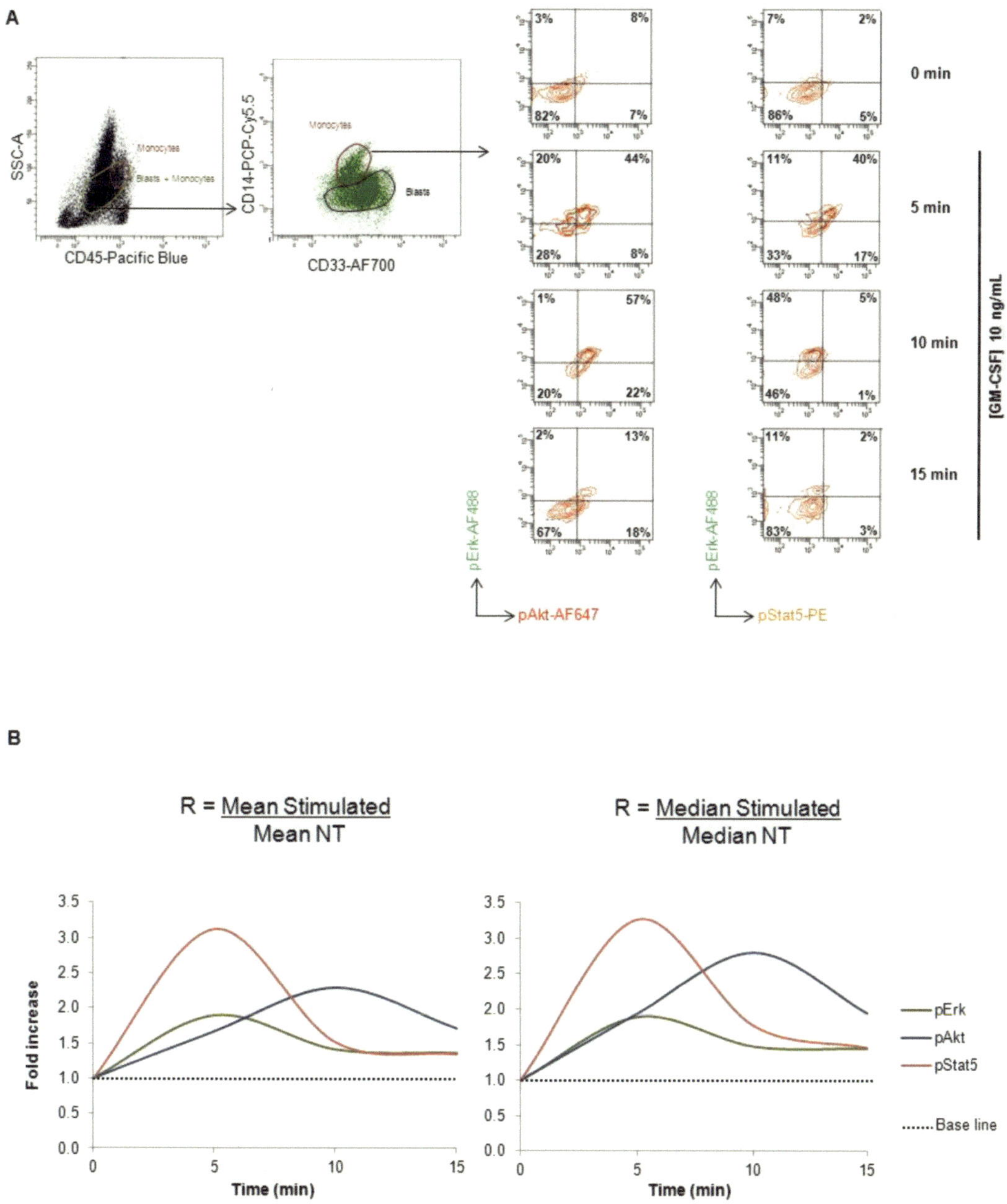

c

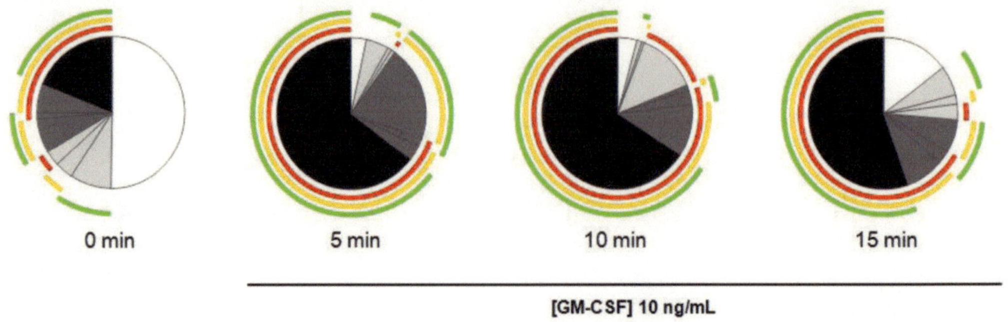

- pAkt
- pErk
- pStat5

pAkt	-	-	-	+	-	+	+	+
pErk	-	-	+	-	+	-	+	+
pStat5	-	+	-	-	+	+	-	+

Fig. 3. Peripheral blood mononuclear cells (PBMC) from bone marrow sample were obtained by Ficoll (AbCyss LymphoPrep, #1114545) gradient (centrifugation at 2500 rpm for 20 min without brake) followed by two washes (centrifugation at 900 rpm for 15 min) in RPMI-1640 medium (Gibco, #21875) added to 2% Fetal Calf Serum (FCS) (Eurobio, #CVFSV F00-01). Cells number was determined by Trypan blue staining. Whole PBMCs were maintained for 16 hrs in RPMI 2% FCS at 2.10^5 cells/mL

For GM-CSF stimulation, 5.10^5 cells were pre incubated 1 min at 37°C, and incubated with 10 ng/mL human GM-CSF (Peprotech # 300-03) in RPMI-1640-2% FCS at 37°C for 5, 10 and 15 min. Cells were fixed by 1,6% paraformaldehyde (PFA) (Sigma Aldrich, # 158127) at room temperature for 10 min. Cells were washed (centrifugation at 1800 rpm for 5 min) twice with phosphate-buffered saline (PBS) (Life Technologies, #70013065). Cells were stained 30 min at 4°C for extracellular lineage markers: CD45 - Pacific Blue (BioLegend, #304029), CD14 - PerCP-Cy5.5 (BD Pharmingen, #550787) and CD33 - AlexaFluor 700 (BD Pharmingen, #561160). After washes in FCM buffer (PBS, 2%, 1mM EDTA) viability was evaluated by Live/Dead Staining (Invitrogen, LIVE/DEAD Fixable Aqua Dead Cell Stain, #L34957) for 15 min at 4°C. Then for intracellular staining, cells were washed twice in FCM buffer and were permeabilized and fixed with Cytofix/Cytoperm (BD Biosciences, #554722) for 10 min at 37°C followed by washes in Perm/Wash buffer (BD Biosciences 10X Perm/Wash Buffer, #554723). Intracellular staining for phosphoflow analysis was performed as previously described (Firaguay & Nunès, 2009). Cells were incubated 30 min at 4°C by adding: i) directly coupled antibodies: anti-phospho-Akt S473 Alexa Fluor 647 (Beckman Coulter, #A88915), anti-phospho-ERK-1/2 T202/Y204 Alexa Fluor 488 (Beckman Coulter, #A88928) and ii) Uncoupled antibodies: anti-phospho-STAT5 (Cell Signaling Technology, #9314). Cells were wash twice in Perm/Wash buffer (BD Biosciences), incubated 20 min at 4°C with biotinylated secondary antibodies (Jackson ImmunoResearch product, Beckman

Coulter, Biotin-SP-AffiniPure F(ab')2 Frag Donkey AntiRabbit IgG (H+L), #711-066-152). After two washes, cells were incubated 15 min at 4°C with Streptavidin conjugated with phycoerythrin (Streptavidin-PE) (Beckman Coulter, #IM3325). Cells were washed twice, re-suspended in PBS and processed on a LSR II SORP 4 lasers flow cytometer (BD Becton Dickinson). Data were collected and analyzed using DIVA software (BD Biosciences) and FlowJo software (Tree Star).

Panel A: Monocyte gating strategy. Monocytes were gated on i) intermediate Side scatter cells and CD45 positive cells and then ii) on both CD14 and CD33 positive cells. Then phospho-Erk, phospho-Akt and phospho-Stat5 were visualized on the monocyte population in resting condition and under 10 ng/mL of human GM-CSF stimulation for different times (5, 10 and 15 min). For this illustration, dot plots were analyzed using DIVA software (BD Biosciences).

Panel B: AKT, ERK1/2 and Stat5 phosphorylation kinetics in monocytes under GM-CSF stimulation. Kinetics Ratio (stimulated / non treated NT) Mean (left) and Median (right) of fluorescence in response to 10 ng/mL human GM-CSF stimulation. As represented, kinetics are similar on both Mean and Median Fluorescence intensity parameters: phospho-Stat5 and phospho-ERK1/2 increase are early: at 5 min of stimulation and they decreased to a constant "sub-basal" level at 10 min, whereas phospho-AKT is increased later: at 10 min of stimulation and decreased at 15 min. For this representation statistical data were extracted using FlowJo software (Tree Star).

Panel C: Statistical representation of phospho-AKT, ERK1/2 and Stat5 negative and positive monocytes populations under GM-CSF stimulation. Color gradation represents percentages of monocytes negative for phospho-ERK1/2, phospho-AKT and phospho-Stat5 (in white), positive for one and two of these parameters (respectively in light and dark grey) and positive for all of them (in black). Colored curves surrounding circles shows positive phospho-proteins represented in each portion of the circle: phospho-ERK1/2, phospho-AKT and phospho-Stat5 are respectively in yellow, red and green. As represented, phopho-Stat5 alone and associated to phospho-ERK alone or with phospho-AKT is the major signaling response of monocytes to GM-CSF stimulation, in particular at 5 min. Phospho-AKT response to stimulation appears to be later since at 10 min the percentage of phospho-AKT positive monocytes is distinctly increased, in particular for proportion only phospho-AKT positive cells at this time of stimulation. For this representation, statistical data were extracted using FlowJo software (Tree Star) and represented with SPICE v5.2 software (Apple Mac U.C. Berkeley, CA, USA).

4. Concluding remarks and recent investigations in phosphoflow analysis

As illustrated by data shown in Figure 3, the phosphoflow analysis permits to use one or multiple signal transduction markers in association with cell surface markers to dissect complex biological processes in heterogeneous populations. This technique is quite rapid, quantitative and a major point: working at the single cell level. However, the investigators must be careful with the buffers used for cell fixation and permeabilization that could affect the binding of the antibodies to the phosphosites (Krutzik et al., 2004). Another major point is a perfect validation of the antibodies used for phosphoflow analysis (see text, paragraph 3.2). In some case, the brightness of a signaling marker will be enhanced by using a sandwich labeling method (Firaguay & Nunès, 2009).

The ability to analyze multiple single-cell parameters is critical for understanding cellular heterogeneity. In the context of oncology, cancer cells harboring a hyperactivation of signaling pathways such PI3K/AKT, Ras/ERK or JAK/Stats pathways can be treated with specific inhibitors of these pathways (Vivanco & Sawyers, 2002; Irish et al., 2006). However, such inhibitors will target the cancer cells but can also affect other cell types that will be involved in the tumor environment (Le Tourneau et al., 2008). Thus, these chemotherapy protocols could affect the homeostasis of the normal cell compartment that could be evaluated by analyzing multiple single-cell parameters. This balance is illustrated by a picture into the Figure 4 (see below).

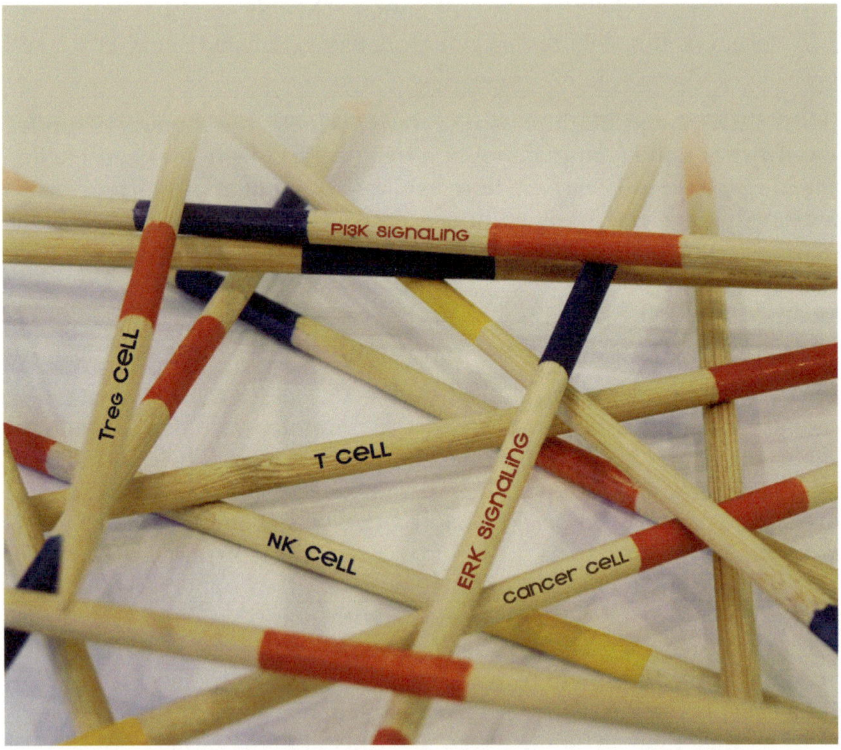

Fig. 4. By targeting Ras/ERK or PI3K/AKT pathways in cancer cells, these treatments could affect for instance immune cells such as Natural Killer (NK) cells or different T cell subsets such as regulatory T cells (Tregs). This cell homeostasis will be affected as illustrated by this picture as a Mikado game where sticks could be a signaling parameter or a cell type. The artwork of this picture has been performed by the STUDIO HULKETTE (*http://www.hulkette.com*)

To analyze a large number of parameters at the single cell level in a heterogeneous population, new apparatus has been developed by Scott Tanner's group, the single-cell mass cytometer (Bandura et al., 2009). In this study, single cell 20 antigen expression assay was performed on cell lines and leukemia patient samples immuno-labeled with lanthanide-tagged antibodies. Recent studies from Gary Nolan's group push this technology to analyze simultaneously 34 cellular parameters, where they compare the consequences of different drug treatments on the immune cells and hematopoiesis (Bendall et al., 2011). The beauty of these new technologies in the field of cell signaling opens a new area on the signal monitoring of treatments in many diseases such as cancers, infectious or autoimmune diseases. However, a brake to the development of these approaches will be the huge number of data that will be generated and how to analyze these data. Some clues of computational approaches were already built such as spanning-tree progression analysis of density-normalized events (SPADE) (Qiu et al., 2011).

Phosphoflow analysis will become an universal technology to investigate cell signaling events at the single cell level. By using validated antibodies for FCM and right protocols of fixation/permeabilization, the phosphoflow analysis will be a standard method in many labs across the world to analyze few parameters at the same time. Moreover, the new technologies are already under the market to analyze more than 30 parameters at the same time.

5. Acknowledgements

We would like to thank Dr. Françoise Gondois-Rey and Dr. Christine Arnoulet for their help on the FCM settings for cell surface markers and le Studio Hulkette for the artwork. This work was supported by grants from Institut National de la Santé et de la Recherche Médicale and the Institut National du Cancer (# PL-06026 and # INCa/DHOS 2009) (to J.A. Nunès). J.A. Nunès is a recipient of a Contrat d'Interface Clinique with the Department of Hematology (Institut Paoli Calmettes). G. Firaguay was supported by fellowships from the Institut National du Cancer. E. Coppin is supported by a fellowship from the Région Provence Alpes Côte d'Azur (PACA) - Innate Pharma.

6. References

Bandura, D.R., Baranov, V.I., Ornatsky, O.I., Antonov, A., Kinach, R., Lou, X., Pavlov, S., Vorobiev, S., Dick, J.E., & Tanner, S.D. (2009). Mass cytometry: technique for real time single cell multitarget immunoassay based on inductively coupled plasma time-of-flight mass spectrometry. *Anal Chem*, 81, pp. 6813-6822, ISSN 1520-6882.

Bendall, S.C., Simonds, E.F., Qiu, P., Amir el, A.D., Krutzik, P.O., Finck, R., Bruggner, R.V., Melamed, R., Trejo, A., Ornatsky, O.I., Balderas, R.S., Plevritis, S.K., Sachs, K., Pe'er, D., Tanner, S.D., & Nolan, G.P. (2011). Single-cell mass cytometry of differential immune and drug responses across a human hematopoietic continuum. *Science*, 332, pp. 687-696, ISSN 1095-9203.

Chow, S., Patel, H., & Hedley, D.W. (2001). Measurement of MAP kinase activation by flow cytometry using phospho-specific antibodies to MEK and ERK: potential for pharmacodynamic monitoring of signal transduction inhibitors. *Cytometry*, 46, pp. 72-78, ISSN 0196-4763.

Firaguay, G., & and Nunes, J.A. (2009). Analysis of signaling events by dynamic phosphoflow cytometry. *Sci Signal*, 2, pl3, ISSN 1937-9145.

Gomperts B.D., Kramer I.M., Tatham P.E.R. (Ed(s).). 2009. *Signal Transduction, 2nd Edition*, Academic Press, ISBN: 978-0-12-369441-6, Maryland Heights, MO, USA.

Irish, J.M., Hovland, R., Krutzik, P.O., Perez, O.D., Bruserud, O., Gjertsen, B.T., & Nolan, G.P. (2004). Single cell profiling of potentiated phospho-protein networks in cancer cells. *Cell*, 118, pp. 217-228, ISSN 0092-8674.

Irish, J.M., Kotecha, N., & Nolan, G.P. (2006). Mapping normal and cancer cell signalling networks: towards single-cell proteomics. *Nat Rev Cancer*, 6, pp. 146-155, ISSN 1474-175X.

Johnson, S.A., & Hunter, T. (2005). Kinomics: methods for deciphering the kinome. Nat Methods 2, 17-25, ISSN 1548-7091.

Krebs, E.G., & Fischer, E.H. (1989). The phosphorylase b to a converting enzyme of rabbit skeletal muscle. 1956. *Biochim Biophys Acta*, 1000, pp. 302-309, ISSN 0006-3002.

Krutzik, P.O., and Nolan, G.P. (2003). Intracellular phospho-protein staining techniques for flow cytometry: monitoring single cell signaling events. *Cytometry A*, 55, pp. 61-70, ISSN 1552-4922.

Krutzik, P.O., Irish, J.M., Nolan, G.P., & Perez, O.D. (2004). Analysis of protein phosphorylation and cellular signaling events by flow cytometry: techniques and clinical applications. *Clin Immunol*, 110, pp. 206-221, ISSN 1521-6616.

Le Tourneau, C., Faivre, S., Serova, M., & Raymond, E. (2008). mTORC1 inhibitors: is temsirolimus in renal cancer telling us how they really work? *Br J Cancer*, 99, pp. 1197-1203, ISSN 1532-1827.

Li, W.X. (2008). Canonical and non-canonical JAK-STAT signaling. Trends Cell Biol, 18, pp. 545-551, ISSN 1879-3088.

Mendoza, M.C., Er, E.E., & Blenis, J. (2011). The Ras-ERK and PI3K-mTOR pathways: cross-talk and compensation. Trends Biochem Sci, 36, pp. 320-328, ISSN 0968-0004.

Nunes, J.A., Collette, Y., Truneh, A., Olive, D., & Cantrell, D.A. (1994). The role of p21ras in CD28 signal transduction: triggering of CD28 with antibodies, but not the ligand B7-1, activates p21ras. *J Exp Med*, 180, 1067-1076, ISSN 0022-1007.

O'Neill, R.A., Bhamidipati, A., Bi, X., Deb-Basu, D., Cahill, L., Ferrante, J., Gentalen, E., Glazer, M., Gossett, J., Hacker, K., Kirby, C., Knittle, J., Loder, R., Mastroieni, C., Maclaren, M., Mills, T., Nguyen, U., Parker, N., Rice, A., Roach, D., Suich, D., Voehringer, D., Voss, K., Yang, J., Yang, T., & Vander Horn, P.B. (2006). Isoelectric focusing technology quantifies protein signaling in 25 cells. *Proc Natl Acad Sci U S A*, 103, pp. 16153-16158, ISSN 0027-8424.

Qiu, P., Simonds, E.F., Bendall, S.C., Gibbs, K.D., Jr., Bruggner, R.V., Linderman, M.D., Sachs, K., Nolan, G.P., & Plevritis, S.K. (2011). Extracting a cellular hierarchy from high-dimensional cytometry data with SPADE. *Nat Biotechnol*, 29, pp. 886-891, ISSN 1546-1696.

Rudolph, M.G., & Wilson, I.A. (2002). The specificity of TCR/pMHC interaction. *Curr Opin Immunol*, 14, pp. 52-65, ISSN 0952-7915.

Towbin, H., Staehelin, T., & Gordon, J. (1979). Electrophoretic transfer of proteins from polyacrylamide gels to nitrocellulose sheets: procedure and some applications. *Proc Natl Acad Sci U S A*, 76, pp. 4350-4354, ISSN 0027-8424.

Vivanco, I., & Sawyers, C.L. (2002). The phosphatidylinositol 3-Kinase AKT pathway in human cancer. *Nat Rev Cancer*, 2, pp. 489-501, ISSN 1474-175X.

Yao, Z., Dolginov, Y., Hanoch, T., Yung, Y., Ridner, G., Lando, Z., Zharhary, D., & Seger, R. (2000). Detection of partially phosphorylated forms of ERK by monoclonal antibodies reveals spatial regulation of ERK activity by phosphatases. *FEBS Lett*, 468, pp. 37-42, ISSN 0014-5793.

Yung, Y., Dolginov, Y., Yao, Z., Rubinfeld, H., Michael, D., Hanoch, T., Roubini, E., Lando, Z., Zharhary, D., & Seger, R. (1997). Detection of ERK activation by a novel monoclonal antibody. *FEBS Lett*, 408, pp. 292-296, ISSN 0014-5793.

17

Gamma Radiation Induces p53-Mediated Cell Cycle Arrest in Bone Marrow Cells

Andrea A. F. S. Moraes et al.*
Universidade Federal de São Paulo – Unifesp,
Universidade Nove de Julho – Uninove,
Universidade Estadual de Santa Cruz – Uesc
Brazil

1. Introduction

The hematopoietic system is organized in a hierarchical manner in which rare hematopoietic stem cells initiate the hierarchy and have the ability to self-renew, proliferate and differentiate into different lineages of peripheral blood cells as well as to intermediate hematopoietic progenitor cells. Most hematopoietic stem cells are quiescent under steady-state conditions and function as a stock population to protect the hematopoietic system from exhaustion due to various stressful conditions. In contrast, hematopoietic progenitor cells are rapidly proliferating cells with limited self-renewal ability. The proliferation and differentiation of hematopoietic progenitor cells fulfills the requirements of normal hematopoiesis allowing the hematopoietic system to react promptly and effectively to meet the demand for increasing the output of mature cells during hematopoietic crisis such as loss of blood, hemolysis, infection, the depletion of HPCs by chemotherapy and/or radiotherapy (Reya, 2003; Weissman *et al.*, 2001; Walkley *et al.*, 2005).

Reactive oxygen species (ROS) are produced in organisms due to radiation, biotransformation of dietary chemicals, some diet components, transient metal ions, inflammatory reactions and during normal cellular metabolism.

The effect of gamma radiation ionization affects the main components of biological material such as carbon, hydrogen, oxygen, nitrogen. Radiobiology is described as the action of ionizing radiation on living things. On the molecular and cellular levels direct ionizing radiation can affect molecules in cells, especially DNA, lipids and proteins, promoting breakage and / or modifications or indirectly acting on water molecules and generating excitation ionization products of water radiolysis which include free radicals present and reactive oxygen species (ROS). Both direct and indirect effects of radiation on cells and tissues have biological effects in the short or long term. Such effects can be mitigated or

* Lucimar P. França, Vanina M. Tucci-Viegas, Fernanda Lasakosvitsch, Silvana Gaiba, Fernanda L. A. Azevedo, Amanda P. Nogueira, Helena R. C. Segreto, Alice T. Ferreira and Jerônimo P. França
Universidade Federal de São Paulo – Unifesp, Brazil
Universidade Nove de Julho – Uninove, Brazil
Universidade Estadual de Santa Cruz – Uesc, Brazil

eliminated by the antioxidant system and cell repair system that work against oxidizable stress and / or cellular stress (Figure 1).

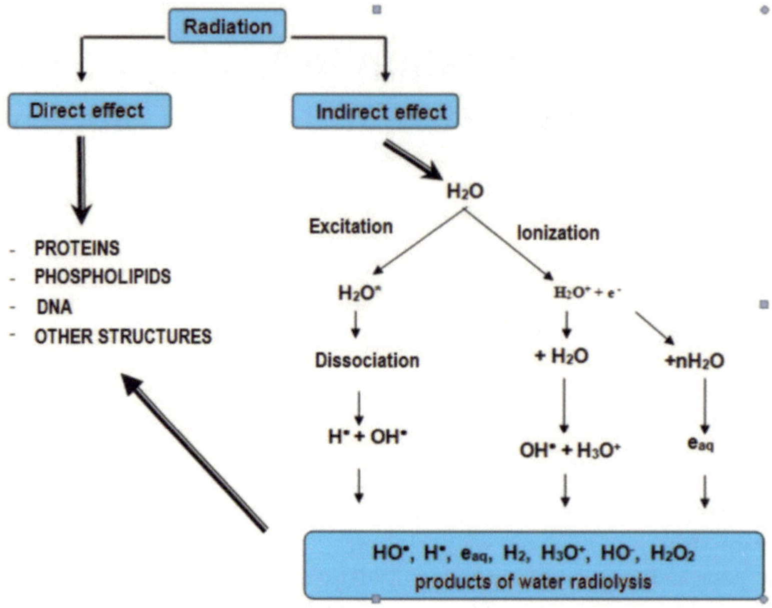

Fig. 1. Direct and indirect effect of radiation produced by free radicals of water radiolysis. Modified scheme of Stark, 1991

The pro-oxidant/antioxidant balance leads to a disturbance which, in turn, results in a condition of oxidative stress subsequently oxidizing cell components, activating cytoplasmic and/or nuclear signal transduction pathways, modulating gene and protein expression and changing both DNA and RNA polymerases activities. Normal cellular metabolism seems to be a primary source for endogenous ROS (such as the participation of oxidatively damaged DNA and repair in aging or cancer development). Oxidative damage to cellular DNA often causes mutagenesis as well as programmed cell death. While mutagenesis might result in carcinogenesis, programmed cell death often causes degenerative disorders (Nakabeppu *et al.*, 2007). Hydroxyl radicals generated from ionizing radiation attack DNA resulting in single strand breaks and oxidative damage to sugar and base residues. Hydroxyl radicals cause ionization of DNA bases as well as of other cellular components. Unsaturated fatty acids play an important role, since lipid peroxidation yields a plethora of stable derivates, which add to nucleic acids forming exocyclic DNA adducts of high miscoding potential, as well as DNA-DNA and DNA-protein cross-links (Bartsch *et al.*, 2004).

Damage of cells by ionizing radiation includes mainly modifications of DNA molecules, such as single and double-strand breaks. While single-strand breaks are quickly repaired in a process that requires poly-(ADP-ribose)-polymerase (PARP), double-strand breaks represent potentially lethal damage and their repair is complicated. Imperfect DNA repair causes mutations and contributes to genome instability. This is mostly manifested as chromosome aberrations, interchromosomal and intrachromosomal rearrangements (dicentric aberrations, translocations, or inversions). Detection of chromosomal aberrations in peripheral lymphocytes is an important indicator of obtained dose of radiation (Kozubek, 2000).

When the DNA is damaged an interconnected network of signaling is activated, resulting in damage repair, temporary or permanent cell cycle arrest or cell death. Cell cycle arrest allows time for DNA damage repair. If the repair is unsuccessful, the cells are removed by apoptosis, necrosis or their proliferation is permanently suppressed by initiation of stress-induced premature senescence (SIPS). Cmielová *et al.*, 2011) reported that it is possible that the major mechanism of response of these tissues to irradiation is not apoptosis, but induction of SIPS. Both pathways often work together to induce replicative and premature senescence. In general, activation of p53 and upregulation of p21 in cells undergoing senescence are transient (Toussaint *et al.*, 2000; Robles & Adami, 1998).

Increased p53 activity and p21 expression usually occur during the onset of senescence and then subside when the expression of p16 starts to rise. Before p16 upregulation, inactivation of p53 can prevent senescence induction in some cells. However, once p16 is highly expressed cell cycle arrest becomes irreversible simply by downregulation of p53 (Campisi *et al.*, 2005; Beausejour *et al.*, 2004; Narita *et al.*, 2004). This suggests that while both p53 and p21 play an important role in the initiation of senescence, only p16 is required for the maintenance of senescence. In agreement with this suggestion, we found that IR-induced activation of p53 and upregulation of p21 occurred prior to the increased expression of p16 and p19 in murine BM HSCs (Meng *et al.*, 2003; Neben *et al.*, 1993; Wang *et al.*, 2006)

Recent studies showed that a majority of murine BM hematopoietic cells including HSCs died by apoptosis after exposure to a moderate dose of IR *in vitro*. However, a subset of these cells survived IR damage up to 35 days in a long-term BM-cell culture although having lost their clonogenic function. These surviving cells exhibited an increased AS β gal activity, a biomarker for senescent cells, and expressed elevated levels of the proteins (p16Ink4a and p19Arf) encoded by the *Ink4a-Arf* locus, whose expression has been implicated in the establishment and maintenance of senescence by direct inhibition of various cyclin-dependent kinases (CDKs), (Meng *et al.*, 2003; Dimri *et al.*, 1995; Lowe *et al.*, 2003; Sharpless *et al.*, 1999).

The main function of mitochondria is ATP production, which occurs during mitochondrial oxidative phosphorylation (ox-phos). In several cell types, mitochondria also act as a very efficient Ca2+ buffer, taking up substantial amounts of cytosolic Ca2+ at the expense of mitochondrial membrane potential (ΔΨm). The pathways of Ca2+ entry into mitochondrial matrix are known as the mitochondrial calcium uniporter (MCU), the "rapid mode" mechanism, and the mitochondrial ryanodine receptor. The main role of mitochondrial Ca2+ is the stimulation of the ox-phos enzymes. In addition to ox-phos, mitochondria are central players in cellular Ca2+ signaling by shaping and buffering cellular Ca2+ signals. As a consequence of Ca2+ uptake, mitochondria can suffer Ca2+ overload, triggering the opening of the permeability transition pore (PTP) which is associated with apoptosis *via* the mitochondrial pathway or necrosis due to mitochondrial damage. PTPs have been shown to be promoted by thiol oxidation and inhibited by antioxidants, supporting a role of ROS in pore opening. In addition, it has been demonstrated that mitochondrial Ca2+ uptake can lead to free radical production. From a thermodynamic point of view, however, it has been noted that Ca2+ uptake occurring at the expense of membrane potential should result in a decrease in ROS production (Crosstalk signaling between mitochondrial Ca2+ and ROS) (Brookes *et al.*, 2004). Mitochondrial PTP is formed from a number of proteins within the matrix, and mitochondrial inner and outer membranes (Ishas & Mazat, 1998; Brookes *et al.*, 2004). One of the processes through which mitochondria contribute to cell death is through PTP opening (Bratton & Cohen, 2001). The PTP precise composition remains unclear, but it is evident that this is a multi-subunit protein channel that spans the mitochondrial inner and outer membrane. Critical components appear to include the mitochondrial VDAC (voltage-dependent anion channel), the ANT (adenine nucleotide translocase), and cyclophilin D (Ishas & Mazat, 1998). It has also been shown that pre-treatment of isolated mitochondria with pro-oxidants can lower the threshold at which the PTP opening occurs (Brookes & Darley-Usmar, 2004). It seems that the opening of this Ca^{2+}-dependent channel plays an important role in controlling the commitment of the cell to death through apoptotic or necrotic mechanisms (Kokoszka *et al.*, 2004; Baines *et al.*, 2005).

2. Objective

The purpose of this work is to evaluate ionizing radiation-induced apoptosis in mice bone marrow cells and the role of p53, p21 and Ca++ in this process, cell cycle alterations and indirect determination of reactive oxygen specimens (ROS).

3. Methods

3.1 Animals

Mice C57BL/10 (3 months) were provided by the Instituto Nacional de Farmacologia (located at Rua Três de Maio 100, Vila Clementino, SP, Brazil). The animals were maintained on standard mouse feed and water *ad libitum*.

3.2 Irradiation

Gamma irradiation was carried out with an Alcyon II ^{60}CO teletherapy unit with the mice at a distance of 80 cm from the source. The dose rate was 1.35 Gy/min. Animals in batches of ten were placed in a well-ventilated acrylic box with an individual cell for each mouse and exposed whole - body to 7Gy (Segreto *et al.*, 1999).

3.3 Preparation procedure of bone marrow cells

The mice were killed by cervical dislocation 4 hours after gamma irradiation, and both femurs were removed from each mouse. After cutting of the proximal and distal ends of the femurs, the bone marrow cells were gently flushed out with 5ml suspension using phosphate buffered saline (PBS) (Segreto *et al.*, 1999).

3.4 Intracellular reactive oxygen species

Intracellular peroxides were determined by incubating $2X10^6$ cells/ml in medium (defined above) with 5 nM 2',7'-dichlorodihydrofluorescein diacetate (DCFH-DA) (Molecular Probes) for 30 min at 37°C, then analyzed using a Becton Dickinson (BD) Bioscience Flow Cytometer - model FACScalibur (San Jose, CA) equipped with an argon laser emitting at 488 nm (Jagetia & Venkatesh, 2007). BD CellQuest Pro software was used for fast reliable acquisition, analysis and presentation of information.

3.5 Measurement of intracellular Ca++

Calcium was measured after incubation of the bone marrow cells with the fluorescence indicator Fura- 2/AM in the form of acetoxymethyl ester (AM). The bone marrow cells at concentration of 10^6 cells/ml were suspended in 2.5 ml of Tyrode's solution (137 mM NaCl, 2.68 KCl, 1.36 mM CaCl2_2H2O, 0.49 mM MgCl2_6H2O, 12 mM NaHCO3, 0.36 mM NaH2PO4, and 5.5 mM D-glucose) for 30 min. The suspension was then centrifuged at 100 g for 4 min, the supernatant was aspirated, and the result pellet was suspended in 2.5 ml of Tyrode and transferred to the quartz cuvette of a SPEX fluorometer (AR CM System) for fluorescence determination. Measurements were made at alternated 340- and 380-nm excitation wavelengths, with emission at 505 nm. The autofluorescence ratio was less than 10% and therefore was not subtracted from the fluorescence measurements before calculation of the fluorescence ratio. The cells were incubated with 0.01% pluronic 127 detergent and 2M Fura-2/AM, and the cuvette was transferred to a PerkinElmer Life Sciences spectrofluorometer (LS 5B, Buckinghamshire, UK) to determine the fluorescence spectrum of the indicator in the excitation range of 300 to 400 nm, with emission at 520 nm. In the esterified form, maximum fluorescence was observed at 390 nm. As the indicator Fura- 2/AM was transformed into the acid form, the fluorescence peak shifted to 350 nm within an average period of 2 h, thus indicating the maximum amount of indicator incorporation into the cell suspension. At that time the cell suspension was washed with 15 ml of Tyrode and centrifuged at 100*g* for 4 min. The supernatant was discarded, and the pellet was suspended in 2.5 ml of Tyrode and transferred to a SPEX fluorometer programmed for excitation at two wavelengths (340 and 380 nm) with emission at 505 nm, under constant stirring at 37 °C. The first reading of this phase corresponded to basal calcium. At the end of each experiment, a control was performed using 50 mM digitonin, 1mM MnCl2, and 2 mM EGTA. The results are calculated by the relative ratio of 340 and 380 nm, considering the reading for digitonin to be 100% (*R*max) and 0% for EGTA (*R*min). Using the ratio *R*max/*R*min, calcium concentration was estimated by the formula of (Grynkiewicz *et al.*, 1985).

3.6 Apoptosis assay

The bone marrow cells were labeled with annexin V-FITC (Roche), binding to phosphatidylserine at the cell surface of apoptotic cells and propidium iodide (PI) provided by Sigma, is used as a marker of cell membrane permeability following manufacturer's instructions. Samples were examined by fluorescence-activated cell sorter (FACS) analysis, and the results were analyzed using Cell-Quest software (Becton Dickinson Model: Facscalibur, San Jose, CA) (Vermes *et al.*, 1995).

3.7 Cell cycle analysis

For cell cycle analysis the cells were washed with cold PBS and fixed with 70% ethanol. For detection of low-molecular-weight fragments of DNA, the cells were incubated for 5 min at room temperature in a buffer (1.92 ml: 0.2 mol/L Na_2HPO_4 + 8 ml: 0. 1 mol/L citric acid, pH 7.8) and then stained with PI in Vindelov's solution for 40 min at 37 °C. The measurements were performed in a Becton Dickinson Flow Cytometer model FACScalibur (San Jose, CA); data were analyzed using Cell Quest software (Vindelov & Christensen, 1990)

3.8 Flow cytometric analysis of p53 and p21

For analysis of p53 and p21 expression and activation, cells were washed once in phosphate-buffered saline (PBS) containing 0.1% sodium azide (Sigma), centrifuged at 1.4G, fixed in 2% paraformaldehyde for 10 minutes at 4°C, washed 3 times in PBS, and washed twice in PBS with 50 mmol/L NH_4Cl. Cells were then permeabilized with 0.1% saponin in PBS containing 10% normal bovine serum for 30 minutes at 22°C. The first primary antibody incubation was performed in PBS containing 10% normal bovine serum and 0.1% saponin. Aliquots were then incubated for 60 minutes with anti-p53 and anti-p21 antibodies (Santa Cruz Biotechnology, Santa Cruz, CA), final dilution 1:800, or rabbit IgG as a control, followed by washing in PBS containing 0.1% saponin 3 times for 5 minutes at 22°C. Cells were then incubated with the first fluorochrome-conjugated secondary antibody Alexa 488 and 594, final dilution 1:1600, for 40 minutes at 37°C in the dark (Danova *et al.*, 1990).

3.9 Immunocytochemistry

After cutting off the proximal and distal ends of the femurs, the bone marrow cells were gently flushed out with 5ml suspension using phosphate buffered saline (PBS) (Segreto *et al.*, 1999). Bone marrow cells were washed 3 times with phosphate-buffered saline (PBS), cytofuged onto glass slides, fixed in 4% paraformaldehyde for 10 minutes at 4°C, washed 3 times in PBS, and washed twice in PBS with 50 mmol/l NH_4Cl. Cells were permeabilized with 0.1% saponin in PBS containing 10% normal bovine serum for 30 minutes at 22°C. The first primary antibody incubation was performed in PBS containing 10% normal bovine serum and 0.1% saponin. Slides were incubated with anti-p53 and anti-p21 antibodies at the dilution 1:100 (Santa Cruz Biotechnology, Santa Cruz, CA) for 2 hours, followed by the nuclear staining dye DAPI (4_6-diamidino-2-phenylindole) 1:10000 (catalog #D1036; Molecular Probes, Invitrogen, Carlsbad, CA) which was diluted in the preparatory solution A of Slowfade Antifade kit (Molecular Probes, Eugene, OR) for a final dilution 1:100 and the fluorescent secondary antibody Alexa 594 and 647, final dilution 1:500 (Invitrogen). Neither one used lectin conjugated with Alexa fluor 488 for the cellular membrane. After an initial primary and secondary antibody staining, the procedure was repeated for the second primary and secondary antibody staining, and the slides were then mounted in the preparatory solution A containing Dapi. Each fluorochrome was analyzed individually by means of an inverted confocal laser scanning Fluorescence Microscope (LSM; Zeiss, Germany).

3.10 Ethics

The present study was performed in accordance with the ethical standards laid down in the updated version of the 1964 Declaration of Helsinki and was approved by the Research Ethics Committee of the Federal University of São Paulo, Brazil (CEP N° 1248/01).

3.11 Statistical analysis

The results obtained were analyzed using a one-way analysis of variance (ANOVA) followed by the Student - Newman - Keuls Multiple Range Test.

4. Results and discussion

Cell exposure to DNA-damaging agents can result in timely repair of the damage and maintenance of genetic fidelity in daughter cells, cell death, or the development of heritable genetic changes in viable daughter cells through replication of damaged DNA or segregation of damaged chromosomes before repair (Nakabeppu *et al.*, 2007; Christine *et al.*, 1995; Szymczyk *et al.*, 2004). The last one could generate the genetic changes that contribute to the development of a malignant phenotype. As a result, the gene products controlling timely repair and appropriate cell death after DNA damage are expected to be critical determinants of neoplastic evolution. Moreover, as most antineoplastic agents are DNA-damaging agents, these same gene products probably influence response and cure rates during the treatment of human tumors (Christine *et al.*, 1995).

The number of cells in apoptosis was determined using Annexin-V and cell viability by propidium iodide using the technique of flow cytometry, Figure 2. These results indicated the loss of transport function or structural integrity of the cytoplasmic membrane, which is crucial to distinguish viable from unviable cells, given the wide variety of cell viability assays using different cationic markers such as (PI, 7 -AAD) or (Hoechst 33342O). These fluorochromes determine the transport characteristics of the plasma membrane (Ormerod *et al.*, 1992, 1993; Poot *et al.*, 1997). In addition, flow cytometry has identified the viability of bone marrow cells (Figure 2) i.e. the number of non-viable cells that characterize death by late apoptosis (Vermes *et al.*, 1995). Contour diagram of FITC-Annexin V/PI flow cytometry of bone marrow cells after 7 Gy irradiation. The lower left quadrants of each panels show the viable cells, which exclude PI and are negative for FITC-Annexin V binding. The upper right quadrants (7.0 ± 1.2) % contain the non-viable, necrotic cells, positive for FITC-Annexin V binding and for PI uptake. The lower right quadrants (50.1 ± 1.2) % represent the apoptotic cells, FITC-Annexin V positive and PI negative demonstrating cytoplasmic membrane integrity.

Ionizing radiation induces G2/M cell cycle arrest and triggers a p53-dependent signaling pathway that, in turn, may induce apoptotic cell death (Szymczyk *et al.*, 2004). Nonetheless, this response may vary and be cell type-dependent because p53 response causes cell cycle arrest in untransformed cells (Bates *et al.*, 1999) and apoptosis in transformed cells (Bates & Vousden, 1999). Cell cycle distribution was determined by propidium iodide staining for both the control group and irradiated group, the latter with cells exposed to 7 Gy radiation (GI). An increase in the percentage of apoptotic cells was observed in the irradiated group 4h after irradiation (Figure 3B) when compared to the control group (Figure 3A). Cells in G2 are more susceptible to ionizing radiation, as this is the moment when the cell must be repaired prior to entering mitosis. It is possible that the increased activity of protein kinase ATM (ataxiatelangiectasia) modifies the p53 levels thereby altering the cell cycle distribution (Figure 3).

Cell cycle progression and cell fate are determined by the dynamic balance between different p53 downstream effectors, including p21 (Waf1/Cip1) (Waldman *et al.*, 1996). DNA damage-induced cell cycle arrest is regulated by the tumor suppressor p53 by direct stimulation of $p21^{WAF1/CIP1}$ expression, an inhibitor of cyclin-dependent kinases (Cdks). Working with the cyclin proteins, Cdks ensure, for example, that DNA replication in the S phase follows from the G_1 resting phase. $p21^{WAF1/CIP1}$ then, inhibits both the G_1/S and the

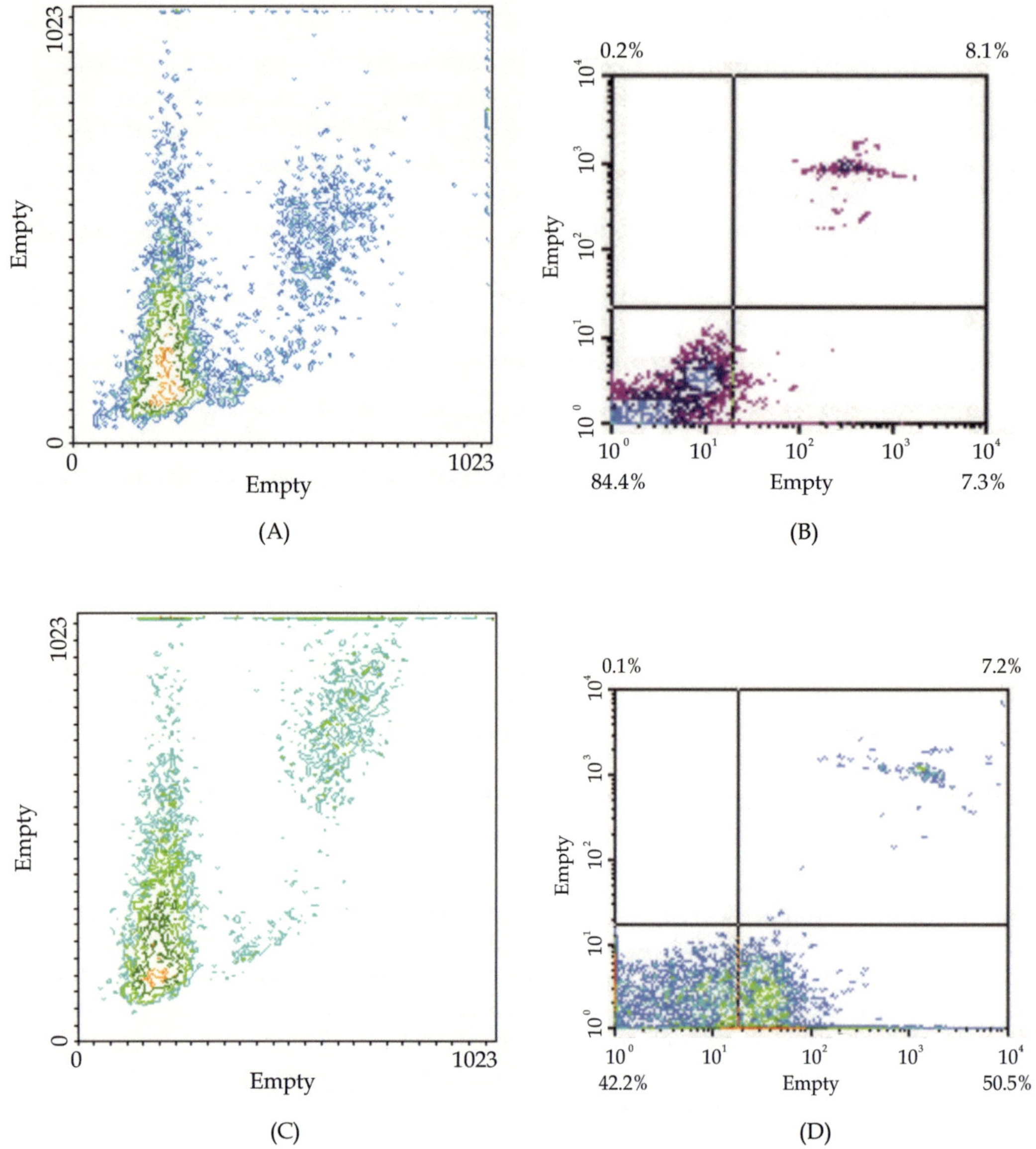

Fig. 2. Flow Cytometric Analysis of control (A and B) and irradiated (C and D) groups to demonstrate the basis for the gating of viable, apoptotic and necrotic cells. The mice were killed by cervical dislocation 4 hours after gamma irradiation. The exposure time was 5.18 minutes in order to achieve 7 Gy of radiation. On Figure 2, A and C, axis X refers to forward scatter and axis Y refers to side scatter. According to the control samples, the following quadrants of the cytograms were defined: - the lower left quadrant showing viable cells; the lower right quadrant representing early apoptotic cells, binding annexin V, but still retaining their cytoplasmic integrity; the upper right quadrant representing nonviable, late apoptotic/necrotic cells, positive for annexin V and the upper left quadrant showing nonviable necrotic cells/nuclear fragments with no annexin V

G_2/mitosis (M) transitions, by exerting its negative effects on various Cdks. For example, according to current theories, by inhibiting cyclin B/Cdc2 (Cdk1) $p21^{WAF1/CIP1}$ induces G_2/M phase arrest. Even without being required for initiating G_2/M cell cycle arrest, p53 and $p21^{WAF1/CIP1}$ seem to be critical for sustaining it as, for instance, cells lacking p53 and $p21^{WAF1/CIP1}$ leave the G_2/M cell cycle arrest prematurely and either enter mitosis or reinitiate DNA replication, causing genomic instability and possibly leading to accumulation of oncogenic mutations (Bork *et al.*, 2009). Changes in the cell cycle in response to ionizing radiation were evaluated using the p53 protein (phosphorylated - serina15). The p53 protein activation is the major route of cellular response after DNA damage in many cell types, as described by Yu & Zhang, 2005. We demonstrated that this machinery is activated when apoptosis is induced by radiation. The signaling pathway after p53 activation leads to an increased expression of p21, which consequently affects the profile of the cell cycle and also leads to cell death by apoptosis. Phosphorylation of serine 15 is a modification that is due to DNA damage induced by radiation. This was evaluated 4h after irradiation, using specific antibodies against p53 and p21 (Figures 4 and 5). We observed the increased expression of p53 and p21 by confocal fluorescence microscopy. These data corroborate the method presented by flow cytometry, which showed an increase in fluorescence intensity of

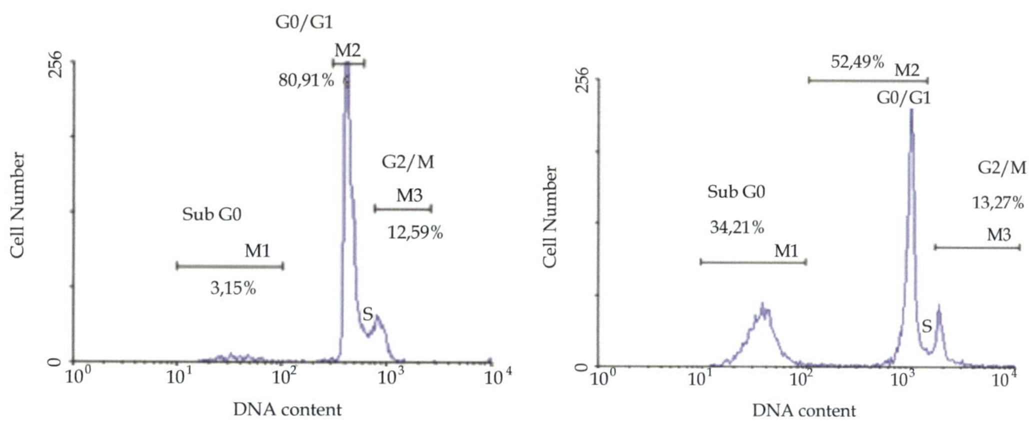

Control group	**Irradiated group**
Sub G0 = 3.3 ± 0.6%	Sub G0 = 32.5 ± 4.1%
G0/G1 = 77.4 ± 5.3%	G0/G1 = 49.2 ± 3.7%
G2/M = 13.6 ± 4.4%	G2/M = 12.1 ± 5.3%

Fig. 3. Analysis of cell cycle distribution: A) Control group and B) Irradiated group. Progression through the cell cycle was monitored 4 h after ionizing radiation. Bone marrow cells were analyzed for DNA content by FACS using PI staining. The histogram was generated using CellQuest software (Alam *et al.*, 2004). Representative histograms are shown from *n*=4 independent experiments. Table show cell percentages quantified by the mean (±SD) of four different peak analyses. Statistical analysis: Anova - Newman Keuls.
$p < 0.05$

these proteins when compared to the control group (Figures 4 and 5). Overlapped images for immunocytochemistry of p53 and p21 proteins and cellular structures (Nuclei: blue-fluorescent DNA and cell membrane: green-fluorescent Lectin). In the irradiated group there is an increase in fluorescence intensity and a change in the distribution of p53 and p21 when compared to the control group (Figures 6 and 7).

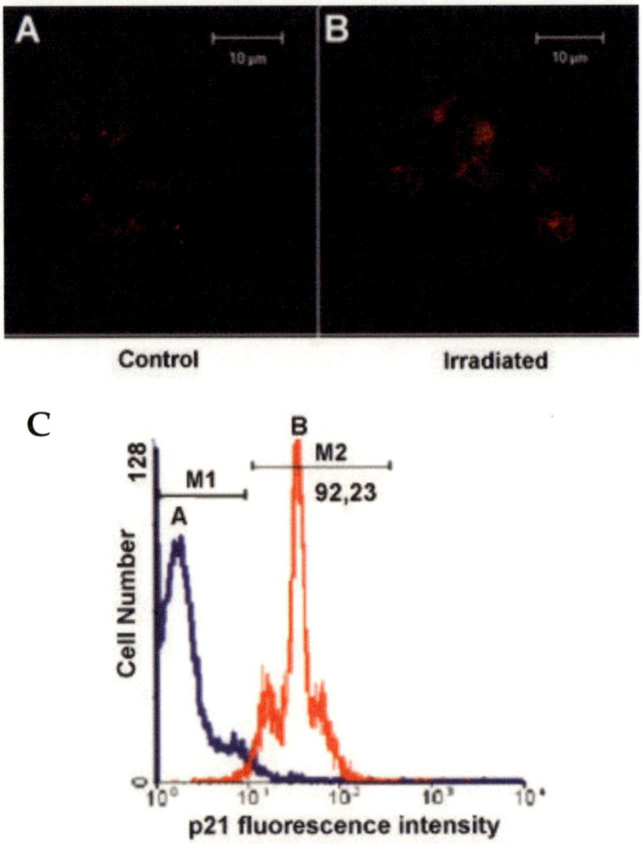

Fig. 4. (above - A and B) Confocal microscopy analysis: bone marrow cells of mice were immunostained in red-fluorescent. Specific staining using antibody p21 (red-fluorescent Alexa Fluor® 594). The irradiated group (B) shows an increase in fluorescence intensity and a change in p21 distribution when compared to the control group (A). (graph below-C) Flow cytometric analysis of p21 protein in paraformaldehyde-fixed cells harvested from mice femurs. Control group A (left) and irradiated group B (right). The bone marrow cells were analyzed 4h after radiation. The cells were pooled, washed, permeabilized with saponin, and stained with anti-p21 antibody and then analyzed by flow cytometry. Histograms were generated and analyzed using CellQuest cell cycle software. Percentage of cells showing fluorescence intensity. Histogram related to gated p21 positive bone marrow cells of GC and GI (89.8 ± 5.3). Statistical analysis: Anova - Newman Keuls. **$p < 0.05$, N = 4.**

Cells with not completely repaired DNA damage entering SIPS instead of being removed by apoptosis cause the selection of a resistant population, creating a risk of developing a population of cells with dangerously damaged genome. Stem cells are currently exhaustively studied due to their self-renewal capability, ability to produce a broad spectrum of cell types and high proliferation potential and they can be used in bone marrow transplantation and peripheral blood stem cell transplantation for patients who had radiation treatment or high dose of chemotherapy in treatment of cancer. Nonetheless, their reaction to DNA damage as a response to genotoxic stress is not widely known, such as ionizing radiation used in the treatment of many cancer types. Hematopoietic stem cells react to irradiation mostly by apoptosis induction, and sometimes by senescence induction. (Vávrová *et al.*, 2002; Meng *et al.*, 2003). Even though mesenchymal stem cells isolated from bone marrow do not die by apoptosis after irradiation, they are notable to proliferate anymore. The irradiation with the dose 2.5-15 Gy do not destruct the cells, but induces telomere shortening, stops cell division and increases the activity of senescence-associated β-galactosidase increases (Serakinci *et al.*,

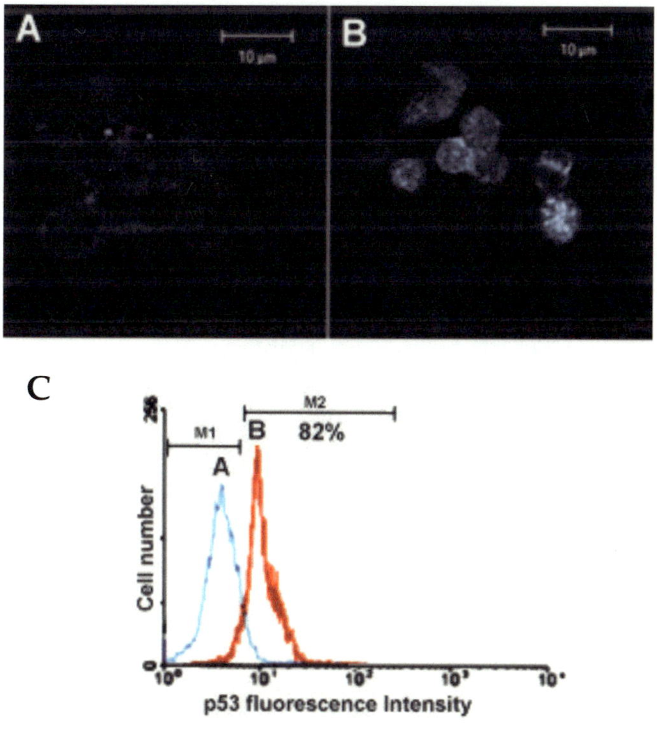

Fig. 5. (above – A and B) Confocal microscopy analysis of mice bone marrow cells. Specific staining using p53 antibody (blue-fluorescent Alexa Fluor® 647). The irradiated group (B) showed an increase in fluorescence intensity and a change in p21 distribution when compared to the control group (A). (graph below - C) Flow cytometric analysis of p53 protein in paraformaldehyde-fixed cells harvested from mice femurs. Control group A (left) and irradiated group B (right). The bone marrow cells were analyzed 4h after radiation. The cells were pooled, washed, permeabilized with saponin, and stained with anti-p53 antibody and then analyzed by flow cytometry. Histograms were generated and analyzed using CellQuest cell cycle software. Percentage of cells showing fluorescence intensity. Histogram related to gated p53 positive bone marrow cells of GC and GI (87.6 ± 5.3). Statistical analysis: Anova - Newman Keuls. **$p < 0.05$, N = 4**

2007). Induction of premature senescence have implicated two major pathways: the p53-p21Cip1/Waf1 or p19Arf-Mdm2-p53- p21Cip1/Waf1 pathway, triggered by DNA damage; and the p16Ink4a-Rb pathway, activated by the Ras-mitogen-activated protein kinase cascade (Livak & Schmittgen, 2001; Takano *et al.*, 2004; Cheng *et al.*, 2000). Activation of either pathway is sufficient to induce senescence, but they frequently work together causing premature senescence. Induction of apoptosis or premature senescence, or both, in HSCs and progenitors can result in inhibition of their hematopoietic function. (Wang *et al.*, 2005).

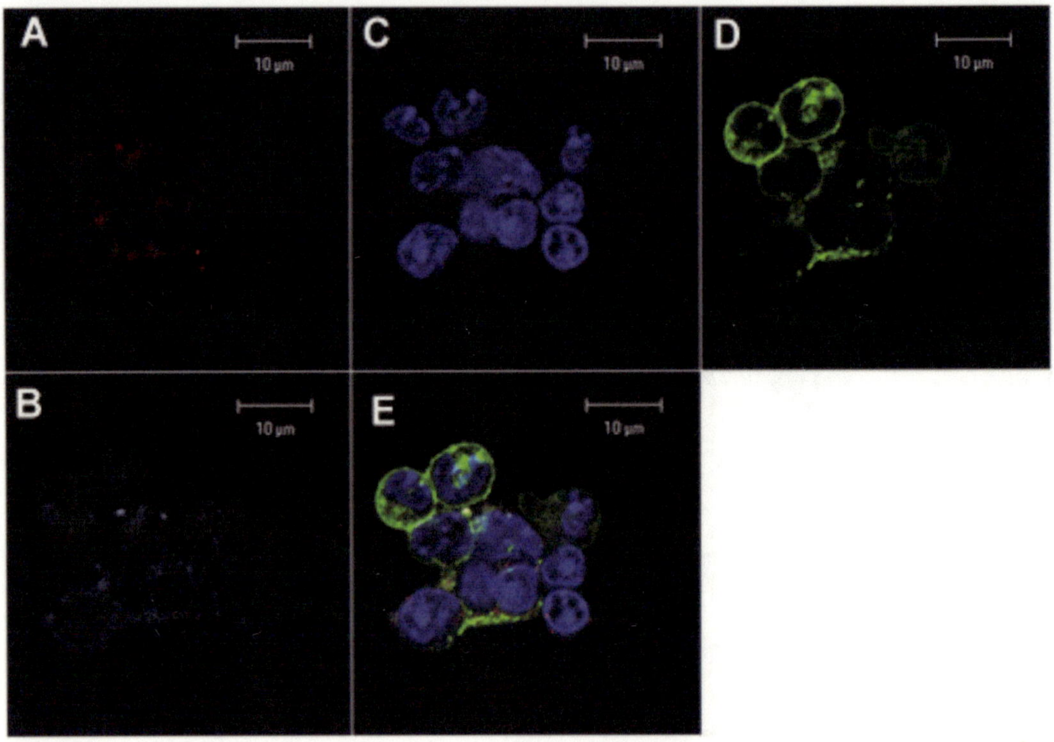

Fig. 6. Laser confocal images of bone marrow cells of the control group mice, were stained by immunofluorescence with combinations of the four fluorophores (red, green, blue and pseudo-colored gray): A) Red channel showing a specific staining using antibody anti-p21 (Alexa fluor 594). B) Pseudo-colored gray channel showing a specific staining using antibody anti-p53 (Alexa fluor 647). C) Blue channel showing nuclei counterstained with the blue-fluorescent DNA stain DAPI (diamidino-2-phenylindole) which is a blue fluorescent probe that fluoresces brightly upon selectively binding to the minor groove of double stranded DNA. D) Green channel showing a Lectin staining using the conjugated with green - fluorescent Alexa fluor 488. Lectin staining using the conjugated with green - fluorescent Alexa fluor 488. E) Specific combination of the four channels reveals overlapped images A, B, C and D. These findings suggest that the bone marrow is more highly susceptible to oxidative damage by radiation ionizing, it also induces alteration in intracellular calcium levels and cell death apoptosis. In summary, the present work demonstrates that radiation induced apoptosis is increase when p53 or p21 responsive G2 arrest being suggestive induction of premature senescence may represent a novel underlying mechanism for radiation

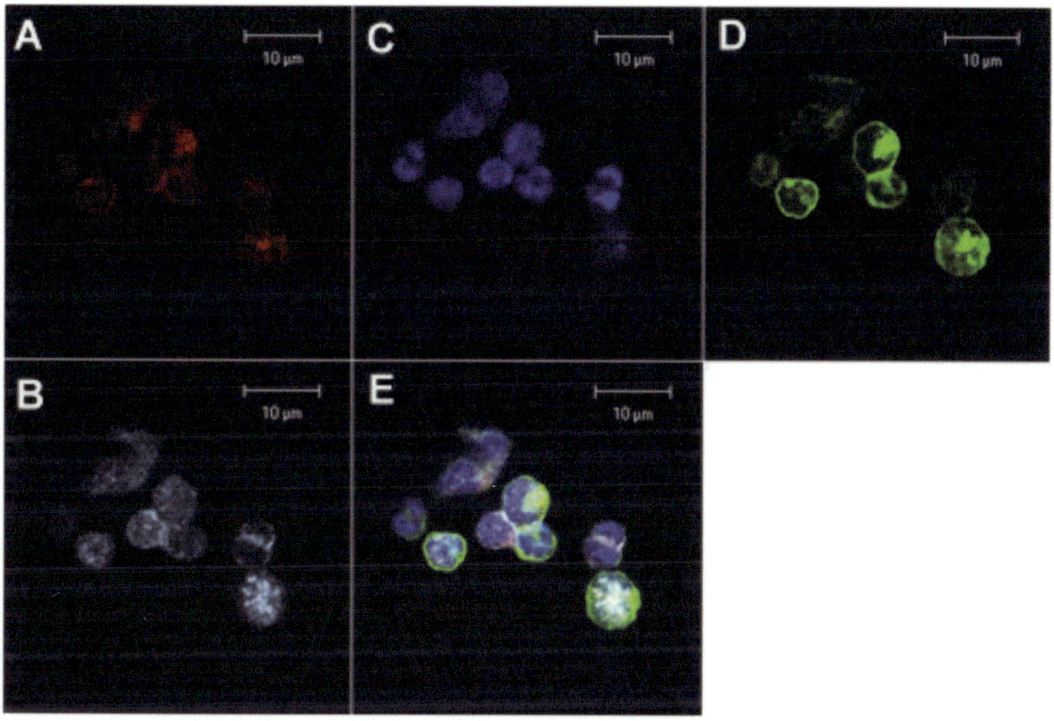

Fig. 7. Laser confocal images of bone marrow cells of the irradiated group mice, were stained by immunofluorescence with combinations of the four fluorophores (red, green, blue and pseudo-colored gray): A) Red channel showing specific staining using antibody anti-p21 (Alexa fluor 594). B) Pseudo-colored gray channel showing a specific staining using antibody anti-p53 (Alexa fluor 647). C) Blue channel showing nuclei counterstained with the blue-fluorescent DNA stain DAPI (diamidino-2-phenylindole) which is a blue fluorescent probe that fluoresces brightly upon selectively binding to the minor groove of double stranded DNA. D) Green channel showing a Lectin staining using the conjugated with green - fluorescent Alexa fluor 488. Lectin staining using the conjugated with green - fluorescent Alexa fluor 488. E) Specific combination of the four channels reveals overlapped images A, B, C and D. In the irradiated group there is an increase in fluorescence intensity and a change in the distribution of p53 and p21 when compared to the control group

In many circumstances, changes in cytosolic Ca2+ concentration may be observed. A surplus of cellular Ca2+ is dangerous for cell life, since it activates many proteases and phospholipases. This Ca2+ surplus can, thus, lead to necrotic cell death. Apoptotic cell death also relies on increased Ca2+ concentrations (Murgia *et al.*, 2009). Both deaths are mediated by endoplasmic reticulum (ER) calcium release and by capacitative Ca2+ influx through Ca2+ release-activated Ca2+ channels (Pinton & Rizzuto, 2006). In Figure 8, we observed the radiation-induced biological effects on cell membranes and the resulting damage which can raise the cytosolic calcium levels triggering cell death by apoptosis, as described by other authors (Starkov *et al.*, 2004). The elevation of cytosolic calcium results in activation of a variety of enzymes sensitive to this ion, such as phosphatases, caspases and calpains, which can be activated from the mitochondria by signaling molecules (Hajnóczky *et al.*, 2003). So it was relevant to determine calcium levels as an indicator of oxidative stress and smooth endoplasmic reticulum stress. Our results showed a significant increase of basal levels of calcium after irradiation (GI). The baseline values of calcium are associated with various cellular responses such as death by necrosis, apoptosis and cell proliferation (Hirota *et al.*, 1998; Anza *et al.*, 1995).

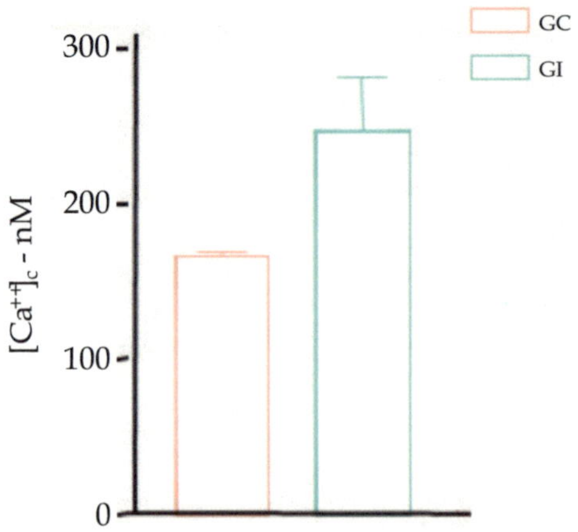

Fig. 8. Effect of γ radiation on basal intracellular Ca^{2+} concentration in mice granulocyte of the control (GC) and irradiated (GI) groups with doses of 700cCy – measured by fura-2 fluorophore. Statistical analysis: Newman Keuls. **p < 0.05, N = 4**

Either necrosis or apoptosis is activated depending on the range of the insult, and consequently on the amount of Ca2+ increase. Ca2+ can establish local concentrations within the cell, due to its low rate of diffusion, when compared to other second messengers and on the dynamic sequestration of this ion by several organelles (Rizzuto & Pozzan, 2006). This unique property allows the cell to decipher various signals, triggering different consequences through a single molecule. ER is crucial to regulate calcium concentration and the sensitivity to apoptosis. Ca2+ accumulated in the ER can be released upon apoptotic stimuli coupled to IP3, and being detected by mitochondria. This process is regulated by Bcl-2 family proteins, strategically located at the ER and mitochondria surfaces. Cells that overexpress Bcl-2 showed a considerable decrease in Ca2+ levels within the ER and the Golgi apparatus. Consequently, reduced Ca2+ concentration increases upon stimuli coupled to IP3 generation were detected both in the cytosol and in the mitochondria (Pinton *et al.*, 2000). In cells in which the pro-apoptotic members of Bcl-2 family, Bax and Bak, were deleted, the same effect was observed. On the other hand, Bax and Bak double knockout cells are protected against apoptotic stimuli (Scorrano *et al.*, 2003). In these cells, ER Ca2+ values were restored to control level through silencing of Bcl-2 (Danial & Korsmeyer, 2004). Stimuli that produce cytosolic Ca2+ increase bring out large Ca2+ influxes in the mitochondria matrix, regardless of the low affinity of mitochondrial Ca2+ carriers for this ion. This is explained by the existence of mitochondria-ER contacts, where microdomains of high Ca2+ concentrations are found and trigger fast accumulation of Ca2+ in the matrix (Hayashi *et al.*, 2009). A variety of responses is caused by mitochondria Ca2+ uptake, from stimulation of metabolism (ATP production) - when they are subject to a transient stimuli, to apoptosis - in case of a more persistent or excessive Ca2+ increase. Additionally, mitochondria Ca2+ accumulation triggered by apoptotic stimuli causes swelling and fragmentation, followed by cytochrome c release. The opening of permeability transition pores (PTP) was also observed upon ceramide-induced apoptosis, which sensitizes mitochondria to the otherwise physiological IP3-mediated Ca2+ signal (Szalai *et al.*, 1999). In which concerns ER calcium concentrations, Bcl-2 family members control this apoptotic pathway. In particular, upon apoptotic stimuli, Bax and Bak localize at the outer mitochondria membrane triggering its permeabilization and release of apoptotic factors in the cytosol (Szalai *et al.*, 1999). Apoptotic cell death may also be caused by mitochondrial malfunction due to ROS-induced mtDNA damage, lipid peroxidation or protein oxidation (Migliaccio *et al.*, 1999).

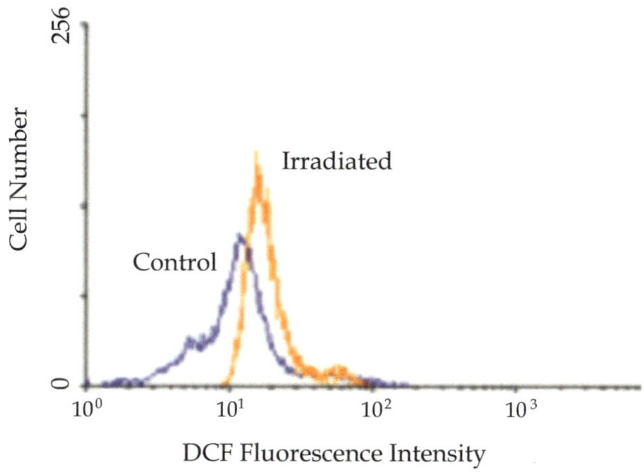

(a)

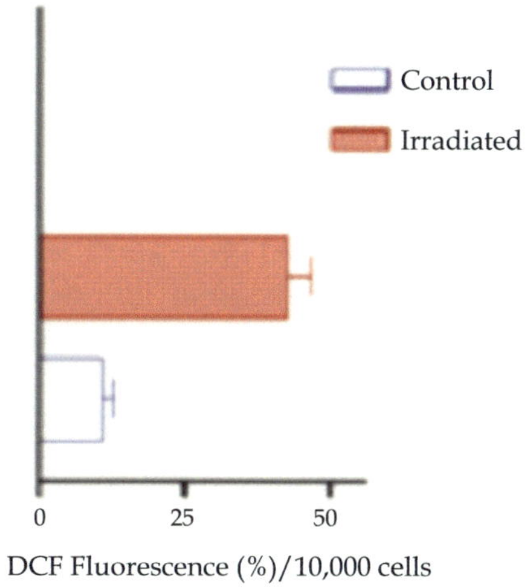

(b)

Fig. 9. Measurement of reactive oxygen species (ROS) induced by ionizing radiation in bone marrow cells. The cells were loaded with DCFH-DA (10μM) for 30 minutes. After conversion of the ester to DCFH by intracellular esterases, the number of cells exhibiting increased fluorescence of oxidized DCF was evaluated by flow cytometry. A- Histograms represent four independent experiments in bone marrow cells for groups control and exposed to ionizing radiation. B- Statistical analysis for groups control and irradiated: Anova - Newman Keuls. **$p < 0.05$, N = 4**

ROS cellular levels induced by ionizing radiation were evaluated by measuring DCFH-fluorescence. DCFH is permeable to membrane cell where it is rapidly hydrolyzed by esterases, thus the production of ROS leads to increased DCF fluorescence. We observed an increase of about 50% in DCF fluorescence induced by radiation in bone marrow cells (Figure 9A) in the irradiated group and with flow cytometry we were able to distinguish differences to this type of analysis (Figure 9B).

However, since the caspases are dependent on a reduced thiol group in their active site to cleave their substrates, apoptosis progression is inhibited by excessive ROS, or reactive oxygen species production (Hengartner, 2000). Once more, it should be pointed out, that a pro-oxidant state is induced in mitochondria by CaCl2 through indirect action, since this molecule did not present an intrinsic capacity to induce oxidative stress directly. As previously reported, the redox effects induced by CaCl2 is very likely to be consequence of CaCl2-dependent MPTP induction (Zamzami & Kroemer, 2001).

5. Conclusion

There is controversy in the literature regarding the use of antioxidants as inhibitor of apoptotic response. In some systems it is almost certain that free radicals and ROS are produced, and in these cases, antioxidants have been shown to reduce or delay apoptosis. Oxidative stress induced by gamma radiation can induce to clonogenic death or apoptosis. Although physical and chemical agents can promote cytotoxicity or genotoxicity action leading to apoptosis independent of production of free radicals, oxidative stress induced by radiation can, without any doubts, elicit cell death, and mild oxidative stress which in turn initiate apoptosis. ROS can cause oxidative stress even though not being essential for the apoptotic processes. A very interesting hypothesis is that perturbation of cellular redox homeostasis may control these key events. p53 protein is widely regarded as an important sensor of genotoxic damage in cells, and mutations in p53 are the most frequent observed in human cancers. After radiation induced damage, a protein expression such as p53 occur, which takes to p21 transcription, leading to cell cycle arrest in G0/G1 in order to repair the DNA damage, irreversible growth arrest, terminal differentiation, or apoptosis. Major processes resulting from oxidative stress include alteration of metabolic pathways, lipid peroxidation and the loss of intracellular calcium homeostasis. Thus, the lethality of gamma radiation is well known as much as cellular radiosensitivity. The syndrome of acute radiation may occur by failure of the bone marrow, gastrointestinal tract or central nervous system. The management of patients suffering from acute radiation syndromes still remains a major challenge. Survival of radiation induced bone marrow failure depends on the dose of radiation received. At radiation doses of 3 to 8 Gy, morbidity and lethality are primarily caused by hematopoietic injury. Our results suggest that bone marrow is highly susceptible to oxidative damage by the gamma radiation dose of 7 Gy, whose mechanism of action is directly related with changes in the intracellular calcium levels, increasing ROS and cell death apoptosis. It was observed that major processes resulting from oxidative stress include alteration of metabolic pathways, lipid peroxidation and the loss of intracellular calcium homeostasis. We demonstrated that this machinery is activated when apoptosis is induced by radiation. The signaling pathway after p53 activation leads to an increased expression of p21, which consequently affects the profile of the cell cycle and also leads to cell death by apoptosis. This confirms the hypothesis that perturbation of cellular redox homeostasis may control these key events in the process of cell death by apoptosis. In summary, our work demonstrates that radiation induced apoptosis is increased when p53 or p21 responsive G2 arrest occur, suggesting induction of premature senescence which may represent a novel underlying mechanism for radiation and may be able to contribute to the treatment of cancer by radiotherapy.

6. Acknowledgements

We would like to thank Unifesp and Uesc (collaborators) for their help in experiments with bone marrow cells mice. The authors gratefully acknowledge the financial support from Fapesp, Fapesb and CNPq grants.

7. References

Alam, S.; Sen, A.; Behie, L.A. & Kallos, M.S. (2004). Cell cycle kinetics of expanding populations of neural stem and progenitor cells in vitro. *Biotechnology and Bioengineering*. Vol.88,No.3,pp.332-347, ISSN 0006-3592

Baines, C.; Kaiser, R.; Purcell, N.; Blair, N.; Osinska, H.; Hambleton, M.; Brunskill, E.; Sayen, M.; Gottlieb, R.; Dorn, G. *et al.* (2005). Loss of cyclophilin D reveals a critical role for mitochondrial permeability transition in cell death. *Nature (London)* Vol.434, pp.658–662, ISSN 0028-0836

Bates, S. & Vousden, K. (1999). Mechanisms of p53-mediated apoptosis. *Cellular and Molecular Life Sciences*, Vol.55, No.1, pp.28–37, ISSN 1420-682X

Bates, S.; Hickman, E. & Vousden, K. (1999). Reversal of p53-induced cell-cycle arrest. *Molecular Carcinogenesis*, Vol.24, No.1, pp. 7–14, ISSN 0899-1987

Beausejour, C.; Krtolica, A.; Galimi, F.; Narita, M.; Lowe, S.; Yaswen, P. & Campisi, J. (2003). Reversal of human cellular senescence: roles of the p53 and p16 pathways. *The EMBO journal*, Vol.22, pp.4212-4222, ISSN 0261-4189

Bratton, S. & Cohen, G. (2001). Apoptotic death sensor: an organelle's alter ego? *Trends in Pharmacological Sciences*, Vol.22, pp.306–315, ISSN 0165-6147

Brookes, P. & Darley-Usmar, V. (2004). Role of calcium and superoxide dismutase in sensitizing mitochondria to peroxynitrite-induced permeability transition. *American Journal of Physiology. Heart and Circulatory Physiology*, Vol.286, pp.H39–H46, ISSN 0363-6135

Brookes, P. & Darley-Usmar, V. (2004). Role of calcium and superoxide dismutase in sensitizing mitochondria to peroxynitrite-induced permeability transition. *American Journal of Physiology. Heart and Circulatory Physiology*, Vol.286, pp.H39–H46, ISSN 0363-6135

Brookes, P.; Yoon, Y.; Robotham, J.; Anders, M. & Sheu, S. (2004). Calcium, ATP, and ROS: a mitochondrial love–hate triangle. *American Journal of Physiology. Cell physiology*, Vol.287, pp.C817–C833, ISNN 0363-6143

Campisi, J. (2005). Senescent cells, tumor suppression, and organismal aging: good citizens, bad neighbors. *Cell*, Vol.120, pp.513-522, ISSN 0092-8674

Canman, C.; Gilmer, T.; Coutts, S. & Kastan, M. (1995). Growth factor modulation of p53-mediated growth arrest versus apoptosis. *Genes & Development*, Vol.1, No.9, pp. 600-611, ISSN 0890-9369

Cmielová, J.; Havelek, R.; Jiroutová, A.; Kohlerová, R.; Seifrtová, M.; Muthná, D.; Vávrová, J. & Řezáčová, M. (2011). DNA Damage Caused by Ionizing Radiation in Embryonic Diploid Fibroblasts WI-38 Induces Both Apoptosis and Senescence. *Physiological Research*, Vol.60, pp.667-677, ISSN 0862-8408

Dimri, G.; Lee, X.; Basile, G. *et al.* A biomarker that identifies senescent human cells in culture and in aging skin in vivo. *Proceedings of the National Academy of Sciences of the United States of America*, Vol.92, pp.9363-9367, ISSN 0027-8424

Grynkiewicz, G.; Poenie, M.; Roger, Y. & Tsien, B. (1985). A New Generation of Ca2+ Indicators with Greatly Improved. Fluorescence Properties. *The journal of Biological Chemistry*, Vol.260, No.6, pp. 3440-3450, ISSN 1067-8816

Hengartner, M. (2000). The biochemistry of apoptosis. *Nature*, Vol.401, pp.770–6, ISSN 0028-0836

Ichas, F. & Mazat, J. (1998). From calcium signaling to cell death: two conformations for the mitochondrial permeability transition pore Switching from low- to highconductance state. *Biochimica et Biophysica Acta*, Vol.1366, pp. 33–50, ISSN 0006-3002

Vermesa, I.; Haanena, C.; Steffens-Nakkena, H. & Reutellingspergerb, C. (1995). A novel assay for apoptosis. Flow cytometric detection of phosphatidylserine expression on early apoptotic cells using fluorescein labelled Annexin V. *Journal of Immunological Methods*, Vol.184, No.1, pp.39-51, ISSN 0022-1759

Jagetia, G. & Venkatesh, P. (2007). .Inhibition of radiation-induced clastogenicity by Aegle marmelos (L.) correa in micebone marrow exposed to different doses of gamma-radiation. *Human & Experimental Toxicology*, Vol.26, No.2, pp.111-24, ISSN 0960-3271

Kokoszka, J.; Waymire, K.; Levy, S.; Sligh, J.; Cai, J.; Jones, D.; MacGregor, G. & Wallace, D. (2004). The ADP/ATP translocator is not essential for the mitochondrial permeability transition pore. *Nature (London)* Vol.427, pp.461–465, ISSN 0028-0836

Lowe, S. & Sherr, C. (2003). Tumor suppression by Ink4a-Arf: progress and puzzles. *Current Opinion in Genetics & Development*. Vol.13, pp.77-83, ISSN 0959-437X

Meng, A.; Wang, Y.; Van Zant, G. & Zhou, D. (2003). Ionizing radiation and busulfan induce premature senescence in murine bone marrow hematopoietic cells. *Cancer Res*earch, Vol.63, pp.5414-5419, ISSN 0008-5472

Nakabeppu, Y.; Tsuchimoto, D.; Yamaguchi, H. & Sakumi, K. (2007). Oxidative damage in nucleic acids and Parkinson's disease. *Journal of Neuroscience Research*, Vol.85, pp. 919–93, ISSN 1097-4547

Narita, M. & Lowe, S. (2004). Executing cell senescence. *Cell Cycle*, Vol.3, pp.244- 246, ISSN 1538-4101

Neben, S.; Hellman, S.; Montgomery, M.; Ferrara, J.; Mauch, P. & Hemman, S. (1993). Hematopoietic stem cell deficit of transplanted bone marrow previously exposed to cytotoxic agents. *Experimental hematology*, Vol.21, pp.156-162, ISSN 0301-472X

Nicoletti, I.; Migliorati, G.; Pagliaci, M.; Grignani, F. & Riccardi, C. (1991). A rapid and simple method for measuring thymocyte apoptosis by propidium iodide staining and flow cytometry. *Journal of Immunological Methods,* Vol.139, pp.271-279, ISSN 0022-1759

Paredes-Gamero, E.; Craveiro, R.; Pesquero, J.; França, J.; Oshiro, M. & Ferreira, A. (2006). Activation of P2Y1 receptor triggers two calcium signaling pathways in bone marrow erythroblasts. *European Journal of Pharmacology,* Vol.534, pp.30–38, ISSN 0014-2999

Poele, R.; Okorokov, A.; Jardine, L.; Cummings, J. & Joel, S. (2002). DNA damage is able to induce senescence in tumor cells in vitro and in vivo. *Cancer Research,* Vol.62, pp.1876-1883, ISSN 0008-5472

Rao, J.; Xu, D.; Zheng, F.; Long, Z.; Huang, S.; Wu, X.; Zhou, W.; Huang, R. & Liu, Q. (2011). Curcumin reduces expression of Bcl-2, leading to apoptosis in daunorubicin-insensitive CD34+ acute myeloid leukemia cell lines and primary sorted CD34+ acute myeloid leukemia cells. *Journal of Translational Medicine,* Vol.9, pp.71, ISSN 1479-5876

Reya, T. (2003). Regulation of hematopoietic stem cell self-renewal. *Recent Progress in Hormone Research,* Vol.58, pp.283-95, ISSN 0079-9963

Robles, S. & Adami, G. (2002). Agents that cause DNA double strand breaks lead to p16INK4a enrichment and the premature senescence of normal fibroblasts. *Oncogene,* Vol.16, pp.1113-1123, ISSN 0950-9232

Segreto, R.; Egami, M.; França, J.; Silva, M.; Ferreira, A. & Segreto, H. (1999). The bone marrow cells radioprotection by amifostine - nn/n ratio, apoptosis, ultrastructural and lipid matrix evaluation. *Interciencia,* Vol. 24, No.2, pp.127-134, ISSN 0378-1844

Sharpless, N. & DePinho, R. (1999). The INK4A/ARF lócus and its two gene products. *Current Opinion in Genetics & Development.* Vol.9, pp.22-30, ISSN 0959-437X

Szymczyk, K.; Shapiro, I. & Adams, C. (2004). Ionizing radiation sensitizes bone cells to apoptosis. *Bone,* Vol.34, No.1, pp. 148–156, ISSN 8756-3282

Toussaint, O.; Medrano, E. & von Zglinicki, T. (2000). Cellular and molecular mechanisms of stressinduced premature senescence (SIPS) of human diploid fibroblasts and melanocytes. *Experimental Gerontology,* Vol.35, pp.927-45, SSN 0531-5565

Vermes, V. I. , Haanen, C; Steffens-Nakken, H & Reutelingsperger, C. (1995). A novel assay for apoptosis - Flow cytometric detection of phosphatidylserine early apoptotic cells using fluorescein labeled expression on Annexin. *Journal of Immunological Methods,* Vol.184, pp. 39-51, ISSN 0022-1759

Vindeløv, L. & Christensen, I. (1990). A review of techniques and results obtained in one laboratory by an integrated system of methods designed for routine flow cytometric DNA analysis. *Cytometry.* Vol.11, pp.753-770, ISSN 1552-4922

Waldman, T.; Lengauer, C.; Kinzler, K. & Vogelstein, B. (1996). Uncoupling of S phase and mitosis induced by anticancer agents in cells lacking p21. *Nature,* Vol.381, No.6584, pp.713–716, ISSN 0028-0836

Walkley, C.; McArthur, G. & Purton, L. (2005). Cell division and hematopoietic stem cells: not always exhausting. *Cell Cycle,* Vol.4, pp.893-896, ISSN 1538-4101

Wang, Y.; Schulte, B.; LaRue, A.; Ogawa, M. & Zhou, D. (2006). Total body irradiation selectively induces murine hematopoietic stem cell senescence. *Blood,* Vol.107, pp.358-366, ISSN 0006-4971

Weissman, I.; Anderson, D. & Gage, F. (2001). Stem and progenitor cells: origins, phenotypes, lineage commitments, and transdifferentiations. *Annual Review of Cell and Developmental Biology*, Vol.17, pp.387-403, ISSN 1081-0706

Zamzami, N. & Kroemer, G. (2001). The mitochondrion in apoptosis: how Pandora's box opens. *Nature Reviews. Molecular Cell Biology*, Vol.2, pp. 67–71, ISSN 1471-0072

18

Early Events in Apoptosis Induction in Polymorphonuclear Leukocytes

Annelie Pichert, Denise Schlorke, Josefin Zschaler,
Jana Fleddermann, Maria Schönberg, Jörg Flemmig and Jürgen Arnhold
Institute for Medical Physics and Biophysics, University of Leipzig, Leipzig
Germany

1. Introduction

Different white blood cells are involved in immune responses to pathogens, environmental stress, alterations in energy and nutrition supply as well as traumata. To find an adequate answer to the myriad of exogenous and endogenous noxes is a high challenge for the human immune system. Chronic inflammatory diseases like rheumatoid arthritis, arteriosclerosis, inflammatory bowel disease, and many others are associated with a disturbed regulation of immune functions (Peng, 2006; Zernecke & Weber, 2010). Despite numerous worldwide investigations regulatory aspects are only scarcely understood in innate and acquired immunity.

Polymorphonuclear leukocytes (PMNs, also called neutrophils) are among the first cells that are rapidly recruited to infected and/or injured tissue. Their infiltration into inflammatory sites is highly regulated and supported by adhesion molecules, cytokines, and extracellular matrix components in both blood vessel wall and adjacent tissue (Muller, 2002; Taylor & Gallo, 2006). These cells, by releasing special proteins and generating reactive metabolites, contribute to pathogen defense, regulation of the inflammatory process, and to tissue injury.

Unperturbed or slightly activated PMNs die by apoptotic cell death (Walker et al., 2005; Erwig & Henson, 2007). The rapid clearance of apoptotic PMNs by macrophages is crucial for efficient resolution of inflammation including the activation of different anti-inflammatory mechanisms that stop the recruitment of novel immune cells, deactivate pro-inflammatory cytokines, depress pro-inflammatory and anti-apoptotic pathways, and promote tissue repair. Apoptosis is induced either by release of mitochondrial constituents or by signalling via death receptors. In these pathways, different initiator and executioner caspases are activated that induce the degradation of molecules of the cytoskeleton, DNA, and others. In the result, numerous apoptotic vesicles will be formed without the release of internal constituents.

Apoptosis induction is mainly counterregulated by signals from phosphoinositide 3-kinase and protein kinase B that suppress caspase activation (Simon, 2003). In PMNs, the anti-apoptotic pathway is activated when the cells phagocytose foreign microorganisms or become attached to other cells or materials. This pathway ensures the functional responsibility of PMNs at inflammatory sites.

Both apoptotic cells/vesicles or cells, in which the anti-apoptotic pathway is activated, can undergo a necrosis that represents a cell death accompanied by cell and organelle swelling, plasma membrane rupture, and release of cytoplasmic content. Besides uncontrolled necrosis due to physical stress, necrotic cell death may be induced and regulated by signalling pathways (Degterev & Yuan, 2008). The uptake of necrotic PMNs by macrophages is associated with the release of pro-inflammatory mediators that further promote the inflammatory process (Vandivier et al., 2006). Thus, the interplay between macrophages and apoptotic/necrotic cells, mostly with PMNs, considerably determines the fate of an inflammation. This scheme, although very simplified, is also supported by the fact that PMN apoptosis is highly delayed and dysregulated in patients with severe sepsis (Jiminez et al., 1997; Fanning et al., 1999).

Special products of apoptotic PMNs apparently contribute to induction of anti-inflammatory signaling pathways in macrophages. Among them, PMN-derived chloramines like taurine chloramine and monochloramine are known to dampen the activation of NFκB in pro-inflammatory cells (Kontny et al., 2003; Ogino et al., 2005). Moreover, the 5-lipoxygenase of PMNs is involved in the transcellular synthesis of lipoxins that are able to stop the invasion of unperturbed PMNs to inflammatory sites (Serhan et al., 2008). However, fine mechanisms of their involvement in regulation of inflammatory processes are only poorly understood.

Thus, the induction of apoptosis in PMNs is an important prerequisite for the successful resolution of immune responses. From this background, we give here an overview about flow cytometry approaches to study early events in activation of PMNs and in apoptosis induction in these cells. These methods enable determination of specific properties of a large number of individual cells in a very short time. Because it is impossible to consider flow cytometry analysis for all PMN constituents, we will focus here on the analysis of those components that are unique to PMNs and highly necessary for specific functions of this type of immune cells.

2. Early activation of PMNs

Recruitment of PMNs from peripheral blood is mediated by selectins and integrins (Springer, 1994). After firm adhesion to the endothelium, PMNs invade into the inflamed tissue. Several chemotactic factors form a gradient for the directed movement of PMNs to the inflammatory loci. The bacterial product fMet-Leu-Phe, soluble immune complexes, leukotriene B_4 and the cytokine interleukin 8 (IL-8) are important chemoattractant agents (Lin et al., 2004). PMNs express specific receptors to these chemotactic factors. Receptor activation by these agents causes local changes in the contractility of cytoskeleton components and favors a directed movement of the cells. As PMNs have to pave their way through the tightly packed vessel wall and adjacent regions filled with different extracellular matrix components, these cells express and release also special proteases helping to degrade tissue and matrix components. Among these proteases are collagenase, gelatinase, different other matrix metalloproteases and the specific PMN serine proteases proteinase 3, cathepsin G, and elastase.

Here we will focus on flow cytometry approaches for binding of IL-8 to PMNs and for the expression of PMN specific serine proteases on the surface of PMNs.

2.1 Binding of IL-8 to PMNs

The cytokine IL-8 (also called CXCL8 according to the chemokine nomenclature) is released at inflammatory sites from fibroblasts, monocytes, endothelial and epithelial cells. It is a strong chemoattractant to PMNs (Rajarathnam et al., 1994). Besides the receptor binding site (the ELR motif near the NH_2-terminus) on IL-8, there are positive charged epitopes on its surface involved in binding to sulfated glycosaminoglycans (Kuschert et al., 1999; Lortat-Jacob et al., 2002; Pichert et al., 2012). Around inflammatory loci, IL-8 is mostly fixed to sulfated extracellular matrix components forming, thus, a gradient for the invading PMNs.

Neutrophils have two kinds of G protein-coupled receptors for IL-8 called CXCR1 and CXCR2 (Stillie et al., 2009). Receptor activation causes phosphorylation of Akt, calcium influx, formation of F-actin, and cytoskeletal rearrangement. These events are important for chemotactic movement. Several factors are known to modulate the binding of IL-8 to its receptors. Alpha-1 antitrypsin and IL-8 form a complex that is unable to interact with CXCR1 (Bergin et al., 2010). Truncation of amino acids at the NH_2-terminus by matrix metalloproteases, CD13, cathepsin L, or proteinase 3 creates a series of natural isoforms of IL-8. Some of them have a higher biological activity than the original IL-8 protein with 77 amino acid residues (Padrines et al., 1994; Mortier et al., 2011).

Oligomerization of chemokines affects also their interaction with receptors. While both monomeric and dimeric IL-8 forms were capable of inducing cell recruitment, the dimeric form induced a stronger migration in a mouse lung model (Das et al., 2010). Binding to sulfated glycosaminoglycans promotes oligomerization of IL-8 (Hoogewerf et al., 1997).

The binding of recombinant IL-8 to PMNs is shown in Fig. 1.

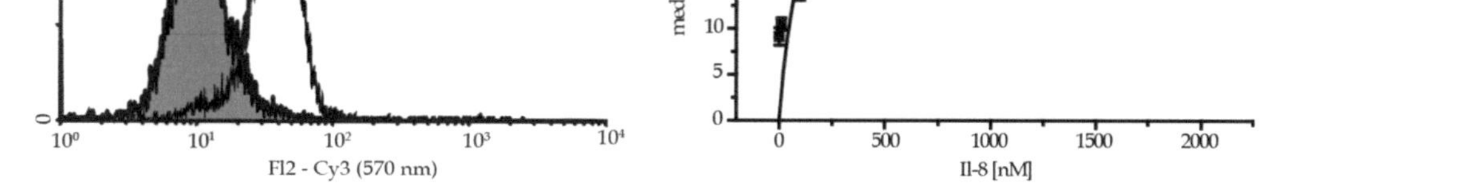

Fig. 1. Binding of IL-8 on the surface of freshly isolated PMNs. PMNs (2 x 10^6) were incubated with varying IL-8 concentrations for 60 min, followed by washing steps to remove unbound protein. After incubation of cells with the primary anti-human IL-8 rabbit antibody (4 µg/ml) for 1 h, PMNs were washed again and the secondary Cy3-conjugated goat anti-rabbit antibody (1.5 µg/ml) was added for 30 min in the dark. A representative example of fluorescence distribution in the presence of 1 µM IL-8 is shown in (a). The control is given in grey. Using median values from three independent measurements a binding curve was created with a K_d value of (112.7 ± 94.3) nM (b)

2.2 Detection of serine proteases on the surface of PMNs

In invading PMNs, the serine proteases proteinase 3, cathepsin G, and elastase are involved in microbicidal activity, penetration of cells through endothelium and adjacent connective tissue, and processing of various cytokines (Meyer-Hoffert, 2009; Kessenbrock et al., 2011). Although all three proteases have striking structural similarities (Korkmaz et al., 2008), there are clear differences in their functional response at inflammatory loci (Fleddermann et al., 2011). Unlike elastase, proteinase 3 and cathepsin G are already released from resting or slightly activated PMNs. While proteinase 3 binds heavily to cell surface epitopes, cathepsin G interacts preferentially with sulfated glycosaminoglycans. Proteinase 3 is apparently involved in both the infiltration of unperturbed PMNs into inflammatory sites and in cell necrosis, while cathepsin G plays most likely an important role in the degradation of specific components of the extracellular matrix during PMN invasion. In contrast, elastase probably contributes to shedding of surface molecules on macrophages helping to induce a pro-inflammatory feature in these cells (Pham, 2006). Examples for the incubation of resting PMNs with proteinase 3, cathepsin G, and elastase are given in Fig. 2.

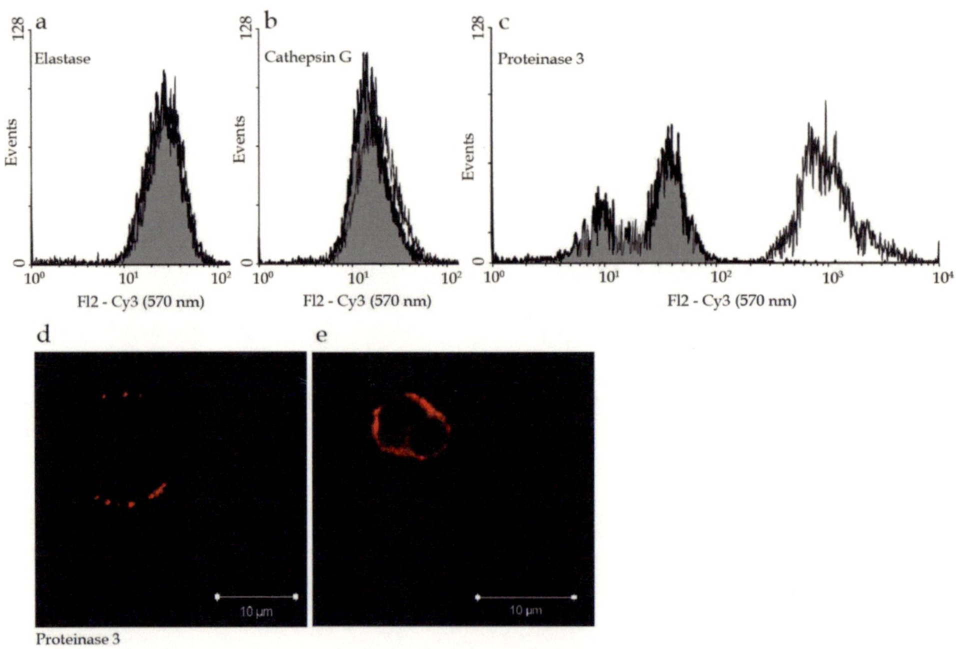

Fig. 2. Binding of externally added serine proteases on the surface of freshly isolated PMNs. Cells (2 x 10^6) were incubated with elastase (0.5 µM), cathepsin G (1.06 µM) and proteinase 3 (1.09 µM) for 1 h. After removal of unbound proteases by washing steps, PMNs were incubated with anti-neutrophil elastase rabbit antibody (134 µg/ml), anti-cathepsin G rabbit antibody (474 µg/ml) or mouse monoclonal proteinase 3 antibody (4 µg/ml) for 60 min. After washing and resuspension, Cy3-conjugated goat anti-mouse or goat anti-rabbit secondary antibodies (1.5 µg/ml) were added and incubated for 30 min in the dark (a-c). Flow cytometry distribution curves with externally added proteases are given in white. Controls are highlighted in grey. Representative confocal fluorescence microscopy images of freshly isolated PMNs treated with Cy3-labeled antibodies against proteinase 3 without (d) or after addition of proteinase 3 (e). Representative data from four measurements are given

As shown in Fig. 2, the difference in the amount of elastase and cathepsin G on the PMN surface is very small after protease addition. However, a drastic shift in fluorescence yield is observed in case of proteinase 3, indicating the existence of a high number of potential binding sites.

3. Alterations in PMNs during apoptosis induction

In contrast to other cell types, systems to resist an apoptosis induction such as glutathione-dependent antioxidant enzymes are expressed to a minor degree in PMNs (Kinnula et al., 2002). In non-affected tissue, PMNs are known to undergo a spontaneous apoptosis (Payne et al., 1994). This type of cell death can be simulated *in vitro* keeping the cells at 37 °C under sterile conditions for several days. Phorbol 12-myristate 13-acetate (PMA) or the calcium ionophore ionomycin accelerate this process and enable investigation of PMN apoptosis within few hours. PMNs activated by 50 nM PMA are characterized by enhanced hydrogen peroxide levels, reduced cell size, condensed nuclei, and enhanced DNA fragmentation (Lundqvist-Gustafsson & Bengtsson, 1999). A late event in apoptosis induction is the breakdown of the original cell into smaller apoptotic vesicles. Their rapid removal by macrophages prevents the release of toxic components due to secondary necrosis of these apoptotic bodies.

We compare sensitive flow cytometry approaches for the detection of changes in the vitality status of PMNs during spontaneous or PMA-mediated apoptosis. PMA was used at very low nanomolar concentrations in order to better visualize early changes during apoptosis induction. Here we present data about forward and sideward scattering of PMNs, binding of fluorescence-labeled annexin V to phosphatidylserine epitopes and the intercalation of propidium iodide into DNA as well as measurement of the integrity of mitochondria using the dye 5,5′,6,6′-tetrachloro-1,1′,3,3′-tetraethylbenzimidazolylcarbocyanine iodide (JC-1).

3.1 Forward and sideward scattering

While the value of the forward scatter depends on the cell size, the sideward scatter is a measure of the cell granularity. In flow cytometry analysis, the first parameter is usually plotted on a linear, the later one on a logarithmic scale.

The assessment of both kinds of scattering already provides a lot of information about the apoptotic process (Fig. 3). After apoptosis induction, a slight increase in the cell size takes place as visualized by a shift in the forward scattering values (Fig. 3b). The granularity remains unaffected. This alteration can be interpreted as a round-up of cells due to the progressive loss of linkages of the actin cytoskeleton with the plasma membrane. An early event in apoptosis induction in PMNs is the degradation of the corresponding link proteins (Kondo et al., 1997). Additionally, parts of the endoplasmic reticulum of the cells will be incorporated into the plasma membrane (Franz et al., 2007).

At later stages of apoptosis (Fig. 3c), enhanced forward scattering values vanished and smaller cell sizes became more prominent. At the same time a broader distribution of sideward scattering values was observed. This indicates the formation of polymorphic apoptotic bodies. The appearance of small apoptotic bodies (low forward and sideward scattering values) can also be seen during later apoptosis. Their appearance is a clear sign for the breakdown of apoptotic cells into smaller vesicles at later stages of apoptosis.

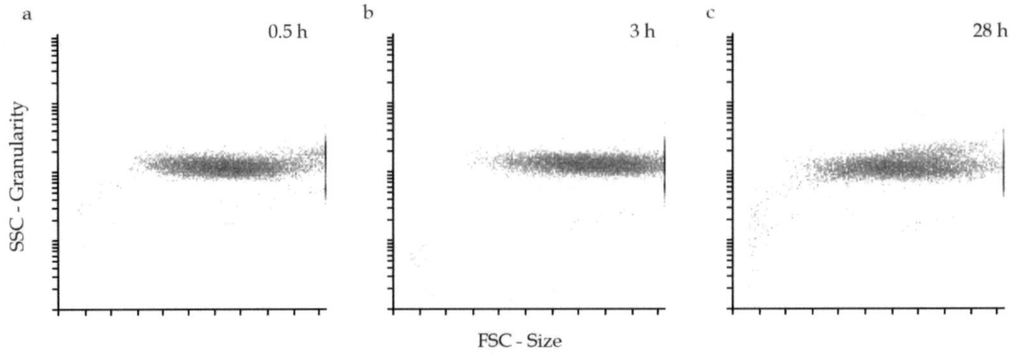

Fig. 3. Changes in cell size and granularity upon spontaneous apoptosis of PMNs. Cells (10^6) were cultivated at 37 °C for 0.5 h (a), 3 h (b), and 28 h (c), respectively. Changes in cell size and granularity were analyzed by flow cytometry using forward scattering (FSC) and sideward scattering (SSC). One representative example from four different cell preparations is shown

3.2 Binding of annexin V and uptake of propidium iodide

This approach is often used to assess the vitality status in a cell population. Vital cells do neither bind annexin V nor incorporate propidium iodide. Apoptotic cells are also unable to take up propidium iodide, but they express phosphatidylserine epitopes on the outer leaflet of the plasma membrane that are able to bind fluorescently labeled annexin V. In necrotic cells, propidium iodide permeates through the damaged plasma membrane and becomes highly fluorescent due to intercalation into DNA.

An example for analysis with both dyes in spontaneous and PMA-induced apoptosis in PMNs is given in Fig. 4.

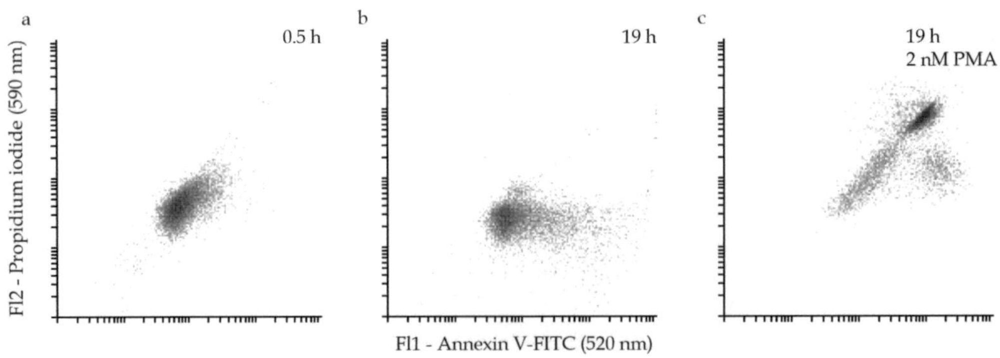

Fig. 4. Detection of apoptosis and necrosis in PMNs by annexin V and propidium iodide. PMNs (10^6) were cultivated at 37 °C for 0.5 h (a), or 19 h (b,c). In (c), cells were additionally activated by 2 nM PMA. Afterwards, PMNs were stained with fluorescently labeled annexin V (annexin V-FITC) and propidium iodide to detect apoptosis and necrosis, respectively. One representative example from four different experiments is shown

Freshly isolated PMNs did neither show any externalization of phosphatidylserine nor an uptake of propidium iodide (Fig. 4a). At prolonged incubation, part of the cells became annexin V-positive, but they did not incorporate propidium iodide (Fig. 4b). Thus, an apoptosis induction was observed. In contrast, the prolonged incubation of PMNs with PMA yielded double-positive cells with enhanced values in both channels (Fig. 4c). From these data necrotic processes in these PMNs can be assumed.

Although this method is very convenient, there are two main problems necessary to consider in its application. An accumulation of phosphatidylserine at the outer leaflet of the plasma membrane is observed in dying cells, where these epitopes serve as a matrix for a number of proteins like annexin 1, thrombospondin, and β_2-glycoprotein 1 and as a signal for cell clearance by macrophages (Lauber et al., 2004; Walker et al., 2005). In apoptotic cells, myeloperoxidase binds also to phosphatidylserine epitopes (Leßig et al., 2007; Flemmig et al., 2008). It is generally assumed that the phosphatidylserine exposure on the cell surface is associated with activation of scramblases and inhibition of translocases (Yoshida et al., 2005). In apoptotic PMNs, there are caspase-dependent and -independent mechanisms in the appearance of annexin V-positive epitopes (Blink et al., 2004; Chen et al., 2006). On the other hand, a transfer of phosphatidylserine from internal granule stores to the cell surface cannot be ruled out during apoptosis (Mirnikjoo et al., 2009).

The second problem concerns changes in the cell size and the breakdown of cells into smaller vesicles during apoptosis. These alterations are already illustrated in forward and sideward scattering (see the previous section). Thus at later stages of apoptosis, the appearance of smaller vesicles and cell debris would affect all fluorescence measurements. It cannot be excluded that these smaller vesicles, even though they are fluorescent, appear in the same gate where originally vital unperturbed cells were found.

3.3 Changes in mitochondria

Neutrophils possess only a few mitochondria that are functionally different in contrast to mitochondria of other cells. Their participation in ATP synthesis and cytochrome *c* content is limited, but they maintain a membrane potential (van Raam et al., 2006). Cellular stress is

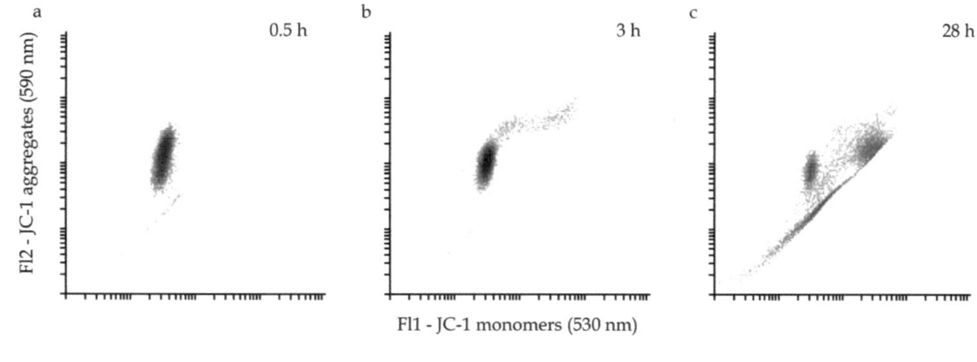

Fig. 5. Application of the dye JC-1 to detect early apoptotic events in PMNs. PMNs (10^6) were cultivated at 37 °C for 0.5 h (a), 3 h (b), or 28 h (c). Afterwards, cells were incubated with JC-1 (0.77 µM) for 10 min. After washing steps, the fluorescence of JC-1 monomers (channel 1) and aggregates (channel 2) was analyzed. Control experiments (not shown) were performed using the mitochondrial membrane ionophore valinomycin. One representative example from five different cell preparations is shown

sensitively reflected at the mitochondrial level leading to a rupture in processes maintaining the mitochondrial potential. In PMNs, pro-apoptotic proteins such as Smac/DIABLO, HtrA2/Omi and cytochrome *c* are released from mitochondria (Maianski et al., 2004). Early changes in mitochondrial integrity can be easily measured by the dye 5,5′,6,6′-tetrachloro-1,1′,3,3′-tetraethylbenzimidazolylcarbocyanine iodide (also called J-aggregate forming cationic dye, JC-1) (Cossarizza et al., 1993). This dye emits a red fluorescence when it accumulates in aggregated form in intact mitochondria. In apoptotic cells with damaged mitochondria, JC-1 is distributed over the whole cell cytoplasm and emits a green fluorescence.

We provide here an example for the application of this dye to PMNs undergoing a spontaneous apoptosis (Fig. 5). In freshly isolated vital PMNs with intact mitochondria, the dye is mainly incorporated in aggregated form with a dominating emission at 590 nm (Fig. 5a). The onset of apoptosis in PMNs was observable by increasing monomer fluorescence (Fig. 5b). At later times, nearly all cells showed a strong fluorescence of JC-1 monomers while the number of JC-1 aggregates was diminished (Fig. 5c).

3.4 Further systems for analysis of apoptosis induction

There are further flow cytometry approaches to detect changes in PMN vitality. As later stages of apoptosis are associated with progressive DNA fragmentation, the appearance of nicks in the DNA can be identified by the terminal deoxynucleotidyl transferase dUTP nick end labeling (TUNEL) assay. The investigation of PMN apoptosis in granulocyte preparations by the TUNEL assay can be affected by eosinophils that yield false positive results (Kern et al., 2000).

Active caspase-3 can be visualized in PMNs by enzyme inhibitors bearing a fluorescence label. This approach has been used to investigate effects of nicotinamide on PMN apoptosis (Fernandes et al., 2011).

4. Generation of oxidants during PMN apoptosis

PMNs are equipped with special enzymes for generation of a large amount of oxidants that are involved in antimicrobial activity, regulation of immune functions and apoptosis induction. These enzymes are NADPH oxidase (Shatwell & Segal, 1996) and myeloperoxidase (Klebanoff, 2005). While the first enzyme generates superoxide anion radicals that further dismutate to hydrogen peroxide, the heme protein myeloperoxidase uses H_2O_2 to oxidize (pseudo)halides to the corresponding (pseudo)hypohalous acids. Under physiological relevant conditions, the production of hypochlorous acid (HOCl) and hypothiocyanite (^-OSCN) is important (van Dalen et al., 1997). As myeloperoxidase is strongly expressed in PMNs (and to a lesser extent in monocytes) there is a great interest to understand specific functions of this enzyme during immune reactions of PMNs (Arnhold & Flemmig, 2010).

In PMNs, reactive oxygen species (ROS) are important for apoptosis induction. Apoptosis is delayed in NADPH oxidase deficiency (Lundqvist-Gustafsson & Bengtsson, 1999) and by scavenging of H_2O_2 by glutathione or catalase (Kasahara et al., 1997; Yamamoto et al., 2002). Interestingly, oxidants down-regulate phosphoinositide 3-kinase γ activity and inhibit actin polymerization during PMN apoptosis (Xu et al., 2010). Myeloperoxidase deficiency suppresses also PMN apoptosis (Tsurubuchi et al., 2001; Milla et al., 2004). Several myeloperoxidase products such as hypothiocyanite, monochloramine and taurine chloramine are potent inducers of apoptosis (Emerson et al., 2005; Lloyd et al., 2008; Ogino et al., 2009).

Here we focused our attention on two sensitive flow cytometry approaches for oxidant generation in close association with apoptosis induction in phorbol ester- and IL-8-activated PMNs. While dihydrorhodamine 123 detects very sensitively but non-specifically the oxidative activity in PMNs (Bizyukin et al., 1995), the combination of the dyes 2-[6-(4′-amino)phenoxy-3H-xanthen-3-on-9-yl]benzoic acid (APF) and 2-[6-(4′-hydroxy)phenoxy-3H-xanthen-3-on-9-yl]benzoic acid (HPF) allows to visualize specifically the generation of the myeloperoxidase product HOCl in PMNs (Setsukinai et al., 2003). Structures of these dyes are given in Fig. 6.

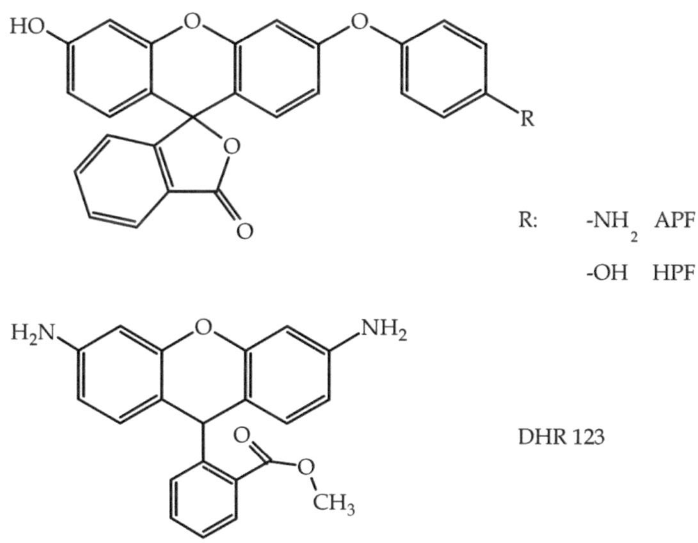

Fig. 6. Chemical structures of dyes applied for oxidant detection in PMNs

4.1 Dihydrorhodamine 123

The non-fluorescent compound dihydrorhodamine 123 is converted intracellularly into the fluorescent rhodamine 123 by several oxidants including superoxide anion radicals, hydrogen peroxide, hydroxyl radicals, hypochlorous acid, but not singlet oxygen (Bizyukin et al., 1995). This selection makes dihydrorhodamine 123 a suitable flow cytometric dye to follow the oxidative activity in neutrophils and other cells. The involvement of given enzymes in oxidant production can be determined by specific enzyme inhibitors.

Here we give an example for the application of dihydrorhodamine 123 to measure the oxidant generation in PMNs activated by the chemokine IL-8 (Fig. 7). In the presence of IL-8 significant higher fluorescence values were observed indicating a more promoted formation of oxidants in stimulated PMNs.

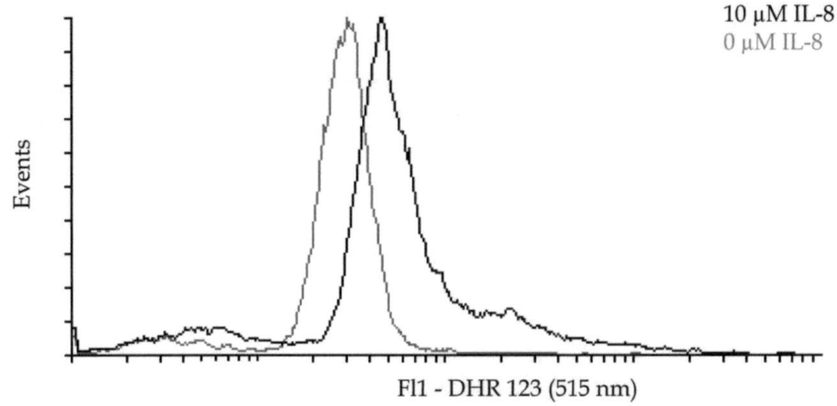

Fig. 7. Application of DHR 123 to detect the oxidative activity in PMNs. PMNs (2 x 10^6) were cultivated for 1 h at 37°C either in the presence (black) or in the absence (grey) of 10 µM IL-8. Afterwards they were stained with 10 µM DHR 123 and analyzed by flow cytometry. One representative example from four different experiments is shown

4.2 The APF/HPF system

In APF and HPF, the fluorescence is quenched by protection of the phenolic hydroxy group at the 6'-position of fluorescein with an electron-rich aromatic ring. The initial reaction with oxidants starts in both dyes by an attack on the aryloxyphenol group resulting in the cleavage of this group and the formation of highly emitting fluorescein. Hydroxyl radicals and peroxynitrite are able to oxidize both HPF and APF. HOCl activates only APF but not HPF. All other biologically relevant oxidants are insensitive against APF and HPF. This oxidant profile allows the application of APF and HPF to detect specifically the formation of HOCl in activated neutrophils (Setsukinai et al., 2003).

We successfully applied APF to visualize the production of HOCl in non-stimulated and PMA-activated neutrophils (Fig. 8). A significant stronger shift in the fluorescence intensity distribution of APF indicates a higher HOCl production in the stimulated cells. In both non-stimulated and PMA-stimulated PMNs the application of the MPO inhibitor 4-aminobenzoic acid hydrazide (4-ABAH) strongly inhibited the HOCl production as can be seen by much lower APF fluorescence values.

4.3 Further systems for oxidant detection

Among other unspecific dyes suitable for flow cytometric analysis of ROS generation in PMNs, we will mention only 2,7-dichlorofluorescein diacetate (Walrand et al., 2003). This non-fluorescent compound is converted by several oxidants into a fluorescent derivative. This system is often used to assess unspecific ROS formation in activated cells.

Besides the APF/HPF method for specific detection of HOCl generation in PMNs, a few further systems have recently been described to visualize the intracellular formation of HOCl. These novel approaches include the use of sulfonaphthoaminophenyl fluorescein (Shepherd et al., 2007), a rhodamin-hydroxamic acid-based system (Yang et al., 2009), and a thiol analogue of hydroxymethyltetramethylrhodamine (Kenmoku et al., 2007).

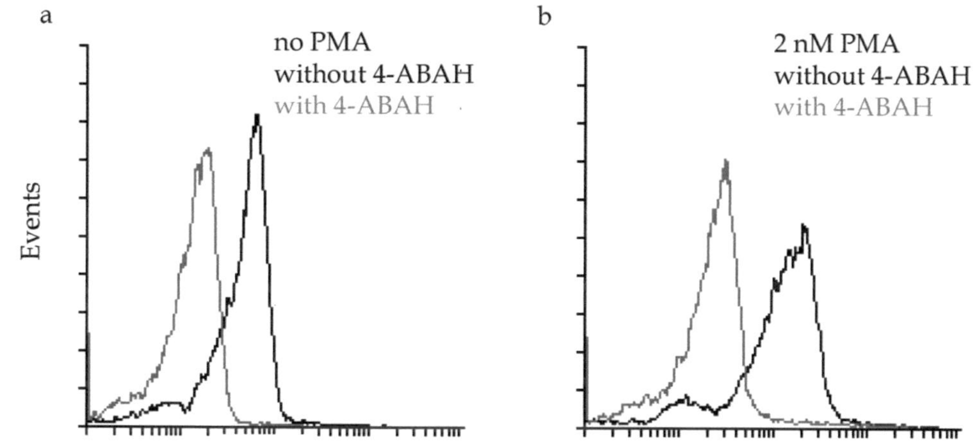

Fig. 8. Detection of HOCl generation in non-stimulated and PMA-stimulated PMNs. PMNs (10^6) were cultivated for 3 h either in the absence (a) or presence (b) of 2 nM PMA. In order to analyze the formation of the myeloperoxidase metabolite HOCl, APF (5 μM) was present during the incubation. In some cases, the myeloperoxidase inhibitor 4-aminobenzoic acid hydrazide (4-ABAH) was also included in the incubation cocktail (grey). One representative example of five different experiments is shown

5. Concluding remarks

Polymorphonuclear leukocytes are key players in innate and acquired immune response. Upon invasion to inflammatory sites, they sense their local environment and contribute to regulation of the further inflammatory process. For successful resolution of inflammation, the initiation of apoptotic cell death in PMNs and the subsequent fast removal of apoptotic bodies by macrophages are crucial. Despite numerous investigations, fine mechanisms of apoptosis induction in PMNs and factors modulating apoptotic pathways are only poorly understood.

Flow cytometry approaches are an important tool in this challenging field. We summarized here advantages and limitations of a number of widely applied methods, but focused also our attention on newly developed approaches for oxidant detection. The myeloperoxidase-hydrogen peroxide-halide system is unique to PMNs and its products are apparently involved in regulation of immune responses. Thus, novel methods for detection of hypochlorous acid generation such as the APF/HPF system are highly necessary for further investigation of modulation of myeloperoxidase activity.

We also directed our focus on enforcement of PMN apoptosis by low-concentrated PMA. This approach allows the convenient study of early changes during cell activation. In granulocytes, mitochondria are mainly responsible for providing pro-apoptotic factors that initiate caspase activation. The application of the dye JC-1 is useful to follow the loss of mitochondria integrity. Mechanisms leading to the appearance of phosphatidylserine epitopes remain puzzling. In this regard, distortions of enzyme reactions maintaining the phospholipid asymmetry and fusion events with internal granule stores are under discussion. Last but not least, the importance of oxidant generation is acknowledged for apoptosis induction in PMNs however, their fine mechanisms are poorly understood.

Detailed knowledge about PMN functions is also necessary to better understand the role of these immune cells in the pathogenesis of diseases and for introducing new therapies helping to terminate inflammatory processes.

6. Acknowledgements

This work was supported by the German Research Foundation (Transregio 67, project A-06) and by the Development Bank of Saxony, Germany.

7. References

Arnhold, J. & Flemmig, J. (2010) Human myeloperoxidase in innate and acquired immunity. *Arch. Biochem. Biophys.* 500, 92-106.

Bergin, D.A.; Reeves, E.P.; Meleady, P.; Henry, M.; McElvaney, O.J.; Carroll, T.P.; Condron, C.; Chotirmall, S.H.; Clynes, M.; O'Neill, S.J. & McElvaney, N.G. (2010) α-1 Antitrypsin regulates human neutrophil chemotaxis induced by soluble immune complexes and IL-8. *J. Clin. Invest.* 120, 4236-4250.

Bizyukin, A.V.; Korkina, L.G. & Velichkovskii, B.T. (1995) Comparative use of 2,7-dichlorofluorescin diacetate, dihydrorhodamine 123, and hydroethidine to study oxidative metabolism in phagocytic cells. *Bull. Exp. Biol. Med.* 119, 347-351.

Blink, E.; Maianski, N.A.; Alnemri, E.S.; Zervos, A.S.; Roos, S. & Kuijpers, T.W. (2004) Intramitochondrial serine protease activity of Omi/Htr2A is required for caspase-independent cell death of human neutrophils. *Cell Death Diff.* 11, 937-939.

Chen, H,-C.; Wang, C.-J.; Chou, C.-L.; Lin, S.-M.; Huang, C.-D.; Lin, T.-Y.; Wang, C.-H.; Lin, H.-C.; Yu, C.-T.; Kuo, H.-P. & Liu, C.-Y. (2006) Tumor necrosis factor-α induces caspase-independent cell death in human neutrophils via reactive oxidants and associated with calpain activity. *J. Biomed. Sci.* 13, 261-273.

Cossarizza, A.; Baccarani-Contri, M.; Kalashnikova, G. & Franceschi, C. (1993) A new method for the cytofluorimetric analysis of mitochondrial membrane potential using the J-aggregate forming lipophilic cation 5,5',6,6'-tetrachloro-1,1',3,3' tetraethylbenzimidazolylcarbocyanine iodide (JC-1). *Biochem. Biophys. Res. Commun.* 197, 40-45.

van Dalen, C.J.; Whitehouse, M.W.; Winterbourn C.C. & Kettle, A.J. (1997) Thiocyanate and chloride as competing substrates for myeloperoxidase. *Biochem. J.* 327, 487-492.

Das, S.T.; Rajagopalan, L.; Guerrero-Plata, A.; Sai, J.; Richmond, A.; Garafalo, R.P. & Rajarathman, K. (2010) Monomeric and dimeric CXCL8 are both essential for in vivo neutrophil recruitment. *PloS One* 5, e11754.

Degterev, A. & Yuan, J. (2008) Expansion and evolution of cell death programmes. *Nat. Rev. Mol. Cell. Biol.* 9, 378-390.

Emerson, D.K.; McCormick, M.L.; Schmidt, J.A. & Knudson, C.M. (2005) Taurine monochloramine activates a cell death pathway involving Bax and caspase-9. *J. Biol. Chem.* 280, 3233-3241.

Erwig, L.-P. & Henson, P.M. (2007) Immunological consequences of apoptotic cell phagocytosis. *Am. J. Pathol.* 171, 2-8.

Fanning, N.F.; Kell, M.R.; Shorten, G.D.; Kirwan, W.O.; Bouchier-Hayes, D.; Cotter, T.G. & Redmond, H.P. (1999) Circulating granulocyte macrophage colony-stimulating factor in plasma of patients with the systemic inflammatory response syndrome delays neutrophil apoptosis through inhibition of spontaneous reactive oxygen species generation. *Shock* 11, 167-174.

Fernandes, C.A.; Fievez, L.; Ucakar, B.; Neyrinck, A.M.; Fillee, C.; Huaux, F.; Delzenne, N.M.; Bureau, F. & Vanbever, R. (2011) Nicotinamide enhances apoptosis of G(M)-CSF-treated neutrophils and attenuates endotoxin-induced airway inflammation in mice. *Am. J. Physiol. Lung Cell. Mol. Physiol.* 300, L354-L361.

Fleddermann, J.; Pichert, A. & Arnhold, J. (2011) Interaction of serine proteases from polymorphonuclear leukocytes with the cell surface and heparin. *Inflammation*, in press.

Flemmig, J.; Leßig, J.; Reibetanz, U.; Dautel, P. & Arnhold, J. (2007) Non-vital polymorphonuclear leukocytes express myeloperoxidase on their surface. *Cell. Physiol. Biochem.* 21, 287-296.

Franz, S.; Herrmann, K.; Führnhorn, B.; Sheriff, A.; Frey, B.; Gaipl, U.S.; Voll, R.E.; Kalden, J.R.; Jäck, H.-M. & Herrmann, M. (2007) After shrinkage apoptotic cells expose internal membrane-derived epitopes on their plasma membranes. *Cell Death Differ.* 14, 733-742.

Hoogewerf, A.J.; Kuschert, G.S.V.; Proudfoot, A.E.I.; Borlat, F.; Clark-Lewis, I.; Power, C.A. & Wells, T.N.C. (1997) Glycosaminoglycans mediate cell surface oligomerization of chemokines. *Biochemistry* 36, 13570-13578.

Jiminez, M.F.; William, R.; Watson, G.; Parodo, J.; Evans, D.; Foster, D.; Steinberg, M.; Rotstein, O. & Marshall, J.C. (1997) Dysregulated expression of neutrophil apoptosis in the systemic inflammatory response syndrome. *Arch. Surg.* 132, 1263-1270.

Kasahara, Y.; Iwai, K.; Yachie, A.; Ohta, K.; Konno, A.; Seki, H.; Miyawaki, T. & Taniguchi, N. (1997) Involvement of reactive oxygen intermediates in spontaneous and CD95 (Fas/APO-1)-mediated apoptosis of neutrophils. *Blood* 89, 1748-1753.

Kenmoku, S.; Urano, Y.; Kojima, H. & Nagano, T. (2007) Development of a highly specific rhodamine-based fluorescence probe for hypochlorous acid and its application to real-time imaging of phagocytosis. *J. Am. Chem. Soc.* 129, 7313-7318.

Kern, P.M.; Herrmann, M.; Stockmeyer, B.; Kalden, J.R.; Valerius, T. & Repp, R. (2000) Flow cytometric discrimination between viable neutrophils, apoptotic neutrophils and eosinophils by double labelling of permeabilized blood granulocytes. *J. Immunol. Meth.* 241, 11-18.

Kessenbrock, K.; Dau, T. & Jenne, D.E. (2011) Tailor-made inflammation: how neutrophil serine proteases modulate the inflammatory response. *J. Mol. Med.* 89, 23-28.

Kinnula, V.L.; Soini, Y.S.; Kvist-Mäkelä, K.; Savolainen, E.-R. & Koistinen, P. (2002) Antioxidant defense mechanisms in human neutrophils. *Antioxid. Redox Signal.* 4, 27-34.

Klebanoff, S.J. (2005) Myeloperoxidase: friend and foe. *J. Leukoc. Biol.* 77, 598-625.

Kondo, T.; Takeuchi, K.; Dori, Y.; Yonemura, S.; Nagata, S.; Tsukita, S. & Tsukita, S. (1997) ERM (ezrin/radixin/moesin)-based molecular mechanism of microvilli breakdown at an early stage of apoptosis. *J. Cell Biol.* 139, 749-758.

Kontny, E.; Maslinki, W. & Marcinkiewicz, J. (2003) Anti-inflammatory activities of taurine chloramine. *Adv. Exp. Med. Biol.* 526, 845-852.

Korkmaz, B.; Moreau, T. & Gauthier, F. (2008) Neutrophil elastase, proteinase 3 and cathepsin G: physicochemical properties, activity and physiopathological functions. *Biochimie* 90, 227-242.

Kuschert, G.S.V.; Coulin, F.; Power, C.A.; Proudfoot, A.E.I.; Hubbard, R.E.; Hoogewerf, A.J. & Wells, T.N.C. (1999) Glycosaminoglycans interact selectively with chemokines and modulate receptor binding and cellular responses. *Biochemistry* 38, 12959-12968.

Lauber, K.; Blumenthal, S.G.; Waibel, M. & Wesselborg, S. (2004) Clearance of apoptotic cells: getting rid of the corpses. *Mol. Cell* 14, 277-287.

Leßig, J.; Spalteholz, H.; Reibetanz, U.; Salavei, P.; Fischlechner, M.; Glander, H.-J. & Arnhold, J. (2007) Myeloperoxidase binds to nonvital spermatozoa on phosphatidylserine epitopes. *Apoptosis* 12, 1803-1812.

Lin; F.; Nguyen, C.M.-C.; Wang, S.J.; Saadi, W.; Gross, S.P. & Jeon, N.L. (2004) Effective neutrophil chemotaxis is strongly influenced by mean IL-8 concentration. *Biochem. Biophys. Res. Commun.* 319, 576-581.

Lloyd, M.M.; van Reyk, D.M.; Davies, M.J. & Hawkins, C.L. (2008) Hypothiocyanous acid is a more potent induced of apoptosis and protein thiol depletion in murine macrophage cells than hypochlorous acid or hypobromous acid. *Biochem. J.* 414, 271-280.

Lortat-Jacob, H.M; Grosdidier, A. & Imberty, A. (2002) Structural diversity of heparan sulfate binding domains in chemokines. *Proc. Natl. Acad. Sci. USA* 99, 1229-1234.

Lundqvist-Gustafsson, H. & Bengtsson, T. (1999) Activation of the granule pool of the NADPH oxidase accelerates apoptosis in human neutrophils. *J. Leukoc. Biol.* 65, 196-204.

Maianski, N.A.; Geissler, J.; Srinivasula, S.M.; Alnemri, E.S.; Roos, D. & Kuijpers, T.W. (2004) Functional characterization of mitochondria in neutrophils: a role restricted to apoptosis. *Cell Death Diff.* 11, 143-153.

Meyer-Hoffert, U. (2009) Neutrophil-derived serine proteases modulate innate immune response. *Front. Biosci.* 14, 3409-3418.

Milla, C.; Yang, S.; Cornfield, D.N.; Brennan, M.-L.; Hazen, S.L.; Panoskaltsis-Mortari, A.; Blazar, B. & Haddad, I.Y. (2004) Myeloperoxidase deficiency enhances inflammation after allogenic marrow transplantation. *Am. J. Physiol. Lung Cell Mol. Physiol.* 287, L706-L714.

Mirnikjoo, B.; Balasubramanian, K. & Schroit, A.J. (2009) Suicidal membrane repair regulates phosphatidylserine externalization during apoptosis. *J. Biol. Chem.* 284, 22512-22516.

Mortier, A.; Gouwy, M.; van Damme, J. & Proost, P. (2011) Effect of posttransitional processing on the in vitro and in vivo activity of chemokines. *Exp. Cell Res.* 317, 642-654.

Muller, W.A. (2002) Leukocyte-endothelial cell interactions in the inflammatory response. *Lab. Invest.* 82, 521-533.

Ogino, T.; Hosako, M.; Hiramatsu, K.; Omori, M.; Ozaki, M. & Okada, S. (2005) Oxidative modification of IkappaB by monochloramine inhibits tumor necrosis factor alpha-induced NFkappaB activation. *Biochim. Biophys. Acta* 1746, 135-142.

Ogino, T.; Ozaki, M.; Hosako, M.; Omori, M.; Okada, S. & Matsukawa, A. (2009) Activation of c-Jun N-terminal kinase is essential for oxidative stress-induced Jurkat cell apoptosis by monochloramine. *Leuk. Res.* 33, 151-158.

Padrines, M.; Wolf, A.; Walz, A. & Baggiolini, M. (1994) Interleukin-8 processing by neutrophil elastase, cathepsin G and proteinase-3. *FEBS Lett.* 352, 231-235.

Payne, C.M.; Glasser, L.; Tischler, M.E.; Wyckoff, D.; Cromey, D.; Fiederlein, R. & Bohnert, O. (1994) Programmed cell death of the normal human neutrophil: an in vitro model of senescence. *Microsc. Res. Tech.* 28, 327-344.

Peng, S.L. (2006) Neutrophil apoptosis in autoimmunity. *J. Mol. Med.* 84, 122-125.

Pham, C.T.N. (2006) Neutrophil serine proteases: specific regulators of inflammation. *Nat. Rev. Immunol.* 6, 541-550.

Pichert, A.; Samsonov, S.; Theisgen, S.; Baumann, L.; Schiller, J.; Beck-Sickinger, A.G.; Huster, D. & Pisabarro M.T. (2012) Characterization of the interaction of interleukin-8 with hyaluronan, chondroitin sulfate, dermatan sulfate, and their sulfated derivatives by spectroscopy and molecular modelling. *Glycobiology*, 22, 134-145.

van Raam, B.J.; Verhoeven, A.J. & Kuijpers, T.W. (2006) Introduction: Mitochondria in neutrophil apoptosis. *Int. J. Hematol.* 84, 199-204.

Rajarathnam, K.; Sykes, B.D.; Kay, C.M.; Dewald, B.; Geiser, M.; Baggiolini, M. & Clark-Lewis, I. (1994) Neutrophil activation by monomeric interleukin-8. *Science* 264, 90-92.

Serhan, C.N.; Chiang, N. & van Dyke, T.E. (2008) Resolving inflammation: dual anti-inflammatory and pro-resolution lipid mediators. *Nat. Rev. Immunol.* 8, 349-361.

Setsukinai, K.; Urano, Y.; Kakinuma, K.; Majima, H.J. & Nagano, T. (2003) Development of novel fluorescence probes that can reliably detect reactive oxygen species and distinguish specific species. *J. Biol. Chem.* 278, 3170-3175.

Shatwell, K.P. Segal, A.W. (1996) NADPH oxidase. *Int. J. Cell Biol.* 28, 1191-1195.

Shepherd, J.; Hilderbrand, S.A.; Waterman, P.; Heinecke, J.W.; Weissleder, R. & Libby, P. (2007) A fluorescent probe for the detection of myeloperoxidase activity in atherosclerosis-associated macrophages. *Chem. Biol.* 14, 1221-1231.

Simon, H.-U. (2003) Neutrophil apoptosis pathways and their modifications in inflammation. *Immunol. Rev.* 193, 101-110.

Springer, T.A. (1994) Traffic signals for leukocyte recirculation and leukocyte emigration: the multistep paradigm. *Cell* 76, 301-314.

Stillie, R.M.; Farooq S.M.; Gordon, J.R. & Stadnyk, A.W. (2009) The functional significance behind expressing two IL-8 receptor types on PMN. *J. Leukoc. Biol.* 86, 529-543.

Taylor, K.R. & Gallo, R.L. (2006) Glycosaminoglycans and their proteoglycans: host-associated molecular pattern for initiation and modulation of inflammation. *FASEB J.* 20, 9-22.

Tsurubuchi, T.; Aratani, Y.; Maeda, N. & Koyama, H. (2001) Retardation of early-onset PMA-induced apoptosis in mouse neutrophils deficient in myeloperoxidase. *J. Leukoc. Biol.* 70, 52-58.

Vandivier, R.W.; Henson, P.M. & Douglas, I.S. (2006) Burying the dead. The impact of failed apoptotic cell removal (efferocytosis) on chronic inflammatory lung disease. *Chest* 129, 1673-1682.

Walker, A.; Ward, C.; Taylor, E.L.; Dransfield, I.; Hart, S.P.; Haslett, C. & Rossi, A.G. (2005) Regulation of neutrophil apoptosis and removal of apoptotic cells. *Curr. Drug Targets Inflamm. Allergy* 4, 447-454.

Walrand, S.; Valeix, S.; Rodriguez, C.; Ligot, P.; Chassagne, J. & Vasson, M.P. (2003) Flow cytometry study of polymorphonuclear neutrophil oxidative burst: a comparison of three fluorescent probes. *Clin. Chim. Acta* 33, 103-110.

Xu, Y.; Loison, F. & Luo, H.R. (2010) Neutrophil spontaneous death is mediated by down-regulation of autocrine signaling through GPCR, PI3Kγ, ROS, and actin. *Proc. Nat. Acad. Sci.* 107, 2950-2955.

Yamamoto, A.; Taniuchi, S.; Tsuji, S.; Hasui, M. & Kobayashi, Y. (2002) Role of reactive oxygen species in neutrophil apoptosis following ingestion of heat-killed Staphylococcus aureus. *Clin. Exp. Immunol.* 129, 479-484.

Yang, Y.-K.; Cho, H.J.; Lee, J.; Shin, I. & Tae, J. (2009) A rhodamine-hydroxamic acid-based fluorescent probe for hypochlorous acid and its application to biological imagings. *Org. Lett.* 11, 859-861.

Yoshida, H.; Kawane, K.; Koike, M.; Uchiyama, Y. & Nagata, S. (2005) Phosphatidylserine-dependent engulfment by macrophages of nuclei from erythroid precursor cells. *Nature* 437, 754-758.

Zernecke, A. & Weber, C. (2010) Chemokines in the vascular inflammatory response of atherosclerosis. *Cardiovasc. Res.* 86, 192-201.

19

New Insights into Cell Encapsulation and the Role of Proteins During Flow Cytometry

Sinéad B. Doherty and A. Brodkorb
Teagasc Food Research Centre Moorepark, Fermoy, Co. Cork, Ireland

1. Introduction

Modern approaches to science tend to follow divergent paths. On one hand, instruments and technologies are developed to capture as much information as possible with the need for complex data analysis to identify problematic issues. On the other hand, formulation focused, minimalistic approaches that gather only the most pertinent data for specific questions also represent a powerful methodology. This chapter will provide many examples of the latter by integrating Flow Cytometry (FACS - Fluorescence-Activated Cell Sorting) technology with high throughput screening (HTS) of encapsulation systems with extensive utility of one-dimensional (1-D) imaging for protein localisation. In this regard, less information is acquired from each cell, data files will be more manageable, easier to analyse and throughput screening will be significantly enhanced beyond traditional HTS analysis, irrespective of the protein concentration present in the background or delivery media.

1.1 Real-time on-line monitoring of bioprocesses

The production of heterologous therapeutic proteins is well established in today's biotechnology industry; however their presence during cytometric screening poses complex analytical obstacles for food and biotechnologists alike. The Process Analytical Technology (PAT) initiative, launched by the Food and Drug Administration (FDA) encourages extensive process understanding to achieve the desired quality of pharmaceutical and bioactive protein products rather than a 'quality-by-testing' approach. Thus, elucidating and monitoring variations within protein production, purification and encapsulation systems is fundamental for quality control, protein detection and localisation (Glassey et al., 2011). One key issue for PAT is the use of on-line process analysers; in this context, 'on-line' is used in the sense of 'fully automatic' or 'without any manual interaction'.

The foundation of early microscopy and its transition to the modern FACS nowadays, proved that cell growth within a population differs significantly from one cell to another. These heterogeneities are caused by either fluctuations in the micro-environment of individual cells (Dunlop and Ye, 1990); phenotypic changes during the cell cycle (Münch et al., 1992); or by mutations resulting in genotypic variations in the population (Hall, 1995) leading to different protein expression levels. Thus, the most important variable in a bioprocess - cell productivity of a heterologous protein product - is distributed over a wide range within the cell population. Protein analytical methods (i.e. SDS-PAGE, Western blot,

MALD-TOF-MS) are off-line, time and cost intensive, require human interaction and are not capable of exhibiting protein expression levels in single cell level. Earlier studies demonstrated that tagging the target protein with a fluorescent reporter molecule (green fluorescent protein GFP) permits detection of low protein concentrations by measuring the reporter molecule's specific fluorescence (Broger et al., 2011). Specific protein fluorescence signals can be measured through on-line, *in situ* fluorescence sensors (Jones et al., 2004, Reischer et al., 2004); but the main drawback of these measuring techniques is that they all result in population averaged data; hence analysis of single cell productivity was not possible. As mentioned FACS is one of the available methods for measurement of population distribution and has been exploited in biotechnology (Rieseberg et al., 2001). To overcome this disadvantage of FACS as an off-line analyser, a number of flow injection (FI) flow cytometer systems have been designed for the determination of proteins (Kelley, 1989). Ruzicka and Lindberg (1992) were the first to utilise FI as an interface between a bioreactor and FACS. Further progress in FI-FACS has been made by Srienc and co-workers (Zhao et al., 1999), examining population dynamics of *Saccharomyces cerevisiae* (Kacmar and Srienc, 2005) and growth dynamics of Chinese Hamster Ovary (CHO) cells and their associated proteins (Sitton and Srienc, 2008a, b). None of them, however, measure single-cell productivity using fluorescent reporter tag co-expressed with target protein, which restricts the purification of secreted protein products.

1.2 Efficacious phenotypic analyses of cell encapsulation systems

Cellular detection and characterization usually involves cell harvesting for more than 20 generations in order to achieve the formation of macro-colonies on solid media. What is more, encapsulation provides an innovative solution for the handling and use of live cells through the use of three-dimensional scaffolds. These scaffolds - commonly known as beads or capsules - can be used in a number of ways, such as for the isolation of individual cells to form clonal populations, for establishing partial barrier for cells from their environment, and for creating a matrix allowing the formation of 3D-cell cultures or clusters. These methods have important implications for the biomedical engineering field and the areas of biomanufacturing and bioprocessing. Nonetheless, a myriad of information remains to be discovered. For example, the chemical composition and engineered functionalities of these scaffolds affect the biology of the encapsulated cells. One particular system that has recently achieved significant recognition are the dairy proteins. A variety of cell types can be enclosed in casein or whey beads scaffolds in a range of sizes. While maintaining their morphology and function, these encapsulated cells can proliferate, form cell clusters, and even lay down extracellular matrix components. Furthermore, cells can be encapsulated in small particles that can then be handled, characterized and analysed with ease. These features make milk proteins an attractive encapsulation material for three dimensional scaffolds of live cells. Meanwhile, HTS of these encapsulated cells is restricted by several practical aspects including low sample throughput, protein matrix limitations and the absence of sorting capability for mixed cell cultures. Hence, a unique reconsideration of conventional cytometric approaches for accelerated food and/ or bioprocess intensification represents a timely research strategy for encapsulation technologists and cytometrists alike. It was recently discovered (Delgado et al., 2010) that microbial growth can be monitored in encapsulated cell systems by following the development of micro-colonies. Therefore, development and dissemination of a FACS technology capable of analysing encapsulated cells within intact micro-capsules encapsulation systems would represent a novel cytometric strategy for academic and industrial applications. This approach would require knowledge management of cytometric control parameters, which would generate reduced capital cost, human error and environmental deterrents associated with conventionally high-throughput screening strategies. However, there is a need for addressing physico-chemical properties of micro-capsules for efficient cytometric screening without i) occlusion of capsular flow in the fluidics system during hydrodynamic focusing or ii) adverse interactions between protein (originating from the micro-capsule or cell metabolic activity) and cytometric buffer media during the screening process.

Delgado et al., (2010) demonstrated that cell proliferation within encapsulation systems can be detected via FACS, provided that the population of capsules exhibit appropriate optical and mechanical properties and are mono-dispersed in size and shape. Encapsulated cells can be further utilized for a variety of applications: from characterizing secreted enzymes to detection of thermo-sensitive mutants. Delgado et al., (2010) successfully revealed the application of Flow Focusing® technology for microencapsulated cells of different types in mono-disperse hydrogel microspheres. Using a CellENA® Flow Focusing® microencapsulator, monodisperse capsules were fabricated containing one single cell with sizes ranging from

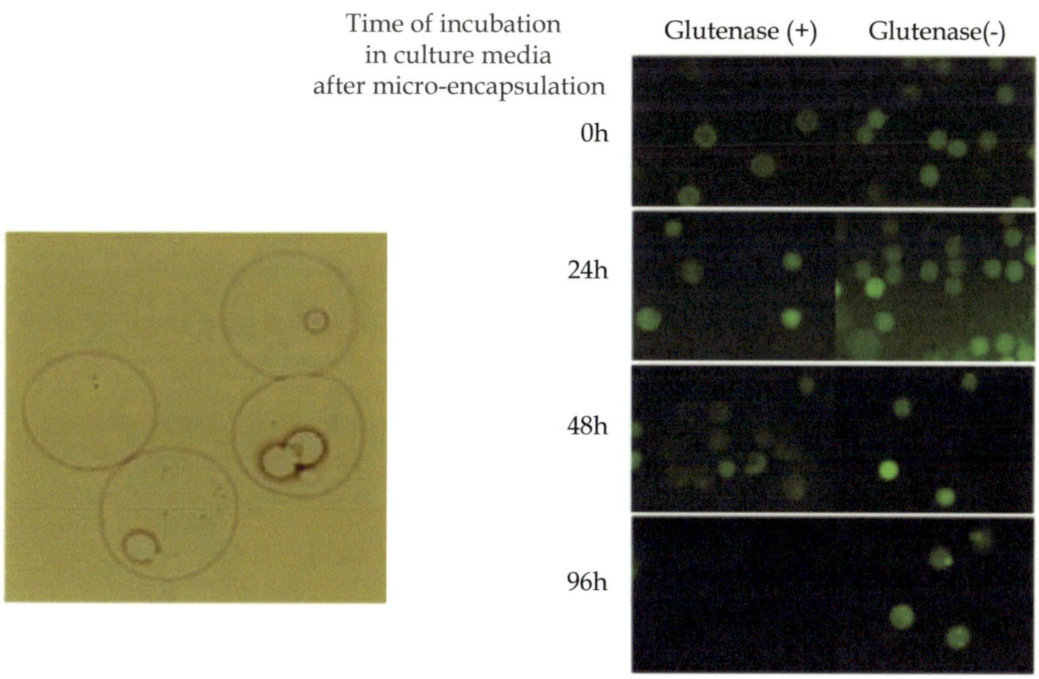

Source: (Delgado et al., 2011). http://www.cellena.net/en/documents/CellenaPoster.pdf

Fig. 1. Data detecting glutenases in micro-encapsulated bacteria. Colonies of bacteria were grown in gliadin-containing capsules. Images on the right illustrate the change in fluorescent intensity as a function of incubation time in culture media after micro-encapsulation. Gliadin content was detected by incubating the particles with the monoclonal antibody G12, conjugated to FITC. The micrograph on the left illustrated colonies of bacteria growing gliadin-containing micorparticles (Delgado et al., 2011)

100 µm to over 600 µm diameter. This offers a plethora of applications including the characterization of secreted therapeutic proteins to detect encapsulated cells or thermo-sensitive mutants. More importantly, cell proliferation inside the micro-capsules was detected by FACS without the need for fluorescent labelling, which represents a significant development (Delgado et al., 2011). Furthermore, bacteria expressing glutenase activity, isolated from agrochemical samples were detected by their ability to degrade gliadin when growing inside capsules as shown in Figure 1. Gliadin content was detected by incubating the particles with the monoclonal antibody G12, conjugated to FITC (Delgado et al., 2010). Further information relating to COPAS analysis can be obtained from Union Biometrica (http://www.unionbio.com/).

Figure 2 illustrates capsules containing yeast colonies incubated for different times. Data revealed that capsules had a similar size (Time of Flight; TOF) but differed in optical complexity (Extinction; EXT). Hence, different yeast concentrations were predicted as a function of time. This Flow Focusing® Technology from Union Biometrica, Belgium, will inevitably bring additional utility and commercial recognition to FACS as an economically viable biochemical application for improved analytical monitoring of downstream processing during fermentation and drug/ protein generation. Figure 3 illustrates the successful analysis of protein capsules based on size (TOF) and extinction (EXT). The best resolution was obtained with the 561nm solid state laser due to higher penetration into the protein capsule, which will depend upon membrane thickness, coating or presence of a

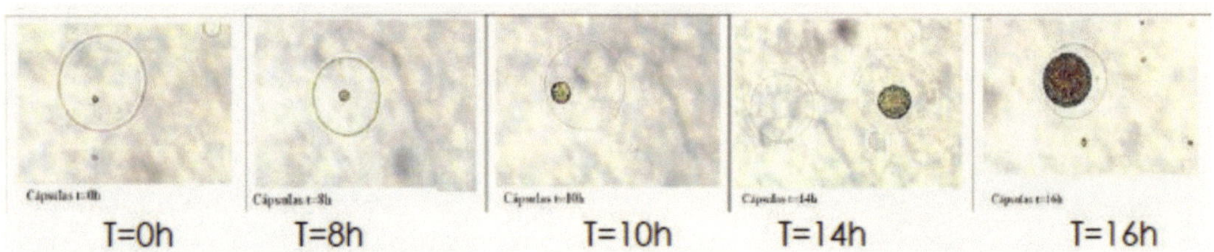

Source: (Delgado et al., 2011). http://www.cellena.net/en/documents/CellenaPoster.pdf

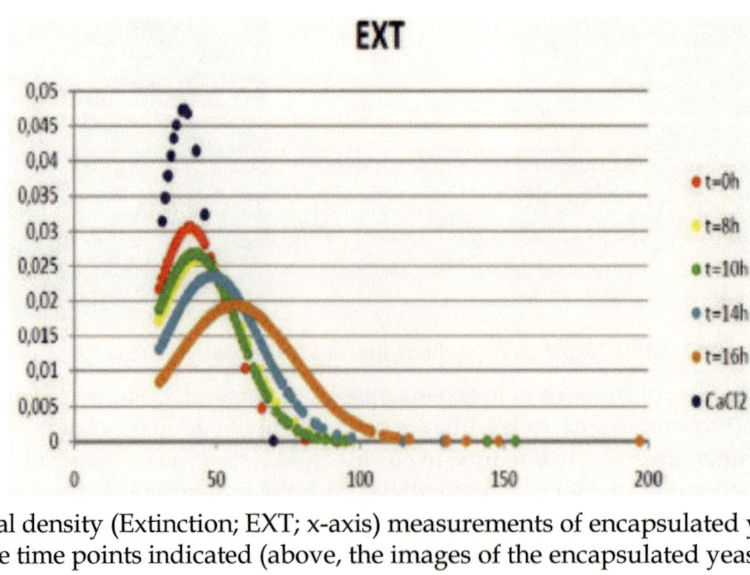

Fig. 2. Optical density (Extinction; EXT; x-axis) measurements of encapsulated yeast following the time points indicated (above, the images of the encapsulated yeast)

surface cross-linker. It was also demonstrated that maximum peak height can be used as a sorting parameter for cytometric sorting of encapsulated cells in protein capsules. Further research is currently being conducted in this promising area of cytometric analysis.

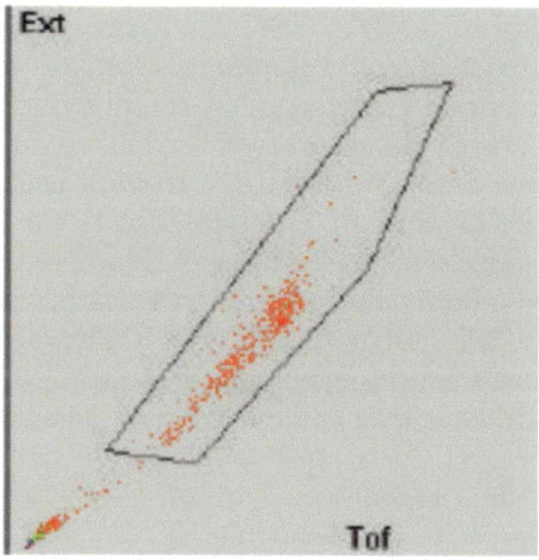

Fig. 3. Displays the dot plots TOF vs. EXT for empty protein capsules. TOF is an indicator of size, while EXT represents the density of the detected object

These developments may aid bioprocessing technology, improve process development and analytical control by sorting cells based on i) micro-capsule size; ii) cell type; iii) cell density; iv) monoclonality and v) protein expression. In this way, fluorescent tagging is not an essential requirement for the characterisation of encapsulated cell cultures and their respective recombinant proteins, which demonstrates a significant development for cost- and time-efficient cytometric screening. Moreover, encapsulation evaluation using Flow Focusing® Technology, can be used for phenotypic analysis of encapsulated cells, such as the expression of specific characteristics of microbial colonies (glutenase expression by bacteria) or growth-related phenotypes (antibiotic resistance and proliferation in thermo-sensitive yeast). Mammalian cells are delicate, difficult to handle and manipulate individually. However, these cells can be encapsulated within a polymer material such as protein or alginate, and these encapsulated scaffolds remain intact throughout all steps of cytometric analysis and dispensing. Furthermore, fragile cells like adipocyte stem cells remain viable for extended periods of time (2 weeks) (Delgado et al., 2010) and can be released and recovered to permit further analysis and use, which endorses an exclusive cytometric development.

1.3 High throughput processing of encapsulated bacterial libraries

Industrial interest in encapsulation has grown exponentially in the fields of bioprocessing, fermentation and elucidation of bacterial libraries, especially in high-throughput environments exceeding 10^6 samples per day. Fundamental pre-requisites reveal the necessity for a one-to-one relationship between individual cells and analytical algorithms. Essentially, each micro-carrier (i.e. capsule) would therefore contain exactly one cell or colony. However, synthesis of larger numbers of capsules containing exactly one cell is not feasible as cells are randomly distributed during capsule production. The problem is clear -

high dilution conditions will yield an adequate degree of monoclonality; however, this will be coupled with the generation of a significant fraction of empty micro-capsules. Conversely, distribution under low dilution conditions will generate unacceptable numbers of polyclonal capsules for whose removal no satisfactory technologies exists to date. Recent finding demonstrated (Walser et al., 2008, 2009) that hydrogel micro-carriers can be applied as growth milieu for individual cell colonies. *Escherichia coli* cells expressing green fluorescent protein (GFP) were encapsulated at low dilution thereby intentionally producing a considerable amount of polyclonal micro-carriers. Empty and polyclonal micro-carriers were then removed from the desired monoclonal fraction using a particle analyzer. Data was compared to model predictions in order to investigate possible limitations in the analysis and sorting of monoclonal micro-carriers. Fluorescent *E. coli* cells (GFP) were randomly distributed throughout the micro-carrier population and cells successfully propagated to colonies in the micro-carrier with enrichment to 95% monoclonality. Interestingly, colony diameter represents a limiting factor for enrichment-efficiency in encapsulation systems. With increasing colony size, two antagonistic effects are associated with the cytometric approach: First, improved sorting efficiency due to increased fluorescence intensity and thus higher detection efficiency, and second, deterioration of sorting efficiency due to occlusion occurring in polyclonal micro-capsules. Hence, encapsulation under low dilution conditions with high-throughput sorting via FACS represents a practical economically viable initiative for isolating large quantities of monoclonal micro-capsules from bacterial libraries and at the same time, keeping the amounts of empty micro-capsules at a moderate level.

1.4 Utilization of micro-capsules for next generation cytometric assays

It is evident that cytometric screening is a pragmatic approach for integration of cell encapsulation within continuous bioprocesses. Subsequent segregation and sorting of microcapsules containing high cell densities of animal cells and associated proteins has recently catalysed interest in cytometric screening. Research performed by Union Biometrica Inc. (www.unionbiometrica.com) applied this technology and found COPAS™ (Complex Object Parametric Analyzer and Sorter) suitable for automated analysis, sorting, and dispensing of 'large' objects such as capsules. The COPAS™ PLUS is capable of analysing particles with diameters of 30 - 800 µm in a continuously flowing stream at a rate of 25-50 objects/second. Physical properties such as size, optical density and intensity of fluorescent markers are taken into consideration. To avoid damaging or changing the fragile biological samples, a gentle pneumatic device located after the flow cell is used for sorting encapsulated cells and therefore makes the instrument suitable for handling live biological materials or sensitive proteins (Figure 4). It is interesting to note that the fluid pressures of the instrument are also significantly lower than those of traditional flow cytometers. The COPAS™ XL instrument has a 2,000 µm flow cell, which allows the analysis of larger beads (30-1,500 µm) compared to the COPAS™ PLUS. If an encapsulated sample contains certain fluorophores that can be excited by light of 488 nm, the emission levels can be detected for each of the objects in the encapsulated system.

Figure 4 details the analysis of intact encapsulation capsules inside the flow cells. Objects are carried through the flow cell by a liquid stream while their physical properties are being measured. Convergence of the sheath and sample fluid allows "hydrodynamic focusing" of the micro-capsules, forcing them to go through the centre of the flow cell along their

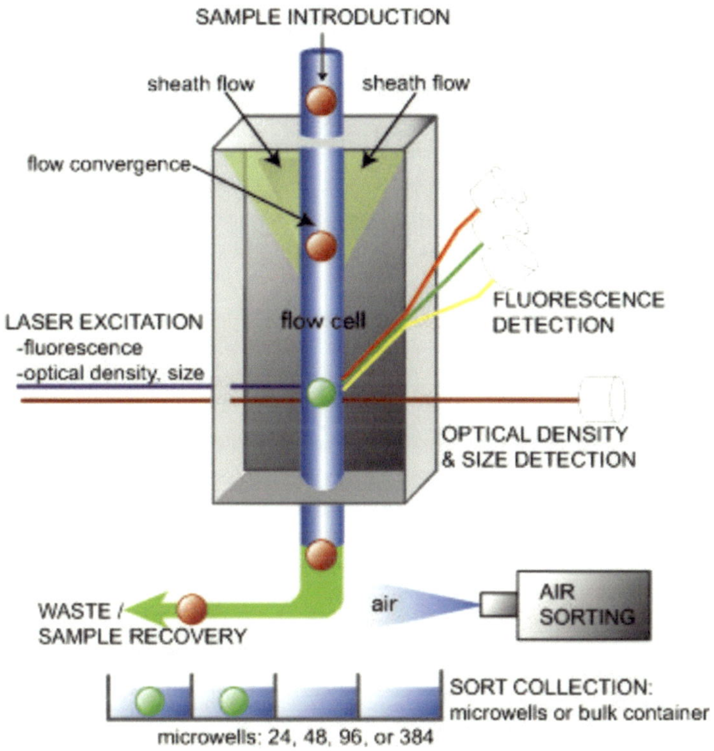

(a)

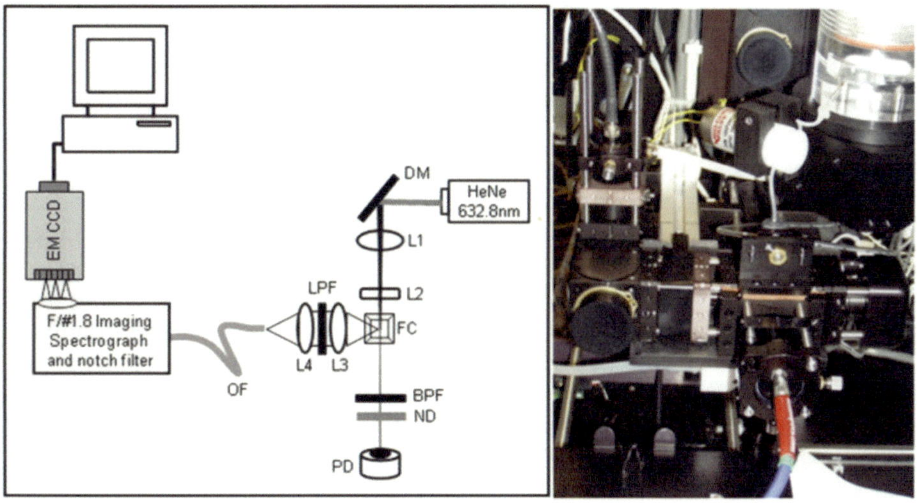

(b)

Fig. 4. Schematic of Flow Focus Technology™ shown in (a). Figure (b) illustrates a schematic (left) and an image (right) of the spectral detection leg constructed on the open face of the COPAS™ flow cell (Watson et al., 2009). DM: dichroic mirror; L1: 80 mm spherical lens; L2: 6 mm cylindrical lens; FC: flow cell; L3, L4: 21 mm aspherical lenses; OF: optical fiber; ND: 0.8 OD neutral density filter longitudinal axes. Inside the flow cell objects are illuminated by two low energy lasers that measure the microcapsule optical properties inclusive of size, optical density and fluorescence. Micro-capsules that meet the sort criteria are permitted to drop into sort collection, while those that do not are diverted to waste recovery using a pneumatic sorting device. Cells may be classified according to their fluorescent intensity or optical density, which will accommodate a greater efficiency for detection of recombinant proteins during encapsulation procedures. Preliminary studies performed using COPAS™ instrumentation has demonstrated the discrimination of hydrogel microcapsules containing mixed cell cultures. During initial sampling, micro-capsules were selected based on their size (TOF), monoclonality and optical density (EXT). Preparation of a standard curve using micro-capsules of known size and TOF measurements provided a practical correlation between TOF measurements generated by the flow cytometer and the actual size. Hence, it is plausible to select micro-capsules that meet specific size and optical density criteria. Furthermore, encapsulated cells can also be chosen to meet criteria of size, optical density and levels of green and red fluorescence. Hence, it is also possible to sort micro-capsules with various magnitudes of cell growth, cell density and recombinant protein content.

Watson et al., (2009) successfully adapted Union Biometrica COPAS™ Plus instrument to allow red excitation and optical fiber-based light collection and spectral analysis using a spectrograph and CCD array detector (Figure 4B). These modifications did not compromise the ability of the instrument to resolve different sized capsules based on their extinction (EXT) and time of flight (TOF) signals. The modified instrument has the sensitivity and spectral resolution to measure the fluorescence and Raman signals from individual particles with signal integration times of 10 usecond. The high speed spectral analysis of individual particles in flow will enable new applications in biological encapsulation systems

2. High content screening – getting more for less

High content screening (HCS) can identify proteins via automated image analysis and, in general, is designed to capture image information regarding cells and associated protein products. The availability of commercial imaging systems has made HCS increasingly practical for protein determination and has placed HCS into a standard tool for protein and drug discovery (Zanella et al., 2010). The value of this protein determination approach is apparent since a vast number of cellular characteristics can be captured in large data files. Over the past decade advances in information technology and biological probes have led to practically automated image analysis with throughput far above that possible by manual cell analysis in protein-rich environments. Several commercial instruments are now available for HCS of proteins, for example the *BD Pathway* (BD Biosciences), *In cell Analyzer* (GE healthcare), *ImageXpress Ultra* (Molecular Devices) and *Scan^R* (Olympus), to name a few. The *Imagestream* (Amnis) is a relatively new instrument that combines aspects of FACS with image analysis, resulting in a device capable of imaging cells at multiple fluorescent wavelengths with a throughput of hundreds of cells per second (Reardon et al., 2009). In HCS devices, the presence of environmental protein presents trade-offs between the quantity (and quality) of data acquired and throughput. Hence, environmental protein is a hindrance to the efficacy of cytometric screening. The *Imagestream*, for example, trades ultrahigh image resolution for speed, and many cellular images are captured in one data file, the size of which can easily exceed 3 gigabytes.

3. Cytometric limitations associated with environmental protein

Contemporary approaches to food fermentations and drug discoveries frequently use HTS to measure the fluorescence of cellular features tagged with fluorochrome-conjugated antibodies or other fluorescent labels in a very rapid manner. This is quite often performed by FACS, a technique well-suited to this purpose. However, tagged cells are often entrapped within a dense protein matrix or lattice, which represents an obstacle against true microbial counts. Hence, applications can be significantly hindered by the presence of proteins since environmental protein particles, matching the size range of cells, are often recognised as cellular bodies during hydrodynamic focusing. An appropriate methodology is therefore required to eliminate interfering environmental protein - non-cellular in origin - from cytometric analysis for successful application of cytometric screening. Traditional FACS can easily capture emissions from ten or more different fluorochromes on a cell at rates exceeding 25,000 cells per second. Although this is appropriate for many assays, FACS cannot provide accurate details on cell morphology or subcellular localisation of fluorescence in the presence of obtrusive environment protein. In the interim, manual microscope examination of fluorescent staining can provide information for these characteristics. However, this approach can be too subjective and lowers throughput substantially. Hence, environmental protein originating from e.g. encapsulation matrices or carrier media may exhibit adverse effects for accurate cytometric analysis.

4. Flow Cytometry for cell viability assessment in complex protein matrices

Proof of principle that product quality can be assessed within complex systems using FACS may raise awareness and further develop cytometric technologies within the industrial domains of quality management and product /process optimization. Rapid and efficient viability assessment is essential for regulation and legislation on therapeutic bioactives or drug product quality. Hence, there is a clear need for real-time cell enumeration techniques. Data procurement in minutes rather than days may identify a problem faster than usual. Within the food industry, FACS represents a major development for high throughput screening (HTS) of high cell density cultures in addition to providing real-time quality control. Numerous technologies, inclusive of FACS have been developed to accelerate data acquisition compared to traditional culture methods. In the food industry, techniques utilizing antibodies for cell labelling prior to FACS analysis have been developed for *Salmonella enterica* serovar Typhimurium and *Listeria monocytogenes* in milk and other dairy products (Patchett et al., 1991). Moreover, Doherty et al., (2010) demonstrated that FACS, coupled with fluorescent techniques, can be successfully applied for the assessment of cell viability in seven different protein matrices ranging in structural complexity. Food containing complex protein matrices can frequently generate unpredictable results regarding cell viability. Cell entrapment within protein networks can severely affect accurate cell enumeration, an issue which requires special attention as it has an impact on both quality and safety of the product. Cell viability can be accurately determined by FACS, specialised for cell encapsulation and protein systems. The distinctive features of this strategy can be summarised as follows: while Delgado et al., (2010) performed cytometric screening on encapsulated cells within intact micro-carriers, Doherty et al., (2010) enumerated cell viability following complete protein matrix digestion. Cell extraction and digestive pre-treatments were designed to liberate cells from the scaffold in order to minimise the protein background, the predominant compositional obstacles for efficient FACS analysis. It is interesting to compare the success of these reverse strategies for use in encapsulation systems. Cell extraction by Doherty et al., (2010) required 40-minute sample preparation and distinct functional cell populations were discriminated based on fluorescent labelling by of Thiazole Orange (TO) and Propidium Iodide (PI). This assay yielded 45–50 samples/hour, a detection range of 10^2–10^{10} cfu mL^{-1} of homogenate and generated correlation coefficients (r) of 0.95, 0.92 and 0.93 in relation to standard plate counts during heat, acid and storage trials, respectively. This cytometric approach could also alleviate problems relating to environmental compatibility during the production of nutraceutical products; a formulation problem generating a strong current of industrial activity. However, uptake of this technology is dependent on cost-efficiency and the scope for extension of product applications. Both of these pre-requisites are satisfactory for food and pharmaceutical manufacture environments due to the i) multi-disciplinary function of the assay for cell viability assessment; ii) minimal personnel training required for instrument commission and iii) rapid, reproducible cytometric signature responses in a variety of encapsulation matrices in the presence of protein. The timely availability of cytometric results also provides manufacturers with the necessary skills to promote problem-solving investigations in bioactive and/ drug development for enhanced performance of therapeutic cultures with subsequent detection and utilisation of recombinant proteins.

4.1 Significance of a protein clearing procedure

Flow Cytometry is commonly associated with inaccuracies due to its basic operating principle involving 'hydrodynamic focusing' whereby each particle, either cell aggregate or single bacterium, is counted as one cell (Maukonen et al., 2006). Hence, fluorescent techniques like FACS are not universal and successful application necessitates detailed tailoring of pre-treatments and buffer compositions for cell lines and product types. Previous research (Bunthof and Abee, 2002, Gunasekera et al., 2000) failed to generate a procedure capable of consistent cellular discrimination within a diverse range of protein environments inclusive of dairy scaffolds, clinical protein supplements and encapsulation polymers. This challenge is associated with the fluctuating proteolysis response of various protein environments due to differing structural orientation and protein complexity. Doherty et al., (2010) optimised sample pre-treatments (Figure 5) buffer composition and probe concentrations in order accurately detect live, injured and dead cells within encapsulation systems. Moreover, this strategy liberated cells from encapsulation and protein networks without any adverse cellular injury as visualised in Figure 6.

The assay advocates rapid, reproducible cell liberation compared to lengthy extraction procedures previously reported for immobilized systems (Sun and Griffiths, 2000). Since cells are in the micron range, the signal-to-noise ratio in FACS analysis is of paramount importance especially in clinical protein supplements, which are normally viscous in nature. More importantly, encapsulation polymers and protein matrices will inevitably generate increased particle scatter due to high concentrations of colloidal particles in the cell size range. It is evident that protein clearing strategy is fundamental for the achievement of reproducible reliable cytometric viability screening in dense environmental milieu commonly encountered in drug and cell delivery models.

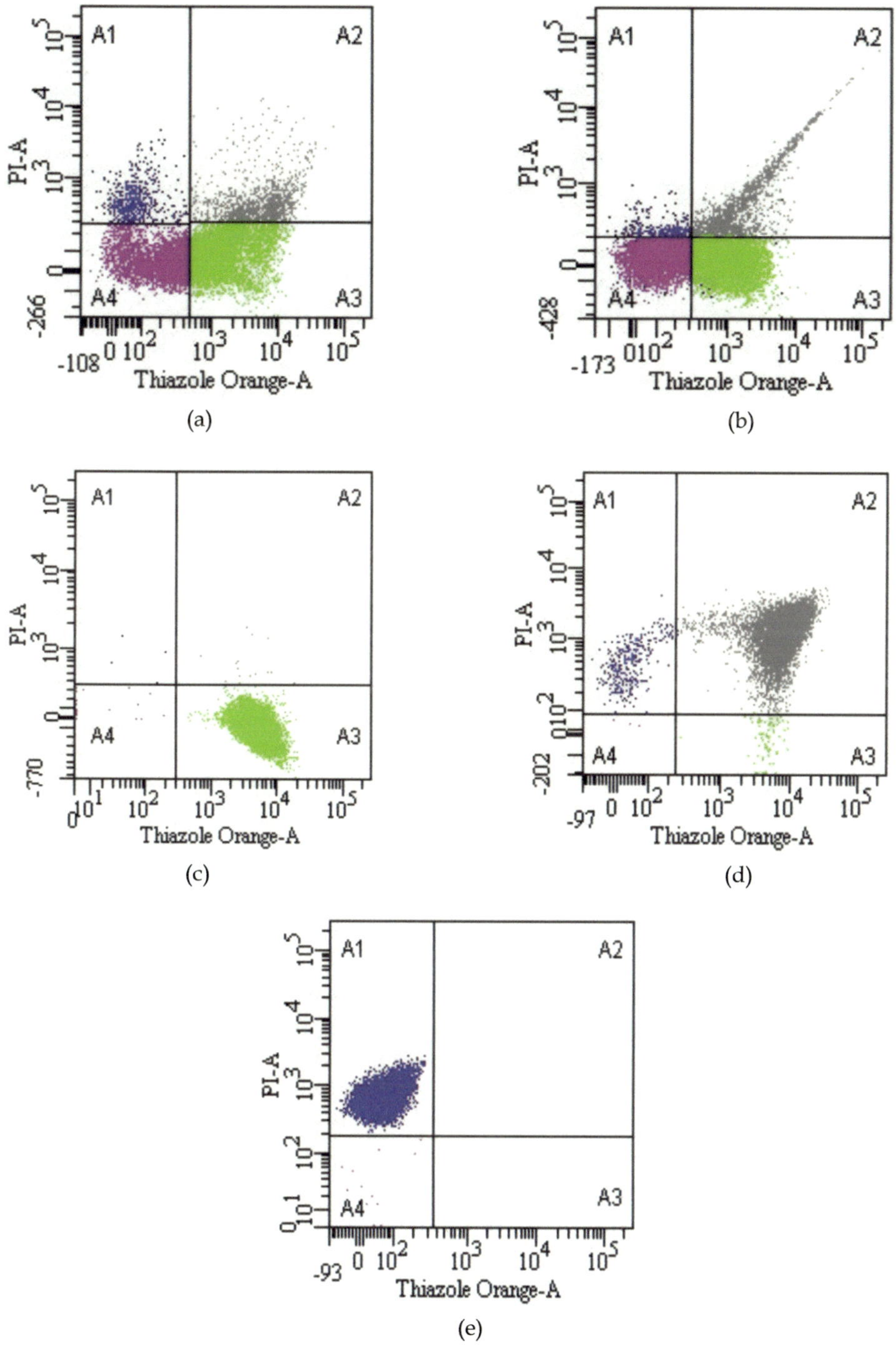

Fig. 5. Flow cytometric dot plots illustrating probiotic bacteria Lb. rhamnosus GG encapsulated in protein gel matrix and pre-sample extraction (a), post-homogenization (b) and after proteolysis digestion of the protein capsule (c). Results also demonstrated the clear distinction between live (c), injured (d) and dead probiotic cells (e)

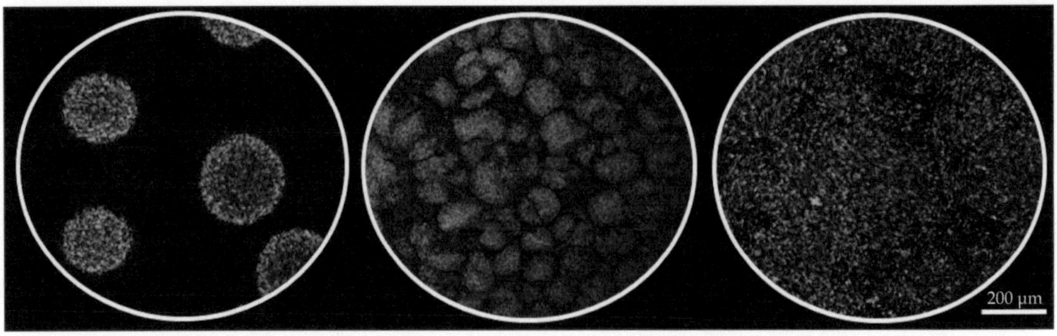

Fig. 6. Confocal image visualising the release of live probiotic bacteria from intact encapsulation scaffolds (left) and their progressive digestion during the protein clearing procedure (left- right)

4.2 Cell release mechanism for enhanced cytometric screening

Current research illustrates a poor correlation between standard plate counts and cytometric screening due to non-specific binding of fluorescent dyes to protein particles (Gunasekera et al., 2000), which failed to be adequately removed by enzymatic treatments or commercial protein-clearing agents (McClelland and Pinder, 1994a, b). Meanwhile, Doherty et al., (2010) further resolved the negative effect of environmental proteins by introducing a mild homogenisation step in order to break-down cellular chains for the provision of true cytometric cell counts. Essentially, this two-stage pre-treatment substantially reduced particle counts or cytometric 'events' that were similar in size to, or larger than typical cellular dimensions i.e. 1 to 5 µm (Figure 7). Interestingly, further physico-chemical analysis e.g. zeta potential and hydrophobicity, provided details of charge interactions within protein-cell systems. This procedure allows to release of clean cell populations from complex or encapsulated protein matrices (Doherty et al., 2010).

4.3 Optimum compensation and fluorescent staining

Spectral overlap of the different fluorochromes used during FACS, if uncorrected, will lead to misinterpretation of data from false positives or artifactual populations. Compensation values in excess of 90% have been reported (Gunasekera et al., 2000, Gunasekera et al., 2003), which can be substantially reduced by pre-treatment to values as low as 28%, which may alleviate distortion of true viable counts. Pre-treatment of the preparations can influence fluorescence compensation values via optimization of instrument settings and equilibration of overlapping spectral channels. Despite dense protein environments in some products, the regression between FACS and plate counts can closely match the guidelines of Feldsine et al., (2002) for validation of qualitative and quantitative microbiological methods. Since all matrix material in the size range of cells can be adequately digested, cell overestimation as a result of matrix staining during FACS analysis was reduced. However, these findings may be interpreted as evidence of a dormant or an active but non-culturable cell condition, since Lahtinen et al., (2005) discovered a subpopulation of non-culturable cells with a functional cell membrane typical of viable cells. Interestingly, non-viable probiotic cells can also illustrate adherence to intestinal mucus for subsequent conveyance of immunomodulatory effects (Ouwehand et al., 2000, Vinderola et al., 2005). Therefore, the detection of compromised

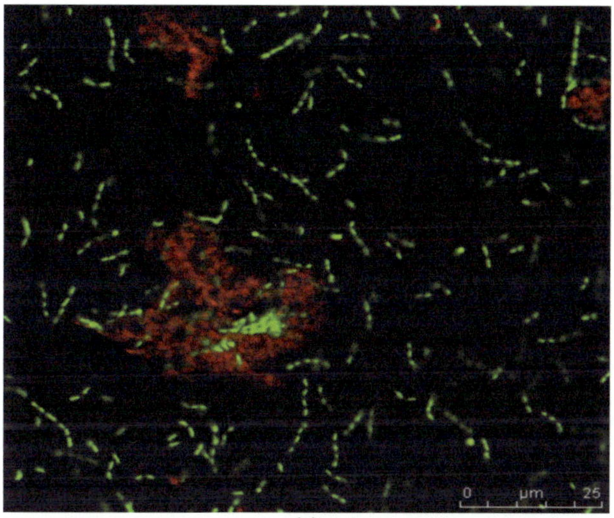

(a)

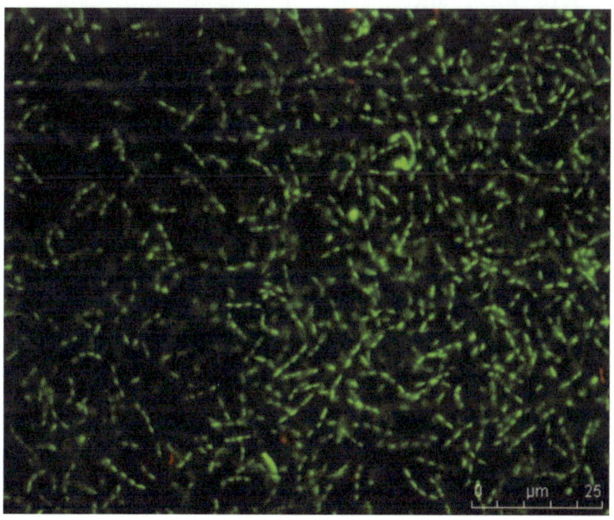

(b)

Fig. 7. Fluorescent Confocal Scanning Laser Microscope (CSLM) images showing the incomplete protein digestion (a) generated after single protein digestion and the homogenous cell suspension generated (b) for FACS analysis following cell extraction and double proteolysis

cells or possibly dead cells may be screened by FACS for the provision of therapeutic cell cultures. Furthermore, Maukonen et al., (2006) highlighted the choice of fluorescent stain, sample pre-treatment and product matrix as additional cytometric factors influencing cell stainability, contrary to general credence based solely on strain characteristics. Retention of fluorescent dyes is synonymous with hydrophilic cell surface properties, both of which were illustrated for probiotic bacteria *Lactobacillus rhamnosus* GG by Doherty et al., (2010). Interestingly, surfaces of lactic acid bacteria studied in literature are also hydrophilic

(Boonaert and Rouxhet, 2000, Pelletier et al., 1997). This acquired knowledge relating to cytometric screening of protein-cell systems will diversify the choice of cell lines and the product range applicable for efficacious cell delivery via encapsulation.

4.4 Next generation flow cytometry for encapsulation applications

As conventional flow cytometers with advanced capabilities mature as large powerful laboratory systems for obtaining highly complex information, a new generation of 'personal flow cytometers' have evolved. These bench-top user-friendly cytometers focus on specific functions (Vignali, 2000) and include less flexible laser selection systems (Shapiro, 1995), less sensitive detectors (www.accuricytometers.com) and/or elimination of sheath fluid (www.millipore.com). These smaller systems can accomplish most customary tasks, including cell counting, measurement of cell viability, antibody quantification and detection of cell death. The Luminex® family of cytometers, in particular, have advanced the use of micro-particle-based assays to provide multiplexed analytical capability while keeping the optics relatively simple. With recent developments in micro-fabrication and microfluidics, such as small, optimised chip design, developers are miniaturising current cytometers even further to create systems for point-of-use applications and some of these systems will continue to employ particle-based assays (Kim et al., 2010).

Micro-particle assays often rely on antibodies as capture molecules on the surface of the capsule. Although, other types of capture molecules can be used, the high specificity and affinity of antibodies in the presence of complex sample matrices has made them a reagent of choice. In 1977, Horan and Wheeless published a manuscript in *Science* detailing the first microsphere-based immunoassay (Horan and Wheeless, 1977). Since then, others have followed with technology of increasing sophistication (Vignali, 2000). Capture antibodies are generally immobilized onto the micro particles using available reactive groups, for example amines, hydroxyls or thiols but carboxyls are the most frequently used. Functionalisation of carboxyl is followed by exposure to ethydimethylaminopropylcarbodiimide and *N*-hydroxysuc-cinimide, which provides a mild procedure for antibody attachment to the surface of micro-particles. The attached antibody can captures antigen from a sample on to the surface for the microsphere. The signal can then be generated as an aggregation event measured using light scattering or electrical or magnetic properties. More frequently, a fluorescent tracer is included in the particle-capture antibody-antigen complex, and fluorescence is measured.

Light scattering in flow cytometers is a staple phenomenon for detecting and characterising particles in FACS and more recently micro-capsules. A light beam directed at a particle can interact through reflective, refractive and diffractive effects. Then, information about the particle, aggregate or micro-capsule can be derived from the change in direction and intensity of a scattered light beam. Collecting scattered light at various angles from the incident beam has been reported to provide different types of information about the particle, e.g. size and density (Zharinov et al., 2001). The diameter of the particle/ capsule should be within the range of 1-50 wavelengths of the incident light beam.

Typically, forward scatter can provide approximate information about size of a protein gel micro-bead or capsule (Shapiro, 2003). It should however, be noted that an increase in the intensity of forward-scattered light does not always correlate with increasing particle size.

Side scattered light is often collected at 90° and provides information about smaller particles and structures within protein particles, scaffold, capsule or gel aggregates. Proportionally more light is scattered by micro-capsules or encapsulated structures at a wide angle than at a small angle, and thus side-scattered light can provide information about the relative roughness or shape of micro-particles and capsules in addition to the granularity of their internal structures. Measuring side-scattered light and forward scattered light has become a standard FACS for biomedical research because this behaviour enables cells to be distinguished by size and granularity, providing insight into mixed populations, viability, or change in internal structure of encapsulation entities.

Using information derived from scatter light at different angles, particles can be classified and studied. Zharinov, et al., (2001) used light scattering data from a scanning FACS to distinguish lymphocytes, erthyrocytes, encapsulation capsules and milk-fat particles of various size and refractive index (Zharinov et al., 2001). These cells and particles generated different scattered light profiles dependent on scattering angle. Steen et al., (1990) custom-built a flow cytometer to characterise viruses of different size using light scattering (Steen et al., 1990).This device could easily distinguish particles with diameters in the range of 30-700 (Steen et al., 1990). In the 1980 Masson and co-workers presented a strong body of work describing particle-counting agglutination immunoassays (PACIA) (Sindic et al., 1981). Initially, PACIA was publicised as a replacement for expensive assay utilizing radioactive labels for characterisation of antigen and antibody interactions. In these assays, polystyrene particles coated with antigens were incubated with antibodies to cause agglutination or aggregation of the particles. Key aspects of this assay were:

- Use of an antibody with multivalent binding sites to enable particle-particle interaction
- Determination of particle concentrations that would allow aggregation; and
- Prevention of non-specific interactions between particles

The samples before and after agglutination were measured in an optical particle counter based on light scattering. The aggregated particles were larger in size than unaggregated particles and resulted in more side-scattered light. In 2003, Pamme, Koyama and Manz described a microfluidic device that used light scattering to analyse agglutination immuno assays (Pamme et al., 2003). The device used a design that focused particles in two dimensions into an optical interrogation region. Particles ranging from 2-9 μm in diameter were distinguished, which is significantly larger than the 70-300 nm range reported previously (Steen et al., 1990). Light scattering is extensively studied with many advantages to developers of microflow cytometry assays for encapsulation purposes. Using just a beam of light of suitable wavelength (relative to the capsule) and detectors at various angles, information regarding size, shape and granularity of a capsule are easily derived. Additionally, scattered light signals tend to be strong and do not need the most advanced or expensive detectors. Yet, distinguishing differing in diameter of a few microns can be challenging and represents the fundamental pre-requisite for encapsulation screening assays.

4.5 High content encapsulation screening

Literature also shows that high resolution two-dimensional (2-D) images consume limited detector bandwidth, introduce a data-acquisition delay that is a barrier for real-time decisions needed for sorting capsules and introduce noise via inaccuracies in image segmentation. This impediment is further addressed to provide the foundation knowledge for a parallel microfluidic cytometer (PMC) using a high-speed scanning photomultiplier-based detector. Development of parallel flow channels within this model PMC would inevitably decouple count rates from signal-to-noise ratio for cytometric analysis of encapsulation systems. Essentially, this approach would demonstrate the feasibility for high throughput visual screening of encapsulated animal cells and stem cell clusters with concomitant determination of recombinant protein generation and localisation.

Imaging flow cytometers based on wide-field-charge-coupled device (CCD) imagers have demonstrated throughput limitations similar to those of microscopes (George et al., 2006). To address these restrictions, industry has developed a multi-channel parallel microfluidic cytometer (PMC) based on analog detection with parallel microfluidics. This design may potentially reduce i) data-buffering and storage requirements and ii) simplify the classification algorithm required to differentiate encapsulated animal or stem cells. Hence, parallel microfluidics will bypass sample-changeover restrictions commonly encountered with single channel flow cytometers. This novel strategy will enhance process efficiency of the PMC detector by increasing the diameter of a laser spot from 1 µm and 4 µm. Furthermore, sample flowing into the focal volume will potentially eliminate the focusing and stage volumes that limit high content screening on a microscope to approx. 2-6 wells min^{-1}. This new cytometric design circumvents many throughput limitations for both high cell density encapsulation and flow cytometer analysis by combining the best features of each technology to achieve efficient cell encapsulation screening.

Although much can be borrowed from the methods of 2-D high content screening (de Vos et al., 2010), 1-D algorithms are fundamentally different. Notably, microscope or flow cytometers draw boundaries around 'primary and secondary objects' (known as segmentation). However, this user-defined aspect of segmentation is a source of assay variability and is often considered the most challenging and time-consuming step. However, the recent application of 1-D cytometric imaging strategy for encapsulation systems integrated resolution issues experience within the standard hardware systems in order to eliminate potential segmentation problems. This was achieved by accepting any resolution element as an 'object'. Hence, this demonstrates the feasibility to develop efficient high content screening algorithms for micro-capsules using relatively low input.

5. Conclusion

Incorporation of bioactive compounds such as probiotics, animal cells and stem cell clusters into encapsulation matrices for food and pharmaceutical purposes can provide a simple way to develop novel nutraceuticals and drug treatment delivery systems with physiological benefits. Exact elucidation of cell proliferation and stability during encapsulation is of utmost importance for industrial or academic application. Hence, this chapter outlines the importance of cytometric analysis of encapsulation systems, in addition to the role of protein during this screening process. Proteins present various challenges for cytometric analysis; however, several techniques have been developed to overcome these limitations for commercial development of this novel technology.

6. Acknowledgements

The support provided by the staff and experts in Union Biometrica, Geel, Belgium is gratefully acknowledged. Some of the cytometric work presented in this chapter was supported by the Irish Dairy Research Trust project NU518 "Probiotic Protection", the Irish National Development Plan 2007 to 2013 and Science Foundation Ireland (SFI). The support provided by C. Stanton and R.P. Ross as well as the National Food Imaging Centre in Moorepark, Teagasc, A.E. Auty, L. Wang and V.L. Gee in particular, is gratefully acknowledged.

7. References

Boonaert, C. J. and P. G. Rouxhet. 2000. Surface of lactic acid bacteria: relationships between chemical composition and physicochemical properties. Applied and environmental microbiology 66(6):2548-2554.

Broger, T., R. P. Odermatt, P. Huber and B. Sonnleitner. 2011. Real-time on-lineflow cytometry for bioprocessmonitoring. Journal of Biotechnology 154(4):240-247.

Bunthof, C. J. and T. Abee. 2002. Development of a flow cytometric method to analyze subpopulations of bacteria in probiotic products and dairy starters. Applied and environmental microbiology 68(6):2934-2942.

de Vos, P., M. M. Faas, M. Spasojevic and J. Sikkema. 2010. Encapsulation for preservation of functionality and targeted delivery of bioactive food components. International Dairy Journal 20(4):292-302.

Delgado, L., G. Jurado, G. Galayo, E. Ogalla, L. Moreno, J. C. Rodríguez-Aguilera, A. Cebolla, M. Flores and S. Chávez. 2010. Encapsulation in monodispersed hydrogel microspheres enables fast and sensitive phenotypic analyses using COPAS large particle flow cytometry. Vol. QTN-019. COPAS™, COPAS™ QUICK TECH NOTES.

Delgado, L., G. Jurado, G. Galayo, E. Ogalla, L. Moreno, J. C. Rodríguez-Aguilera, A. Cebolla, C. Sousa, C. Flores and S. Chávez. 2011. Microbial encapsulation in monodisperse hydrogel microspheres enables fast and sensitive phenotypic analyses using flow cytometers. in Application of Flow Cytometry in Microbiology. Geel, Belgium.

Doherty, S. B., L. Wang, R. P. Ross, C. Stanton, G. F. Fitzgerald and A. Brodkorb. 2010. Use of viability staining in combination with flow cytometry for rapid viability assessment of Lactobacillus rhamnosus GG in complex protein matrices. Journal of Microbiological Methods 82(3):301-310.

Dunlop, E. H. and S. J. Ye. 1990. Micromixing in fermentors: Metabolic changes in Saccharomyces cerevisiae and their relationship to fluid turbulence. Biotechnology and Bioengineering 36(8):854-864.

Feldsine, P., C. Abeyta and W. H. Andrews. 2002. AOAC International methods committee guidelines for validation of qualitative and quantitative food microbiological official methods of analysis. Journal of AOAC International 85(5):1187-1200.

George, T. C., S. L. Fanning, P. Fitzgeral-Bocarsly, R. B. Medeiros, S. Highfill, Y. Shimizu, B. E. Hall, K. Frost, D. Basiji, W. E. Ortyn, P. J. Morrissey and D. H. Lynch. 2006. Quantitative measurement of nuclear translocation events using similarity analysis of multispectral cellular images obtained in flow. Journal of Immunological Methods 311(1-2):117-129.

Glassey, J., K. V. Gernaey, C. Clemens, T. W. Schulz, R. Oliveira, G. Striedner and C.-F. Mandenius. 2011. Process analytical technology (PAT) for biopharmaceuticals. Biotechnology Journal 6(4):369-377.

Gunasekera, T. S., P. V. Attfield and D. A. Veal. 2000. A flow cytometry method for rapid detection and enumeration of total bacteria in milk. Applied and Environmental Microbiology 66(3):1228-1232.

Gunasekera, T. S., D. A. Veal and P. V. Attfield. 2003. Potential for broad applications of flow cytometry and fluorescence techniques in microbiological and somatic cell analyses of milk. International Journal of Food Microbiology 85(3):269-279.

Hall, B. G. 1995. Adaptive mutations in Escherichia coli as a model for the multiple mutational origins of tumors. Proceeedings of the National Academy of Sciences of the United States of America 92(12):5669-5673.

Horan, P. K. and L. L. Wheeless. 1977. Quantitative single cell analysis and sorting. Science 14(198(4313):):149-157.

Jones, J. J., A. M. Bridges, A. P. Fosberry, S. Gardner, R. R. Lowers, R. R. Newby, P. J. James, R. M. Hall and O. Jenkins. 2004. Potential of real-time measurement of GFP-fusion proteins. Journal of Biotechnology 109(1-2):201-211.

Kacmar, J. and F. Srienc. 2005. Dynamics of single cell property distributions in Chinese hamster ovary cell cultures monitored and controlled with automated flowcytometry. Journal of Biotechnology 120(4):410-420.

Kelley, K. A. 1989. Sample station modification providing on-line reagent addition and reduced sample transit time for flow cytometers. Cytometry 10(6):796-800.

Kim, J. Y., W. Choi, Y. H. Kim, G. T. Tae, S. Y. Lee, K. Kim and I. C. Kwon. 2010. In-vivo tumor targeting of pluronic-based nano-carriers Journal of Controlled Release 147(1):109-117.

Lahtinen, S. J., M. Gueimonde, A. C. Ouwehand, J. P. Reinikainen and S. J. Salminen. 2005. Probiotic bacteria may become dormant during storage. Applied and Environmental Microbiology 71(3):1662-1663.

Maukonen, J., H. L. Alakomi, L. Nohynek, K. Hallamaa, S. Leppämäki, J. Mättö and M. Saarela. 2006. Suitability of the fluorescent techniques for the enumeration of probiotic bacteria in commercial non-dairy drinks and in pharmaceutical products. Food Research International 39(1):22-32.

McClelland, R. G. and A. C. Pinder. 1994a. Detection of low levels of specific Salmonella species by fluorescent antibodies and flow cytometry. The Journal of applied bacteriology 77(4):440-447.

McClelland, R. G. and A. C. Pinder. 1994b. Detection of Salmonella typhimurium in dairy products with flow cytometry and monoclonal antibodies. Applied and environmental microbiology 60(12):4255-4262.

Münch, T., B. Sonnleitner and A. Fiechter. 1992. The decisive role of the Saccharomyces cerevisiae cell cycle behaviour for dynamic growth characterization. Journal of Biotechnology 22:329-352.

Ouwehand, A. C., S. Tolkko, J. Kulmala, S. Salminen and E. Salminen. 2000. Adhesion of inactivated probiotic strains to intestinal mucus. Letters in Applied Microbiology 31(1):82-86.

Pamme, N., R. Koyama and A. Manz. 2003. Counting and sizing of particles and particle agglomerates in a microfluidic device using laser light scattering: application to a particle-enhanced immunoassay Lab on chip 3(3):187-192.

Patchett, R. A., J. P. Back, A. C. Pinder and R. G. Kroll. 1991. Enumeration of bacteria in pure cultures and in foods using a commercial flow cytometer. Food Microbiology 8(2):119-125.

Pelletier, C., C. Bouley, C. Cayuela, S. Bouttier, P. Bourlioux and M. N. Bellon-Fontaine. 1997. Cell surface characteristics of Lactobacillus casei subsp. casei, Lactobacillus paracasei subsp. paracasei and Lactobacillus rhamnosus strains. Applied and environmental microbiology 63(5):1725-1731.

Reardon, A. J., J. A. W. Elliott and L. E. McGann. 2009. Fluorescence as a better approach to gate cells for cryobiological studies with flow cytometry. Crybiology 63(3):317-329.

Reischer, H., I. Schotola, G. Striedner, F. Pötschacher and K. Bayer. 2004. Evaluation of the GFP signal and its aptitude for novel on-linemonitoring strategies of recombinant fermentation processes. Journal of Biotechnology 108(2):115-125.

Rieseberg, M., C. Kasper, K. F. Reardon and T. Scheper. 2001. Flowcytometry in biotechnology. Applied Microbiology and Biotechnology 56(3-4):350-360.

Ruzicka, J. and W. Lindberg. 1992. Flow injection cytoanalysis. Analytical Chemistry 69(9):A537-A545.

Shapiro, H. M. 1995. Practical Flow Cytometry. Vol. 3. No. 3. A.R. Liss, New York.

Sindic, C. J. M., M. P. Chalon, C. L. Cambiaso, D. Collet-Cassart and M. P.L. 1981. Particle counting immunoassay (PACIA)—VI. The determination of rabbit IgG antibodies against myelin basic protein using IgM rheumatoid factor. Molecular Immunology 18(293-299).

Sitton, G. and F. Srienc. 2008a. Growth dynamics of mammalian cells monitored with automated cell cycle staining and flowcytometry. Cytometry A 6:538-545.

Sitton, G. and F. Srienc. 2008b. Mammalian cell culture scale-up and fed-batch control using automated flowcytometry. Journal of Biotechnology 32(2):174-180.

Steen, P. D., E. R. Ashwood, K. Huang, R. A. Daynes, H. T. Chung and W. E. Samlowski. 1990. Mechanisms of pertussis toxin inhibition of lymphocyte-HEV interactions: I. Analysis of lymphocyte homing receptor-mediated Cellular Immunology 131(1):67-85.

Sun, W. and M. W. Griffiths. 2000. Survival of bifidobacteria in yogurt and simulated gastric juice following immobilization in gellan-xanthan beads. International Journal of Food Microbiology 61(1):17-25.

Vignali, D. A. A. 2000. Multiplexed particle-based flow cytometric assays Journal of Immunological Methods 243(1-2):243-255.

Vinderola, G., C. Matar and G. Perdigon. 2005. Role of intestinal epithelial cells in immune effects mediated by gram-positive probiotic bacteria: involvement of toll-like receptors. Clinical and Diagnostic Laboratory Immunology 12(9):1075-1084.

Walser, M., R. M. Leibundgut, R. Pellaux, S. Panke and M. Held. 2008. Isolation of monoclonal microcarriers colonized by fluorescent E. coli. Cytometry 73(9):788-798.

Walser, M., R. Pellaux, A. Meyer, M. Bechtold, H. Vanderschuren, Reinhardt R., J. Magyar, S. Panke and M. Held. 2009. Novel method for high-throughput colony PCR screening in nanoliter-reactors. Nucleic Acid Research 37(8):e57/51-e57/58.

Watson, D. A., D. F. Gaskill, L. O. Brown, S. K. Doorn and J. P. Nolan. 2009. Spectral Measurements of Large Particles by Flow Cytometry. Cytometry A 75(5):460-464.

Zanella, F., J. B. Lorens and W. Link. 2010. High content screening: seeing is believing Trends in Biotechnology 28(5):237-245.

Zhao, R., A. Natarajan and F. Srienc. 1999. A flow injection flowcytometry system for on-linemonitoring of bioreactors. Biotechnology and Bioengineering 65(5):609-617.

Zharinov, A., P. Tarasov, A. Shvalov, K. Semyanov, D. R. van Bockstaele and V. Maltsev. 2001. A study of light scattering of mononuclear blood cells with scanning flow cytometry Journal of Quantitative Spectroscopy and Radiative Transfer 102(1):121-128.

20

Median Effect Dose and Combination Index Analysis of Cytotoxic Drugs Using Flow Cytometry

Tomás Lombardo, Laura Anaya, Laura Kornblihtt and Guillermo Blanco
Laboratory of Immunotoxicology (LaITo), Hospital de Clínicas San Martín,
University of Buenos Aires
Argentina

1. Introduction

Targeted therapy is a strategy of anticancer treatment that aims to interfere with processes of tumorigenesis, cancer progression and metastasis by selectively affecting key molecules of tumor cells (Armand et al., 2007; Favoni & Florio, 2011; Gross-Goupil & Escudier, 2010). Targeted therapies are directed to small molecules participating in different mechanisms that control cell survival through cellular proteins or signalling pathways (Mueller et al., 2009; Zahorowska et al., 2009). Targeted therapies may offer enhanced efficacy, enhanced selectivity, and less toxicity. However, targeting selective molecules and pathways often induces the activation of redundant mechanisms and enhances the emergence of resistant cells due to selective pressure (Woodcock et al., 2011). This is one of the reasons why the effects of targeted agents are not durable when used alone, and often result in drug resistance and clinical relapse.

Except for specific cases the use of these targeted drugs as monotherapy is often discouraged due to lack of efficacy. However, combined therapy with drugs targeting several mechanisms of tumor cell death can greatly improve efficacy and may overcome resistance. Several genomic and epigenetic alterations have been identified in tumor cells that lead to unrestrained proliferation, evasion of proapoptotic signals, metastasis, and resistance to drug-induced cell death. These alterations are critical for cancer progression and therefore combination strategies employing multiple targeted agents can be a successful therapeutic strategy. In vertical combination strategies two or more drugs target a same pathway at two different points, while in horizontal combinations drugs are directed towards different intracellular signalling pathways and have the potential advantage of combining agents with non-overlapping toxicities (Gross-Goupil & Escudier, 2010).

Novel treatments require the investigation of mechanisms of action and synergy of combination treatments to enhance the role of the targeted pharmacological agents (Carew et al., 2008; Mitsiades et al., 2011). Evaluating combinations of targeted drugs, including investigational agents, are an essential part of this effort (Dancey & Chen, 2006). An interesting example is represented by Bortezomib, a drug currently effective as single agent in multiple myeloma and mantle cell lymphoma (Bross et al., 2004; Kane et al., 2007; Wright,

2010). Bortezomib is a proteasome inhibitor that selectively triggers apoptosis in various types of neoplastic cells. It has been tested in a wide variety of solid tumors but has generally been ineffective as monotherapy (Boccadoro et al., 2005). However Bortezomib has shown increased activity when combined with several novel targeted agents including protein deacetylase inhibitors, kinase inhibitors, farnesyltransferase inhibitors, HSP-90 inhibitors, pan-Bcl-2 family inhibitors, and other classes of targeted inhibitors (Dai et al., 2003; Karp & Lancet, 2005; Pei et al., 2004; Perez-Galan et al., 2008; Trudel et al., 2007; Workman et al., 2007; Yanamandra et al., 2006). Thus, Bortezomib in combination with novel targeted therapies increase antitumor activity and overcome specific cellular antiapoptotic mechanisms (Wright, 2010).

Two-drug combination therapies are being assessed in a variety of tumors, usually testing agents that have different targets, nonoverlapping toxicity, and some rationale for evaluation (Belinsky et al., 2011; Castaneda & Gomez, 2009; Eriksen et al., 2009; Klosowska-Wardega et al., 2010). An increase in the number of these studies is expected in coming years, on the basis of emerging data with new agents, which is expanding our understanding of the molecular pathways important in cancer progression. (Woodcock et al., 2011). Tumor intracellular signalling pathway dependencies are being increasingly analyzed, and patients treated on the basis of resistance profile detected for specific drug combinations (Busch et al.; Derenzini et al., 2009; Michiels et al., 2011). This approach may facilitate the development of combination regimens optimized for specific tumor subtypes, thus providing the potential for tailored therapy in individual patients on the basis of certain molecular and genetic characteristics of their disease.

1.1 Targeted drugs often induce programmed cell death as their main mechanism of anti-tumor activity

Many of the classic chemotherapeutic agents (alkylating agents, antimetabolites, antibiotics, topoisomerase inhibitors) are known to block cell division by compromising DNA replication and halting cell cycle progression, or inhibit mitosis, eventually leading to cell death (Foye, 1995; Goodman et al., 2010; Shuck & Turchi, 2010). Indicators of cell proliferation are suitable effect biomarkers to assess whether a combination of these agents is synergic, additive or antagonistic. Biomarkers frequently used for this purpose include incorporation of nucleotide analogues such as bromodeoxyuridine, or metabolic indicators of cell number such as tetrazolium salt-based assays (Karaca et al., 2009; Olszewska-Slonina et al., 2004; Sims & Plattner, 2009). However many of the new targeted agents interfere with constitutively active survival pathways or initiate apoptosis by directly influencing pro-apoptotic signals (Citri et al., 2004; Kim et al., 2005; Larsen et al., 2011; Vega et al., 2009; Zhang et al., 2009). In addition autophagic cell death and programmed necrosis are being actively investigated as alternative and pharmacologically relevant forms of programmed cell death (Berghe et al., 2010; Bijnsdorp et al., 2011; Duan et al., 2010; Gozuacik & Kimchi, 2007; McCall, 2010; Notte et al., 2011; Paglin et al., 2005; Platini et al., 2010). Combination studies should be conducted using effect biomarkers that are as close as possible to the known mechanisms targeted by single agents, and biomarkers specifically related to drug-induce tumor cell death appear more adequate for the assessment of new targeted agents (Cameron et al., 2001; Facoetti et al., 2008; Wesierska-Gadek et al., 2005). A straightforward approach is to determine the proportion of live and dead cells in viability studies scoring thousands of cells through flow cytometry which ensures exceptional precision for dose-effect cytotoxicity studies.

2. Assessment of viability through flow cytometry

The strength of flow cytometry when compared to other methods available to assess the proportion of live and dead cells is the accuracy and precision brought by single cell multiparametric assessment. A variety of fluorescent probes may be chosen to use in viability assessment through flow cytometry. These probes are based on cell functions and biological conditions that are differentially preserved in live cells and lost in dead cells. It is usual to select at least two probes measuring independent functional conditions. For example, a probe evaluating membrane integrity of cells and another probe evaluating enzymatic activity. Probes should be selected to match specific experimental requirements such as biological variability, duration of the experiments, whether cells exposed to drugs are adherent or non-adherent, and illumination lines available in the flow cytometer. Some probes may be released after being retained within the cells for a short time and require immediate assessment through the flow cytometer after labelling, while others may be retained for several hours or may be even retained indefinitely by being covalently linked to cellular components. In addition some specimens may require fixation due to biohazard issues, so another kind of probes should be chosen and combined in these cases (De Clerck et al., 1994).

2.1 Fluorescent staining of live and dead cells

Viability is not easily defined in terms of a single physiological or morphological parameter. No single parameter fully defines cell death in all systems; therefore, it is often advantageous to use more than one cell death indicators based on different parameters such as membrane damage, and enzymatic or metabolic activity. A considerably large number of fluorescent probes have been introduced in the recent years that are dedicated to the assessment of viability on a single cell basis. Many of these new probes have features that are useful under specific experimental circumstances. The two conditions most often detected are increased cell membrane permeability in dead cells and the presence of enzymatic activity in live cells. The former is assessed with probes that become fluorescent when bound to DNA but are not able to pass through cell membrane if selective permeability is preserved, while the later is determined by fluorogenic substrates. However other conditions occurring only in live cells may be used to demonstrate viability such as enzymatic oxidation, reduction and mitochondrial membrane potential (Callewaert et al., 1991). It is important to underscore this concept because these probes are often used for assessment of specific cellular functions and it may be erroneously assumed that they have no contribution to the assessment of viability.

2.2 Enzymatic activity in live cells, use of tracker dyes

One of the first probes introduced and most frequently used to stain live cells has been fluorescein-diacetate (FDA) (Jones & Senft, 1985; Ross et al., 1989). This non-fluorescent cell-permeant esterase substrate penetrates the cell and is converted by nonspecific intracellular esterases into fluorescein.

Thus it becomes a more polar compound and is retained within those cells that have intact plasma membranes. In contrast, nonfluorescent FDA and fluorescein rapidly leak from those cells that have a damaged cell membrane because it is no longer retained due to increased permeability (Prosperi et al., 1986). This property ensures that dead cells will never retain FDA or fluorescein, even if cell death occurs after the labelling procedure. This is one of the reasons why it is recommended to analyze cells rapidly through the flow cytometer after staining with FDA and why they should be kept in low incubation temperatures to minimize potential fluorescein leakage.

Calcein-acetoxymethyl-ester (Calcein-AM) is a derivative of calcein that has several improvements over FDA (Duan et al., 2010; Papadopoulos et al., 1994). Calcein-AM is also a substrate of nonspecific intracellular esterases. The fluorescent product is calcein and is better retained in cells because it is a polyanionic compound that has six negative charges and two positive charges at pH 7. Calcein-Blue-AM and Calcein-Violet-AM are similar to Calcein-AM but have different excitation and emission wavelengths (Fuchs et al., 2007). Calcein-Blue-AM is excited with UV lasers while Calcein-Violet-AM is excited with 405 nm violet diode lasers, although both dyes emit blue fluorescence (Prowse et al., 2009). They can be used when the green fluorescence channel from the 488 nm excitation line is needed for other purpose and a UV or violet illumination line is available. Chloromethyl-fluorescein-diacteate (CM-FDA), is a FDA derivative that is retained within the cell even after damage to the plasma membrane due to its ability to bind thiol groups (Lantz et al., 2001; Sarkar et al., 2009). The weakly thiol-reactive chloromethyl moieties of this compound react with intracellular thiols and the acetate groups are cleaved by cytoplasmic esterases (West et al., 2001). This compound will not stain dead cells but the label will be preserved in those cells that die after the labelling procedure because the fluorescent product will be bound to SH groups within the cells (Sebastia et al., 2003). Chloromethyl SNARF-1 acetate is similar to CM-FDA but exhibits red fluorescence when excited with 488 nm blue laser. Thus it can be used when the green fluorescence channel is needed for other purpose and a UV or violet illumination line is not available (Hamilton et al., 2007). Carboxi-fluorescein-succinimidyl-ester (CFSE) is converted to fluorescent compound by intracellular esterases but covalently

Probe	Excitation line	Fluorescence emission	Intracellular retention
FDA	Blue	Green	Poor
Calcein-AM	Blue	Green	Good
Calcein Blue-AM	UV	Blue	Good
Calcein Violet-AM	Violet	Blue	Good
5-Cl-M-FDA	Blue	Green	Excellent
5-Cl-M-SNARF	Blue	Orange	Excellent
CFSE	Blue	Green	Excellent

Table 1. Fluorogenic substrates of intracellular esterases that are commonly used as viability probes

binds amino groups of proteins and is completely retained within cells, even after damage of cell membrane (Fujioka et al., 1994; Li et al., 2003). This dye is also used as cell tracker because it is retained in daughter cells after several rounds of cell division (Parish & Warren, 2002). It is worth to note that probes like FDA may give poor results with trypsinized cells owing to potential leakage of fluorescein during the staining and washing procedures (Zamai et al., 2001). Thus probes like CM-FDA, CM-SNARF-1, and CFSE may be a better choice for staining adherent cells.

2.3 DNA labelling in live and dead cells

Many polar nucleic acid stains are able to enter eukaryotic cells only when the plasma membrane is damaged. These stains are known as cell-impermeant dyes and include propidium iodide (PI) which is the most frequently used probe for assessing viability in flow cytometry (Yeh et al., 1981). This dye is excluded from live cells because it is negatively charged but readily penetrates the membrane of damaged cells and binds DNA. When excited at 488 nm DNA-bound PI increases orange-red fluorescence emission more than 1000 fold. Another commonly used cell-impermeant dye excited with 488 nm laser is 7-aminoactinomycin-D (7AAD). This dye binds DNA only in dead cells but emits fluorescence beyond 610 nm and allows the usage of the yellow-orange fluorescence channel for other purpose (Pallis et al., 1999).

Both PI and 7AAD have large Stokes shifts and can be used in 488 nm laser flow cytometers with green fluorescent tracker dyes such as FDA, CM-FDA, Calcein-AM and CFSE. Cells with damaged membranes may be identified with other cell-impermeant DNA fluorescent dyes that emit fluorescence in different wavelengths than that of PI.

The SYTOX series includes SYTOX-green (excited with 488 nm laser), SYTOX-red (excited with 633 and 635 nm lasers) and SYTOX-blue (excited with UV or 405 nm violet diode laser) (Haase, 2004; Lebaron et al., 1998; Yan et al., 2005). In contrast to SYTOX dyes, the SYTO series of nucleic acid stains can enter live cells and are thus cell-permeant DNA dyes (Ullal et al., 2010). The SYTO probes bind DNA with low affinity in live or dead cells (Eray et al., 2001; Poot et al., 1997). They are combined with high affinity cell-impermeant dyes to discriminate live from dead cells (Wlodkowic & Skommer, 2007). For example cell-permeant SYTO-red will stain live and dead cells with red fluorescence binding with low affinity to DNA, but if used together with SYTOX-green dead cells will be green fluorescent, because SYTOX-green has much higher affinity for DNA and will displace the low affinity SYTO-red. In addition, SYTOX-green will never stain live cells because it is cell-impermeant.

2.4 Biohazardous specimens

Viability staining of biohazardous specimens often requires fixation procedures that inactivate pathogens but produce minimal distortion of cellular characteristics. Some combinations of cell permeant and cell impermeant DNA dyes can be treated with fixatives such as 4% glutaraldehyde or formaldehyde to allow safer handling during analysis, without disrupting the distinctive staining pattern. An example is provided by cell-permeant, green-fluorescent DNA probe SYTO-10 and the cell-impermeant, red-fluorescent DNA probe ethidium homodimer-2 (Barnett et al., 2004; Poole et al., 1996). Using these two probes cells can be stained and fixed at various times during an experiment, and the results can be analyzed several hours later. This method may be applied to viability assessment of any non-adherent cells, as well as trypsinized adherent cells. Tables 1, 2, and 4 summarize the main features of viability probes based on enzymatic activity and DNA labelling discussed above that may be considered to meet specific experimental requirements.

Probe	Excitation line	Fluorescence emission	Membrane Permeant	DNA Affinity	Fixable
SYTOX-Blue	UV-Violet	Blue	NO	High	NO
SYTOX-Green	Blue	Green	NO	High	NO
SYTOX-Red	Red	Red	NO	High	NO
Propidium iodide	Blue	Orange-Red	NO	High	NO
7AAD	Blue	Red	NO	High	NO
SYTO-10	Blue	Green	YES	Low	YES
SYTO-Red	Blue	Red	YES	Low	NO
Ethidium homodimer-2	Blue	Green	NO	High	YES

Table 2. DNA probes used for viability assessment

2.5 Two parameter assessment of viability through flow cytometry

Identification of live and dead cells is often conducted with simultaneous use of two probes. The combination may include a cell-impermeant DNA probe and either a fluorogenic substrate or a cell-permeant DNA probe. It should be highlighted that viability may be also indicated by probes that have been designed to assess other cellular functions. For example generation of hydrogen peroxide and superoxide anion occurs in live cells due to normal function of mitochondrial electron transport chain and does not occur in dead cells. The superoxide anion probe dihydroethidine (HE) and the hydrogen-peroxide probe dihydro-dichloro-fluoresceindiacetate (DH-DCFDA) will stain live cells red fluorescent and green fluorescent respectively (Eruslanov & Kusmartsev, 2010; Zanetti et al., 2005). Both probes may be appropriately combined with cell-impermeant DNA dyes to discriminate between live and dead cells.

Similarly potentiometric dyes stain live cells with preserved mitochondrial membrane potential, but not dead or compromised live cells where the mitochondrial membrane potential has collapsed (Marchetti et al., 2004). Thus they may also be combined with cell-impermeant DNA dyes to discriminate live and dead cells. For example, rhodamine 123 has been used in combination with propidium iodide for viability assessment with two-color flow cytomety (Darzynkiewicz et al., 1982). Metabolically active cells undergo normal oxidation-reduction reactions and thus can also reduce a variety of probes, providing a measure of cell viability and overall cell health (Callewaert et al., 1991; Radcliff et al., 1991). Resazurin and dodecylresazurin (C12-resazurin) have been extensively used as oxidation–reduction indicators to detect viable cells (Czekanska, 2011). Reduction of resazurin yields the red fluorescent product resorufin while C12-resazurin yields C12-resorufin which is better retained by single cells (Talbot et al., 2008).

Again these probes may be combined with cell-impermeant DNA probes like SYTOX-green to discriminate live and dead cells with two color flow cytometry.

2.6 Viability assessment with single-color fixable dyes

In some experimental circumstances only one fluorescence channel may be dedicated to assessment of cell viability. In this case amine-reactive fluorescent dyes can be used to evaluate mammalian cell viability.

In cells with compromised membranes, these dyes react with free amines both in the cell interior and on the cell surface, yielding intense fluorescent staining. In viable cells, the dyes only stain cell-surface amines, resulting in less intense fluorescence (Elrefaei et al., 2008). The difference in intensity between the live and dead cell populations is preserved following formaldehyde fixation, using conditions that inactivate pathogens (Burmeister et al., 2008). There are several options of fluorescence excitation (UV, violet, blue, and red lasers) and emission wavelength (blue, green, yellow, red).

Probe	Excitation line	Fluorescence emission
LIVE/DEAD® fixable Blue	UV	Blue-450 nm
LIVE/DEAD ® Fixable Aqua	UV	Green-526 nm
LIVE/DEAD ® Fixable Yellow	Violet	Yellow-575 nm
LIVE/DEAD ® Fixable Violet	Violet	Blue-450 nm
eFluor® 450	Violet	Blue-450 nm
Fixable Viability Stain 450 ®	Violet	Blue-450 nm
LIVE/DEAD ® Fixable Green	Blue	Green-520 nm
eFluor® 506	Blue	Green-506 nm
LIVE/DEAD ® Fixable Red	Red	Red-615 nm
LIVE/DEAD ® Fixable Far Red	Red	Far Red-665 nm
eFluor® 660	Red	Far Red-660 nm

Table 3. Fixable amine-reactive fluorescent probes used for single-color assessment of cell viability. The wavelengths indicated correspond to the emission peaks as specified by the probe manufacturer

2.7 Viability vs. apoptosis

Most targeted cytotoxic drugs have been shown to induce apoptosis or other modes of programmed cell death, including autophagic cell death or programmed necrosis. These mechanisms of cell death are often contrasted to necrosis where a passive, sudden and uncontrolled disintegration of the cell occurs. Physiological consequences of apoptosis and passive necrosis are different, and thus it is important to determine the cell death phenotype. When assessed through flow cytometry, cells undergoing apoptosis or other forms of programmed cell death show a decrease in cell volume and forward light scatter (FSC), and an increase in side light scatter (SSC) mainly due to cytoplasmic and nuclear changes such as blebbing, and nuclear fragmentations (Dive et al., 1992; Pheng et al., 2000). In contrast necrosis often shows increased cell volume and FSC without changes in SSC (Healy et al., 1998). Viability assessment after cytotoxic drug exposure does not address the cell death phenotype, thus any kind of cell death phenotype may be induce by drug treatment including passive necrosis (Healy et al., 1998). However studies determining the median cytotoxic dose will require exposure to increasing doses from sub-lethal levels to the minimal doses approaching 100% cell death. In this scenario, programmed cell death phenotypes are more frequently observed than passive necrosis.

Probe	Membrane Permeant	Excitation line	Fluorescence emission
YOYO-1	NO	Blue	Green
TOTO	NO	Blue	Green
TO-PRO	NO	Blue	Green
POPO-1	NO	UV-Violet	Blue
BOBO-1	NO	UV-Violet	Blue
YOYO-3	NO	Red	Red
TOTO-3	NO	Red	Far Red
BOBO-3	NO	Red	Red
JOJO-1	NO	Green	Orange
JO-PRO-1	NO	Green	Orange

Table 4. Membrane–impermeant dimeric and monomeric cyanine dyes are nonfluorescent unless bound to nucleic acids and have extinction coefficients 10–20 times greater than that of DNA-bound propidium iodide

2.8 FDA-PI staining and the "cell death pathway": Frequency distributions of graded and abrupt transitions

When two fluorescent probes are used to determine the proportion of live and dead cells after exposure to cytotoxic drugs over an extended dose range data analysis would be better analyzed on a bivariate plot.

An example is the pair represented by FDA as an indicator of esterase activity in live cells and PI as an indicator of cell membrane damage (Fig. 1). In this case a bivariate plot of green fluorescence against red fluorescence will aid in determining the percentage of live and dead cells (Fig. 1A,C). In addition, the bivariate plot will provide useful data about the biological processes evaluated with FDA and PI.

A concept frequently present in flow cytometry, particularly when analyzing bivariate plots, is the presence of graded transitions or abrupt changes (Shapiro, 2003). These patterns in bivariate distributions are determined by the underlying biological process that is being studied. For example damage of cell membrane allows staining by PI probe so that cells may be classified as dead with a permeable membrane or live having preserved selective permeability, depending on whether they are red fluorescent or not. Cells are observed to be bright stained or having no stain at all, but very rarely they are observed to have dim red fluorescence. Thus membrane damage and PI staining is an example of an abrupt transition or discrete process represented by membrane damage that produces a sudden change in the frequency distribution. This frequency distribution is symmetric, bell-shaped, and has low variability around the peak (Fig. 1C,E.).

By contrast when analyzing drug-induced effects on esterase activity through green fluorescence we will observe a graded transition from bright fluorescence to dim fluorescence (Fig. 1C). Thus a graded biological process represented by progressively decreased esterase activity determines a skewed frequency distribution with higher variability around the peak (Fig. 1F). In this case there will be a higher probability of observing cells within any level of metabolic activity represented by the amount of green fluorescence: bright, intermediate and dim. Note also that cells with damaged membrane no longer retain fluorescein (very few events are seen in upper right quadrant, Fig. 1C).

When analysis is restricted to live cells without damaged membrane (PI negative) it is more evident that the probability of finding live cells with low metabolic activity in the drug-treated population decreases gradually (Fig. 1H). By contrast, when the analysis is restricted to cells without metabolic activity a narrow bell-shape distribution is observed meaning that the probability of finding cells with damaged membrane in cells without metabolic activity increases abruptly (Fig. 1G). When combined in a bivariate plot the gradual decrease in metabolic activity in live cells is observed as a continuous distribution or pathway, while the abrupt transition from membrane-impermeable to membrane-permeable is observed as a discrete transition to a main single cluster of PI-positive cells with very low or no metabolic activity (Fig. 1C). The probability of finding cells with low or no metabolic activity is very low as shown by the few cells in an intermediate position along this "death-pathway". Changes in FSC and SSC are also graded transitions and define a "death-pathway" in bivariate plots (Fig. 1D). Most cells having membrane damage have low FSC and high SSC, those cells without membrane damage and with metabolic activity have high FSC and low SSC, while intermediate positions may be occupied by either of these populations (Fig. 1D). Thus the death pathway defines a whole range of changes occurring in all four parameter FSC, SSC, FDA, and PI. However the main result is characterizing cells as either dead or alive and this difference is brought by PI staining and membrane damage. Thus applying quadrant analysis we would add the fraction of cells in both upper quadrants and the fraction of cells in the lower quadrants as live cells (Fig 1C). The remaining parameters will work as internal quality controls.

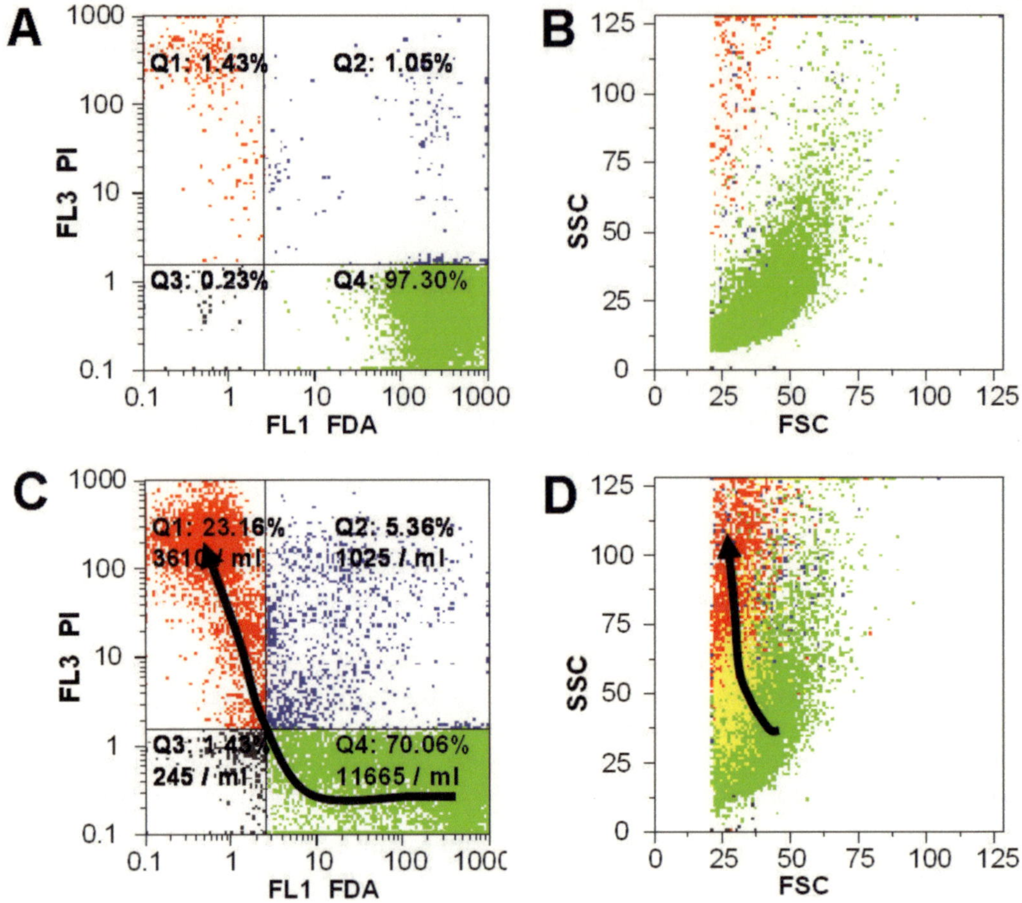

Fig. 1. (continues on next page) The FDA vs. PI bivariate plot and the cell death pathway. A. Sample of human U937 leukemic cells labelled with FDA and PI. Lower right quadrant shows that most cells (97.30%) have esterase enzymatic activity and preserved membrane permeability because they exclude PI staining. Only 1.43% of cells have PI staining without FDA fluorescence, while 1.05% are double positive indicating both enzymatic activity and damaged membrane. B. FSC-SSC profile of live cells is show in green and corresponds to the 97.30% of cells shown in the lower right quadrant of panel A. The small amount of single PI positive (red) and double positive cells (blue) are also observed. C. Sample of human U937 cells exposed to 5 μM sodium arsenite (AsNaO2) for 72h stained with FDA and PI showing a "slow" transition from high FDA fluorescence to low FDA fluorescence (green) and a further "abrupt" transition to a PI positive FDA negative cluster of dead cells (red). A minority of cells are double positive (blue). The whole transition is indicated with the black arrow. D. FSC vs. SSC plot of the sample shown in C. Green color represents FSC-SSC paired values only occupied by live cells (lower right quadrant shown in C), red color represents FSC-SSC paired values only occupied by dead cells (upper left quadrant in C), while yellow color represents FSC-SSC paired values occupied by both live and dead cells. The black arrow shows the graphical death pathway transition in the FSC SSC plot. The FSC-SSC values of the minority of double positive cells are shown in blue

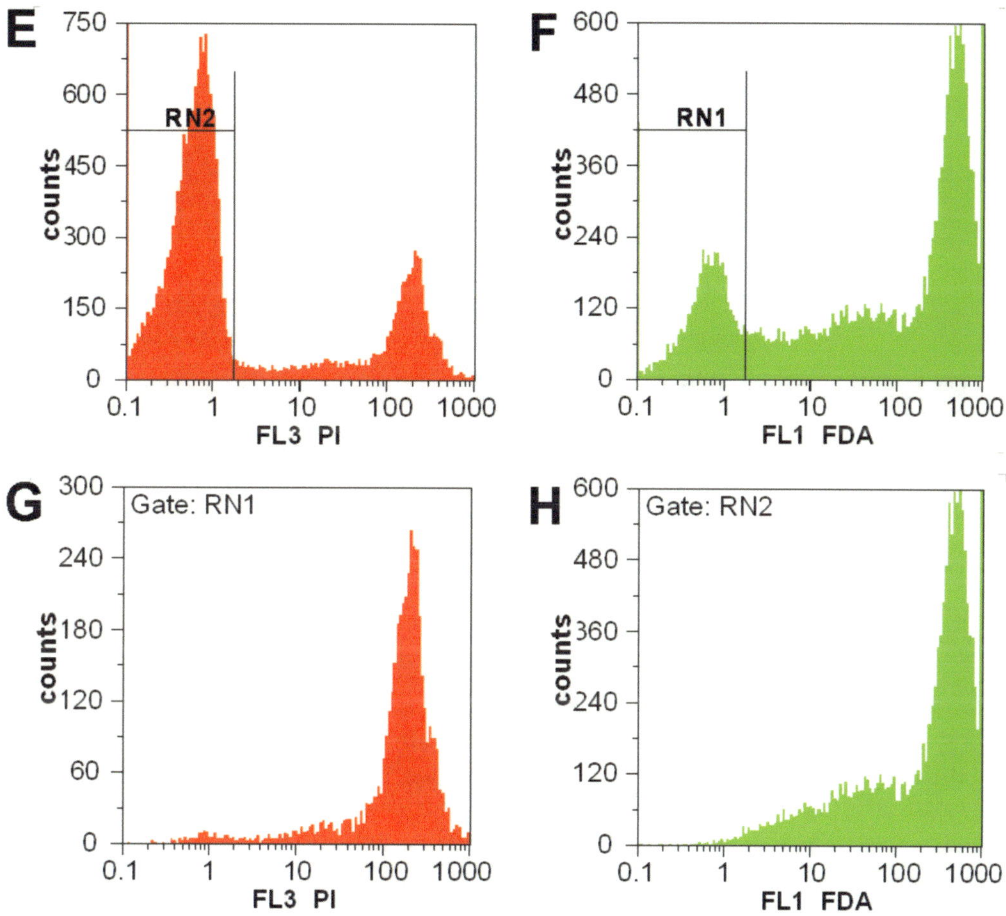

Fig. 1. (continued) E. Frequency distribution of PI fluorescence corresponding to the sample shown in C and D. Note that positive and negative cell populations are bell-shaped, symmetrical, with low variability around the peaks, and well separated from each other F. Frequency distribution of FDA fluorescence of the same sample shown in C and D. The population of positive cells shows asymmetrical left-skewed distribution with great variability to the left of the peak. G. The sample shown in E with live cells excluded. The probability of finding positive cells with intermediate and dim PI fluorescence decreases abruptly to the left. H. The sample shown in F with dead cells excluded. The probability of finding positive cells with intermediate and dim FDA fluorescence decreases slowly to the left

3. Building a cytotoxic dose response curve

Theoretically, if a population of cells were homogenously sensitive to cell death induced by a certain drug there would be a single dose D at which 100% cell death would be observed (Casarett et al., 2008; Goodman et al., 2010). However in any given sample of drug-treated cells a random proportion of cells will die at doses lower or higher than D due to experimental and biological variability. This random divergence from D follows a Gaussian distribution (Fig. 2A,C).

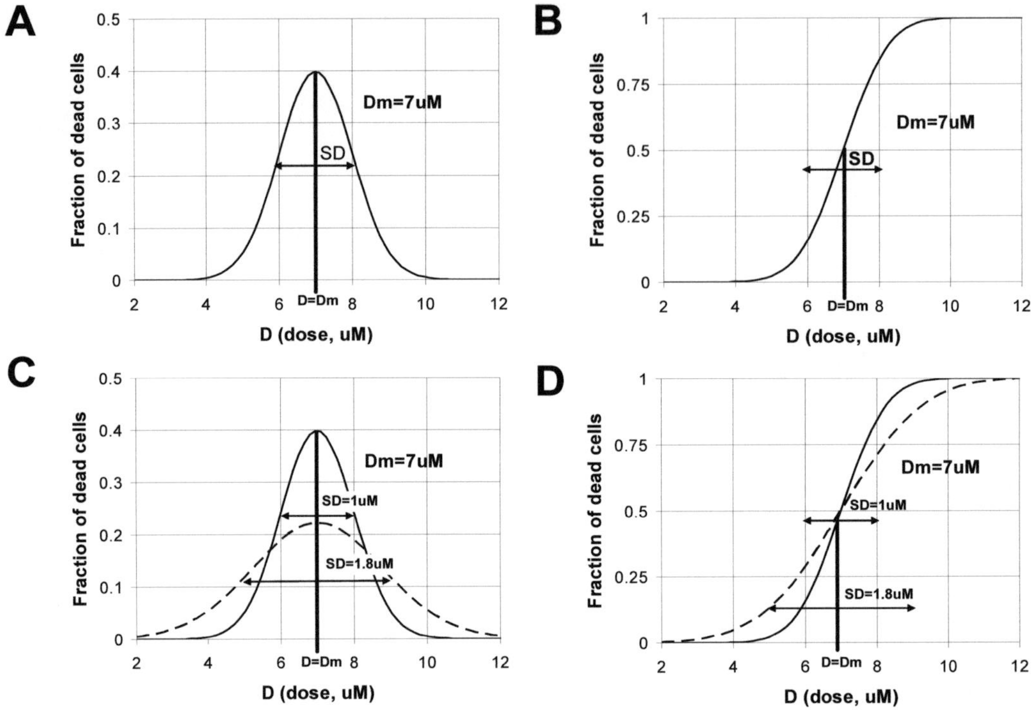

Fig. 2. Quantal dose response model. A. Single cells will show differences on the minimal drug dose required to induce cell death. Dm is the most frequent minimal dose required to elicit cell death. Variations around this value have a normal distribution. In this particular example Dm is 7uM and the standard deviation (SD) is 1uM. B. Dm is the drug dose that is estimated to kill half of the cells in a sample. When running experiments exposing cells to incremental doses of a cytotoxic drug the fraction of dead cells observed will follow a normal cumulative function. C. Differences between two cytotoxic drugs in the variability observed around Dm. The drug represented by the dotted line has larger variability (SD=1.8 uM) than the drug represented in full line (SD=1 uM). D. Increased variability around Dm is observed as a dose response curve with a smaller slope as shown by the dotted line of the cumulative normal distribution

The median dose Dm represents a dose D where half of the cells are killed and half of the cells remain live (Fig. 2 B). However, as indicated by the bell shape of the Gaussian distribution many of the 50% of cells killed at a dose Dm may have required less than Dm to be killed. In fact as shown in figure 2A only a fraction of cells will require strictly a dose Dm (those in the bell peak), while a minority of cells will require a dose much lower than Dm to be killed (those in the left tail of the bell-shaped curve). If we conduct experiments evaluating the cytotoxic effect of increasing doses we will observe a sigmoid curve that follows a cumulative Gaussian frequency distribution (Fig. 2B). Doses lower than Dm will show decreased probability of cell death approaching 0% while doses higher than Dm will show increased probability of cell death approaching 100% (Fig. 2B). This model is known as quantal dose-response because it is based on the scoring of all members of a sample population for having or not having a certain condition at a given applied dose (Casarett et al., 2008). This is precisely what is done through flow cytometry assessing a sample on a cell by cell basis for being dead or alive. Using flow cytometry we can measure the fraction of cells killed (fa) at a dose D with high accuracy and precision due to the large number of cells analyzed which ensures an extremely low standard error (SE). However, high accuracy and precision apply to a single sample and not to replicates. The source of variability between replicates will be both biological and experimental. For example cells overgrown in culture may respond with higher variability than cells in exponential growth when estimated from replicates. Similarly any problems around drug exposure or the staining procedure will add to the variability of replicates although the precision and accuracy of each sample determination will be very high due to the large amount of cells scored in each sample tube. Regarding calculation of the median cytotoxic dose Dm this replicates will have a critical impact on the statistical precision of the Dm estimate.

3.1 Calculating the median dose: The median effect equation

Cells cultured in vitro can be exposed to increasing doses of a cytotoxic drug during a certain time interval (e.g., 48h or 72h) to determine a median cytotoxic dose Dm. Several doses should be tested to extend over a dose range. The lower doses should induce a fraction of dead cells close to that of unexposed cells, while the higher doses should induce death values approaching 100% or achieve a plateau of maximal effect. In between these boundary doses the more intervals assessed the more precision we will get in the estimates. For example seven doses assessed in triplicate that yield cell death fractions between 5% and 95% would be enough to obtain regression estimates with an adequate precision. The dose response sigmoidal curve can be fit to a two parameter logistic function of the type:

$$fa= 1 / [1+1/(D/Dm)^m] \quad (1)$$

where D is the dose, Dm is the dose required to achieve the median cytotoxic effect, fa is the fraction of dead cells, and m is a measurement of the sigmoidicity of the curve. When m=1 the dose-effect curve is hyperbolic, when m>1 the curve is sigmoidal, while m<1 indicates a negative sigmoidal shape (Fig. 3A).

To estimate Dm and m the median effect equation is written as:

$$fa/(1-fa) = (D/Dm)^m \quad (2)$$

The factor (1-fa) is the fraction of live cells. Applying a log transformation the following linear function is obtained:

$$\log (fa/(1-fa) = m \,.\, \log (D) - m \,.\, \log (Dm) \quad (3)$$

Thus plotting log values of experimental doses against log values of the ratio of dead/live cells will show a linear trend that is often referred to as median effect plot (Fig. 3B).

This is a linear function of the type y= m.x + b, where y=fa/(1-fa), x=log(D), and b=-m.log (Dm). A linear regression can be applied to these data to obtain estimates for m and Dm. The m coefficient can be readily determined by the slope of the regression, and Dm is derived from the estimate of the intercept -m.log(Dm).

The squared correlation coefficient or R2 value is an estimate of the precision of the overall regression (Fig. 3B). In this particular application to data representing cell death vs. dose of cytotoxic drug, R2 is affected mainly by the scattering of replicate values, which in turn depend on the experimental and biological variability, and also on the number of sample doses in between the lowest and highest effect values. The standard error (SE) of m and the intercept can also be obtained from regression analysis to get a 95% confidence interval around log(Dm). The formula for manual calculation is rather complicated and involves computing SE(log(D)) when D=Dm (shown in eq. 14, Table 5) but may be obtained using any software that implements this calculation such as Calcusyn or Compusyn (Bijnsdorp et al., 2011; Ikeda et al., 2011; Ramachandran et al., 2010).

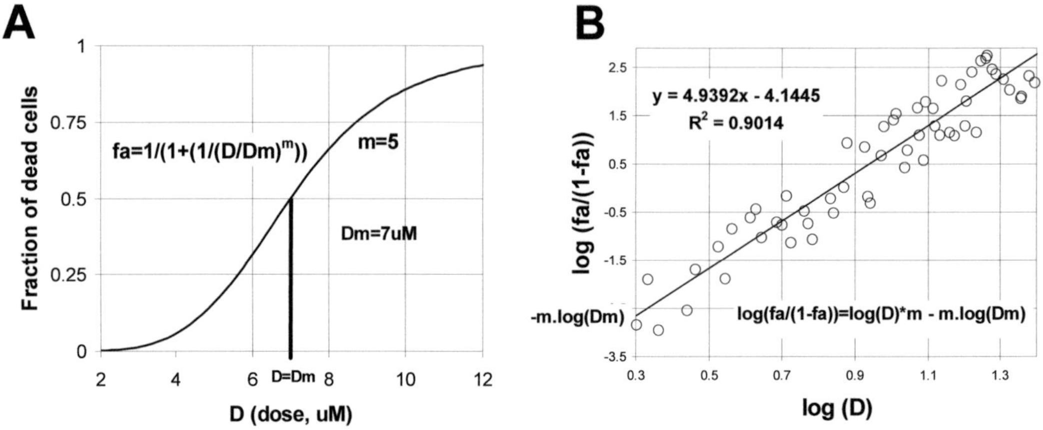

Fig. 3. Median effect plot. A. The two parameter dose-response sigmoidal curve for a particular example with Dm=7uM and m=5. B. Algebraic and log transformation to obtain a linear function. A linear regression can be applied to experimental data in order to obtain estimates of the two parameters Dm and m. The squared correlation coefficient R2 is a measure of the overall precision of the linear regression and thus the Dm and m estimates

3.2 Threshold, median dose and maximal efficacy

Analysis of the dose-effect plot can be informative about threshold values and maximal efficacy values.

In practice the threshold value will be the minimal dose where the fraction of dead cells is higher than that of untreated cells. The maximal efficacy would be the fraction of dead cells where the sigmoidal curve approaches a plateau. Quite often the maximal efficacy approaches 100%. However a cell population may exhibit a differential response and a fraction of cells may require quite larger doses. In these cases the maximal efficacy will be much less than 100%.

3.3 Comparing two drugs

To compare two drugs and evaluate whether combination results in synergy or not a first step is to calculate Dm for the two drugs. Thus, the same approach described above should be applied to the second drug. The procedure will include evaluating several doses in replicates with the same exposure time interval as the first drug, obtaining data to create a median effect plot and estimating m and Dm by linear regression (Chang et al., 1987; Chou & Talalay, 1984; Sugiyama et al., 1998).

Results from assessment of the two drugs can be analyzed together in a combined median effect plot where log doses (in molar units) are depicted against log (fa/1-fa). In this plot the relative potency of the two drugs can be easily appreciated (Fig. 4A). A drug a is said to be more potent than a second drug b regarding the cytotoxic effect when less dose of dug a is needed to achieve the same cytotoxic effect with drug b on a molar basis. In addition when the slopes of the two drugs are different it suggests that the drugs have different mechanisms to induce cytotoxicity.

The dose effect equation can be re-written to calculate the dose required to induce a given cytotoxic effect:

$$D=Dm\ (fa/(1-fa))^{1/m} \quad (4)$$

For example the effective cytotoxic dose 50% (EC50) is the dose D that is estimated to kill 50% of the cells. In this case fa=0.5 and EC50 is coincident with the median dose Dm. Similarly EC25 is the dose D that is estimated to kill 25% of the cells.

3.3.1 Assessing the combined effect of two drugs under fixed molar ratio

Once obtained the dose-response curve for two drugs a and b, a third experiment with combination of a + b will be needed to determine if the interaction of these drugs is additive, synergic or antagonistic.

Assuming that the drug b is less potent than the drug a, fixed molar ratio could be used in the combination based on the relative potency EC50(a)/EC50(b). For example if EC50(a) is 10μM and EC50(b) is 30μM, the molar ratio of the combination would be 1/3. An empirical approach is to start the combination experiment with a combination of a+b calculated as

$$EC50(a+b)=10^{\{[\log(EC50(a))+\log(EC50(b))]/2\}} \quad (5)$$

In this example this estimated value would be 17.3 μM. Assuming the fixed molar ratio 1/3 this combination would have 4.3μM of drug a and 13.0 μM of drug b.

Next we should treat this combination as a new drug a+b and evaluate several doses above and below 17.3μM in replicates to span a dose range of the combination. Thus, we will experimentally obtain a new data set of doses and cytotoxic effects that we should evaluate by the same procedure with the median effect plot, and conduct a linear regression to obtain estimates for m and Dm with the combination of a+b.

In particular we will obtain an effect-dose equation as shown above (eq. 4) to determine the dose of the combination a+b to achieve a desired cytotoxic effect level (EC)

$$D= Dm_{a+b}\ (fa/(1-fa))^{1/m_{a+b}} \quad (6)$$

For example applying (eq.5) EC50 (a+b) will be equal to the median dose estimated from the regression in the combined experiment (Dm_{a+b})

3.4 Graphical analysis

A first approach is to plot this result together with results of single drug effects to depict some relevant information (Pegram et al., 1999). When the combined-drug curve lies in a midpoint between the two single drug curves it suggests an additive effect (Fig. 4A). It indicates that the potency of the combined drugs is at an intermediate point between the potency of each drug. When the combined drug curve is shifted to the left it would be closer to the more potent single drug and thus suggests synergism (Fig. 1B). On the other side when the combined drug curve is shifted to the right and closer to the low potency drug it is suggestive of antagonism (Fig. 1C). Another hint that could aid in generating hypothesis is the curve shape and particularly the slope. The variability around Dm is represented by the standard deviation (SD) of the Gaussian distribution underlying the quantal dose-response model discussed above. A large SD is in accordance with a flat curve while a small SD is in accordance with a steep curve (Fig. 2C,D). This variability has a biological significance and two drugs having different mechanisms of inducing cell death in a certain cell line may have different slopes.

3.5 Calculating the combination index (CI)

The graphical analysis gives some clues about what kind of interaction results from the combination of drugs a and b and depicts useful information but is less conclusive in quantitative terms. A more thorough conclusion can be derived from computing the combination index for each cytotoxic effect level (Chou, 2008; 2010). Computing the combination index (CI) for each effect level provides an answer to what kind of interaction occurs between drug a and drug b throughout the whole dose range.

The combination index method takes data provided by single and combined dose-effect equations to provide an estimate at the whole range of cytotoxic effects. The combination index is defined for a given effect level i by the following equation:

$$CI(i) = Dac(i) / Das(i) + Dbc(i) / Dbs(i) + \alpha\, Dac(i) \,.\, Dbc(i) / Das(i) \,.\, Dbs(i) \quad (7)$$

Where Dac(i) and Dbc(i) are the doses of drugs a and b respectively required in the combination a+b to produce an effect level i.

Das(i) and Dbs(i) are the doses of drug a and b respectively, required to produce an effect level i when used as single drugs. For any level i, these values are obtained from the three dose response curves defined by (eq. 4) (two single and one combined) obtained with parameters Dm and m that in turn were obtained from regression analysis with (eq.3) applied to experimental data. It is often assumed the conservative criteria that cytotoxic drugs are mutually non exclusive and $\alpha=1$. If the three lines are strictly parallel and both drugs have a similar molecular target it could be assumed that they are mutually exclusive and in that case $\alpha=0$. If the fixed molar ratio of drug a and b in the combined treatment is p/q, then for an effect level i:

$$Das(i)=Dm_a\,(fa(i)/(1-fa(i)))^{1/m_a} \quad (8)$$

$$Dbs(i)=Dm_b\,(fa(i)/(1-fa(i)))^{1/m_b} \quad (9)$$

$$Dac(i)=p/(p+q)\; Dm_{a+b}\,(fa(i)/(1-fa(i)))^{1/m_{a+b}} \quad (10)$$

$$Dbc(i)=q/(p+q)\; Dm_{a+b}\,(fa(i)/(1-fa(i)))^{1/m_{a+b}} \quad (11)$$

Where fa(i) is the fraction of dead cells at effect level i, Dm_a and m_a are the median dose and the slope estimated for drug a, Dm_b and m_b are the median dose and the slope estimated for drug b, and Dm_{a+b} and m_{a+b} are the median dose and the slope estimated for the combined treatment with drugs a and b. Thus the combination index is calculated for any effect level above 0 and below 1.

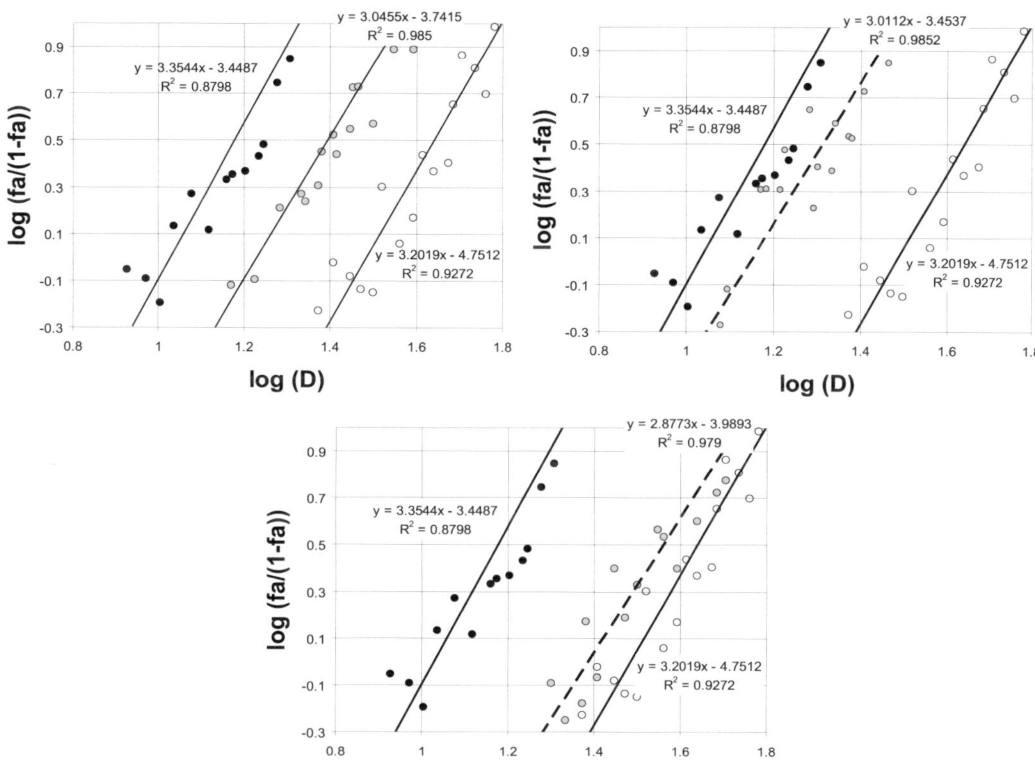

Fig. 4. Drug interaction and median effect plot. A. In this example experimental values are represented by circles and linear regression is applied to obtain estimates for Dm and m. Experimental values obtained for a drug a are shown in black circles. The values of Dm and m for drug a were 10 μM and and 3.0 respectively. Experimental values for a less potent drug b are shown in open circles. The values of Dm and m for drug a were 30 uM and and 3.0 respectively. A combined experiment was run with a+b with a constant mass ratio of 1/3 based on EC50(a)/EC50(b) and assuming that under additive effect EC50(a+b)=10{[log(EC50(a))+log(EC50(b))]/2}. Experimental values for the combination are shown in grey circles. The values of Dm and m for the combination a+b were 17.0 uM and and 3.0 respectively. In this example drugs a and b have an additive interaction and the median effect plot of the combination lies in a mid position between the lines corresponding to the single drugs. B. The same experiment shown in A, but in this case the drugs a and b have synergic effect. The values of Dm and m for the combination a+b were 14.0 uM and and 3.0 respectively. The median effect plot of the combination is shifted towards the drug a, which has the highest potency. C. The same experiment shown in A, but in this example the drugs a and b have antagonistic effect. The values of Dm and m for the combination a+b were 24.4 uM and and 2.9 respectively. The median effect plot of the combination in this case is shifted towards the drug b which has the lowest potency

			Three alternative results of the experimental assay with combination *a+b* (considering α=1, mutually non-exclusive condition)		
			Additive	**Synergic**	**Antagonistic**
	Single drug a	Single drug b	Combined drugs a+b	Combined drugs a+b	Combined drugs a+b
Dm (uM) #(1)	10	30	17	14	24.4
m #(1)	3	3	3	3	3
fa(i)	0.5				
Das(i) #(2)	10				
Dbs(i) #(3)		30			
Dac(i) #(4)			4.25	3.5	6.1
Dbc(i) #(5)			12.75	10.5	18.3
p/(p+q) #(6)			0.25	0.25	0.25
q/(p+q) #(6)			0.75	0.75	0.75
CI (i) #(7)			1.03	0.82	1.59

$SE(CI(i))=\{\{ Dac(i)/ Das(i) . [SE(Dac(i)/ Dac(i)+ SE(Das(i)/ Das(i)]\}^2 +\{ Dbc(i)/ Dbs(i) . [SE(Dbc(i)/ Dbc(i)+ SE(Dbs(i)/ Dbs(i)]\}^2\}^{1/2}$ **(eq. 12)**

$SE(D) = 1/2 . \{10^{[log(D)+SE(log(D)]} - 10^{[log(D)-SE(log(D)]}\}$ **(eq. 13)**

$SE(log (D)) =\{log(D) . [SE(b)/log(fa/(1-fa)-b]^2+[SE(m)/m]^2+2[-(logD)^{1/2} . SE(m)/SE/(b)] . SE(b)/b . SE(m)/m\}^{1/2}$ **(eq. 14)**

where b=-m.log(Dm)

A 95% confidence interval around D in general and around Dm in particular, can be computed using the formulas for standard error (SE, eq. 13 and eq. 14).

A 95% confidence interval around CI at any effect level i can be computed from the standard error formulas presented in eq. 12, 13, and 14.

\# (1) Obtained from linear regression of experimental data

\# (2) $Das(i)=Dm_a (fa(i)/(1-fa(i)))^{1/m}a$

\# (3) $Dbs(i)=Dm_b (fa(i)/(1-fa(i)))^{1/m}b$

\# (4) $Dac(i)=p/(p+q) Dm_{a+b} (fa(i)/(1-fa(i)))^{1/m}a+b$

\# (5) $Dbc(i)=q/(p+q) Dm_{a+b} (fa(i)/(1-fa(i)))^{1/m}a+b$

\# (6) Molar ratio p/q = Dm(a) /Dm(b) = 10/30 = 1/3

\# (7) CI(i) = Dac(i) /Das(i) +Dbc(i) /Dbs(i) + α Dac(i) . Dbc(i) / Das(i) . Dbs(i)

Table 5. CI calculation between two drugs a and b at the 50% effect level under three alternative conditions: additive, synergic, antagonistic. To obtain CI as a function of the effect level i, the calculation has to be repeated for each arbitrary level i between 0 and 1. A 95% confidence interval around D in general and around Dm in particular, can be computed using the formulas for standard error (SE, eq. 13 and eq. 14). A 95% confidence interval around CI at any effect level i can be computed from the standard error formulas presented in eq. 12, 13 and 14

Table 5 summarizes a manual calculation of CI of two drugs a and b using these formulas for the 50% effect level under three hypothetical results: additive, synergic or antagonistic effect.

The same calculation can be applied to any effect level to plot CI as a function of effect level. When the interaction is additive CI =1. In this case it can be interpreted that one of the drugs (the less potent one, i.e. drug b in the example) is acting as though it is merely a diluted form of the other (drug a in the example). When CI<1 the combination of a+b is synergic while CI>1 indicates antagonism. Synergy, implies that the combination of the two drugs achieves a cytotoxic effect greater than that expected by the simple addition of the effects of the drugs a and b, while antagonism achieves a cytotoxic effect lower than that expected by additive effects of drugs a and b.

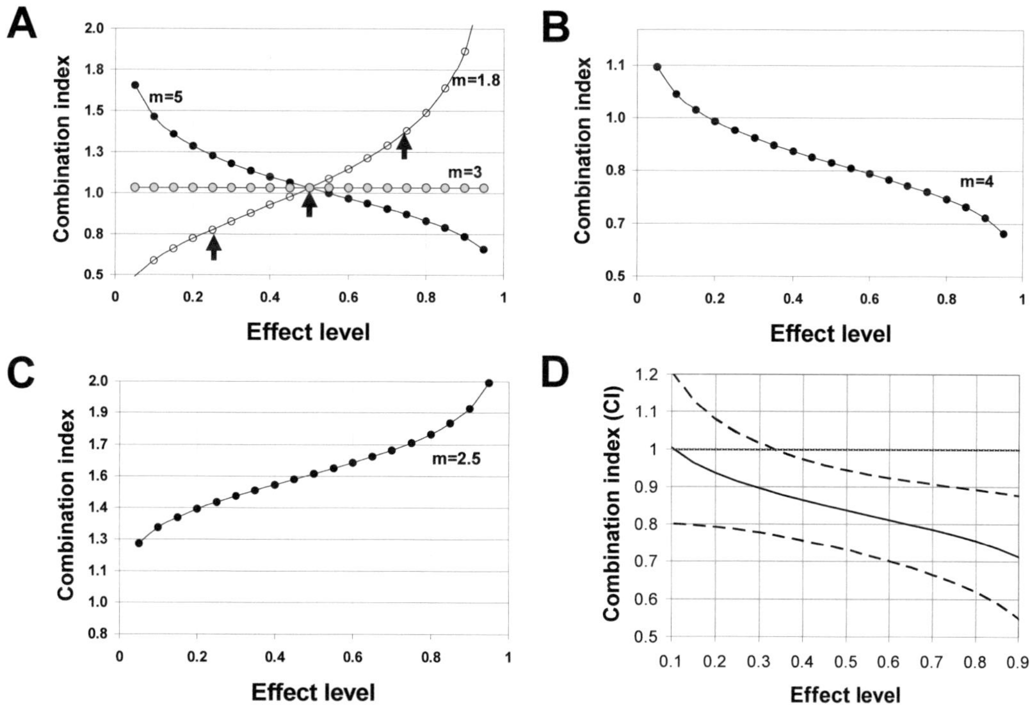

Fig. 5. Drug interaction and CI calculation. A. Only rarely the combination index obtained is constant for all effect levels. Here it is shown how different values of the slope m obtained through linear regression in the combination experiment (a+b) would affect the shape of the curve representing the CI as a function of the effect level. Similarly, differences between the slopes obtained for drugs a and b through the single drug experiments will contribute to the uneven shape of the CI function. Note that depending on the effect level the interaction a+b with m=1.8 would be synergism, additive or antagonism at EC25. EC50, and EC75 respectively (arrows). B. Results of CI calculation for the example where a+b results in synergism considering m=4 in the regression of the combined-drug experiment. C. Results of CI calculation for the example where a+b results in antagonism considering m=2.5 in the regression of the combined-drug experiment. D. 95% confidence level intervals around CI, using an algebraic approximation (eq. 12, Table 5) in an example where combination of a+b is synergic

The horizontal line corresponding to CI(i)=1, where i is any effect level in the interval (0,1), is often call the additive effect line. A combination of drugs a and b may result in CI values above or below the additive line at different effect levels. Thus, the CI as a function of effect level is not constant or linear and it may be decreasing or increasing (Fig 5A). If data from the combination experiment in the example of figure 4A resulted in m_{a+b}=5 or m_{a+b}=1.8, even still with Dm_{a+b} =17 the CI line would be inclined downwards or upwards respectively (Fig. 5A). Only at effect levels close to EC50 the result would be strictly additive. An important conclusion is that for some drug combinations, experiments conducted at different single dose-effect levels may yield opposing results. For example if the combination a+b with m=1.8 shown in figure 5A were experimentally evaluated only at effect level 0.25 the single dose analysis would conclude on synergism. However if it were evaluated at effect level 0.75 it would conclude on antagonism (Fig. 5A). This exemplifies why the assessment of combination index over the whole dose range will show all kinds of interactions that may result from combination at different effect levels.

Computing a standard error of CI allows plotting confidence intervals at all effect levels providing a further assurance over the computation. A 95% confidence interval will indicate that if we repeat the experiment 100 times, 95 out 100 times the CI would be within this interval. For example, observing whether or not confidence limits are above or below the additive line will allow concluding with further statistical support on antagonism or synergism respectively. Computation of the standard error of CI and confidence intervals at all levels should be better obtained through specialized software such as Calcusyn or Compusyn (Bijnsdorp et al., 2011; Chou, 2010). It may also require approaches such as Monte Carlo simulation based on the estimated parameter for m and Dm in single and combined equations.

4. Concluding remarks

A thorough assessment of drug interaction is an essential step in targeted combined therapy. The new targeted agents are seldom useful as single agents but may be effective when used in specific combinations. The median effect and combination index calculation are well founded methods traditionally used in pharmacological and toxicological studies. Since new cytotoxic drugs target mechanisms eliciting cell death, biomarkers related to viability assessment are preferred to biomarkers of cell proliferation. Flow cytometry is an ideal technology to provide massive data from cell death biomarkers to build dose response curves of cytotoxic effect. When these data is further used to determine the combination index a full characterization of drug interaction over the cytotoxic effect is obtained at all effect levels. This approach can be applied to tumor cell lines in preclinical studies and also in patient-derived tumor cells, thus providing useful information as prospective indicators of the potential therapeutic response to combined-drug antitumor treatment.

5. References

Armand, J. P., Burnett, A. K., Drach, J., Harousseau, J. L., Lowenberg, B. & San Miguel, J. (2007). The emerging role of targeted therapy for hematologic malignancies: update on bortezomib and tipifarnib. Oncologist Vol. 12, No. 3, (Mar, 2007), pp. 281-290

Barnett, M. J., McGhee-Wilson, D., Shapiro, A. M. & Lakey, J. R. (2004). Variation in human islet viability based on different membrane integrity stains. Cell Transplant Vol. 13, No. 5, 2004), pp. 481-488

Belinsky, S. A., Grimes, M. J., Picchi, M. A., Mitchell, H. D., Stidley, C. A., Tesfaigzi, Y., Channell, M. M., Liu, Y., Casero, R. A., Jr., Baylin, S. B. et al. (2011). Combination therapy with vidaza and entinostat suppresses tumor growth and reprograms the epigenome in an orthotopic lung cancer model. Cancer Res Vol. 71, No. 2, (Jan 15, 2011), pp. 454-462

Berghe, T. V., Vanlangenakker, N., Parthoens, E., Deckers, W., Devos, M., Festjens, N., Guerin, C. J., Brunk, U. T., Declercq, W. & Vandenabeele, P. (2010). Necroptosis, necrosis and secondary necrosis converge on similar cellular disintegration features. Cell Death Differ Vol. 17, No. 6, (Jun, 2010), pp. 922-930

Bijnsdorp, I. V., Giovannetti, E. & Peters, G. J. (2011). Analysis of drug interactions. Methods Mol Biol Vol. 731, No., 2011), pp. 421-434

Boccadoro, M., Morgan, G. & Cavenagh, J. (2005). Preclinical evaluation of the proteasome inhibitor bortezomib in cancer therapy. Cancer Cell Int Vol. 5, No. 1, (Jun 1, 2005), pp. 18

Bross, P. F., Kane, R., Farrell, A. T., Abraham, S., Benson, K., Brower, M. E., Bradley, S., Gobburu, J. V., Goheer, A., Lee, S. L. et al. (2004). Approval summary for bortezomib for injection in the treatment of multiple myeloma. Clin Cancer Res Vol. 10, No. 12 Pt 1, (Jun 15, 2004), pp. 3954-3964

Burmeister, Y., Lischke, T., Dahler, A. C., Mages, H. W., Lam, K. P., Coyle, A. J., Kroczek, R. A. & Hutloff, A. (2008). ICOS controls the pool size of effector-memory and regulatory T cells. J Immunol Vol. 180, No. 2, (Jan 15, 2008), pp. 774-782

Busch, C., Geisler, J., Knappskog, S., Lillehaug, J. R. & Lonning, P. E. Alterations in the p53 pathway and p16INK4a expression predict overall survival in metastatic melanoma patients treated with dacarbazine. J Invest Dermatol Vol. 130, No. 10, (Oct, pp. 2514-2516

Callewaert, D. M., Radcliff, G., Waite, R., LeFevre, J. & Poulik, M. D. (1991). Characterization of effector-target conjugates for cloned human natural killer and human lymphokine activated killer cells by flow cytometry. Cytometry Vol. 12, No. 7, 1991), pp. 666-676

Cameron, D. A., Ritchie, A. A. & Miller, W. R. (2001). The relative importance of proliferation and cell death in breast cancer growth and response to tamoxifen. Eur J Cancer Vol. 37, No. 12, (Aug, 2001), pp. 1545-1553

Carew, J. S., Giles, F. J. & Nawrocki, S. T. (2008). Histone deacetylase inhibitors: mechanisms of cell death and promise in combination cancer therapy. Cancer Lett Vol. 269, No. 1, (Sep 28, 2008), pp. 7-17

Casarett, L. J., Doull, J. & Klaassen, C. D. (2008). Casarett and Doull's toxicology: the basic science of poisons. 7th Edition. McGraw-Hill. ISBN (9780071470513-0071470514) New York

Castaneda, C. A. &Gomez, H. L. (2009). Targeted therapies: Combined lapatinib and paclitaxel in HER2-positive breast cancer. Nat Rev Clin Oncol Vol. 6, No. 6, (Jun, 2009), pp. 308-309

Citri, A., Kochupurakkal, B. S. & Yarden, Y. (2004). The achilles heel of ErbB-2/HER2: regulation by the Hsp90 chaperone machine and potential for pharmacological intervention. Cell Cycle Vol. 3, No. 1, (Jan, 2004), pp. 51-60

Czekanska, E. M. (2011). Assessment of cell proliferation with resazurin-based fluorescent dye. Methods Mol Biol Vol. 740, No., 2011), pp. 27-32

Chang, T. T., Gulati, S., Chou, T. C., Colvin, M. & Clarkson, B. (1987). Comparative cytotoxicity of various drug combinations for human leukemic cells and normal hematopoietic precursors. Cancer Res Vol. 47, No. 1, (Jan 1, 1987), pp. 119-122

Chou, T. C. (2008). Preclinical versus clinical drug combination studies. Leuk Lymphoma Vol. 49, No. 11, (Nov, 2008), pp. 2059-2080

Chou, T. C. (2010). Drug combination studies and their synergy quantification using the Chou-Talalay method. Cancer Res Vol. 70, No. 2, (Jan 15, 2010), pp. 440-446

Chou, T. C. &Talalay, P. (1984). Quantitative analysis of dose-effect relationships: the combined effects of multiple drugs or enzyme inhibitors. Adv Enzyme Regul Vol. 22, No., 1984), pp. 27-55

Dai, Y., Rahmani, M. & Grant, S. (2003). Proteasome inhibitors potentiate leukemic cell apoptosis induced by the cyclin-dependent kinase inhibitor flavopiridol through a SAPK/JNK- and NF-kappaB-dependent process. Oncogene Vol. 22, No. 46, (Oct 16, 2003), pp. 7108-7122

Dancey, J. E. &Chen, H. X. (2006). Strategies for optimizing combinations of molecularly targeted anticancer agents. Nat Rev Drug Discov Vol. 5, No. 8, (Aug, 2006), pp. 649-659

Darzynkiewicz, Z., Traganos, F., Staiano-Coico, L., Kapuscinski, J. & Melamed, M. R. (1982). Interaction of rhodamine 123 with living cells studied by flow cytometry. Cancer Res Vol. 42, No. 3, (Mar, 1982), pp. 799-806

De Clerck, L. S., Bridts, C. H., Mertens, A. M., Moens, M. M. & Stevens, W. J. (1994). Use of fluorescent dyes in the determination of adherence of human leucocytes to endothelial cells and the effect of fluorochromes on cellular function. J Immunol Methods Vol. 172, No. 1, (Jun 3, 1994), pp. 115-124

Derenzini, M., Brighenti, E., Donati, G., Vici, M., Ceccarelli, C., Santini, D., Taffurelli, M., Montanaro, L. & Trere, D. (2009). The p53-mediated sensitivity of cancer cells to chemotherapeutic agents is conditioned by the status of the retinoblastoma protein. J Pathol Vol. 219, No. 3, (Nov, 2009), pp. 373-382

Dive, C., Gregory, C. D., Phipps, D. J., Evans, D. L., Milner, A. E. & Wyllie, A. H. (1992). Analysis and discrimination of necrosis and apoptosis (programmed cell death) by multiparameter flow cytometry. Biochim Biophys Acta Vol. 1133, No. 3, (Feb 3, 1992), pp. 275-285

Duan, X. F., Wu, Y. L., Xu, H. Z., Zhao, M., Zhuang, H. Y., Wang, X. D., Yan, H. & Chen, G. Q. (2010). Synergistic mitosis-arresting effects of arsenic trioxide and paclitaxel on human malignant lymphocytes. Chem Biol Interact Vol. 183, No. 1, (Jan 5, 2010), pp. 222-230

Elrefaei, M., Baker, C. A., Jones, N. G., Bangsberg, D. R. & Cao, H. (2008). Presence of suppressor HIV-specific CD8+ T cells is associated with increased PD-1 expression on effector CD8+ T cells. J Immunol Vol. 180, No. 11, (Jun 1, 2008), pp. 7757-7763

Eray, M., Matto, M., Kaartinen, M., Andersson, L. & Pelkonen, J. (2001). Flow cytometric analysis of apoptotic subpopulations with a combination of annexin V-FITC, propidium iodide, and SYTO 17. Cytometry Vol. 43, No. 2, (Feb 1, 2001), pp. 134-142

Eriksen, K. W., Sondergaard, H., Woetmann, A., Krejsgaard, T., Skak, K., Geisler, C., Wasik, M. A. & Odum, N. (2009). The combination of IL-21 and IFN-alpha boosts STAT3 activation, cytotoxicity and experimental tumor therapy. Mol Immunol Vol. 46, No. 5, (Feb, 2009), pp. 812-820

Eruslanov, E. &Kusmartsev, S. (2010). Identification of ROS using oxidized DCFDA and flow-cytometry. Methods Mol Biol Vol. 594, No., 2010), pp. 57-72

Facoetti, A., Ranza, E. & Nano, R. (2008). Proliferation and programmed cell death: role of p53 protein in high and low grade astrocytoma. Anticancer Res Vol. 28, No. 1A, (Jan-Feb, 2008), pp. 15-19

Favoni, R. E. &Florio, T. (2011). Combined chemotherapy with cytotoxic and targeted compounds for the management of human malignant pleural mesothelioma. Trends Pharmacol Sci Vol. 32, No. 8, (Aug, 2011), pp. 463-479

Foye, W. O. (1995). Cancer chemotherapeutic agents.American Chemical Society. ISBN (9780841229204-0841229201) Washington, DC

Fuchs, T. A., Abed, U., Goosmann, C., Hurwitz, R., Schulze, I., Wahn, V., Weinrauch, Y., Brinkmann, V. & Zychlinsky, A. (2007). Novel cell death program leads to neutrophil extracellular traps. J Cell Biol Vol. 176, No. 2, (Jan 15, 2007), pp. 231-241

Fujioka, H., Hunt, P. J., Rozga, J., Wu, G. D., Cramer, D. V., Demetriou, A. A. & Moscioni, A. D. (1994). Carboxyfluorescein (CFSE) labelling of hepatocytes for short-term localization following intraportal transplantation. Cell Transplant Vol. 3, No. 5, (Sep-Oct, 1994), pp. 397-408

Goodman, L. S., Brunton, L. L., Chabner, B. & Knollmann, B. C. (2010). Goodman & Gilman's pharmacological basis of therapeutics.12th Edition.McGraw-Hill. ISBN (9780071624428-0071624422) New York

Gozuacik, D. &Kimchi, A. (2007). Autophagy and cell death. Curr Top Dev Biol Vol. 78, No., 2007), pp. 217-245

Gross-Goupil, M. &Escudier, B. (2010). [Targeted therapies: sequential and combined treatments]. Bull Cancer Vol. 97, No., 2010), pp. 65-71

Haase, S. B. (2004). Cell cycle analysis of budding yeast using SYTOX Green. Curr Protoc Cytom Vol. Chapter 7, No., (Nov, 2004), pp. Unit 7 23

Hamilton, D., Loignon, M., Alaoui-Jamali, M. A. & Batist, G. (2007). Novel use of the fluorescent dye 5-(and-6)-chloromethyl SNARF-1 acetate for the measurement of intracellular glutathione in leukemic cells and primary lymphocytes. Cytometry A Vol. 71, No. 9, (Sep, 2007), pp. 709-715

Healy, E., Dempsey, M., Lally, C. & Ryan, M. P. (1998). Apoptosis and necrosis: mechanisms of cell death induced by cyclosporine A in a renal proximal tubular cell line. Kidney Int Vol. 54, No. 6, (Dec, 1998), pp. 1955-1966

Ikeda, H., Taira, N., Nogami, T., Shien, K., Okada, M., Shien, T., Doihara, H. & Miyoshi, S. (2011). Combination treatment with fulvestrant and various cytotoxic agents (doxorubicin, paclitaxel, docetaxel, vinorelbine, and 5-fluorouracil) has a synergistic effect in estrogen receptor-positive breast cancer. Cancer Sci Vol., No., (Jul 30, 2011),

Jones, K. H. &Senft, J. A. (1985). An improved method to determine cell viability by simultaneous staining with fluorescein diacetate-propidium iodide. J Histochem Cytochem Vol. 33, No. 1, (Jan, 1985), pp. 77-79

Kane, R. C., Dagher, R., Farrell, A., Ko, C. W., Sridhara, R., Justice, R. & Pazdur, R. (2007). Bortezomib for the treatment of mantle cell lymphoma. Clin Cancer Res Vol. 13, No. 18 Pt 1, (Sep 15, 2007), pp. 5291-5294

Karaca, B., Atmaca, H., Uzunoglu, S., Karabulut, B., Sanli, U. A. & Uslu, R. (2009). Enhancement of taxane-induced cytotoxicity and apoptosis by gossypol in human breast cancer cell line MCF-7. J Buon Vol. 14, No. 3, (Jul-Sep, 2009), pp. 479-485

Karp, J. E. &Lancet, J. E. (2005). Development of the farnesyltransferase inhibitor tipifarnib for therapy of hematologic malignancies. Future Oncol Vol. 1, No. 6, (Dec, 2005), pp. 719-731

Kim, D., Cheng, G. Z., Lindsley, C. W., Yang, H. & Cheng, J. Q. (2005). Targeting the phosphatidylinositol-3 kinase/Akt pathway for the treatment of cancer. Curr Opin Investig Drugs Vol. 6, No. 12, (Dec, 2005), pp. 1250-1258

Klosowska-Wardega, A., Hasumi, Y., Ahgren, A., Heldin, C. H. & Hellberg, C. (2010). Combination therapy using imatinib and vatalanib improves the therapeutic efficiency of paclitaxel towards a mouse melanoma tumor. Melanoma Res Vol., No., (Oct 21, 2010),

Lantz, R. C., Lemus, R., Lange, R. W. & Karol, M. H. (2001). Rapid reduction of intracellular glutathione in human bronchial epithelial cells exposed to occupational levels of toluene diisocyanate. Toxicol Sci Vol. 60, No. 2, (Apr, 2001), pp. 348-355

Larsen, A. K., Ouaret, D., El Ouadrani, K. & Petitprez, A. (2011). Targeting EGFR and VEGF(R) pathway cross-talk in tumor survival and angiogenesis. Pharmacol Ther Vol. 131, No. 1, (Jul, 2011), pp. 80-90

Lebaron, P., Catala, P. & Parthuisot, N. (1998). Effectiveness of SYTOX Green stain for bacterial viability assessment. Appl Environ Microbiol Vol. 64, No. 7, (Jul, 1998), pp. 2697-2700

Li, X., Dancausse, H., Grijalva, I., Oliveira, M. & Levi, A. D. (2003). Labeling Schwann cells with CFSE-an in vitro and in vivo study. J Neurosci Methods Vol. 125, No. 1-2, (May 30, 2003), pp. 83-91

Marchetti, C., Jouy, N., Leroy-Martin, B., Defossez, A., Formstecher, P. & Marchetti, P. (2004). Comparison of four fluorochromes for the detection of the inner mitochondrial membrane potential in human spermatozoa and their correlation with sperm motility. Hum Reprod Vol. 19, No. 10, (Oct, 2004), pp. 2267-2276

McCall, K. (2010). Genetic control of necrosis - another type of programmed cell death. Curr Opin Cell Biol Vol. 22, No. 6, (Dec, 2010), pp. 882-888

Michiels, S., Potthoff, R. F. & George, S. L. (2011). Multiple testing of treatment-effect-modifying biomarkers in a randomized clinical trial with a survival endpoint. Stat Med Vol. 30, No. 13, (Jun 15, 2011), pp. 1502-1518

Mitsiades, C. S., Davies, F. E., Laubach, J. P., Joshua, D., San Miguel, J., Anderson, K. C. & Richardson, P. G. (2011). Future directions of next-generation novel therapies, combination approaches, and the development of personalized medicine in myeloma. J Clin Oncol Vol. 29, No. 14, (May 10, 2011), pp. 1916-1923

Mueller, M. T., Hermann, P. C., Witthauer, J., Rubio-Viqueira, B., Leicht, S. F., Huber, S., Ellwart, J. W., Mustafa, M., Bartenstein, P., D'Haese, J. G. et al. (2009). Combined targeted treatment to eliminate tumorigenic cancer stem cells in human pancreatic cancer. Gastroenterology Vol. 137, No. 3, (Sep, 2009), pp. 1102-1113

Notte, A., Leclere, L. & Michiels, C. (2011). Autophagy as a mediator of chemotherapy-induced cell death in cancer. Biochem Pharmacol Vol. 82, No. 5, (Sep 1, 2011), pp. 427-434

Olszewska-Slonina, D., Drewa, T., Musialkiewicz, D. & Olszewski, K. (2004). Comparison of viability of B16 and Cl S91 cells in three cytotoxicity tests: cells counting, MTT and flow cytometry after cytostatic drug treatment. Acta Pol Pharm Vol. 61, No. 1, (Jan-Feb, 2004), pp. 31-37

Paglin, S., Lee, N. Y., Nakar, C., Fitzgerald, M., Plotkin, J., Deuel, B., Hackett, N., McMahill, M., Sphicas, E., Lampen, N. et al. (2005). Rapamycin-sensitive pathway regulates mitochondrial membrane potential, autophagy, and survival in irradiated MCF-7 cells. Cancer Res Vol. 65, No. 23, (Dec 1, 2005), pp. 11061-11070

Pallis, M., Syan, J. & Russell, N. H. (1999). Flow cytometric chemosensitivity analysis of blasts from patients with acute myeloblastic leukemia and myelodysplastic syndromes: the use of 7AAD with antibodies to CD45 or CD34. Cytometry Vol. 37, No. 4, (Dec 1, 1999), pp. 308-313

Papadopoulos, N. G., Dedoussis, G. V., Spanakos, G., Gritzapis, A. D., Baxevanis, C. N. & Papamichail, M. (1994). An improved fluorescence assay for the determination of lymphocyte-mediated cytotoxicity using flow cytometry. J Immunol Methods Vol. 177, No. 1-2, (Dec 28, 1994), pp. 101-111

Parish, C. R. &Warren, H. S. (2002). Use of the intracellular fluorescent dye CFSE to monitor lymphocyte migration and proliferation. Curr Protoc Immunol Vol. Chapter 4, No., (Aug, 2002), pp. Unit 4 9

Pegram, M., Hsu, S., Lewis, G., Pietras, R., Beryt, M., Sliwkowski, M., Coombs, D., Baly, D., Kabbinavar, F. & Slamon, D. (1999). Inhibitory effects of combinations of HER-2/neu antibody and chemotherapeutic agents used for treatment of human breast cancers. Oncogene Vol. 18, No. 13, (Apr 1, 1999), pp. 2241-2251

Pei, X. Y., Dai, Y. & Grant, S. (2004). Synergistic induction of oxidative injury and apoptosis in human multiple myeloma cells by the proteasome inhibitor bortezomib and histone deacetylase inhibitors. Clin Cancer Res Vol. 10, No. 11, (Jun 1, 2004), pp. 3839-3852

Perez-Galan, P., Roue, G., Lopez-Guerra, M., Nguyen, M., Villamor, N., Montserrat, E., Shore, G. C., Campo, E. & Colomer, D. (2008). BCL-2 phosphorylation modulates sensitivity to the BH3 mimetic GX15-070 (Obatoclax) and reduces its synergistic interaction with bortezomib in chronic lymphocytic leukemia cells. Leukemia Vol. 22, No. 9, (Sep, 2008), pp. 1712-1720

Pheng, S., Chakrabarti, S. & Lamontagne, L. (2000). Dose-dependent apoptosis induced by low concentrations of methylmercury in murine splenic Fas+ T cell subsets. Toxicology Vol. 149, No. 2-3, (Aug 21, 2000), pp. 115-128

Platini, F., Perez-Tomas, R., Ambrosio, S. & Tessitore, L. (2010). Understanding autophagy in cell death control. Curr Pharm Des Vol. 16, No. 1, (Jan, 2010), pp. 101-113

Poole, C. A., Brookes, N. H., Gilbert, R. T., Beaumont, B. W., Crowther, A., Scott, L. & Merrilees, M. J. (1996). Detection of viable and non-viable cells in connective tissue explants using the fixable fluoroprobes 5-chloromethylfluorescein diacetate and ethidium homodimer-1. Connect Tissue Res Vol. 33, No. 4, 1996), pp. 233-241

Poot, M., Gibson, L. L. & Singer, V. L. (1997). Detection of apoptosis in live cells by MitoTracker red CMXRos and SYTO dye flow cytometry. Cytometry Vol. 27, No. 4, (Apr 1, 1997), pp. 358-364

Prosperi, E., Croce, A. C., Bottiroli, G. & Supino, R. (1986). Flow cytometric analysis of membrane permeability properties influencing intracellular accumulation and efflux of fluorescein. Cytometry Vol. 7, No. 1, (Jan, 1986), pp. 70-75

Prowse, A. B., Wilson, J., Osborne, G. W., Gray, P. P. & Wolvetang, E. J. (2009). Multiplexed staining of live human embryonic stem cells for flow cytometric analysis of pluripotency markers. Stem Cells Dev Vol. 18, No. 8, (Oct, 2009), pp. 1135-1140

Radcliff, G., Waite, R., LeFevre, J., Poulik, M. D. & Callewaert, D. M. (1991). Quantification of effector/target conjugation involving natural killer (NK) or lymphokine activated killer (LAK) cells by two-color flow cytometry. J Immunol Methods Vol. 139, No. 2, (Jun 3, 1991), pp. 281-292

Ramachandran, C., Resek, A. P., Escalon, E., Aviram, A. & Melnick, S. J. (2010). Potentiation of gemcitabine by Turmeric Force in pancreatic cancer cell lines. Oncol Rep Vol. 23, No. 6, (Jun, 2010), pp. 1529-1535

Ross, D. D., Joneckis, C. C., Ordonez, J. V., Sisk, A. M., Wu, R. K., Hamburger, A. W. N. R. E. & Nora, R. E. (1989). Estimation of cell survival by flow cytometric quantification of fluorescein diacetate/propidium iodide viable cell number. Cancer Res Vol. 49, No. 14, (Jul 15, 1989), pp. 3776-3782

Sarkar, A., Mandal, G., Singh, N., Sundar, S. & Chatterjee, M. (2009). Flow cytometric determination of intracellular non-protein thiols in Leishmania promastigotes using 5-chloromethyl fluorescein diacetate. Exp Parasitol Vol. 122, No. 4, (Aug, 2009), pp. 299-305

Sebastia, J., Cristofol, R., Martin, M., Rodriguez-Farre, E. & Sanfeliu, C. (2003). Evaluation of fluorescent dyes for measuring intracellular glutathione content in primary cultures of human neurons and neuroblastoma SH-SY5Y. Cytometry A Vol. 51, No. 1, (Jan, 2003), pp. 16-25

Shapiro, H. M. (2003). Practical flow cytometry. 4th Edition. Wiley-Liss. ISBN (9780471411253-0471411256) Hoboken, N.J.

Shuck, S. C. & Turchi, J. J. (2010). Targeted inhibition of Replication Protein A reveals cytotoxic activity, synergy with chemotherapeutic DNA-damaging agents, and insight into cellular function. Cancer Res Vol. 70, No. 8, (Apr 15, 2010), pp. 3189-3198

Sims, J. T. & Plattner, R. (2009). MTT assays cannot be utilized to study the effects of STI571/Gleevec on the viability of solid tumor cell lines. Cancer Chemother Pharmacol Vol. 64, No. 3, (Aug, 2009), pp. 629-633

Sugiyama, K., Shimizu, M., Akiyama, T., Ishida, H., Okabe, M., Tamaoki, T. & Akinaga, S. (1998). Combined effect of navelbine with medroxyprogesterone acetate against human breast carcinoma MCF-7 cells in vitro. Br J Cancer Vol. 77, No. 11, (Jun, 1998), pp. 1737-1743

Talbot, J. D., Barrett, J. N., Barrett, E. F. & David, G. (2008). Rapid, stimulation-induced reduction of C12-resorufin in motor nerve terminals: linkage to mitochondrial metabolism. J Neurochem Vol. 105, No. 3, (May, 2008), pp. 807-819

Trudel, S., Li, Z. H., Rauw, J., Tiedemann, R. E., Wen, X. Y. & Stewart, A. K. (2007). Preclinical studies of the pan-Bcl inhibitor obatoclax (GX015-070) in multiple myeloma. Blood Vol. 109, No. 12, (Jun 15, 2007), pp. 5430-5438

Ullal, A. J., Pisetsky, D. S. & Reich, C. F., 3rd. (2010). Use of SYTO 13, a fluorescent dye binding nucleic acids, for the detection of microparticles in in vitro systems. Cytometry A Vol. 77, No. 3, (Mar, 2010), pp. 294-301

Vega, M. I., Martinez-Paniagua, M., Huerta-Yepez, S., Gonzalez-Bonilla, C., Uematsu, N. & Bonavida, B. (2009). Dysregulation of the cell survival/anti-apoptotic NF-kappaB pathway by the novel humanized BM-ca anti-CD20 mAb: implication in chemosensitization. Int J Oncol Vol. 35, No. 6, (Dec, 2009), pp. 1289-1296

Wesierska-Gadek, J., Gueorguieva, M., Ranftler, C. & Zerza-Schnitzhofer, G. (2005). A new multiplex assay allowing simultaneous detection of the inhibition of cell proliferation and induction of cell death. J Cell Biochem Vol. 96, No. 1, (Sep 1, 2005), pp. 1-7

West, C. A., He, C., Su, M., Swanson, S. J. & Mentzer, S. J. (2001). Aldehyde fixation of thiol-reactive fluorescent cytoplasmic probes for tracking cell migration. J Histochem Cytochem Vol. 49, No. 4, (Apr, 2001), pp. 511-518

Wlodkowic, D. & Skommer, J. (2007). SYTO probes: markers of apoptotic cell demise. Curr Protoc Cytom Vol. Chapter 7, No., (Oct, 2007), pp. Unit7 33

Woodcock, J., Griffin, J. P. & Behrman, R. E. (2011). Development of novel combination therapies. N Engl J Med Vol. 364, No. 11, (Mar 17, 2011), pp. 985-987

Workman, P., Burrows, F., Neckers, L. & Rosen, N. (2007). Drugging the cancer chaperone HSP90: combinatorial therapeutic exploitation of oncogene addiction and tumor stress. Ann N Y Acad Sci Vol. 1113, No., (Oct, 2007), pp. 202-216

Wright, J. J. (2010). Combination therapy of bortezomib with novel targeted agents: an emerging treatment strategy. Clin Cancer Res Vol. 16, No. 16, (Aug 15, 2010), pp. 4094-4104

Yan, X., Habbersett, R. C., Yoshida, T. M., Nolan, J. P., Jett, J. H. & Marrone, B. L. (2005). Probing the kinetics of SYTOX Orange stain binding to double-stranded DNA with implications for DNA analysis. Anal Chem Vol. 77, No. 11, (Jun 1, 2005), pp. 3554-3562

Yanamandra, N., Colaco, N. M., Parquet, N. A., Buzzeo, R. W., Boulware, D., Wright, G., Perez, L. E., Dalton, W. S. & Beaupre, D. M. (2006). Tipifarnib and bortezomib are synergistic and overcome cell adhesion-mediated drug resistance in multiple myeloma and acute myeloid leukemia. Clin Cancer Res Vol. 12, No. 2, (Jan 15, 2006), pp. 591-599

Yeh, C. J., Hsi, B. L. & Faulk, W. P. (1981). Propidium iodide as a nuclear marker in immunofluorescence. II. Use with cellular identification and viability studies. J Immunol Methods Vol. 43, No. 3, 1981), pp. 269-275

Zahorowska, B., Crowe, P. J. & Yang, J. L. (2009). Combined therapies for cancer: a review of EGFR-targeted monotherapy and combination treatment with other drugs. J Cancer Res Clin Oncol Vol. 135, No. 9, (Sep, 2009), pp. 1137-1148

Zamai, L., Canonico, B., Luchetti, F., Ferri, P., Melloni, E., Guidotti, L., Cappellini, A., Cutroneo, G., Vitale, M. & Papa, S. (2001). Supravital exposure to propidium iodide identifies apoptosis on adherent cells. Cytometry Vol. 44, No. 1, (May 1, 2001), pp. 57-64

Zanetti, M., d'Uscio, L. V., Peterson, T. E., Katusic, Z. S. & O'Brien, T. (2005). Analysis of superoxide anion production in tissue. Methods Mol Med Vol. 108, No., 2005), pp. 65-72

Zhang, N., Wu, Z. M., McGowan, E., Shi, J., Hong, Z. B., Ding, C. W., Xia, P. & Di, W. (2009). Arsenic trioxide and cisplatin synergism increase cytotoxicity in human ovarian cancer cells: therapeutic potential for ovarian cancer. Cancer Sci Vol. 100, No. 12, (Dec, 2009), pp. 2459-2464

21

Flow Cytometry Analysis of Intracellular Protein

Irena Koutná[1], Pavel Šimara[1], Petra Ondráčková[2] and Lenka Tesařová[1]
Masaryk University/ Centre for Biomedical Image Analysis, FI
Veterinary Reasearch Institute/ Department of Immunology
Czech Republic

1. Introduction

The technique of measuring intracellular protein levels using flow cytometry is a very rapid method to detect protein on a single-cell level.

The demand for determining protein levels in a continuously decreasing amount of input cells is currently being developed by scientists and medical doctors. Another demanding area is the splitting of active and inactive (phosphorylated and unphosphorylated, respectively) forms of the protein being monitored, e.g., during different phases of the cell cycle, differentiation or carcinogenesis. The Western blot technique has been typically used for this purpose. The utilization of multi color flow cytometry allows for measurements of multiple proteins in parallel, regardless of the protein length. As the technique evolves, it is possible to obtain information on over 13 parameters per cell (Krutzik et al., 2004).

Measuring the phosphorylation status of specific proteins using this technique is very efficient. It eliminates a number of problems related either to Western blotting or ELISA.

Compared to the Western blot, this progressive method has much lower requirements on the number of input cells (only 1×10^4 cells are needed for determining the concentration of a given protein), it requires less time for processing and, last but not least, is also much more cost effective. Furthermore, it allows researchers to distinguish the various cell populations in the sample without complicated cell separation, if the appropriate antibodies are used. This is beneficial for searching for cell populations and their reactions on external stimuli, such as changed cultivation conditions during in vitro experiments or influencing the organism during in vivo experiments.

In this chapter, the application and pitfalls of flow cytometric intracellular protein measurements are illustrated by the data of our original research of porcine monocytes and CD34+ hematopoietic stem/progenitor cells. In short, a successful utilization of this progressive technique depends on correctly performing the 4 following steps:

1. Precise experimental planning to obtain a defined cell population using this technique.
2. Effective fixation and permeabilization of the cell population.
3. Choosing the optimal isotype control.
4. Selecting the optimal system of primary and secondary antibodies.

2. Fixation and permeabilization

Intracellular flow cytometry, in comparison with conventional cell surface labeling methods, requires fixation and permeabilization of the cells before staining of intracellular antigens (Robinson et al., 1993). Moreover, a variety of commercial kits for fixation and permeabilization are available.

The first step in the population analysis is high quality fixation. A crosslinking reagent (typically formaldehyde) could be used for this purpose. For every given cell population, it is necessary to test the adequate concentration of the solution. The most common formaldehyde concentration is about 4%. Other fixation limiting factors are time and temperature. The incubation time, according to the cell population type, varies between 8 and 15 minutes. The incubation temperature is 37 °C. A variety of commercial kits for fixation and permeabilization are available.

The following step is for permeabilization with detergents (Triton X 100 or saponin) or alcohol (ethanol or methanol). Although the protocols that have been used to stain phosphoepitopes for flow cytometry differ from one to another, they rely on two primary permeabilization reagents - saponin or methanol.

Saponin permeabilization

Saponin is a mixture of terpenoid molecules and glycosides that permeabilize cells by interacting with cholesterol present in the cell membrane (Melan et al. 1999). This creates pores in the plasma membrane that are large enough for entry of fluorophore-conjugated antibodies. Because the intracellular proteins can leak out of saponin-treated cells, they must be first exposed to a crosslinking reagent, such as formaldehyde, to cross-link proteins and nucleic acids into a cohesive unit within the cell. Saponin has become the detergent of choice for cytokine staining, and several groups have utilized it for permeabilization in phospho-epitope staining protocols (Pala et al., 2000). It is typically used at concentrations ranging from 0.1% to 0.5%, similar to cytokine-staining procedures.

Three commercially available kits (Leukoperm, Serotec, UK; Fix & Perm, An Der Grub, Austria; IntraStain, DAKO Cytomation, Denmark) along with combinations of 2 or 4% paraformaldehyde with 0.1 or 0.05% saponin were tested for fixation and permeabilization of isolated pig's peripheral blood mononuclear cells or whole blood leukocytes (Zelnickova et al., 2007).

The fixation and permeabilization process could lead to non-specific binding of primary or secondary antibodies. In comparison to all three tested commercial kits, a combination of paraformaldehyde and saponin caused an increase in non-specific binding of antibodies. The intensity of fluorescence of the negative peak of paraformaldehyde/saponin fixed cells was evidently higher in comparison with the negative peak of cells fixed with the use of commercial kits.

The fixation and permeabilization process could lead to elevation of autofluorescence of cells. The autofluorescence of cells was at the lowest level in all tested kits. In contrast, the combination of paraformaldehyde and saponin in all concentrations caused an increase of autofluorescence. The autofluorescence in samples fixed with 4% paraformaldehyde was higher than with 2% paraformaldehyde.

The fixation and permeabilization process could damage the light scatter properties of the cells. The light scatter characteristics of all tested cells were comparable after any type of fixation and permeabilization. The light scatter characteristics were always changed in comparison with fresh preparations. However, well distinguishable and bounded subpopulations of mononuclear cells and neutrophils were obtained by adjusting the settings in the side and forward scatters.

Some protocols use labeling of intracellular molecules in the whole blood instead of isolated blood leukocytes. In our laboratory, the lysis of red blood cells (RBC) is always performed before starting the staining procedure. However, in order to make the processing of large amounts of samples as quick as possible, the hemolysis is commonly performed in the 96-well plate in which the cultivation was previously performed. The volume of the hemolytic reagent is therefore relatively small and the hemolysis is not complete. Therefore, it is advantageous if the fixation and permeabilization procedure leads to the lysis of these contaminating erythrocytes. It was found that only the IntraStain kit and paraformaldehyde/saponin fixation and permeabilization completely lysed RBC in the samples. The other two kits did not induce a lysis of porcine RBC (although complete lysis of human RBC was obtained by these kits in preliminary experiments, which is in accordance with the manufacturer's instructions).

The problem can occur when the lysis of RBC is performed before fixation and permeabilization. The lysis of RBC induced by ammonium chloride solution (the lysing reagent commonly used in our laboratory to lyse porcine RBC) before fixation and permeabilization with commercial kits strongly changed the light scatter characteristics of white blood cells (WBC). This was apparent, especially in neutrophils, which completely fused with the lymphocyte population. Moreover, the population of lymphocytes was much more dispersed as shown by the side scatter measurements. If the lysis of RBC was performed before their fixation and permeabilization with the IntraStain kit, and the cells were washed twice in CWS solution immediately after lysis, the scatters were not altered. If these washing steps were tested with the other two kits, the light scatters were changed. Thus, the lysis of RBC cannot be achieved with the Fix&Perm or Leukoperm kits without alteration of light scatter characteristics of WBC.

Finally, the effect of different fixation/permeabilization reagents on IFN-γ and TNF-α staining was tested. Generally, we can say that commercial kits mostly gave better results compared with paraformaldehyde/saponin. IntraStain and Leukoperm gave better results than Fix&Perm in some cases. If the use of a combination of paraformaldehyde/saponin is considered, 0.05% saponin should be avoided, especially in combination with 2% paraformaldehyde. Saponin in a concentration of 0.1% in combination with 4% paraformaldehyde slightly increased the percentages of positive cells in comparison with 2% paraformaldehyde. However, these differences were nonsignificant.

Consistent with the above mentioned parameters, the IntraStain kit gave the best results compared to the other two tested kits, as well as when compared to paraformaldehyde/saponin. Therefore, this kit was chosen for fixation and permeabilization of porcine leukocytes for experimentation.

Since a wide range of different fixation and permeabilization reagents that were not tested in our study are currently available, the above mentioned parameters can serve as a particular protocol of intracellular cytokine detection and also as a suggestion for optimization of the fixation, permeabilization and cell surface labeling procedures for any laboratory.

2.1 Methanol permeabilization

Alcohol permeabilization has typically been used for the analysis of DNA by flow cytometry (Ormerod et al., 2002), but can be successfully applied to phospho-epitope staining as well (Krutzik et al., 2003). It is thought that alcohols fix and permeabilize cells by dehydrating them and solubilizing molecules out of the plasma membrane. Proteins may be made more accessible to antibodies during the process and cells are permeabilized to a greater extent than with saponin, allowing efficient access to the nuclear antigens.

Another option is to use commercially available kits. Currently, there are a large number of them available on the market. A fact that needs to be taken into account when using the commercial kits is that even if the kit works well, the method cannot be excessively modified. This could be reflected in the scale of results.

By using one of the best available kits for permeabilization, BD Fix&Perm, with methanol permeabilization during "The decrease in p-CrkL levels upon imatinib treatment" experiment, we came to the following conclusion:

The method (permeabilization using BD Fix&Perm) is less sensitive. It does not recognize the difference between 0 μM and 5 μM imatinib (IM). The speed (2 hours) is an advantage and there is a smaller amount of necessary input material (cells) as well. Although the peaks are sharp, it seems to be more difficult for the antigens to get into the cell, because of less aggressive permeabilization. The methanol permeabilization is much more sensitive. It is able to recognize differences between 0 μM and 5 μM IM. It is more time consuming (5 hours) and requires a higher amount of input material (cells). The significant advantage is the customizability of the method according to user needs (Figure 1).

3. Isotype control

The selection of the appropriate isotype control is an important element in flow cytometry experiments. Isotype controls are antibodies of the same isotype as the target primary antibody. They are of unknown specificity or are raised against antigens known to be absent in target cells. Isotype controls are used to estimate non-specific staining of primary antibodies. Several factors can contribute to the levels of this "background" staining, including Fc receptor binding, non-specific protein interactions, and cell autofluorescence. These factors may vary depending on the target cell type and the isotype of the primary antibody. Therefore, isotype controls need to be properly chosen. Isotype control antibodies ideally match the primary antibody's host species, isotype, and conjugation format. For example, if the primary antibody is an APC-conjugated mouse IgG2a, then it will be necessary to choose an APC-conjugated mouse IgG2a isotype control. Thus, isotype control is supposed to have all the non-specific characteristics of the target primary antibody and it is able to accurately determine the level of specific staining. Various monoclonal antibody idiotypes are used in flow cytometry applications: most frequently, IgG1, IgG2a, IgG2b, IgG3, IgM, and IgA; less frequently IgD, IgE, IgG2c, Ig kappa, and Ig lambda are applied. Designing the experiment, this isotype and origin species of the primary antibody must be known to find a suitable isotype control. The appropriate isotype control is subsequently looked up in a company product list according to the desired isotype (IgG1, IgG2a, IgM, etc.), reactivity (mouse, human, rat, etc.), and conjugate (FITC, PE, APC, etc.). In addition, recommended isotype controls can often be found on the Data Sheets for primary

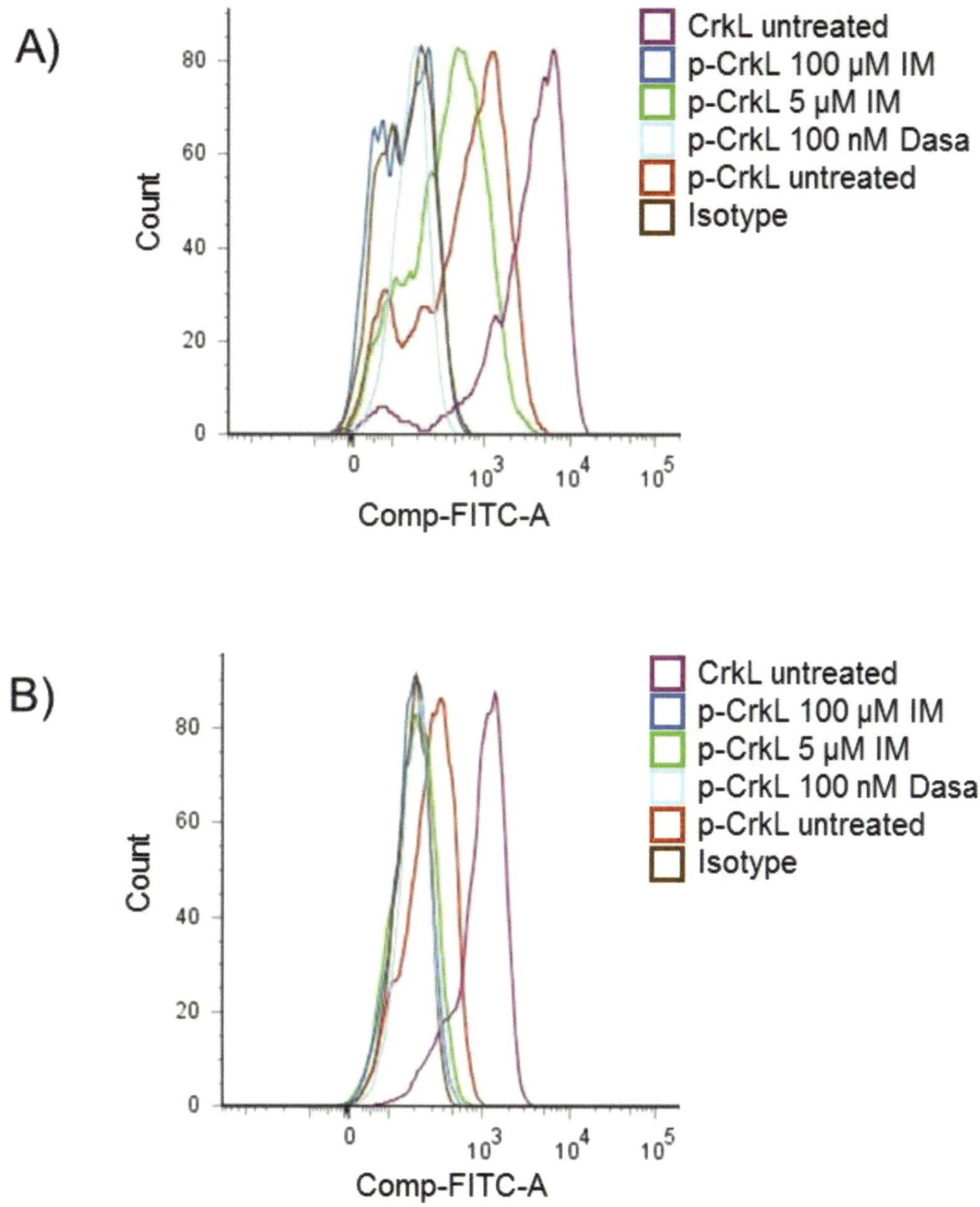

Fig. 1. The difference between permeabilization protocols using (A) methanol and (B) the BD Fix&Perm kit. Permebilization with methanol is more sensitive and allows researchers to distinguish between individual MFI peaks. Fix&Perm kit is less time consuming with relatively low sensitivity

antibodies. Isotype control antibodies are commercially available for both direct and indirect immunofluorescence in the form of fluorochrome-conjugated antibodies and unconjugated antibodies, respectively. During the flow cytometry analysis, the idiotype control antibody is diluted to the same concentration as the specific primary antibody, and is used to stain the sample of negative control cells. This negative control serves to determine the amount of non-specific "background" fluorescence. It allows for setting a threshold of negativity of stained cells. Any event generating a signal above this baseline is considered to be specifically labeled with the target primary antibody.

The isotype control plays an important role during the processing of final measurements. The level of monitored protein is determined as the geometric mean of fluorescent intensity (MFI) of labeled sample, minus the isotype control (O'Gorman et al., 1999, Holden et al., 2006,Hulspas et al., 2009).

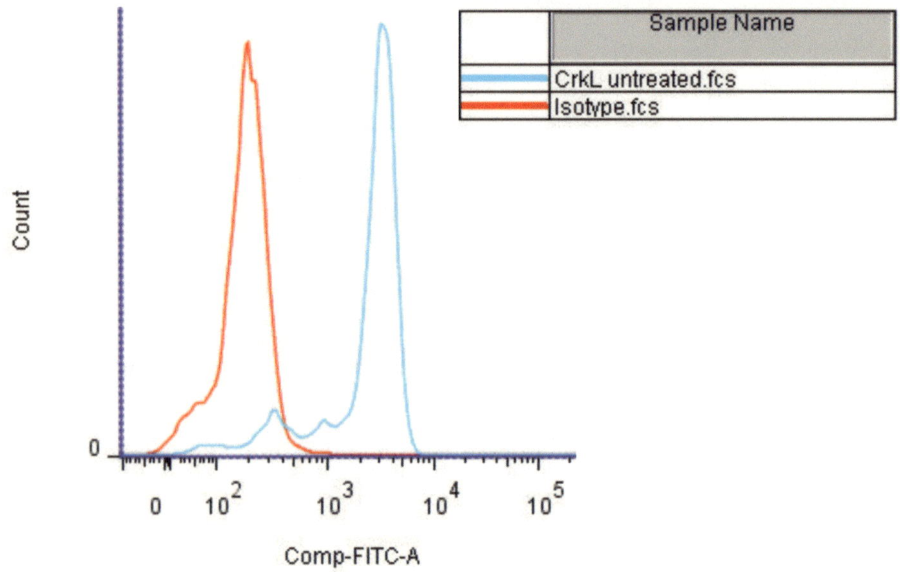

Fig. 2. Representative FACS plot showing isotype and CrkL MFI peaks visualized by a FITC-conjugated secondary antibody in CD34+ cells isolated from peripheral blood of a newly diagnosed CML patient. The MFI peak of isotype indicates the FITC unspecific background fluorescence. These were visualized using FlowJo software

4. Intracellular antigens for flow cytometry

The most common way to visualize of the complex between a monoclonal antibody and an antigen in flow cytometry is to covalently bind the antibody to different fluorescent molecules (fluorophores). After exposure to radiation from an excitation source, these fluorophores emit photons with longer wavelengths. Currently, there is a wide range of commercially available fluorophores starting from the small polycyclic molecules, such as fluorescein isothiocyanate (FITC), cyanines, and dyes of the Alexa series, through fluorescent phycobilipoproteins whose best-known representatives are phycoerythrin (PE), allophycocyanin (APC). New way in flow cytometry is also Qdot® nanocrystals –

nanometer-scale semiconductor particles with unique fluorescence properties (eBioscience , Molecular Probes®)..

The world leader in bringing innovative diagnostic and research tools to different specialists are Beckman Coulter and eBioscience as the major companies producing unconjugated and conjugated antibodies for flow cytometry. BD Biosciences offers a number of Alexa Flouro (AF®) 488/647/700-, APC-, FITC-, PE-, and Pacific BlueTM- conjugated antibodies of BD PharmingenTM and BD PhosflowTM brands used for multicolor flow cytometry (BD Biosciences, 2011).

A particularly strong area of leukemia immunophenotyping that contains a broad panel of research products has been built up by (DAKO, 2010). DAKO offers various types of reagents for use in flow cytometry, including primary single-color antibodies conjugated with a single fluorochrome; MultiMix™ Dual-Color Reagents based on the combination of two or more antibodies labeled with FITC and RPE; and MultiMix™ Triple-Color Reagents based on the combination of three antibodies labeled with fluorescein isothiocyanate (FITC), R-phycoerythrin (RPE) and allophycocyanin (APC) or FITC, RPE and RPE-Cy5. Other products for use in flow cytometry are isotype reagents, secondary antibody conjugates, streptavidine conjugates and other accessories. There are also several kits available, e.g. an apoptosis kit used for flow cytometric distinction between viable cells in single cell suspensions or an Enumeration of Stem Cells Kit used for optimal enumeration of CD34+ hematopoietic stem / progenitor cells (DAKO, 2010).

Another strong company in the production of high-quality activation-state antibodies is Cell Signaling Technology. They offer a number of primary and conjugated antibodies as well as antibody-related kits. Conjugated antibodies are conjugated with AF®, PE or biotin (Cell Signaling Technology, 2011)

There are many other companies not mentioned in the table, including R&D Systems, Miltenyi Biotec and BioLegend, that offer a wide range of unconjugated and conjugated monoclonal antibodies and kits. For example, R&D Systems offers a wide range of biotin-, fluorescein-, PE-, PerCP-, AF® 488-, or APC- conjugated monoclonal antibodies specifically designed to monitor protein expression by flow cytometry (R&D Systems, 2011).

Generally, the problem with labeling various molecules for flow cytometry in animal species other than mice is the poor availability of directly conjugated primary antibodies. Therefore, indirect labeling is commonly used. This includes labeling cells with a non-conjugated antibody and subsequent visualization with a secondary fluorochrome-conjugated antibody. This indirect labeling is limited by the subclasses of primary antibodies, which should not share the same subclass. This limits the use of the antibodies, especially in the case of multicolor labeling.

When intracellular labeling is combined with cell surface marker labeling in pigs, the problem with sharing the same subclasses is more noticeable since all the anti-porcine cytokine antibodies used share the most common mouse IgG1 subclass. The cell surface molecules are always labeled prior to the labeling of the intracellular cytokine in our protocol. Accordingly, the anti-cytokine antibody must be directly conjugated with fluorochrome (such as anti-TNF-α or anti-IFN-γ) or it must be biotinylated (such as anti-IL-2 or anti-IL-10) or pre-labeled in some other way (Zelnickova et al., 2008).

Intracellular marker	Type	Clone name	Isotype	Reactivity	Labelling	Source	Ref.
Cytokines							
IL-2, IL-4, TNF- α, etc.	mAb	5344.111, 3010.211, 6401.1111, …	Ms IgG_1,κ	Hu	FITC/ PE/APC/…	BD Biosciences	Karanikas et al., 2000
IFN- γ	mAb	P2G10	Ms IgG_1,κ	Pig	PE-conjugate	BD Biosciences	Gerner et al., 2008
Cell cycle or Apoptosis							
p53	mAb	DO7	Ms IgG_2b	Hu	nonconjugated	Dako	Millard et al., 1998
bcl-2	mAb	124	Ms IgG_1	Hu	FITC-conjugated	Dako	Millard et al., 1998
rb	mAb	G3-245	Ms IgG_1	Ms, Qua, Mn, Mk, Rat, Hu	nonconjugated	BD Biosciences	Millard et al., 1998
MDR1	mAb	JSB-1	Ms IgG_1	Hu, Rat, Ms	nonconjugated	Millipore	Millard et al., 1998
PCNA	mAb	PC10	Ms IgG_{2a}	Hu	nonconjugated	Dako	Millard et al., 1998
caspases	pAb	-	Rab IgG	Hu, Rat, Ms	PE-conjugated	BD Biosciences	Belloc et al., 2000
perforin	mAb	dG9	Ms IgG_{2b}	Hu	PE-conjugated	BD Biosciences	Gerner et al., 2008
Ki67	mAb	B56	Ms IgG_1,κ	Ms	FITC-conjugated	BD Biosciences	Gerner et al., 2008
Bax, Bcl-x_L, Mcl-1	pAb	-	Rab IgG	Ms/ Rab/ Hu	unconjugated	Santa Cruz Biotechnology	van Stijn et al., 2003
Viral particles							
HIV	mAb	unknown	MsIgG_{1b12}	Hu	unknown	Denis Burton	Mascola et al., 2002
Receptors or their proteins, enzymes							
Steroid hormone receptor proteins	mAb pAb	*(various)*	*(various)*	*(various)*	*(various)*	Affinity bioreagents	Butts et al., 2007
Cox1/2	mAb	AS70, AS67	Ms IgG_1,κ	Hu	FITC, PE	BD Biosciences	Ruitenberg et al., 2003
Estrogen Receptor α	mAb	1D5	Ms IgG_1	Hu	unconjugated	Dako	Cao et al., 2000
Phospho-proteins							
Akt	mAb	5G3	Ms IgG_1	Hu, Ms, Rat, Hm	unconjugated	Cell Signaling Technology	Tazzari et al., 2002
	pAb	-	Rab IgG	Hu, Ms, Rat, Hm, Mk, Chick, Dm, Bov, Pig, Dog			
MEK1/2	pAb	-	Rab IgG	Hu, Ms, Rat, Mk, Sc	unconjugated	Cell Signaling Technology	Chow et al., 2001
ERK1/2	mAb	20A	Ms IgG_1	Hu, Ms, Rat	AF-conjugated	BD Biosciences	Krutzik et al., 2003
JNK	mAb	41	Ms IgG_1	Hu	unconjugated	BD Biosciences	Krutzik et al., 2003
p38 MAPK	mAb	30	Ms IgG_1	Hu, Rat, Ms	unconjugated	BD Biosciences	Krutzik et al., 2003
Stat1	mAb	14	Ms IgG_1,κ	Hu, Ms	unconjugated	BD Biosciences	Krutzik et al., 2003
Stat3	mAb	D3A7	Rab IgG	Hu, Ms, Rat, Mk	AF-conjugated	Cell Signaling Technology	Kalaitzidis et al., 2008
Stat4	pAb	-	Rab IgG	Hu, Ms	unconjugated	Invitrogen	Uzel et al., 2001

Table 1. continues on next page

Intracellular marker	Type	Clone name	Isotype	Reactivity	Labelling	Source	Ref.
Stat5	mAb	47	Ms IgG_1	Hu	AF-conjugated	BD Biosciences	Krutzik et al., 2003
Stat6	mAb	18	Ms IgG_{2a}	Hu	PE-conjugated	BD Biosciences	Krutzik et al., 2003
CD79a	mAb	HM57	Ms IgG_1	Hu	PE-conugated	Dako	Gerner et al., 2008
mTOR	mAb	D9C2	Rab IgG	Hu, Ms, Mk, (Rat)	unconjugated	Cell Signaling Technology	Kalaitzidis et al., 2008

Hu - human; Ms - mouse; Mk - monkey; Hm - hamster; Dm - drosophila melanogaster; Bov - bovine; Sc - saccharomyces cerevisiae; Mk - mink; Qua - quail

Table 1. Intracellular antigens for flow cytometry

A method for the direct labeling of antibodies that share the same subclass was tested. Because it was necessary to label relatively small amounts of antibodies, the Zenon-labeling technology was chosen.

The Zenon reagents are provided by Invitrogen. This labeling involves the binding of Fab fragments of the fluorochrome-labeled, subclass-specific secondary antibody to the primary antibody, prior to the labeling of the cells. The excess of the fluorochrome-labeled secondary antibody is neutralized by addition of irrelevant mouse antibody in excess, which is supplied within the Zenon kit. The disadvantage of these reagents is the relatively high price. The price is the same for all fluorochromes; however, the number of reactions that can be performed by the kit differ among fluorochromes. Packages with Alexa Fluor, FITC, Texas Red and Pacific dyes contain reagents for 50 rounds of labeling, packages with phycobiliprotein dyes such as R-PE or APC contain reagents for 25 rounds of labeling, and packages with tandem dyes contain reagents for only 10 rounds of labeling. Therefore, it is advantageous to choose Zenon reagents containing Alexa Fluor dyes.

The other disadvantage of the Zenon labeling is that the fluorescence yield of Zenon-labeled antibodies is slightly lower compared to classical indirect labeling. Therefore, antibodies against strongly expressed markers should be preferably stained with the Zenon reagents. (Ondrackova et al., 2010, 2011)

General protocol for cell surface staining followed by intracellular labeling

1. Place the samples of cell suspensions into a U-bottom 96-well plate, spin the plate, remove as much supernatant as possible, and vortex the plate.
   If viability staining with permanent dye combined with intracellular staining is performed, then:
2. Add the viability staining dye, incubate according the manufacturer's instructions, vortex the plate, and wash once.
   The cell surface staining is performed as follows:
3. Add the cocktail of primary antibodies against cell surface molecules in a total volume of 10 µl (dilute antibodies in CWS) + 10 µl of heat-inactivated, filtered goat serum, vortex the plate, incubate for 15 min at 4°C, and wash twice.
4. Add a secondary antibody cocktail in total volume of 25 µl (dilute antibodies in CWS), vortex the plate, and incubate for 20 min at 4°C.
   If the cell surface molecules are to be labeled with Zenon reagents or if intracellular staining follows, then:

5. Wash once and vortex the plate thoroughly because the plate in the next step cannot be vortexed due to the risk of the samples overflowing into the neighboring wells.
6. Add 100 µl of heat-inactivated, filtered mouse serum diluted 1:10 in CWS, incubate for 20 min at 4°C, and wash once.
   Labeling cell surface molecules with Zenon-labeled antibodies now follows, but this step can be omitted if it is not required:
7. Add the cocktail of Zenon-labeled antibodies against cell surface molecules in a total volume of 10 µl, incubate for 15 min at 4°C, vortex the plate, and wash –twice.
   Staining of intracellular molecules with directly-labeled, Zenon-labeled, or unlabeled antibodies follows, but these steps can be omitted if they not required:
8. Add 30 µl of Solution A from the IntraStain kit, vortex thoroughly to allow complete hemolysis of contaminating red blood cells, incubate for 15 min at room temperature, and wash –twice.
9. Add primary antibodies against intracellular molecules (directly-labeled, Zenon-labeled, or unlabeled) diluted in Solution B from the IntraStain kit in a total volume of 20 µl, vortex the plate, incubate for 20 min at room temperature, and wash twice.
10. Add secondary antibodies diluted in Solution B from the InraStain kit and CWS (ratio of Solution B and CWS 1:1) in total volume of 25 µl, incubate for 20 min at room temperature, wash twice.
11. Resuspend samples in CWS in the volume that is required for the subsequent measurement and measure by the appropriate method.

CWS solution: PBS containing 1.84 g/l EDTA, 1 g/l NaN3, 4 ml/l gelatin from cold water fish skin

Wash definition: Add as much CWS into each well as possible, spin 3 min at 500 g, remove much supernatant as possible, and vortex.

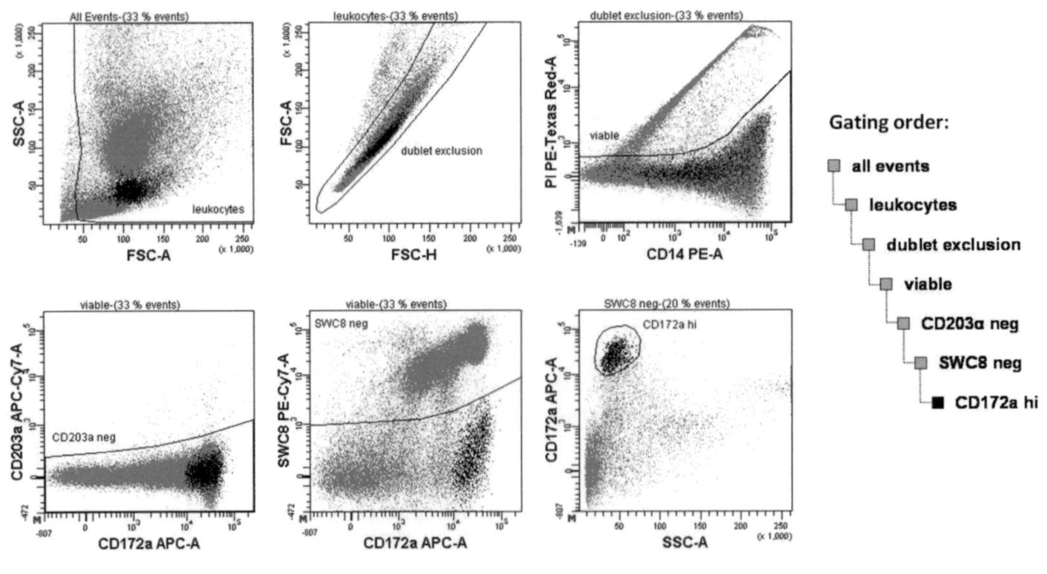

(a)

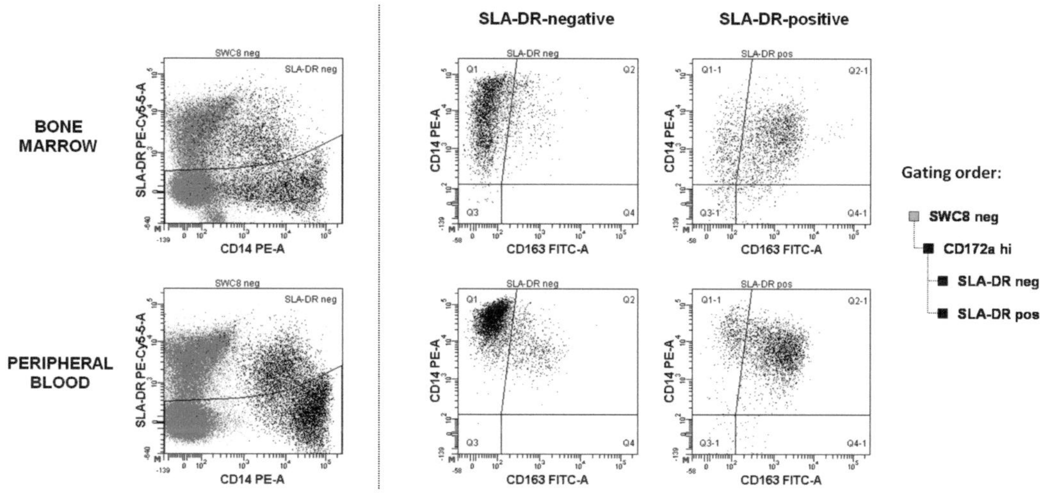

(b)

Fig. 3. Seven color flow cytometry for identification of porcine monocyte subpopulations using two Zenon-labeled antibodies

The red blood cells from the whole peripheral blood or from the bone marrow sample were lysed with ammonium chloride solution. The following fluorescent staining was performed:

Excitation wavelength	Primary antibody					Secondary antibody / Zenon reagent / viability stain				
	Target molecule	Clone	Manufacturer	Amount per well	Stained at point	Class/ subclass	Fluorochrome	Manufacturer	Dilution	Stained at point
488	CD163	2A10/ 11	VMRD, USA	0.1 µl	3)	IgG1	AlexaFluor488	Invitrogen, USA	1:750	4)
488	CD14	MIL-2	Serotec, UK	1 µl	3)	IgG2b	AlexaFluor647	Invitrogen, USA	1:750	4)
488						Propidium iodide				11)
488	SLA-DR	MSA3	VMRD, USA	0.05 µl	3)	IgG2a	PE-Cy5.5	Invitrogen, USA	1:100	4)
488	SWC8	MIL-3	Dr. J.K. Lunney *	1 µl	3)	IgM	DyLight405	GeneTex, USA	1:500	4)
640	CD172α	DH59 B	VMRD, USA	0.1 µl	7)	Zenon IgG1 **	AlexaFluor647	Invitrogen, USA		
640	CD203α	PM 18-7	Serotec, UK	0.1 µl	7)	Zenon IgG1 ***	APC-AlexaFluor750	Invitrogen, USA		

* a generous gift from Dr. J.K. Lunney, Animal Parasitology Institute, Beltsville, MO, USA
** labeling with the Zenon® AlexaFluor647 Mouse IgG1 Labeling Kit perform as follows: 0.1 µl of anti-CD172α and 0.5 µl of Solution A of the Zenon Kit, mix well, incubate 10 min at 4°C, then add 0.5 µl of Solution B of the Zenon kit, mix well, incubate 10 min at 4°C
*** labeling with the Zenon® APC-AlexaFluor750 Mouse IgG1 Labeling Kit perform as follows: 0.1 µl of anti- CD203α and 0.5 µl of Solution A of the Zenon kit, mix well, incubate 10 min at 4°C, then add 0.5 µl of Solution B of the Zenon kit, mix well, incubate 10 min at 4°C
The measurement was performed by using BD FACSAria I flow cytometer (Becton Dickinson, USA).

The gating strategy for identification of monocytes in the bone marrow is depicted (A). Briefly, the leukocytes were gated according their light scatter properties (upper left dot-plot). The dublets of cells were excluded from the further analysis (upper middle dot-plot). The viable (propidium iodide-negative) cell were gated (upper right dot-plot). The CD203α-positive macrophages were excluded (lower left dot-plot). The monocytes were identified as SWC8-negative (lower middle dot-plot) CD172α-positive cells (lower right dot-plot).

Then monocyte subpopulations from the bone marrow and peripheral blood were identified based on expression of SLA-DR, CD14 and CD163 (B). The SLA-DR-positive and negative monocytes were gated (left dot-plots). Then SLA-DR-negative (middle dot-plots) and SLA-DR-positive (right dot-plots) monocyte subpopulations were depicted in CD163 vs. CD14 dot-plots.

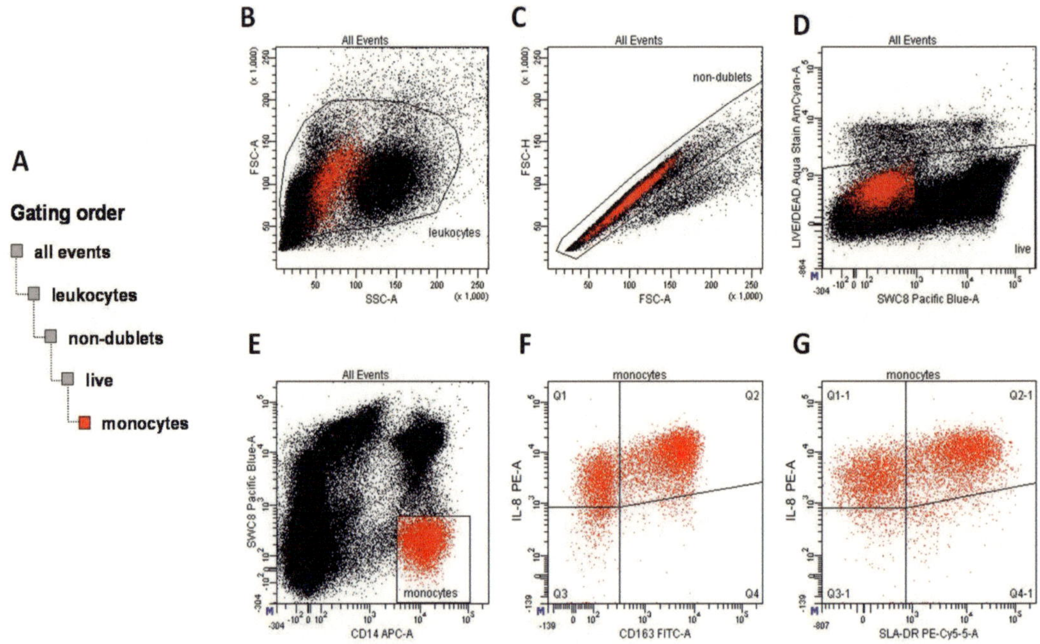

Fig. 4. Six color flow cytometry for measurement of IL-8 production by monocyte subpopulations using the Zenon-labeled anti-IL-8 antibody

The gating order for evaluation of IL-8 production by monocyte subpopulations is depicted (A). Briefly, the leukocytes were gated according their light scatter properties (B). The dublets of cells were excluded excluded from the further analysis (C). The viable (LIVE/DEAD® Fixable Aqua Dead Cell Stain-negative) cell were gated (D). The monocytes were identified as SWC8-negative CD14-positive cells (E). The IL-8 production by CD163-positive and negative monocytes (F) and by SLA-DR-positive and negative monocytes (G) was then evaluated.

The whole peripheral blood diluted 1:1 with RPMI 1640 was stimulated for 2 hours with LPS (1 μg/ml) in the presence of brefeldin A (10 μg/ml). The red blood cells were lysed with ammonium chloride solution. The following fluorescent staining was performed:

Excitation wavelength	Primary antibody					Secondary antibody / Zenon reagent / viability stain				
	Target molecule	Clone	Manufacturer	Amount per well	Stained at point	Class/subclass	Fluorochrome	Manufacturer	Dilution	Stained at point
405	SWC8	MIL-3	Dr. J.K. Lunney *	1 µl	3)	IgM	DyLight405	GeneTex, USA	1:500	4)
405						LIVE/DEAD® Fixable Aqua Dead Cell Stain Kit **				2)
488	CD163	2A10/11	VMRD, USA	0.1 µl	3)	IgG1	AlexaFluor488	Invitrogen, USA	1:750	4)
561	IL-8	8M6	Serotec, UK	0.2 µl	9)	Zenon IgG1 ***	R-PE	Invitrogen, USA		
561	SLA-DR	MSA3	VMRD, USA	0.05 µl	3)	IgG2a	PE-Cy5.5	Invitrogen, USA	1:100	4)
640	CD14	MIL-2	Serotec, UK	1 µl	3)	IgG2b	AlexaFluor647	Invitrogen, USA	1:750	4)

* a generous gift from Dr. J.K. Lunney, Animal Parasitology Institute, Beltsville, MO, USA
** diluted 1:1000 in PBS, 10 µl / well, incubation15 min at 4°C
*** labeling with the Zenon® R-Phycoerythrin Mouse IgG1 Labeling Kit perform as follows: 0.2 µl of anti-IL-8 and 4 µl of Solution A of the Zenon kit, mix well, incubate 10 min at 4°C, then add 4 µl of solution B of the Zenon kit, mix well, incubate 10 min at 4°C, then add 11.8 µl of Solution B of IntraStain kit
The measurement was performed by using BD LSRFortessa flow cytometer (Becton Dickinson, USA)

5. Intracellular measurement of the p-CrkL and CrkL levels using flow cytometry

5.1 Theoretical background

Chronic myeloid leukemia (CML) is a myeloproliferative disorder of hematopoietic stem cells that is characterized by the presence of the BCR-ABL fusion gene, which encodes the constitutively active BCR-ABL tyrosine kinase (Daley et al., 1990). Currently, the tyrosine kinase inhibitor imatinib (IM) (a potent inhibitor of BCR-ABL) is used as a first line therapy for CML patients (Baccarani et al., 2009).

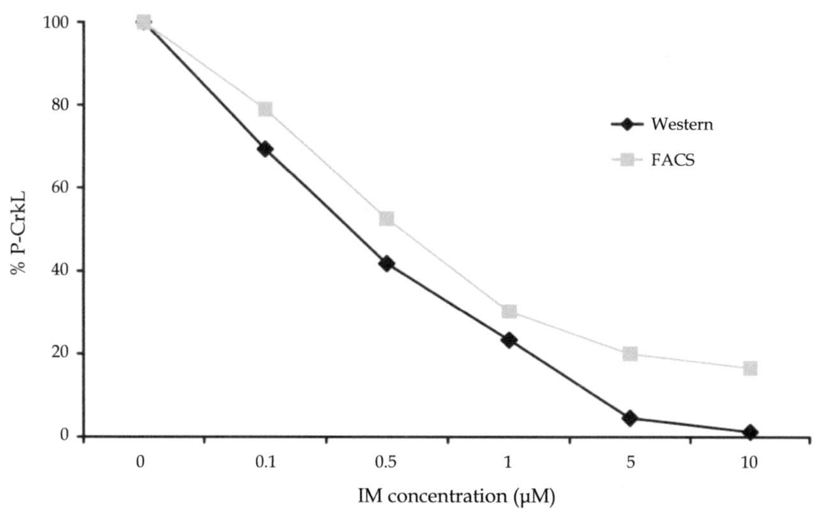

Fig. 5. The equivalence between flow cytometry and Western blot methods, in p-CrkL reduction in a BCR-ABL positive K562 cell line after 48 h treatment with imatinib (Hamilton et al., 2006)

The CrkL protein is a downstream signaling substrate of BCR-ABL, and its tyrosine phosphorylation (p-CrkL) serves as a specific indicator of BCR-ABL kinase activity in CML cells (Nichols et al., 1994; Patel et al., 2006). Recent studies have revealed that p-CrkL can act as a prognostic marker for imatinib treatment response of CML patients using either western blotting (White et al., 2005) or flow cytometry (Lucas et al., 2010). However, certain discrepancies have been found in the literature concerning the predictive value of p-CrkL in different cell types (mononuclear cells or CD34+ cells) used for analysis (Khorashad et al., 2009).

The technique for measuring p-CrkL levels using flow cytometry was originally described by Hamilton et al., (Hamilton et al., 2006) and the equivalence between flow cytometry and western blot methods was demonstrated (Figure 5).

5.2 The technique of intracellular p-CrkL and CrkL measurement by flow cytometry

Mononuclear cells (MNCs) were isolated from PB of newly diagnosed CML patients using Histopaque-1077 density gradient centrifugation (Sigma–Aldrich, St. Louis, MO, USA) and subsequently enriched for CD34+ cells using magnetic-activated cell sorting (MACS) with a CD34 MicroBead Kit (Miltenyi Biotec, Bergisch Gladbach, Germany) according to the manufacturer's instructions. CD34+ cells ($5x10^4$) were incubated for 16 h with 0, 0.5, 1.5, and 5 µM imatinib in 1 ml of serum-free medium (SFEM), supplemented with StemSpan CC100 cytokine mixture (StemCell Technologies, Köln, Germany) as previously described (Koutna et al., 2011). Then the cells were washed in phosphate buffered saline (PBS) and fixed with 4% formaldehyde for 10 min at 37°C, then washed in PBS and permeabilized by 90% methanol at 4°C for 30 min.

After permeabilization, the cells were washed in PBS and incubated with primary unlabeled antibody for 30 min at 4°C in 100 µl of FACS incubation buffer (0.5% bovine serum albumin in PBS). The concentration of primary antibodies was 12 µg/ml (p-CrkL, Cell Signaling Technology, Danvers, MA, USA; CrkL, Santa Cruz biotechnology, Santa Cruz, CA, USA; isotype control anti-normal-rabbit IgG G, R&D Systems, Minneapolis, MN, USA). The cells were washed in FACS incubation buffer and incubated with FITC-conjugated anti-rabbit IgG secondary antibody (Sigma-Aldrich) in a concentration of 10 µl/ml.

All samples were measured on a FACSCanto II Flow Cytometer (Becton Dickinson). For data analysis, BD FACSDiva (Becton-Dickinson) and FlowJo (Tree Star, Ashland, USA) software were used. The viable cell population was gated according to forward scatter and side scatter parameters. The level of p-CrkL and CrkL in the viable cells was determined as the geometric mean fluorescence intensity (MFI) of the p-CrkL- or CrkL-labeled sample minus the MFI of the isotype control (Figure 6).

The $IC50^{imatinib}$ was defined as the concentration of imatinib that caused a 50% decrease in the amount of p-CrkL compared to the untreated control (Figure 7) (White et al., 2005). The p-CrkL/CrkL ratio was calculated by dividing the concentrations of p-CrkL by those of CrkL and multiplying by 100 in untreated cells (Lucas et al., 2010). The p-CrkL ratio was assessed as a percentage of p-CrkL in the samples treated with a maximal imatinib concentration (5 µM) relative to the untreated control (Figure 7) (Khorashad et al., 2009).

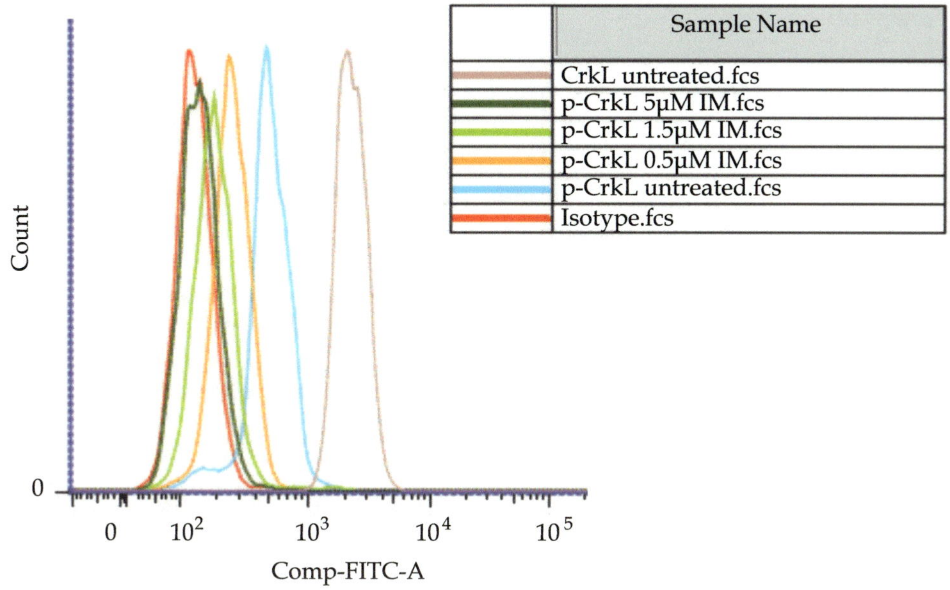

Fig. 6. Representative FACS plot showing isotype, p-CrkL and CrkL MFI peaks in CD34+ cells isolated from peripheral blood of a newly diagnosed CML patient. Changes in p-CrkL MFI peaks following *in vitro* imatinib (IM) treatment are detectable and were visualized using FlowJo software

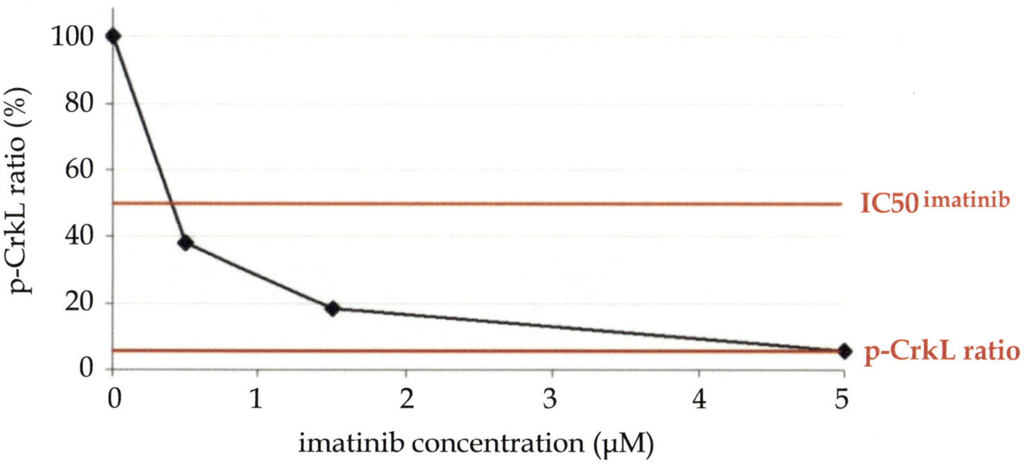

Fig. 7. The graph of p-CrkL decrease upon *in vitro* imatinib treatment. MFI peaks quantification was calculated in FlowJo software

6. Acknowledgment

This work was generously supported by grant of the Ministry of Education of the Czech Republic MSM 0021622430, grant and Ministryof Health NS-9681 and Ministry of Agriculture of the Czech Republic MZE0002716202

7. References

Baccarani, M., Cortes, J., Pane, F., Niederwieser, D., Saglio, G., Apperley, J., Cervantes, F., Deininger, M., Gratwohl, A., Guilhot, F., Hochhaus, A., Horowitz, M., Hughes, T., Kantarjian, H., Larson, R., Radich, J., Simonsson, B., Silver, R., Goldman, J., Hehlmann, R., & LeukemiaNet, E. (2009). Chronic myeloid leukemia: an update of concepts and management recommendations of European LeukemiaNet. J Clin Oncol, 27, 35, 6041-51, 1527-7755

Belloc, F., Belaud-Rotureau, M. A., Lavignolle, V., Bascans, E., Braz-Pereira, E., Durrieu, F., & Lacombe, F. (2000). Flow cytometry detection of caspase 3 activation in preapoptotic leukemic cells. Cytometry, 40, 2, 151-60, 0196-4763

Butts, C. L., Shukair, S.A., Duncan, K. M., Harris, C. W., Belyavskaya, E., & Sternberg, E.M. (2007). Evaluation of steroid hormone receptor protein expression in intact cells using flow cytometry. Nucl Recept Signal, 5, e007, 1550-7629

Cao, S., Hudnall, S.D., Kohen, F., & Lu, L. J. (2000). Measurement of estrogen receptors in intact cells by flow cytometry. Cytometry, 41, 2, 109-14, 0196-4763

Chow, S., Patel, H., & Hedley, D.W. (2001). Measurement of MAP kinase activation by flow cytometry using phospho-specific antibodies to MEK and ERK: potential for pharmacodynamic monitoring of signal transduction inhibitors. Cytometry, 46, 2, 72-8, 0196-4763

Daley, G. Q., Van Etten, R. A., & Baltimore, D. (1990). Induction of chronic myelogenous leukemia in mice by the P210bcr/abl gene of the Philadelphia chromosome. Science, 247, 4944, 824-30, 0036-8075

Gerner, W., Käser, T., Pintaric, M., Groiss, S., & Saalmüller, A. (2008). Detection of intracellular antigens in porcine PBMC by flow cytometry: A comparison of fixation and permeabilisation reagents. Vet Immunol Immunopathol, 121, 3-4, 251-9, 0165-2427

Hamilton, A., Elrick, L., Myssina, S., Copland, M., Jørgensen, H., Melo, J., & Holyoake, T. (2006). BCR-ABL activity and its response to drugs can be determined in CD34+ CML stem cells by CrkL phosphorylation status using flow cytometry. Leukemia, 20, 6, 1035-9, 0887-6924

Hulspas, R., O'Gorman, M. R., Wood, B. L., Gratama, J.W., & Sutherland, D. R. (2009). Considerations for the control of background fluorescence in clinical flow cytometry. Cytometry B Clin Cytom, 76, 6, 355-64, 1552-4957

Kalaitzidis, D., & Neel, B. G. (2008). Flow-cytometric phosphoprotein analysis reveals agonist and temporal differences in responses of murine hematopoietic stem/progenitor cells. PLoS One, 3, 11, e3776, 1932-6203

Karanikas, V., Lodding, J., Maino, V. C., & McKenzie, I. F. (2000). Flow cytometric measurement of intracellular cytokines detects immune responses in MUC1 immunotherapy. Clin Cancer Res, 6, 3, 829-37, 1078-0432

Khorashad, J., Wagner, S., Greener, L., Marin, D., Reid, A., Milojkovic, D., Patel, H., Willimott, S., Rezvani, K., Gerrard, G., Loaiza, S., Davis, J., Goldman, J., Melo, J., Apperley, J., & Foroni, L. (2009). The level of BCR-ABL1 kinase activity before treatment does not identify chronic myeloid leukemia patients who fail to achieve a complete cytogenetic response on imatinib. Haematologica, 94, 6, 861-4, 1592-8721

Koutna, I., Peterkova, M., Simara, P., Stejskal, S., Tesarova, L., & Kozubek, M. (2011). Proliferation and differentiation potential of CD133+ and CD34+ populations from the bone marrow and mobilized peripheral blood. Ann Hematol, 90, 2, 127-37, 1432-0584

Krutzik, P. O., & Nolan, G. P. (2003). Intracellular phospho-protein staining techniques for flow cytometry: monitoring single cell signaling events. Cytometry A, 55, 2, 61-70, 1552-4922

Lucas, C., Harris, R., Giannoudis, A., Knight, K., Watmough, S., & Clark, R. (2010). BCR-ABL1 tyrosine kinase activity at diagnosis, as determined via the pCrkL/CrkL ratio, is predictive of clinical outcome in chronic myeloid leukaemia. Br J Haematol, 149, 3, 458-60, 1365-2141

Maecker, H. T., & Trotter, J. (2006). Flow cytometry controls, instrument setup, and the determination of positivity. Cytometry A, 69, 9, 1037-42, 1552-4922

Mascola, J. R., Louder, M. K., Winter, C., Prabhakara, R., De Rosa, S. C., Douek, D. C., Hill, B. J., Gabuzda, D., & Roederer, M. (2002). Human immunodeficiency virus type 1 neutralization measured by flow cytometric quantitation of single-round infection of primary human T cells. J Virol, 76, 10, 4810-21, 0022-538X

Melan, M. A. (1999). Overview of cell fixatives and cell membrane permeants. Methods Mol Biol, 115, 45-55, 1064-3745

Millard, I., Degrave, E., Philippe, M., & Gala, J. L. (1998). Detection of intracellular antigens by flow cytometry: comparison of two chemical methods and microwave heating. Clin Chem, 44, 11, 2320-30, 0009-9147

Nichols, G., Raines, M., Vera, J., Lacomis, L., Tempst, P., & Golde, D. (1994). Identification of CRKL as the constitutively phosphorylated 39-kD tyrosine phosphoprotein in chronic myelogenous leukemia cells. Blood, 84, 9, 2912-8, 0006-4971

O'Gorman, M. R., & Thomas, J. (1999). Isotype controls--time to let go? Cytometry, 38, 2, 78-80, 0196-4763

Ondrackova, P., Nechvatalova, K., Kucerova, Z., Leva, L., Dominguez, J., & Faldyna, M. (2010). Porcine mononuclear phagocyte subpopulations in the lung, blood and bone marrow: dynamics during inflammation induced by Actinobacillus pleuropneumoniae. Vet Res, 41, 5, 64, 0928-4249

Ormerod, M. G. (2002). Investigating the relationship between the cell cycle and apoptosis using flow cytometry. J Immunol Methods, 265, 1-2, 73-80, 0022-1759

Pala, P., Hussell, T., & Openshaw, P. J. (2000). Flow cytometric measurement of intracellular cytokines. J Immunol Methods, 243, 1-2, 107-24, 0022-1759

Patel, H., Marley, S., & Gordon, M. (2006). Detection in primary chronic myeloid leukaemia cells of p210BCR-ABL1 in complexes with adaptor proteins CBL, CRKL, and GRB2. Genes Chromosomes Cancer, 45, 12, 1121-9, 1045-2257

Ruitenberg, J. J., & Waters, C. A. (2003). A rapid flow cytometric method for the detection of intracellular cyclooxygenases in human whole blood monocytes and a COX-2 inducible human cell line. J Immunol Methods, 274, 1-2, 93-104, 0022-1759

Tazzari, P. L., Cappellini, A., Bortul, R., Ricci, F., Billi, A. M., Tabellini, G., Conte, R., & Martelli, A. M. (2002). Flow cytometric detection of total and serine 473 phosphorylated Akt. J Cell Biochem, 86, 4, 704-15, 0730-2312

Uzel, G., Frucht, D. M., Fleisher, T. A., & Holland, S. M. (2001). Detection of intracellular phosphorylated STAT-4 by flow cytometry. Clin Immunol, 100, 3, 270-6, 1521-6616

van Stijn, A., Kok, A., van der Pol, M. A., Feller, N., Roemen, G. M., Westra, A. H., Ossenkoppele, G. J., & Schuurhuis, G. J. (2003). A flow cytometric method to detect apoptosis-related protein expression in minimal residual disease in acute myeloid leukemia. Leukemia, 17, 4, 780-6, 0887-6924

White, D., Saunders, V., Lyons, A., Branford, S., Grigg, A., To, L., & Hughes, T. (2005). In vitro sensitivity to imatinib-induced inhibition of ABL kinase activity is predictive of molecular response in patients with de novo CML. Blood, 106, 7, 2520-6, 0006-4971

Zelnickova, P., Faldyna, M., Stepanova, H., Ondracek, J., & Kovaru, F. (2007). Intracellular cytokine detection by flow cytometry in pigs: fixation, permeabilization and cell surface staining. J Immunol Methods, 327, 1-2, 18-29, 0022-1759

Zelnickova, P., Leva, L., Stepanova, H., Kovaru, F., & Faldyna, M. (2008). Age-dependent changes of proinflammatory cytokine production by porcine peripheral blood phagocytes. Vet Immunol Immunopathol, 124, 3-4, 367-78, 0165-2427

BD Biosciences; http://www.bdbiosciences.com

Beckman Coulter https://www.beckmancoulter.com

Cell Signaling Technology; http://www.cellsignal.com

Dako; http://www.dako.com

eBioscience (2011) http://www.ebioscience.com

R&D Systems http://www.rndsystems.com

22

Biological Effects Induced by Ultraviolet Radiation in Human Fibroblasts

Silvana Gaiba et al*,
Universidade Federal de São Paulo – Unifesp,
Universidade Estadual de Santa Cruz – Uesc
Universidade Nove de Julho – Uninove
Brazil

1. Introduction

As the most superficial body organ, skin plays an important role in protecting the body from environmental damage. The skin is composed of three layers: the epidermis, dermis and subcutaneous tissue. The epidermis, the outermost layer, has as main functions to protect the body against harmful environmental stimuli and to reduce fluid loss. It is a stratified squamous epithelium with several layers and its major cell type is the keratinocyte. This tissue is constantly being renewed by keratinization, a process of detachment of cornified cells (Blumenberg & Tomic-Canic, 1997). Located under the epidermis are the dermis and the dermal connective tissue, with extracellular matrix proteins such as collagen, elastic fibers, fibronectin, glycosaminoglycans and proteoglycans, which are produced and secreted into the extracellular space by fibroblasts, the major cell type found in this tissue (Makrantonaki & Zouboulis, 2007). The extracellular matrix proteins in the dermal connective tissue contribute for maintaining skin preservation and integrity (Hwang *et al.*, 2011). Stromal fibroblasts play an important role in tissue homeostasis regulation and wound repair via protein synthesis and secretion of growth factors or cytokines of paracrine action with direct effect on proliferation and differentiation of adjacent epithelial tissues (Andriani *et al.*, 2011). Solar ultraviolet (UV) radiation is a predictable epidemiologic risk factor for melanoma and non-melanoma skin cancers. (Katiyar *et al.*, 2011). UV irradiation can impair cellular functions by directly damaging DNA to induce apoptosis (Wäster & Ollinger, 2009). Among other things, longer UV wavelengths (UVB, UVA) induce oxidative stress and protein denaturation whereas short wavelength UV radiation (UVC) causes predominantly DNA damage to cells in the form of pyrimidine dimers, 6-4 photoproducts and apoptosis (Armstrong & Kricker, 2001; Gruijl *et al.*, 2001). UVB irradiation damages skin cells by the formation of ROS (Reactive Oxygen Species) resulting in oxidative stress, an important mediator of damage to cell structures, including lipids and membranes, proteins, and DNA (Wäster & Ollinger, 2009). However, it has less penetrating power than UVA and acts mainly on the epidermal basal layer of the skin. UVC, on the other hand, is extremely damaging to the skin because its wavelengths have enormous energy and induce genotoxic

* Vanina M. Tucci-Viegas, Lucimar P. França, Fernanda Lasakosvitsch, Fernanda L. A. Azevedo, Andrea A. F. S. Moraes, Alice T. Ferreira and Jerônimo P. França

stress. Fortunately, UVC is prevented from reaching the earth, as it is largely absorbed by atmospheric ozone layer (Afag, 2011). It has already been proposed that programmed cell death (apoptosis) can be induced by UV light in various cell types (reviewed in Schwarz, 1998). The cellular responses to injuries or stresses are important in determining cell fate (Aylon & Oren, 2007). Many signaling pathways participate in this process, with the mitogen-activated protein kinase (MAPK) cascades and p53 pathway being two of the major pathways implicated (Aylon & Oren, 2007; Li *et al.*, 2009). The cellular response to DNA damage is focused on p53, which can induce the cell to apoptosis by the protein PUMA (p53 up-regulated modulator of apoptosis), a member of the Bcl-2 homology (BH)3-only Bcl-2 family proteins. Recent studies suggest that Bcl-2 family members play an essential role in regulating apoptosis initiation through the mitochondria (Zhang *et al.*, 2009). UV irradiation induces permeabilization of the lysosomal membrane with release of cathepsin B and D to the cytosol, translocation of the proapoptotic Bcl-2 proteins Bax and Bid to mitochondrial-like structures. Subsequently, there is cytochrome c release and activation of caspase-3 (Bivik *et al.*, 2006). p38 MAPK, one of the four MAPK subfamilies in mammalian cells, is activated by proinflammatory cytokines and environmental stress (Brown & Benchimol, 2006; Johnson & Lapadat, 2002). p38 is not only reported to be phosphorylated and activated to mediate cell apoptosis and the differentiation process (Thornton & Rincon, 2009), but also to have cell protective effects under certain circumstances (Chouinard *et al.*, 2002). MAPK pathways mediate cellular responses to many different extracellular signaling molecules such as the ones involved in differentiation, gene expression, regulation of proliferation, apoptosis, development, motility or metabolism. The typical MAPK pathways, characterized by the ERK1/2, ERK5, JNK, and $p38^{MAPK}$ components, comprise a cascade of three successive phosphorylation events exerted by a MAPK kinase kinase (MAPKKK), a MAPK kinase (MAPKK), and a MAPK (Kostenko *et al.*, 2011).

Ultraviolet UVA light absorption after solar exposure is responsible for photoactivation of DNA and other biomolecules. Additionally, UVA radiation (320-400 nm) induces photoaddition, oxidative stress and DNA damage, which may be continuous. The cell is also unable to replicate in case of severe DNA damage. This way, DNA repair must be considered essential for genetic information preservation and transmission in any life form. UVA light generates mutagenic DNA lesions in the skin. Exposure to solar UVB radiation is responsible for skin inflammation and tumorigenesis.

Besides that, oxidative stress induced by solar radiation could be responsible, as well, for the increased frequency of DNA mutations in photoaged human skin. Genomic DNA damage triggers the activation of a network of pathways that rapidly modulate several cellular activities. ROS and hydrogen peroxide can damage DNA. Furthermore, it has been recently shown that increased oxidative stress is correlated to DNA alterations. ROS are deleterious to DNA, membranes and proteins although their exact role in mutagenesis and lethality is still unclear in the many skin cell types. In addition, repair ability and defense mechanisms may differ a lot from one cellular type to another.

Epidermal and dermal cells are targets for UVA oxidative stress and their antioxidant defenses can be defeated. Keratinocytes and fibroblasts may respond differently to UV radiation depending on their localization in the body or their functional and metabolic characteristics. Cell culture models have helped to describe the cytotoxic action of UVA and the role of ROS in UVA-induced cellular damage (Tyrrell, 1990). p53 stabilization and activation, an essential outcome of the DNA damage response pathway, leads to cell cycle arrest and DNA repair, apoptosis, or cellular senescence. More specifically, initial genomic insults lead to p53 stabilization and nuclear localization where transient cell cycle arrest can be quickly activated, allowing damaged DNA repair prior to replication. A signaling cascade can be activated by p53 in case of extreme and irreversible DNA damage to induce programmed cell death through transcription of different proapoptotic factors.

UV radiation induces phospholipids peroxidation in cellular membrane. Lipid peroxidation is a consequence of free primary radicals (ROS). This, in turn, leads to the generation of polar products and increase the membrane dielectric constant and capacitance. An important consequence of this phenomenon is the alteration of transport particles across the membrane (Strässle *et al.*, 1991)

During the Fenton reaction, singlet oxygen directly initiates lipid peroxides and hydrogen peroxides indirectly initiate hydroxyl radicals (Halliwell & Gutteridge, 1999).

Cellular responses that lead to cell cycle arrest, DNA repair, apoptosis or senescence are induced by the p53 tumor suppressor pathway upon activation by genotoxic stress. This pathway works mostly through transactivation of different downstream targets, for example, p21 cell cycle inhibitor, required for short-term cell cycle arrest or long-term cellular senescence, or other proapoptotic genes such as p53 upregulated modulator of apoptosis (PUMA) (Tavana *et al.*, 2010). Yet, the mechanism that regulates the switching from cell cycle arrest to apoptosis is still unknown. In case of extreme or irreversible damage, p53 can additionally activate a signaling cascade to induce apoptosis through transcription of pro-apoptotic genes, most particularly p53-upregulated modulator of apoptosis (PUMA) and trans-repression of anti-apoptotic genes including Bcl-2. Programmed cell death directly protects cells against the accumulation of genomic instability that could lead to tumorigenesis.

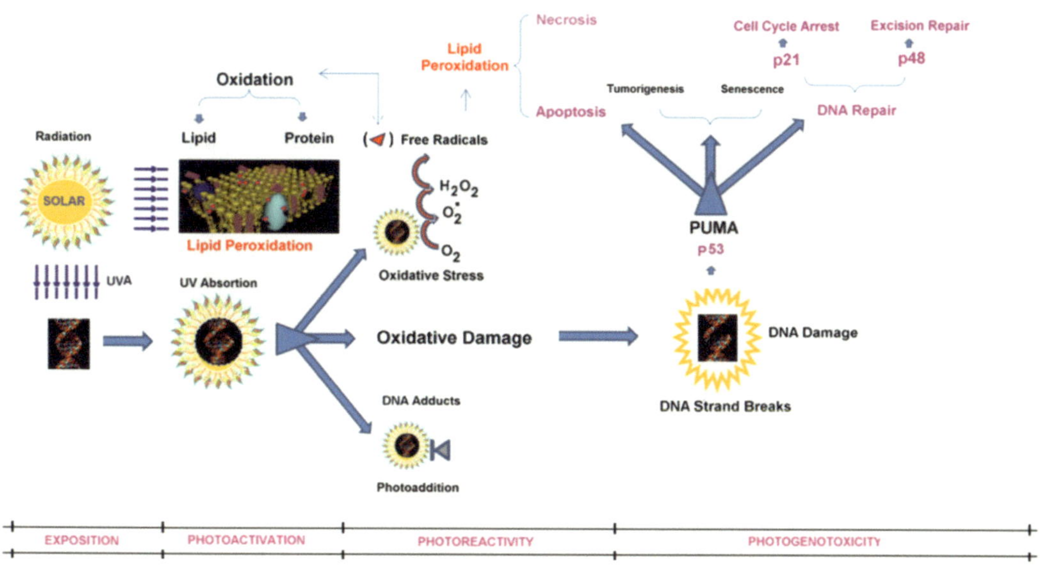

Fig. 1. Schematic representation. Photobiological effects of ultraviolet radiation on human skin cells

Senescence, an irreversible cell cycle arrest, can also be induced by DNA damage. p21, the cyclin-dependent kinase inhibitor, plays an important role in cell cycle checkpoint regulation and induction of cellular senescence, thus being one key p53 target. After DNA damage, p21 is commonly transactivated and induces G1arrest by inhibiting the cyclinE/CDK2 complex. (Campisi, 2009). Many different stimuli can induce cellular senescence including telomere shortening (replicative senescence), oncogenic signaling (oncogene-induced senescence), or stress/DNA damage irrespectively of the two previous signaling pathways (premature senescence) (Campisi, 2009). Despite the stimuli, cellular senescence and apoptosis are somewhat equivalent in preventing genomic instability and consequently inhibiting tumor formation (Van Nguyen, 2007). Upon UV exposure, p48 mRNA levels strongly depended on basal p53 expression and increased even more after DNA damage in a p53-dependent manner thus pointing as the link between p53 and the nucleotide excision repair apparatus (Hwang *et al.*, 1999).

2. Objective

The objective of this study was to investigate modifications in cytoskeleton through the formation of blebs and apoptosis in cultured human fibroblasts by confocal microscopy and flow cytometry.

3. Methods

This study was performed in accordance with the ethical standards laid down in the updated version of the 1964 Declaration of Helsinki and was approved by the Research Ethics Committee of the Federal University of São Paulo. All patients signed a free and informed consent form. Samples of normal adult human skin (6 women, 18-50 years, skin phototype Fitzpatrick class. III-IV) were obtained as discarded tissue from trunk cosmetic surgery.

3.1 Fibroblast culture

Primary human skin fibroblast culture was done by explant. Fragments were placed in 15 ml conic tubes and exhaustively rinsed (six times) with 10 ml PBS (Phosphate-Buffered Saline, Cultilab, Campinas, SP, Brazil) containing penicillin (100 Ul/ml, Gibco, Carlsbad, CA, USA) and streptomycin (100µg/ml, Gibco) under vigorous agitation, changing tubes and PBS at each repetition. Then, fragments were transferred to 60 mm^2 diameter Petri dishes, in grid areas scratched with a scalpel. Dishes were left semi-opened in the laminar flow for 20 min, for the fragments to adhere to its surface. Then, 6 ml of DMEM (Dulbecco's Modified Eagle's Medium, Cultilab) supplemented with 10% FBS (Fetal Bovine Serum, Cultilab), 1% glutamine, penicillin (100 UI/ml, Gibco) and streptomycin (100 µg/ml, Gibco) were carefully added to each plate. Plates were kept in humidified incubator (37°C, 95% O_2, 5%CO_2).

Culture medium was changed every two days and a few days after establishing the primary culture, spindle-like cells were seen proliferating from the edges of the explanted tissue, regarded as culturing fibroblasts. Fibroblast satisfactory proliferation was observed in approximately 7-14 days and subculturing (passage) was performed when cellular confluence reached approximately 80% at the Petri dish. For all experiments, cells from passages one to five (Figure 2) were used after harvesting by trypsinization [0.025% trypsin,

0.02% ethylene diamine tetra acetic acid (EDTA; Sigma Chemical Co., Saint Louis, MO, USA) in PBS].

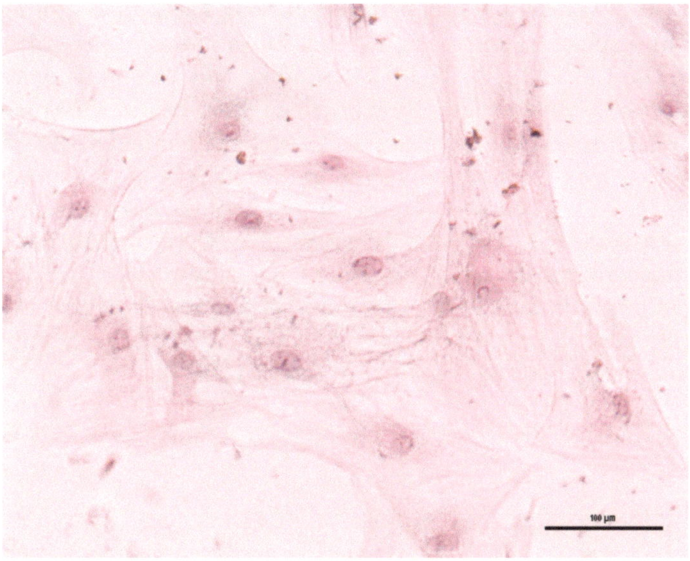

Fig. 2. Optical microscopy. Primary human skin fibroblast culture. Hematoxilin and eosin staining

3.2 Ultraviolet irradiation

Cells were rinsed in PBS. The PBS was then removed and a thin layer of buffer was left on top of the coverslip. Fibroblasts were irradiated in culture dishes in a $10cm^2$ field using a UV chamber (with 6 UV F40 Philips lamps) in exposure times of 30 and 60 minutes.

3.3 Immunofluorescence labeling

Primary human skin fibroblast culture were used after harvesting by trypsinization [0.025% trypsin, 0.02% ethylene diamine tetra acetic acid (EDTA; Sigma Chemical Co., Saint Louis, MO, USA) in PBS]. The cells were washed 3 times with phosphate-buffered saline (PBS). Human fibroblasts were plated on glass coverslips, fixed in 2% paraformaldehyde for 10 minutes at 4°C, washed 3 times in PBS, and washed twice in PBS with 50 mmol/L NH_4Cl. Cells were permeabilized with 0.1% saponin in PBS containing 10% normal bovine serum for 30 minutes at 22°C and stained with a combination of fluorescent dyes. Filaments of cytoskeleton immunostained with phalloidin conjugated fluorescent with Alexa Fluor 594 (red) - Molecular Probe, were used to identify actin filaments F inside the cells. Phalloidin (1:500) incubation was performed in PBS containing 10% normal bovine serum and 0.1% saponin. Nuclei were counter stained with blue - fluorescent DNA stain DAPI (4_6-diamidino-2-phenylindole) 1:10000 (catalog #D1036; Molecular Probes, Invitrogen, Carlsbad, CA), and excited using a 750nm multiphoton source (two simultaneous photon excitations at 375nm). The images are a composite of three images acquired using filter sets appropriate for blue and red fluorescence, on a Zeiss confocal microscope (LSM 510, Germany).

3.4 Determination of MDA-TBA levels

Taking the 1h time-point, which proved to be optimal for the determination of MDA increase, we then studied dose kinetics. Fibroblasts were exposed to a series of single doses UV irradiation in exposure times of 30 and 60 minutes. Markedly elevated MDA concentrations in the UV and TBARs–MDA complex concentrations were determined by high-performance liquid chromatography (HPLC) as described by Gueguen *et al.*, 2002. The MDA-TBA test, which is the colorimetric reaction of malondialdehyde and thiobarbituric acid in acid solution, was used to determine the MDA levels. HPLC was used after the formation of the MDA-TBA complex (Figure 3) to assess the concentration of the complex based on a known standard curve. After heating at 95 °C for 60 min, the MDA-TBA chromogen was fluorometrically analyzed using a reversed-phase C18 column HPLC and a wavelength of 532 nm. The MDA-TBA method was previously described by Chirico *et al.* (1993). MDA levels were expressed in relation to the total cellular lysate protein amount, which was assessed using Bradford's method (Bradford, 1976).

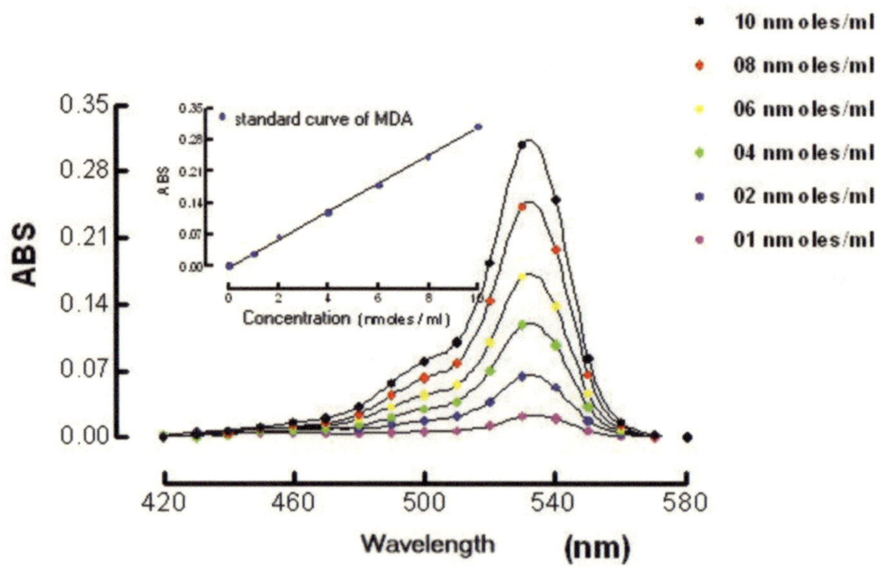

Fig. 3. Absorbance spectra for MDA – TBA chromogen complex standards in Thiobarbituric Acid Reactions (TBARs). Malondialdehyde (MDA) is a very effective method for determining lipid peroxidation levels in fibroblasts exposed to ultraviolet radiation. The standards absorption peaks of the inserted curve were highly linear in the range of 0 to 10nmoles/mL with maximum absorption at 532nm

3.5 Apoptosis assay

Flow cytometry technique, using propidium iodide, was used to detect apoptosis in fibroblast culture of human skin exposed to UV radiation (Nicoletti *et al.*, 1991).

Human fibroblasts were labeled with annexin V-FITC (Roche), which bind to phosphatidylserine at the cell surface of apoptotic cells, and propidium iodide (PI; Sigma Aldrich), was used as a marker of cell membrane permeability according to manufacturer's directions. Samples were examined by fluorescence-activated cell sorter (FACS) analysis, and the results were analyzed using Cell-Quest software (Becton Dickinson, San Jose, CA) (Vermes *et al.*, 1995).

3.6 Flow cytometric analysis of caspase 3 and p53

Briefly, normal human fibroblast cells from cultures with increasing passage number were collected and re-suspended in a buffer saline (PBS) containing 0.1% sodium azide (Sigma) containing 20 mM HEPES (pH 7.5), the cells were homogenized and centrifuged at 10,000 x g for 5 min. For analysis of caspase 3 and p53 expression, cells were fixed in 2% paraformaldehyde for 10 minutes at 4°C, washed 3 times in PBS, then washed twice in PBS with 50 mmol/L NH_4Cl. Cells were permeabilized with 0.1% saponin in PBS containing 10% normal bovine serum for 30 minutes at 22°C. The first primary antibody incubation (anti-p53 (SER 15) or anti-cleaved caspase 3) was performed in PBS containing 10% normal bovine serum and 0.1% saponin. Aliquots were then incubated for 60 minutes with anti-caspase 3 and p53 antibodies (Santa Cruz Biotechnology, Santa Cruz, CA), final dilution 1:800, or rabbit IgG as a control, followed by washing in PBS containing 0.1% saponin 3 times for 5 minutes each at 22°C. Cells were then incubated with the first fluorochrome-conjugated secondary antibodies Alexa 488 and 594 diluted 1:1600, and incubation was performed for 40 minutes at 37°C in the dark (Danova *et al.*, 1990).

3.7 Statistical analysis

The results obtained were analyzed using a one-way analysis of variance (ANOVA) followed by the Student–Newman–Keuls Multiple Range Test. Data were analyzed by GraphPad Prism v.3.0 software.

4. Results and discussion

Skin cells exposure to solar radiation may result in biological consequences, one of the most important being skin DNA photodamage due to sunlight ultraviolet (UV) radiation. Wavelengths in the UVB range are absorbed by DNA and can induce mutagenesis. It has been suggested that p53-independent mechanisms of killing tumor cells may not involve programmed cell death and could be a result of induced mechanical damage, rather than apoptosis (Funkel, 1999).

Ultraviolet A radiation (UVA, 320–400 nm), an oxidizing component of sunlight, exerts its biological effect mainly by producing reactive oxygen species (ROS) which cause biological damage in exposed tissues, including the lipid bilayer, via iron-catalyzed oxidative reactions (Halliwell & Gutteridge, 1999; Tyrrell, 1990). Membrane alterations induced by UV irradiation were determined, such as MDA concentration increase, which indicates lipid peroxidation levels (methods previously described -Figure 3). The UV radiation effects in the cellular production of ROS were indirectly determined by the ratio: (MDA concentration / total amount of fibroblasts) at the sample. Analyses of the lipid peroxidation by measuring the products that react with Tiobarbituric Acids (TBARs) normalizing the obtained MDA (malondialdehyde) results by the number of cells in the sample (Figure 4). A significant MDA increase was observed, of about 45.0 % after 30 min of UV exposure and 130% after 60 min of UV exposure.

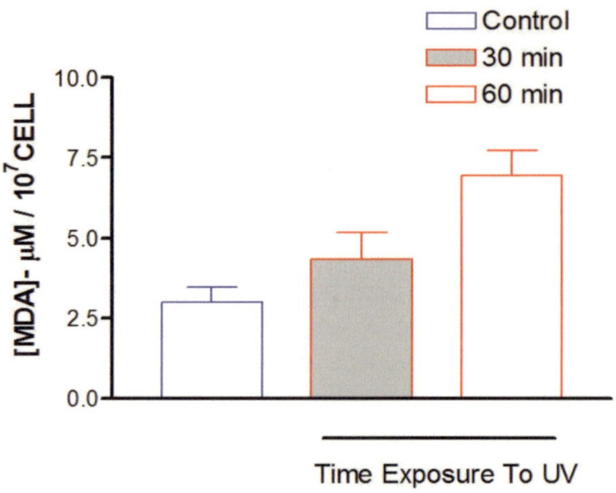

Fig. 4. Effect of UV radiation in the cellular production of oxygen reactive species measured by ratio: MDA concentration by total number of fibroblast in the sample. Histograms values differ significantly from each other. *Data analyzed with one-way ANOVA followed by Newman Keuls (significance level $p < 0.05$). Values represent the mean ± SEM of at least four different experiments

Similar results are also described by several studies demonstrating that low UVA radiation doses can induce lipid peroxidation in membranes of both human fibroblasts and keratinocytes via pathways involving singlet oxygen and iron (Morliere *et al*, 1991).

Looking from a different angle, cells also have repair mechanisms to respond to DNA damage, and at least two different mechanisms are responsible for UVA-induced DNA damage repair. The primary process that removes bulky damage is the nucleotide excision repair pathway. Small lesions induced by ROS are mostly processed by base excision repair pathway. On the other hand, highly damaged cells may undergo cell cycle arrest, apoptosis and senescence (Hazane *et al.*, 2006). Our results are consistent with those of Shindo *et al.* (1994) who investigated antioxidant molecules in crude extracts of human epidermis and dermis. In addition, Moysan *et al.* (1995), using cells from the same biopsy, found no link between UVA cytotoxicity and antioxidant capacity since SOD, catalase and GSH were identical in both cells and GSH-Px was higher in fibroblasts (Degterev *et al.*, 2008). Other authors, however, have found more antioxidant molecules in fibroblasts than in keratinocytes. Yohn *et al.* (1991), using cells from different donors, found increased GSH-Px, SOD and catalase in fibroblasts compared to keratinocytes, and in keratinocytes compared to melanocytes (Huang *et al.*, 2008).

Several *in vitro* and *in vivo* studies on skin cells have demonstrated that UV radiation can damage many molecules and structures (Matsumura & Ananthaswamy, 2004). Corroborating these results, morphological analysis by confocal fluorescence microscopy of fibroblasts group control showed characteristics of nuclear and cytoskeleton integrity. High cellularity was also observed (Figure 5). In contrast, exposed to UV for 30 and 60 minutes showed changes in the actin filaments arrangement of the cellular cytoskeleton. Groups irradiated for 30 and 60 min presented disruption of the actin filaments, with the formation of blebbing and nuclear fragmentation as a consequence of the ultraviolet radiation (Figure 6).

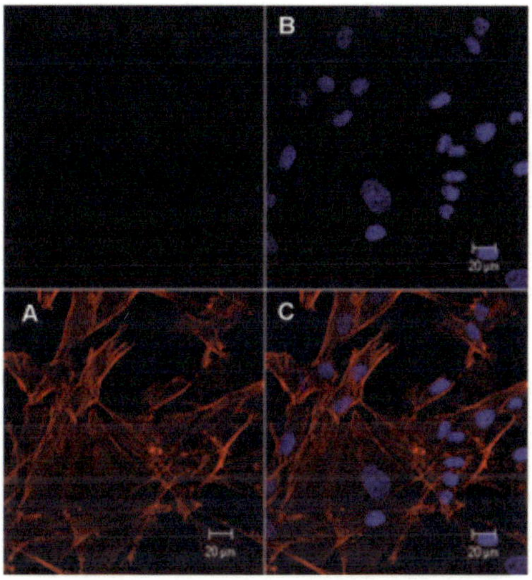

Fig. 5. Confocal microscopy. Cultured human skin fibroblasts. Control group. Cellular localization of actin filaments and nuclei. A) Actin filaments immunostained with phalloidin conjugated with Alexa Fluor 594 (red). B) Cell nuclei stained with DAPI (blue), showing characteristics of nuclear and cytoskeleton integrity. High cellularity was also observed. C) Overlapped images A and B

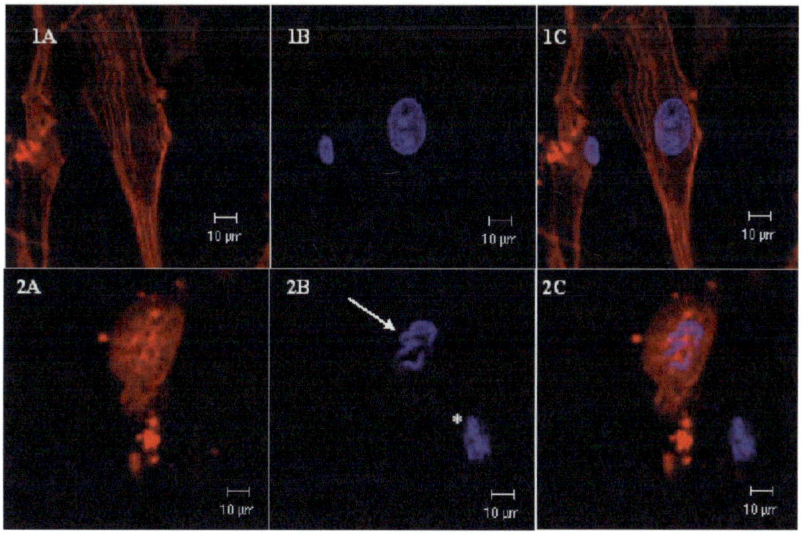

Fig. 6. Confocal microscopy. Cultured human skin fibroblasts. Cellular localization of actin filaments and nuclei. Cells exposed to UV radiation for 30 min (1A, 1B, 1C) or 60 min (2A, 2B, 2C). 1A) Actin filaments immunostained with phalloidin conjugated with Alexa Fluor 594 (red). The occurrence of blebbing can be observed. 1B) Cell nuclei stained with DAPI (blue), showing characteristics of nuclear and cytoskeleton integrity. 1C) Overlapped images A and B. 2A) Actin filaments immunostained with phalloidin conjugated with Alexa Fluor 594 (red). 2B) Pyknotic nuclei (*) and nuclear fragmentation (arrow) were observed. 2C) Overlapped images A and B

In addition, skin fibroblasts viability, stained by propidium iodide (PI), was analyzed by flow cytometry. Viable cells were characterized by a structurally intact cell membrane and no PI uptake. In contrast, dead cells (necrosis or late apoptotic cells) were characterized by loss of the integrity of their membranes and were stained by PI. At all UV radiation tested doses, the amount of viable cells was reduced, as verified by PI staining. The amount of viable fibroblasts was dramatically reduced by UV radiation at all tested doses/exposure times, about 80% after 30 min of exposure and 30% after 60 min of exposure (Figures 7A and 8A).

There are strong evidences that skin cancer can be developed as a result of ultraviolet radiation, which is directly associated to the TP53-gene tumor mutation.

To further investigate whether p53 is involved in the apoptosis induced by UV, cells were first stained for membrane-exposed phosphatidylserine using annexin-V conjugated to fluorescein (FITC). There was a significant increase of the number of apoptotic cells: about 21.0 % (30 min) and 50% (60 min) after irradiation (Figures 7B and 8B) and (Figures 7C and 8C), respectively.

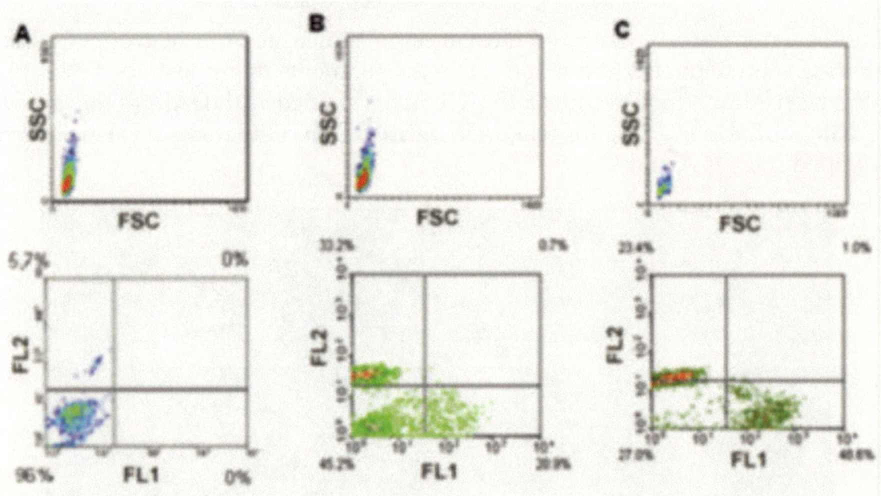

Fig. 7. Contour diagram of PI flow cytometry of cultured fibroblasts for groups: A) Control; B) UV irradiated for 30 min and C) UV irradiated for 60 min. The lower left quadrant of the cytograms shows the viable cells, which excluded PI. The upper right quadrants represent the apoptotic cells showing PI uptake. Panel (B) shows cells number (%) for apoptosis and necrosis 30 minutes after exposure to ultraviolet radiation. Panel (C) shows cells number (%) for apoptosis and necrosis 60 minutes after exposure to ultraviolet radiation. Data are representative of 04 independent experiments

Ultraviolet radiation is a carcinogenic agent for the skin. Even though being a tumor suppressor gene, details are still needed in order to understand the signaling mechanisms of skin cell death induced by UV radiations, which can lead to cancer and/or cell aging.

DNA alteration can ultimately lead to the development of skin cancer, so DNA itself is a critical target (Matsumura *et al.*, 2004). Skin DNA photodamage activates the signaling pathway of cell death by apoptosis. Apoptosis is a crucial mechanism in eliminating cells with unrepaired DNA damage and preventing carcinogenesis.

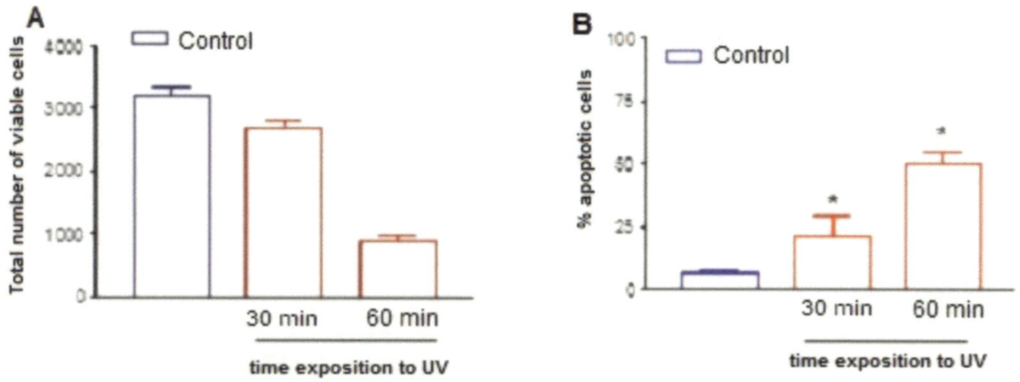

Fig. 8. Mean percentage ± of apoptotic cells in groups control and 30min and 60min after exposure to UV radiation. Data are the means of triplicate assays of one experiment representative of three that gave similar results. A) Total number of viable cells and B) Percentage of apoptotic cells. *Data analyzed with one-way **ANOVA** followed by Newman Keuls (significance level $p < 0.05$). Values represent the mean ± SEM of at least four different experiments

DNA is a critical target because its alteration can ultimately lead to the development of skin cancer (Matsumura *et al.*, 2004). In addition, Skin DNA photodamage activates the signaling pathway of cell death by apoptosis. Apoptosis is a crucial mechanism in eliminating cells with unrepaired DNA damage and preventing carcinogenesis (or preventing the formation of malignant tumors).

Apoptosis is characterized by a p53-dependent induction of pro-apoptotic proteins, leading to permeabilization of the outer mitochondrial membrane, release of apoptogenic factors into the cytoplasm, activation of caspases (cysteine-aspartic proteases) and subsequent cleavage of various cellular proteins. Apoptogenic effects include chromatin condensation and exposure of phosphatidylserine on the cell membrane surface (Meier *et al.*, 2007).

p53 levels increased about 40% after 30 min of UV exposure and about 60% after 60 min of UV exposure (Figure 9).

Previous studies indicated that BimL was involved in UV-induced apoptosis, but it remains unclear whether Bim directly activates Bax or if this activation occurs via the release of pro-survival factors (antiapoptotic) such as Bcl-xL. In recent studies, Wang *et al.* (2009) determined the interactions between BimL and Bax/Bcl-xL during UV-induced apoptosis.

Caspases have a major role in apoptosis. They are synthesized as inactive proenzymes that become activated by cleavage. Procaspase 3 is a constitutive proenzyme activated by cleavage during apoptosis. (Cohen, 1997). Caspase-3 is the most important protease in the caspase-dependent apoptosis pathway, as it is required for chromatin condensation and fragmentation (Porter & Jänicke, 1999). Poly-ADP ribose polymerase (PARP-1) is a major target of caspase-3, since cleavage-mediated inactivation of PARP-1 preserves cellular ATP that is required for apoptosis (Bouchard *et al.*, 2003).

Regarding the caspases, the resulting enzyme is able to cleave several aspartate residues of many target proteins, after a DEVD sequence common to all caspases 3 and 7 substrates

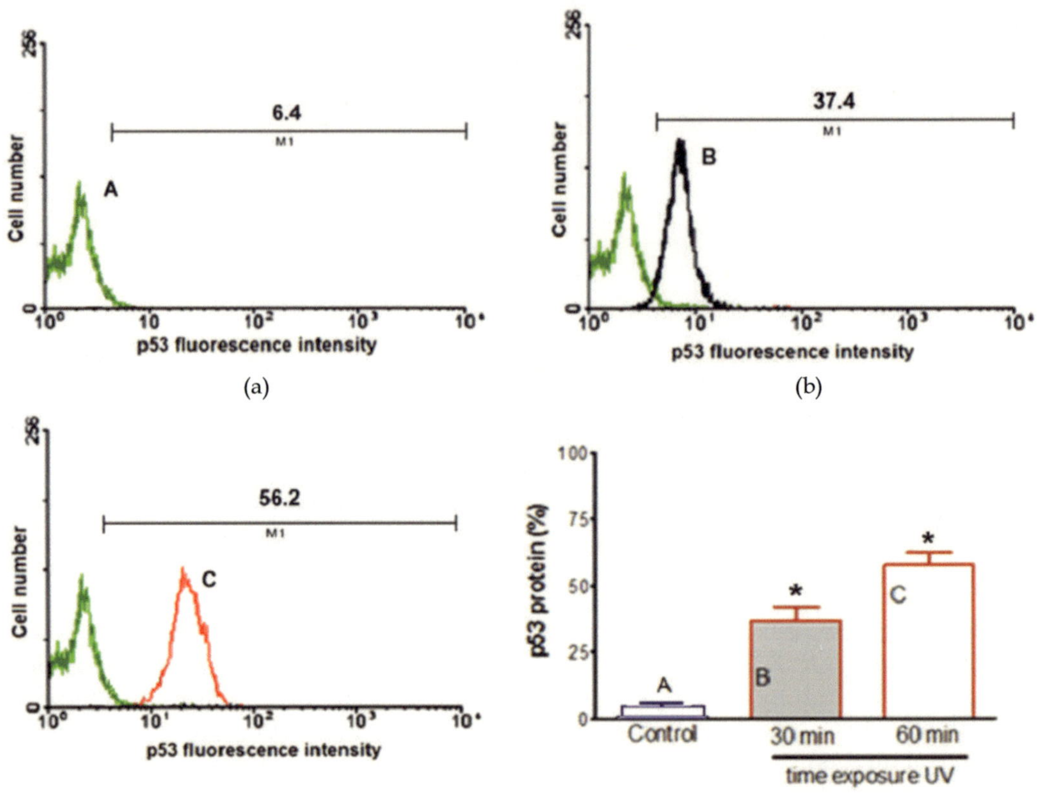

Fig. 9. Flow cytometry (FCM) analysis of p53 protein accumulation control (upper left set of panel - figure 9A - green line) and / or activation by UV can be followed of cultured fibroblasts for groups: UV irradiated for 30 min (right set of figure 9B - Black line) and UV irradiated for 60 min (right set of figure 9C - red line). The fibroblasts treated in 2% paraformaldehyde are the same as those shown in Figure 05 (control group) and figure 06 (UV irradiated groups). Cells were permeabilized with 0.1% saponin in PBS containing 10% normal bovine serum for 30 minutes at 22°C and stained with anti-p53 (SER 15) antibodies at figures (9A), (9B), and (9C) after the beginning of the experiment and analyzed by FCM. A control performed with an irrelevant antibody is shown figure 9A. The percentage of cells exhibiting active p53 conjugated with FITC is indicated on each histogram. The results from one representative experiment of four experiments performed are shown. The numbers indicate the percentages of positive cells and fluorescence intensity. Histogram overlays show the FL1 (green fluorescence) intensity corresponding to a given p53 (black line - UV irradiated for 30min and red line - UV irradiated for 60min) compared to the intensity for the control (green line). 9D Mean percentage ± of cells exhibiting active p53 in groups control (figure 9A - green line) and groups UV irradiate for 30 min (figure 9B - Black line) and UV irradiated for 60 min (figure 9C - red line). Data are the means of triplicate assays of one experiment representative of three that gave similar results. A) Total number cells fibroblasts exhibiting active p53 antibodies at figures (9A), (9B), and (9C). Histograms values differ significantly from each other. *Data analyzed with one-way ANOVA followed by Newman Keuls (significance level $p < 0.05$). Values represent the mean ± SEM of at least four different experiments

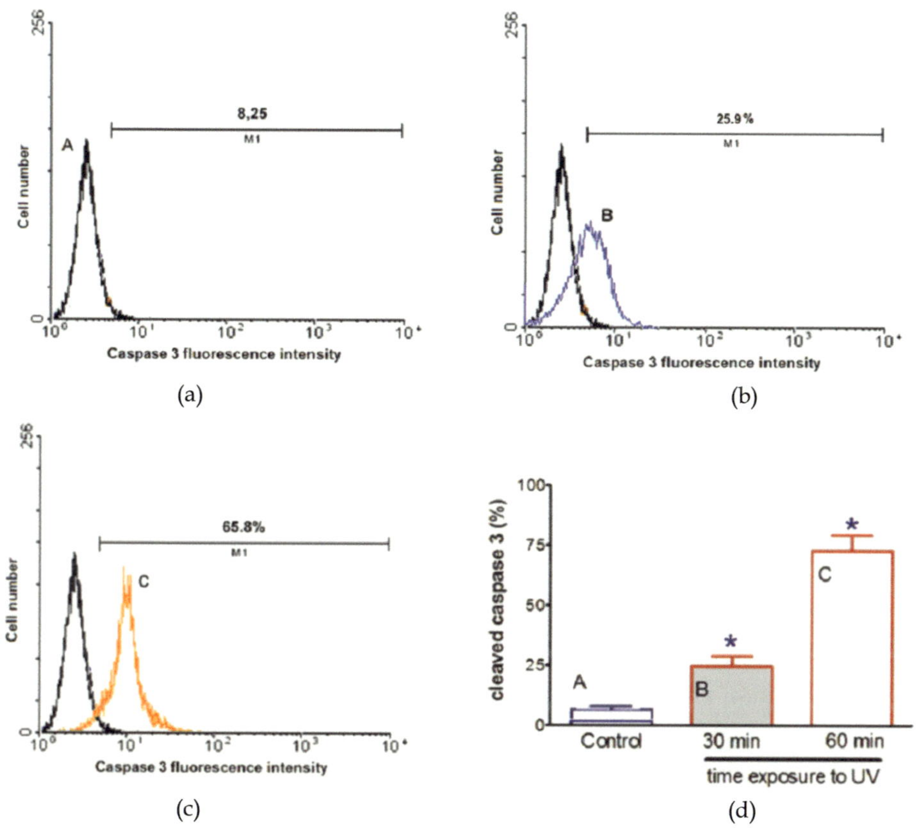

Fig. 10. Activation of caspase 3 by UV can be followed by flow cytometry (FCM) of cultured fibroblasts for groups: A) control (upper left set of panel - figure 10A - Black line) and UV irradiated for 30 min (right set of figure 10B – Blue line) and UV irradiated for 60 min (right set of 10C - orange line). The fibroblasts treated in 2% paraformaldehyde are the same as those shown in figure 05 (control group) and figure 06 (UV irradiated groups). Cells were permeabilized with 0.1% saponin in PBS containing 10% normal bovine serum for 30 minutes at 22°C and stained with anti–cleaved caspase 3 antibodies at figures (10A), (10B), and (10C) after the beginning of the experiment and analyzed by FCM. A control performed with an irrelevant antibody is shown 10A. The percentage of cells exhibiting active caspase 3 conjugated with FITC is indicated on each histogram. The results from one representative experiment of four experiments performed are shown. The numbers indicate the percentages of positive cells and fluorescence intensity. Histogram overlays show the FL1 (green fluorescence) intensity corresponding to a given caspase 3:(blue line - UV irradiated for 30min and red line - UV irradiated for 60min compared to the intensity for the control (black line). 10D Mean percentage ± of cells exhibiting active caspase 3 in groups control (figure 9A – green line) and groups UV irradiated for 30 min (figure 9B – Black line) and UV irradiated for 60 min (figure 9C – red line). Data are the means of triplicate assays of one experiment representative of three that gave similar results. A) Total number cells fibroblasts exhibiting active caspase 3 antibodies at figures (10A), (10B), and (10C). Histograms values differ significantly from each other. *Data analyzed with one-way ANOVA followed by Newman Keuls (significance level $p < 0.05$). Values represent the mean ± SEM of at least four different experiments

(DEVDase). Thus, active caspase 3 is a common effector protein in several apoptotic pathways, and it may be a good marker to detect (pre-) apoptotic cells by flow cytometry (Porter & Jänicke, 1999). Taking this into consideration, apoptosis was confirmed by determining the increased expression of cleaved caspase 3 after fibroblasts exposure to UV radiation. In this work we could verify a significant increase of cleaved caspase 3 levels, about 25.0 % after 30 min of UV exposure and 75% after 60 min of UV exposure (Figure 10).

Although caspases represent a significant component of the apoptotic pathway, there is indication that a caspase-independent apoptosis pathway also exists (Broker *et al.*, 2005). This pathway involves the Apoptosis-Inducing Factor (AIF), which translocates from the mitochondria to the nucleus to cause chromatin condensation (Daugas *et al.*, 2000).

Then again, genotoxic effects of solar UVA are mediated essentially by the activation of endogenous photosensitizers which generate a local oxidative stress. Depending on the dose and duration of exposure, UV-induced effects may occur, and DNA damage can lead to mutations and genetic instability. This is one of the reasons why sunlight overexposure increases the risk of skin cancer and DNA photolesions can also be involved in other skin-specific responses to UV radiation: erythema, immunosuppression, and melanogenesis (Matsumura & Ananthaswamy, 2004).

5. Conclusion

Damages occurring on DNA molecules not always induce mutagenesis. We should take in consideration many strong scientific evidences showing that specific activation molecular signaling pathways promote several different answers. Both the prolonged exposure time and the increase in the UV radiation dose were able to induce lipid peroxidation and cell death by apoptosis. Our results suggest that the major part of UV induced apoptosis cell death is caspase-dependent, although a minority of cells may die by a caspase-independent pathway, presumably apoptotic. In this work we also showed that p53 levels increased after UV exposure. In these circumstances, the action of UV radiation on skin cells still involves many issues depending on the cell type and on different cellular response pathways induced by phototoxic stress. Skin fibroblasts are surely sensitive to UV radiation, thus, from a better understanding of the molecular mechanisms triggered by the action of UV radiation on skin cells, it will be possible to work on improving skin radioprotection and attenuating the effects of sunlight exposure.

6. Acknowledgment

We would like to thank UNIFESP and UESC (collaborators) for their help in experiments with fibroblast cell culture. The authors gratefully acknowledge the financial support from FAPESP, FAPESB and CNPq grants.

7. References

Abbas, T & Dutta, A. (2009). p21 in cancer: intricate networks and multiple activities. *Nature reviews. Cancer*, Vol.9, pp.400-414, ISSN 1759-4782

Afag, F. (2011). Natural agents: cellular and molecular mechanisms of photoprotection. *Archives of Biochemistry and Biophysics*, Vol.508, pp. 144-151, ISSN 0003-9861

Andriani, F.; Marquelis, A.; Lin, N.; Griffey, S. & Garlick, J. A. (2003). Analysis of microenvironmental factors contributing to basement membrane assembly and normalized epidermal phenotype. *Journal of Investigative Dermatology*, Vol.120, pp. 923-931, ISSN 0022-202X

Armstrong, B. K. & Kricker, A. (2001). The epidemiology of UV induced skin cancer. *Journal of Photochemistry and Photobiology B*, Vol.63, pp.8-18, ISSN 1011-1344

Aylon & Oren. (2007). Living with p53, dying of p53. *Cell*, Vol. 130, No.4, pp. 597-600, ISSN 1097-4172

Bivik, C. A.; Larsson P. K.; Kadegal, K. M.; Rosdah, l. K. & Ollinger, K. M. (2006). UVA/B – induced apoptosis in human melanocytes involves translocation of cathepsins and Bcl-2 family members. *Journal of Investigative Dermatology*, Vol.126, pp. 1119-1127, ISSN 0022-202X .

Blumenberg, M. & Tomić-Canić M. (1997). Human epidermal keratinocyte: keratinization processes. *EXS*, Vol.78, pp.1-29, ISSN 1023-294X

Bouchard, V. J.; Rouleau, M.; Poirier, G. G. (2003). PARP-1, a determinant of cell survival in response to DNA damage. *Experimental Hematology*, Vol.31, pp.446–454, ISSN 0301-472X

Bradford, M. M. (1976). A rapid and sensitive method for the quantification of microgram quantities of protein utilizing the principle of protein-dye binding. *Analytical Biochemistry*, Vol.72, pp.248–254, ISSN0003-2697

Broker, L. E.; Kruyt, F. A. E & Giaccone, G. (2005). Cell death independent of caspases: a review. *Clinical Cancer Research*, Vol.11, pp.3155–3162, ISSN: 1078-0432

Brown, L & Benchimol, S. (2006). The involvement of MAPK signaling pathways in determining the cellular response to p53 activation: cell cycle arrest or apoptosis. *The Journal Of Biological Chemistry*, Vol.281, No.7, pp.:3832-3840, ISSN 1083-351X

Campisi, J. (2005). Senescent cells, tumor suppression and organismal aging: good citizens, bad neighbors. *Cell*, Vol.120, pp.513-522, ISSN 1097-4172

Canman, C. E. & Kastan, M. B. (1996). Signal transduction. Three paths to stress relief. *Nature*, Vol.384, pp.213-214, ISSN 0028-0836

Chirico, S.; Smith, C.; Marchant, C.; Mitchinson, M. J. & Halliwell, B. (1993). Lipid peroxidation in hyperlipidaemic patients. A study of plasma using an HPLC-based thiobarbituric acid test. *Free radical research communications*, Vol.19, pp.51-57, ISSN 8755-0199

Chouinard, N.; Valerie, K.; Rouabhia, M & Huot J. (2002). UVB-mediated activation of p38 mitogen-activated protein kinase enhances resistance of normal human keratinocytes to apoptosis by stabilizing cytoplasmic p53. *Biochemical Jounal*, Vol.365, pp.133-134, ISSN · 0264-6021

Chung, J. H.; Hanft, V. N. & Kang, S. (2003). Aging and photoaging. *Journal of the American Academy of Dermatology*. Vol.49, pp.690–697, ISSN 0190-9622

Chung, J. H.; Seo, J. Y.; Choi, H. R.; Lee, M. K.; Youn, C. S.; Rhie, G.; Cho, K. H.; Kim, K. H.; Park, K. C. & Eun, H. C. (2001). Modulation of skin collagen metabolism in aged and photo-aged human skin in vivo. *Journal of Investigative Dermatology*, Vol.117, pp. 1218-1224, ISSN 0022-202X

Chung, J. H.; Seo, J. Y.; Lee, M. K.; Eun, H. C.; Lee, J. H.; Kang, S.; Fisher, G. J. & Voorhees, J. J. (2002). Ultraviolet modulation of human macrophage metalloelastase in human skin in vivo. *Journal of Investigative Dermatology,* Vol.119, pp.507-512, ISSN 0022-202X

Cohen, G. (1997). Caspases: the executioners of apoptosis. *Biochemical Jounal,* Vol.326, pp.1–16, ISSN 0264-6021

Danova, M.; Giordano, M; Mazzini, G. & Riccardi, A. (1990). Expression of p53 protein during the cell cycle measured by flow cytometry in human leukemia. Leukemia Research, Vol.14, pp.417–422, ISSN 0145-2126

Daugas, E.; Nochy, D.; Ravagnan, L.; Loeffler, M.; Susin, S. A.; Zamzami, N. & Kroemer, G. (2000). Apoptosis inducing factor (AIF): a ubiquitous mitochondrial oxidoreductase involved in apoptosis. *FEBS Letters,* Vol.476, pp.118–123, ISSN 0014-5793

Degterev, A.; Hitomi, J.; Germscheid, M.; Chen, I. L.; Korkina, O. *et al.* (2008). Identification of RIP1 kinase as a specific cellular target of necrostatins. *Nature Chemical Biology,* Vol.5, pp.313–321, ISSN 1552-4450

Florence, H.; Sauvaigo, S.; Douki, T.; Favier, A. & Beani, J-C. (2006). Age-dependent DNA repair and cell cycle distribution of human skin fibroblasts in response to UVA irradiation. Journal of *Photochemistry and Photobiology* B, Vol.82, pp.214–223, ISSN 0031-8655

Funkel, E. (1999). Does cancer therapy trigger cell suicide? *Science,* Vol.286, pp.2256–2258, ISSN 0036-8075

Gruijl, F. R. (1999). Skin cancer and solar UV radiation. *European Journal of Cancer,* Vol.35, pp.2003-2009, ISSN 1359-6349

Gruijl, F. R.; Van Kranen, H. J. & Mullenders, L. H. (2001). UV-induced DNA damage, repair, mutations and oncogenic pathways in skin cancer. *Journal of Photochemistry and Photobiology B,* Vol.63, pp.19-27, ISSN 1011-1344

Gueguen, S.; Herbeth, B.; Siest, G. & Leroy P. (2002). An isocratic liquid chromatographic method with diode-array detection for the simultaneous determination of alpha-tocopherol, retinol, and five carotenoids in human serum. *Journal of Chromatographic Science,* Vol.40, No.2, pp.69-76, ISSN 1570-0232

Halliwell, B. & Gutteridge, J. M. (1999). Measurement of reactive species, In: *Free Radicals in Biology and Medicine,* pp.284 -313, Oxford University Press, Inc., ISBN 019-8568-69-X New York

Huang, H.; Fletcher, L.; Beeharry, N.; Daniel, R.; Kao, G.; Yen, T. J. & Ruth J. Muschel, R. J. (2008). Abnormal cytokinesis after X-irradiation in tumor cells that override the G2 DNA damage checkpoint. *Cancer Research,* Vol.68, pp.3724–3732, ISSN 0008-5472

Hwang, B. J; Ford, J.M.; Hanawallt, P.C.; Chu, G. (1999). Expression of the p48 xeroderma pigmentosum gene is p53-dependent and is involved in global genomic repair. *Proceedings of the National Academy of Sciences of the United States of America. Biochemistry,* Vol.96, pp.424–428, ISSN 0027-8424

Hwang, K. A.; Yi, B. R. & Choi, K. C. (2011). Molecular mechanisms and in vivo mouse models of skin aging associated with dermal matrix alteration. *Laboratory Animal Research,* Vol.27, pp.1-8, ISSN 1738-6055

Janicke, R. U.; Sprengart, M. L.; Wati, M. R. & Porter, A. G. (1998). Caspase-3 is required for DNA fragmentation and morphological changes associated with apoptosis. *Journal of Biological Chemistry,* Vol.273, pp.9357–9360, ISSN 0021-9258

Johnson, G. L. & Lapadat, R. Mitogen-activated protein kinase pathways mediated by ERK, JNK, and p38 protein kinases. (2002). *Science,* Vol.298, pp.1911-1912, ISSN 0036-8075

Katiyar, S. K.; Mantena, S. K. & Meiran, S. M. (2011). Silymarin protects epidermal keratinocytes from ultraviolet radiation-induced apoptosis and DNA damage by nucleotide excision repair mechanism. *PLoS One*, Vol.6, pp.1-11, ISSN 1932-6203

Kostenko, S.; Shiryaev, A.; Gerits, N.; Dumitriu, G.; Klenow, H.; Johannessen, M. & Moens, U. (2011). Serine residue 115 of MAPK- activated protein kinase MK5 is crucial for its PKA- regulated nuclear export and biological function. *Cellular and Molecular Life Sciences*, Vol.68, pp.847-862, ISSN 1420-682X

Li, G.; Mongillo, M.; Chin, K. T.; Harding. H.; Ron, D.; Marks, A. R. & Tabas, I. (2009). Role of ERO1-α–mediated stimulation of inositol 1,4,5-triphosphate receptor activity in endoplasmic reticulum stress–induced apoptosis. The Journal of Cell Biology, Vol.186, pp.783–792, ISSN 0021-9525

Makrantonaki, E. & Zouboulis, C. C. (2007). The skin as a mirror of the aging process in the human organism-state of the art and results of the aging research in the German National Genoma Research Network 2 (NGFN-2) *Experimental Gerontology*, Vol.42, pp.879-886, ISSN 0531-5565

Matsumura, Y. & Ananthaswamy, H. N. (2004). Toxic effects of ultraviolet radiation on skin. *Toxicology and Applied Pharmacology*, Vol.195, pp.298-308, ISSN 0041-008X

Meier, P. & Vousden, K. H. (2007). Lucifer's labyrinth - ten years of path finding in cell death. *Molecular Cell*, V.28, pp. 746–754, ISSN 1097-2765

Morliere, P.; Moysan, A.; Santus, R.; Huppe, G.; Maziere, J. C. & Dubertret, L. (1991). UVA-induced lipid peroxidation in cultured human fibroblasts. *Biochimica et Biophysica Acta*, Vol.084, pp.261–268, ISSN 0006-3002

Moysan, A.; Clement-Lacroix, P. M.; Dubertret. L. & Morliere, P. (1995). Effects of ultraviolet A and antioxidant defense in cultured fibroblasts and keratinocytes. *Photodermatology, photoimmunology & photomedicine*, Vol.11, pp.192-197, ISSN 0905-4383

Nicoletti, I.; Migliorati, G.; Pagliaci, M. C.; Grignani, F. & Riccardi, C. (1991). A rapid and simple method for measuring thymocyte apoptosis by propidium iodide staining and flow cytometry. *Journal of Immunological Methods*, Vol.139, pp.271-279, ISSN 1872-7905

Porter, A. G. & Janicke, R. U. (1999). Emerging roles of caspase-3 in apoptosis. *Cell Death & Differentiation*,Vol.6, pp.99–104, ISSN 1350-9047

Schwarz, T. (1998). UV light affects cell membrane and cytoplasmic targets. *Journal of Photochemistry and Photobiology B*, Vol.44, pp.91-96, ISSN 1011-1344

Shindo, Y.; Witt, E.; Han, D.; Epstein, W. & Packer, L. (1994). Enzymic and non-enzymic antioxidants in epidermis and dermis of human skin. *Journal of Investigative Dermatology*, Vol.102, pp.122-124, ISSN 0022-202X

Shreeram, S.; Hee, W. K. & Bulavin, D. V. (2008). Cdc25A serine 123 phosphorylation couples centrosome duplication with DNA replication and regulates tumorigenesis. *Molecular and Cell Biology*. Vol.28, No.24, pp.7442-7450, ISSN 0270-7306

Strässle, M.; Wilhelm, M. & Stark, G. (1991). The Increase of Membrane Capacitance as a Consequence of Radiation-induced Lipid Peroxidation. *International Journal of Radiation Biology*, Vol. 59, No.1, pp.71-83, INSS 0360-3016

Tavana, O.; Benjamin, C. L.; Puebla-Osorio, N.; Sang, M.; Ullrich, S. E.; Ananthaswamy, H. N. & Zhu, C. (2010). Absence of p53-dependent apoptosis leads to UV radiation hypersensitivity, enhanced immunosuppression and cellular senescence. *Cell Cycle*, Vol.9, pp.3328-3336, ISSN 1551-4005

Tyrrell, R. M. & Keyse, S. M. (1990). New trends in photobiology. The interactions of UV-A radiation with cultured cells *Journal of Photochemistry and Photobiology B*, Vol.4, pp.349-361, ISSN 1011-1344

Thornton, T.M. & Rincon, M. (2009). Non-Classical P38 Map Kinase Functions: Cell Cycle Checkpoints and Survival. *International Journal of Biological Scienses*, Vol.1, pp.44-52, ISSN 1449-2288

Van Nguyen, T.; Puebla-Osorio, N.; Pang, H.; Dujka, M. E. & Zhu, C. (2007. DNA damage-induced cellular senescence is sufficient to suppress tumorigenesis: a mouse model. *The Journal of experimental medicine*, Vol.204 pp.1453-1461, ISSN 1540-9538

Varani, J.; Perone, P.; Fligiel, S. E.; Fisher, G. J. & Voorhees, J. J. (2002). Inhibition of type I procollagen production in photodamage: correlation between presence of high molecular weight collagen fragments and reduced procollagen synthesis. *Journal of Investigative Dermatology*, Vol.119, pp. 122-129, ISSN 0022-202X

Vermes, I.; Haanen, C.; Steffens-Nakken, H. & Reutelingsperger, C. (1995). A novel assay for apoptosis. Flow cytometric detection of phosphatidylserine expression on early apoptotic cells using fluorescein labelled Annexin V. *Journal of Immunological Methods*, Vol.184, pp.39–51, ISSN 0022-1759

Wang, X.; Xing, D.; Liu, L. & Chen, W. R. (2009). BimL directly neutralizes Bcl-xL to promote Bax activation during UV-induced apoptosis. *FEBS Letters*, Vol.583, pp.1873-1879, ISSN

Wäster, P. K. & Ollinger, K. M. (2009). Redox-dependent translocation of p53 to mitochondria or nucleus in human melanocytes after UVA- an UVB- induced apoptosis. *Journal of Investigative Dermatology*, Vol.129, pp.1769-1781, ISSN 0022-202X

Wäster, P. K. & Ollinger, K. M. (2009). Redox-dependent translocation of p53 to mitochondria or nucleus in human melanocytes after UVA- an UVB- induced apoptosis. *Journal of Investigative Dermatology*, Vol.129, pp. 1769-1781, ISSN 0022-202X

Yohn, J. J.; Norris, D. A.; Yrastorza, D. G.; Buno, I. J,. Leff, J. A.; Hake, S. S. & Repine, J. E. (1991). Disparate antioxidant enzyme activities in cultured human cutaneous fibroblasts, keratinocytes and melanocytes. *Journal of Investigative Dermatology*, Vol.97, pp.405-409. ISSN, 0022-202X

Zhang, Y.; Xing, D. & Liu, L. (2009). PUMA promotes Bax translocation by both directly interacting with Bax and by competitive binding to Bcl-XL during UV- induced apoptosis. *Molecular Biology of the Cell*, Vol.20, pp.3077-3087, ISSN 1936-4586

23

Immunophenotypic Characterization of Normal Bone Marrow Stem Cells

Paula Laranjeira, Andreia Ribeiro, Sandrine Mendes,
Ana Henriques, M. Luísa Pais and Artur Paiva
Histocompatibility Center of Coimbra
Portugal

1. Introduction

Despite of being described more than one decade ago (Pittenger et al., 1999), the immunophenotypic profile of bone marrow mesenchymal stem cells (MSC) still not well documented. The difficulty in achieving a detailed phenotypic characterization is common in less-represented cell populations and/or populations lacking a specific known cell marker, like bone marrow MSC.

The recent advances in flow cytometry technology and the emergence of new high-speed flow cytometers have given a valuable contribute to diminish this problem in two different (but complementary) aspects: 1) by reducing dramatically the acquisition time period, making it more reasonable to study minor cell populations; and 2) by increasing the number of parameters that can be analyzed per cell at the same time, which is critical to improve the immunophenotypic characterization of those not-well characterized cell populations that lack a specific known marker.

A good example of the practical usefulness of such technical developments is the description of different cell compartments in the bone marrow CD34+ hematopoietic stem cell (HSC) population. Detailed studies on this minor bone marrow cell population demonstrated that each compartment is committed to a different hematopoietic cell lineage. An extensive immunophenotypic characterization of those CD34+ compartments allowed the development of protocols to easily and quickly identify, quantify and evaluate phenotypic aberrations and maturational blocks in those cells, which is decisive to the diagnosis, prognosis, or follow-up of a variety of hematological clonal diseases (del Cañizo et al., 2003; Lochem et al., 2004; Matarraz et al., 2008; Orfao et al. 2004).

2. Bone marrow mesenchymal stem cells

After the identification of a plastic-adherent bone marrow stromal cell population in 1976 by Friedenstein and colleagues and the first evidence of their multilineage potential (Pittenger et al., 1999) with subsequent confirmation of their stem cell nature, an increasing interest on these bone marrow MSC has emerged, mainly because of their promising therapeutic applications.

By definition, a stem cell is an undifferentiated cell with the potential ability of self-renewal and the capability of differentiation along different cell lineages (multipotency). MSC can be found on a great variety of adult tissues, where they play an important role in tissue regeneration, such as: bone marrow, adipose tissue, umbilical cord blood, umbilical cord matrix, menstrual blood, endometrium, placenta, dental pulp, skin and thymus, among others (Chamberlain et al., 2007; Ding et al. 2011; Kolf et al., 2007; Martins et al., 2009; Musina et al., 2005; Pittenger et al., 1999).

In addition to their presence in numerous adult tissues, MSC are relatively easy to isolate and have the capability to expand manyfold in culture without lose their stem cell properties. Moreover, when MSC are systemically transplanted, they are able to migrate to sites of injury and promote tissue repair, by producing growth factors or other soluble factors important to tissue regeneration, as well as by undergoing cellular differentiation (Chamberlain et al., 2007, Kolf et al., 2007; Mafi et al., 2011); such features explain the success of MSC transfusion therapy in genetic disorders affecting mesenchymal tissues (Horwitz et al., 2002; Undale et al., 2009). Furthermore, those cells have the ability of suppressing the immune response of a wide variety of immune cells, including T, B and NK lymphocytes, and antigen-presenting cells (Chamberlain et al., 2007; Stagg, 2007), and their importance in patients' clinical outcome has already been proven in severe acute graft-versus-host disease (Remberger et al., 2011; von Bahr et al., 2011). Moreover, the results achieved in animal models of autoimmune diseases are promising and encouraged the beginning of phase I clinical trials in multiple sclerosis (Constantin et al., 2009; Darlington et al., 2011; Siatskas et al., 2009).

2.1 Identification and quantification of bone marrow MSC

As referred previously, the study of minor cell populations with no known specific cell marker toke great advantage on the development of high-speed multi-parameter flow cytometers. The use of an 8-color FACSCanto II (Becton Dickinson Biosciences, BDB) flow cytometer allowed us to identify MSC in bone marrow, quantify them and further characterize their immunophenotypic profile. We employed a monoclonal antibody panel with a backbone of 3 common markers (CD13, CD45 and CD11b) for the identification of MSC (known to be CD13+CD45-CD11b-) in each tube that, at the same time, permitted the study of the expression of five more proteins on MSC per tube.

MSC are rare in bone marrow, being reported that they represent approximately 0,01% of all nucleated bone marrow cells (Chamberlain et al., 2007; Mafi et al., 2011), although is known that their number declines with aging (Caplan, 2007). Our data point to a percentage ranging between 0,01% and 0,03% of all nucleated bone marrow cells (Martins et al., 2009).

2.2 Immunophenotypic characterization of bone marrow MSC

2.2.1 Flow cytometer quality control, compensation setup strategies and other technical issues

According to the manufacturer's recommendations, it is done a daily quality control using the Rainbow Beads (BDB). In what concerns to cytometer's compensation setup, it is made once per month by setting up the Rainbow Beads (BDB) values according to the EuroFlow consortium's guidelines and then by doing a general compensation for stable fluorochromes and a specific compensation for each monoclonal antibody conjugated with tandem fluorochromes. Although the compensation is automatic, it is always revised by experienced staff at the end of the process.

In order to detect cellular autofluorescence, a negative control was made for each sample, where the bone marrow sample was only stained for CD45 PO and CD34 PerCPcy5.5.

SSC and FSC light dispersion properties allow a good discrimination between viable and dead cells and the doublets were excluded based on FSC-Area *versus* FSC-Height characteristics.

2.2.2 Material and methods

The immunophenotypic characterization of bone marrow MSC were performed in fresh EDTA-collected bone marrow samples from healthy individuals. After collection the samples were stored at 4 °C and processed within 24 hours.

Whole bone marrow samples were stained for surface cell markers using a stain-lyse-and-then-wash direct immunofluorescence technique. 200 µl of whole bone marrow were aliquoted in different tubes and stained with the following combinations of monoclonal antibodies in an 8-color staining protocol, detailed in table 1.

	FITC	PE	PerCPcy5.5	PEcy7	APC	APCH7	PB	PO
Tube 1	CD49e (SAM1) Beckman Coulter	CD73 (AD2) BD Pharmingen	CD34 (8G12) BDB	CD13 (Immu103.44) Beckman Coulter	CD90 (5E10) BD Pharmingen	HLA-DR (L243) BDB	CD11b (ICRF44) BD Pharmingen	CD45 (HI30) Invitrogen
Tube 2	CD31 (WM59) BD Pharmingen	NGFR (C40-1457) BD Pharmingen	CD14 (M5E2) BD Pharmingen	CD13	CD133 (293C3) Miltenyi Biotec	-	CD11b	CD45
Tube 3	CD15 (HI98) BDB	CD146 (P1H12) BD Pharmingen	CD24 (ALB9) Beckman Coulter	CD13	CD90	CD29 (TS2/16) BioLegend	CD11b	CD45
Tube 4	CD106 (51-10C9) BD Pharmingen	CD105 (1G2) Beckman Coulter	-	CD13	HLA-A, B, C (G46-2.6) BD Pharmingen	-	CD11b	CD45
Tube 5	-	CD73	CD24	CD13	CD90	-	CD11b	CD45

Table 1. Panel of monoclonal antibodies used for the bone marrow MSC characterization. FITC - fluorescein isothiocyanate; PE – phycoerythrin; PerCPcy5.5 - peridinin chlorophyll protein cyanine 5.5; PEcy7 - R-phycoerythrin cyanine 7; APC – allophycocyanin; APCH7 - allophycocyanin H 7; PB - pacific blue; PO - pacific orange

Data acquisition was performed in a FACSCanto II flow cytometer (BDB), using FACSDiva acquisition software (BDB). The total bone marrow cellularity of the whole sample was acquired (5 x 10^6 events, minimum) for each tube. Bone marrow MSC were identified as $CD13^+/CD45^-/CD11b^-$, as shown in Figure 1.

Data analysis was performed using Infinicyt software (Cytognos, Salamanca, Spain).

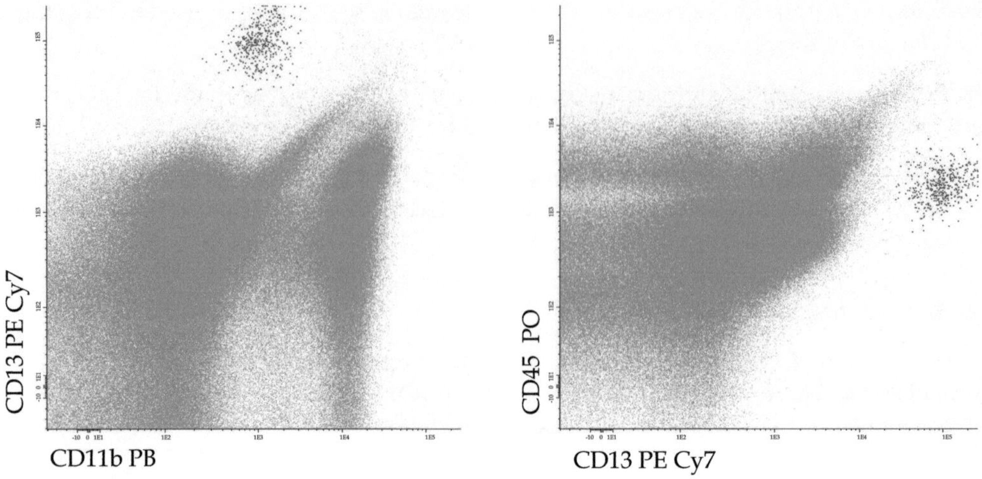

Fig. 1. Identification of bone marrow MSC (blue) present in a whole bone marrow sample, phenotypically characterized as CD13$^+$CD45$^-$CD11b$^-$

2.2.3 Results and discussion

Bone marrow MSC showed to be uniformly positive to CD13, CD29, CD49e, CD90, CD106, CD146, CD73, NGFR, CD105 and HLA-A, B, C (Figure 1 and Figure 2); and negative to CD24, CD31, CD11b, CD14, CD15, CD34, CD45, CD133 and HLA-DR, which is in agreement with previous studies described in the literature (Chamberlain et al., 2007; Delorme et al., 2008; Ehninger & Trumpp, 2011; Fox et al., 2007; Jones & McGonagle, 2008; Kolf et al., 2007; Martins et al., 2009; Pittenger et al., 1999; Tormin et al., 2011). Based on the expression profile of these markers, bone marrow MSC behave as one sole cell population, as all the studied markers were homogeneously expressed inside the MSC population.

Several studies on adhesion molecules and chemokine receptors expression have been made in order to shed light on MSC migratory and homing ability. CD29 (integrin β_1-subunit) and CD106 (vascular cell adhesion molecule 1, VCAM-1) seem to be important in the adhesion of MSC to endothelial cells (Chamberlain et al., 2007; Kolf et al., 2007; Stagg, 2007) and CD29, which when dimerized with CD49e (integrin α_5-subunit) forms a receptor that binds to fibronectin and invasin, is likely to promote MSC-extracellular matrix interaction (Gu et al., 2009). CD146 (Muc18) plays an important role in cell-cell and cell-extracellular matrix adhesion and an increased expression of these marker on tumor cells is associated with an increased cell motility and invasiveness/ metastasis capability (Bardin et al., 2001; Zeng et al., 2011). The glycoprotein CD90 (Thy-1) regulates as well cell-cell and cell-extracellular matrix interactions, being involved in adhesion to endothelial cells, migration, metastasis and tissue regeneration (Jurisic et al., 2010; Rege & Hagood, 2006).

The enzyme CD73 is an ecto-5'-nucleotidase that produces extracellular adenosine. In animal tumor models, CD73-generated adenosine inhibits both homing and expansion of T cells via adenosine-receptor signaling. In fact, recent research shows that adenosine suppresses T cell immune response both in activation and effector phases, as well as NK cell immune activity (Wang et al., 2011; Zhang et al., 2010).

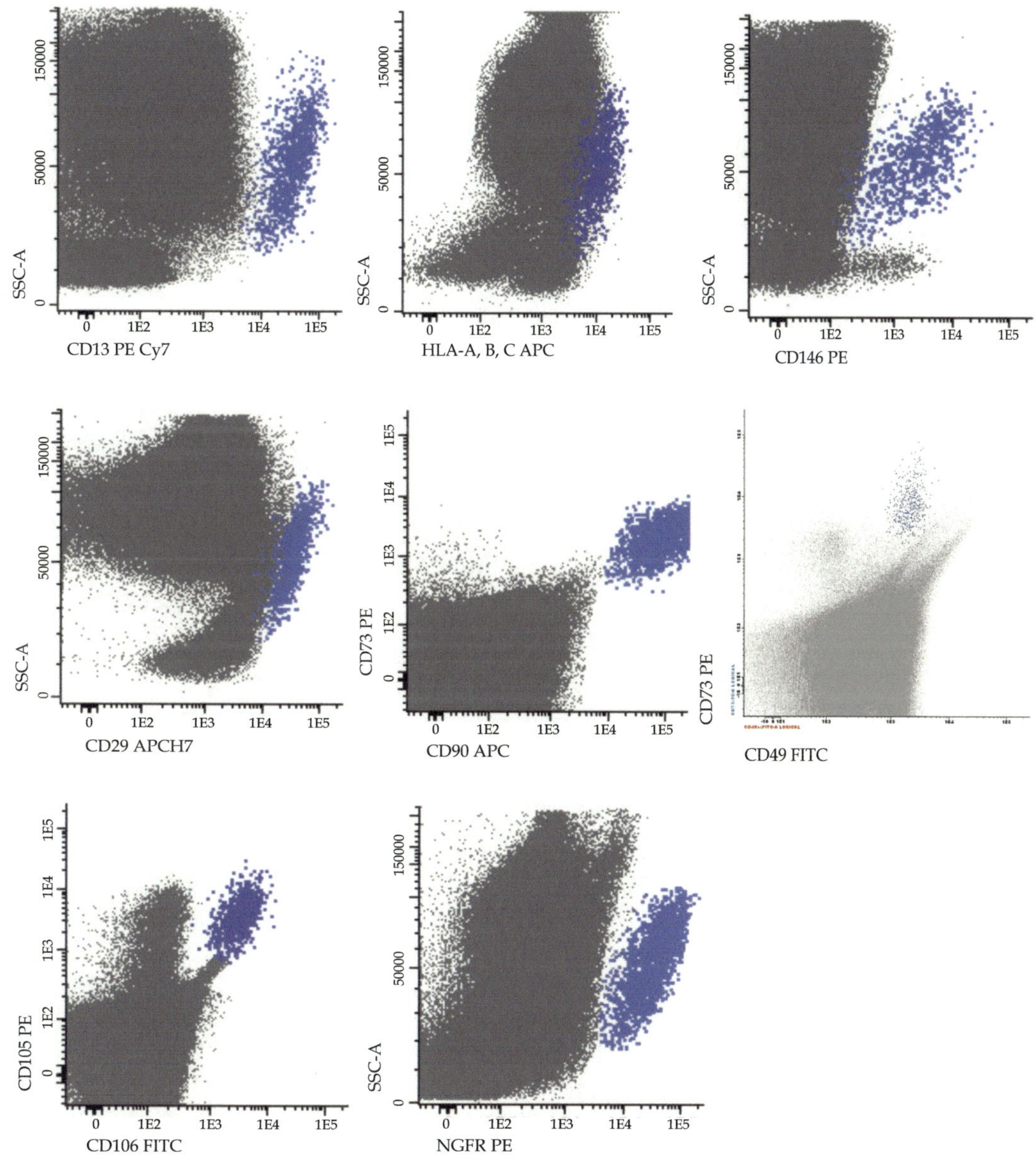

Fig. 2. Immunophenotypic characteristics of bone marrow MSC (blue). The remaining bone marrow nucleated cells are represented as grey events

In what concerns to growth factor receptors, NGFR (nerve growth factor receptor, CD271) is expressed in a wide variety of tissues and, depending on the cell type, signaling through this receptor regulates NF-kB activation, apoptosis, tissue regeneration, immune cell activation, proliferation and cell differentiation (Micera et al., 2007; Rogers et al., 2010). Finally, CD105 (endoglin) is one of the receptors for TGF-β, a growth factor involved in the regulation of development, maintenance and proliferation of MSC (Stagg, 2007), and also known to play an important role in tissue repair.

Some discrepancies described in the expression of adhesion molecules, chemokine receptors and other proteins, may be the reflex of the microenvironmental differences present in different studies. Although there are a great similitude in the phenotypic profile of MSC isolated from different tissues, differences do exist (Chamberlain et al., 2007; Kolf et al., 2007; Martins et al., 2009). As well as different cultures conditions can also change the MSC phenotype (Chamberlain et al., 2007; Halfon et al., 2011; Stagg, 2007; Tormin et al., 2011). This could be a clue of MSC highly sensitiveness to microenvironment alterations, and their potential to change their protein expression profile could be of great importance in giving an appropriate response to physiological or pathological challenges: by changing their migratory pattern, by initiating an immunomodulatory or immunosuppressive response, by modifying the production and release of soluble factors, or by undergoing cell differentiation.

As a minor bone marrow cell population easy to expand in vitro, it is attractive to characterize the MSC immunophenotype after culture cell expansion. Nevertheless, characterizing these cells directly (without previous culture) enables an analysis closest to their physiological conditions, excluding the phenotypic alterations induced by factors present in the culture medium. Moreover, this direct approach allows an accurate quantification of MSC in bone marrow. Also, this same strategy can be applied to MSC from other tissues.

3. Bone marrow hematopoietic stem cells

The multipotent hematopoietic stem cell is mainly located in the bone marrow of adult animals and has the ability to differentiate along all hematopoietic cell lineages. A number of studies based on in vitro cell culture, xeno-transplantation of hematopoietic human cells in immunodeficient mice and in pre-immune animal fetuses, were carried out to identify the human hematopoietic stem cell and unveil the hematopoietic precursors hierarchy (Nimer, 2008; Yin et al., 2007), becoming clear that CD34-positive cells were able to differentiate and give rise to all blood cells. There are evidences that, within this heterogeneous population, the more immature CD34+ HSC expresses CD133 and are CD38-negative/dim. It is also known that the CD34+CD133+ subpopulation can arise from the CD133+CD34-CD38- subset (Goussetis et al., 2006; Nimer, 2008; Yin et al., 1997).

3.1 Identification and quantification of the different bone marrow CD34+ HSC cell compartments

As already referred, CD34-positive cells are an heterogeneous bone marrow cell population, consisting in various cell compartments differing in immunophenotype, size and lineage commitment. The immunophenotypic pattern of each compartment is well described and, with a relatively low number of markers, the majority of those subsets can be accurately and easily identified.

Attending only to the immunophenotypic features, is possible to identify the following bone marrow CD34+ cell subsets by flow cytometry: uncommitted (more immature) precursors, neutrophil precursors, B cell precursors, monocytic precursors, plasmacytoid dendritic cells precursors, erythroid precursors, basophil precursors and mast cell precursors.

A detailed immunophenotypic description of human bone marrow CD34+ cells was published, few years ago, by Matarraz and colleagues (Matarraz et al., 2008) and Lochem and colleagues (Lochem et al., 2004), along with the frequency of each CD34+ cell subpopulation in normal hematopoiesis (Matarraz et al. 2008), presented on table 2.

Bone marrow CD34+ HSC compartments	Mean ± Standard deviation	Range
% Bone marrow CD34+ HSC (of total bone marrow)	0,9 ± 0,3	(0,2-1,6)
Immature CD34+ precursor (%) (within CD34+ cells)	52 ± 12	(19-66)
CD34+ neutrophil precursors (%) (within CD34+ cells)	34 ± 7	(15-47)
CD34+ B cell precursors (%) (within CD34+ cells)	14 ± 10	(1-36)
CD34+ monocytic precursors (%) (within CD34+ cells)	10 ± 7	(0-26)
CD34+ plasmacytoid dendritic cell precursors (%) (within CD34+ cells)	5 ± 2	(0-9)
CD34+ erythroid precursors (%) (within CD34+ cells)	18 ± 8	(1-36)
CD34+ basophil precursors (%) (within CD34+ cells)	0,7 ± 0,4	(0-1,5)
CD34+ mast cell precursors (%) (within CD34+ cells)	0 ± 0,005	(0-0,02)

Table 2. Distribution of the different cell compartments of bone marrow CD34+ HSC. The results are expressed as mean ± standard deviation (range). Adapted from Matarraz et al. Leukemia 2008

The most immature CD34+ subset can be identified based on CD133 expression (Goussetis et al., 2006; Pastore et al., 2008; Yin et al., 1997). When other markers are concerned, these cell are $CD34^{hi}/CD45^{int}/HLA\text{-}DR^{hi}/cyMPO^{-}/nTdT^{-}/CD117^{hi}$ and have intermediate side scatter (SSC) and forward scatter (FSC) light dispersion properties (Matarraz et al., 2008). As previously described by Matarraz and colleagues, the phenotypic profile of CD34+ B cell precursors is $CD34^{int}/CD45^{int/dim}/HLA\text{-}DR^{hi}/cyMPO^{-}/nTdT^{int}/CD117^{-}$ and these cells present the lowest SSC and FSC of all CD34+ subpopulations (Lochem et al., 2004; Matarraz et al., 2008); the CD34+ neutrophil precursors present $CD34^{hi}/CD45^{int/dim}/HLA\text{-}DR^{hi}/cyMPO^{int/hi}/nTdT^{-}/CD117^{hi}$, along with the highest values for SSC and FSC of all CD34+ subsets; the CD34+ plasmacytoid dendritic cell precursors are identified based on the expression of $CD34^{+}/CD123^{hi/int}/HLA\text{-}DR^{hi}$; CD34+ monocytic precursors display $CD34+/HLA\text{-}DR^{hi}/CD64^{hi}/CD45^{hi}/CD117^{-}$ immunophenotype; basophil precursors are described as being $CD34^{+}/CD123^{int/hi}/HLA\text{-}DR^{-/+}$; and CD34+ mast cell precursors are $CD34+/CD117^{hi}/HLA\text{-}DR^{-/int}$ (Matarraz et al., 2008). Finally, CD34+ erythroid precursors are characterized by $CD34^{+}/CD36^{+}/CD64^{-}/CD45^{lo}$ immunophenotype (Matarraz et al., 2008) and by CD105 expression (Buhring et al., 1991; Rokhlin et al., 1995). As a matter of fact, CD105 and TGF-β_1 have a pivotal role in the regulation of the differentiation in the erythroid lineage (Fortunel et al., 2000; Moody et al., 2007).

3.2 A single-tube protocol to identify the different bone marrow CD34+ HSC compartments

Recently, we developed an 8-color single-tube protocol to identify the different bone marrow CD34+ HSC subsets by flow cytometry.

The single-tube protocol we propose here was constructed to allow an accurate, quick and easy identification and quantification of those cellular compartments. Attending to the monoclonal antibodies and fluorochrome-conjugation available on the market and to compensation issues, and based on our experience and knowledge on the hematopoietic maturation dynamics, we elected the best markers to identify with precision the cell populations of interest.

3.2.1 Material and methods

The immunophenotypic characterization of bone marrow CD34+ precursors were performed in fresh EDTA-collected bone marrow samples from healthy individuals. After collection, the samples were stored at 4 °C and processed within 24 hours. The quality control and compensation strategies are described in detail in section 2.2.1.

A stain-lyse-and-then-wash direct immunofluorescence protocol was used, and the monoclonal antibodies were combined as presented on table 3.

	FITC	PE	PerCPcy 5.5	PEcy7	APC	APCH7	PB	PO
Single Tube Protocol	CD35 (E11) BDB Pharmingem	CD123 (SSDCL Y107D2) Beckman Coulter	CD34 (8G12) BDB	CD117 (PN IM3698) Beckman Coulter	CD133 (293C3) Miltenyi Biotec	HLA-DR (L243) BDB	CD44 (IM7) Biolegend	CD45 (HI30) Invitrogen

FITC - fluorescein isothiocyanate; PE – phycoerythrin; PerCPcy5.5 - peridinin chlorophyll protein cyanine 5.5; PEcy7 - R-phycoerythrin cyanine 7; APC – allophycocyanin; APCH7 - allophycocyanin H 7; PB - pacific blue; PO - pacific orange.

Table 3. Panel of monoclonal antibodies used for the identification and quantification of the different subpopulations found in bone marrow CD34+ HSC

Data acquisition was performed on a FACSCanto II flow cytometer (BDB), using FACSDiva acquisition software (BDB). In a first step of acquisition, the whole bone marrow cellularity was stored (100.000 events). In a second step, only events within the CD34+ electronic gate were acquired (5.000 to 10.000 CD34+ events).

Data analysis was performed using Infinicyt software (Cytognos, Salamanca, Spain).

3.2.2 How to identify the different CD34+ HSC compartments with the single-tube protocol?

1. The most immature (uncommitted) compartment of bone marrow C34+ HSC
   The most immature compartment can be easily identified based on their positivity to CD133 marker ($CD133^{hi}$). To differentiate this subset from CD34+ neutrophil precursors and CD34+ plasmacytoid dendritic cell precursors, also expressing CD133 ($CD133^{int}$),

other important phenotypic characteristics have to be taken into account: CD35⁻/CD34ʰⁱ/HLA-DRʰⁱ/CD117ʰⁱ/FSCⁱⁿᵗ/SSCⁱⁿᵗ/CD123⁻. Figure 3 presents a detailed immunophenotype of this compartment considering all the markers used in this protocol.

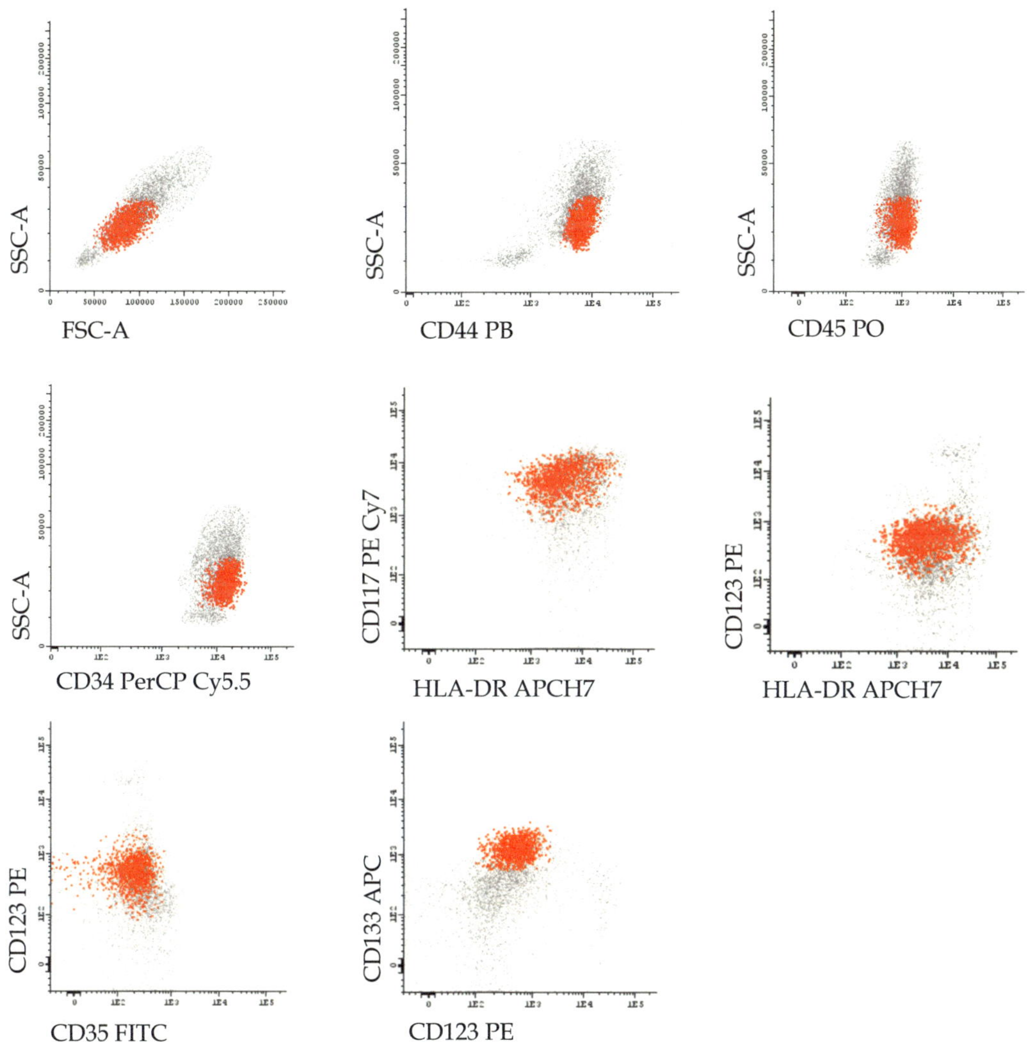

Fig. 3. Uncommitted bone marrow CD34+ HSC (red) immunophenotype. The remaining bone marrow CD34+ cell compartments are presented in grey

2. Bone marrow CD34+ erythroid precursors
   Both CD34+ erythroid precursors and monocytic precursors express CD35. The two CD34+ subpopulations can be distinguished in this protocol by the expression of CD117 and HLA-DR. The erythroid precursors are $CD117^{+}$/HLA-DR^{int} and the monocytic precursors are $CD117^{dim/-}$/HLA-DR^{hi}. Moreover, the erythroid precursors are characterized by a dim expression of CD34, CD45 and CD44 (Figure 4).

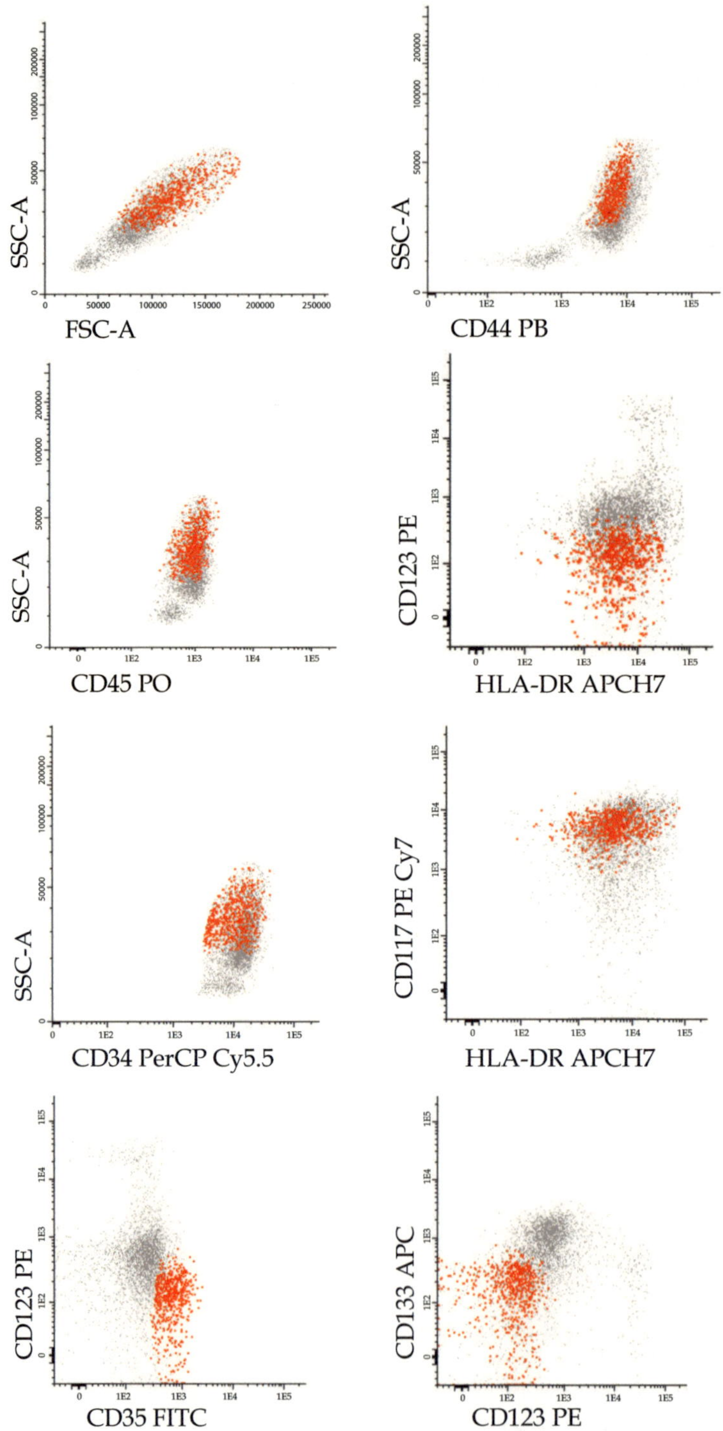

Fig. 4. Erythroid-committed bone marrow CD34+ precursors (red) immunophenotype. The remaining bone marrow CD34+ cell compartments correspond to the grey events

It is worth mentioning that our previous studies with simultaneous staining of CD105 and CD35 proved that the two markers were co-expressed in the same subset of CD34+ bone marrow cells and CD35 appears slightly before CD105 (Figure 5)[1].

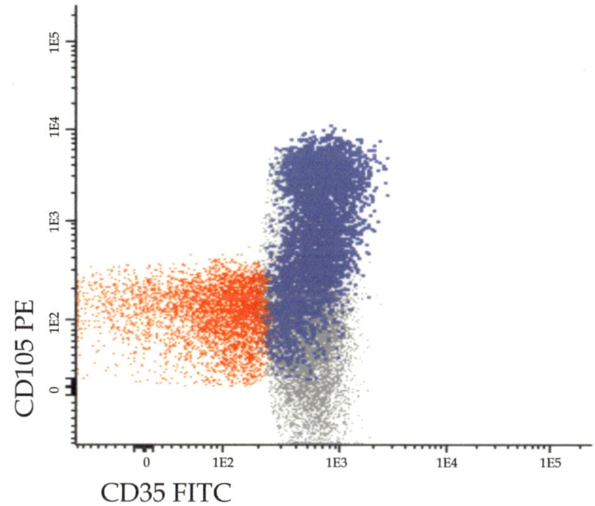

Fig. 5. Expression of CD105 and CD35 in bone marrow erythroid lineage: uncommitted CD34+ cells (red), CD34+erythroid precursors (blue) and CD34- erythroid precursors (grey)

3. Bone marrow CD34+ neutrophil precursors
   Neutrophil precursors show high reactivity to CD44 antigen, as the plasmacytoid dendritic cell precursors (CD44^{hi}), but in the absence of CD123 marker. Other important immunophenotypic features of this CD34+ compartment are: CD133^{int}/CD35^{-}/HLA-DR^{hi}/CD117^{hi}/CD45$^{int/dim}$/FSC^{hi}/SSC^{hi} (Figure 6).

4. Bone marrow CD34+ monocyte precursors
   Using this single-tube approach, the monocyte precursors are primarily identified by exclusion of all the other myeloid CD34+ precursors. Is noteworthy that a large percentage of monocyte-committed CD34+ precursors express CD35, being discriminated from CD34+ erythroid precursors by their CD117$^{dim/-}$/HLA-DR^{+}/CD45^{hi} phenotype. Although classically the identification of this CD34+ subset was made focusing on the expression of CD64, this marker seems to be also present on CD34+ plasmacytoid and myeloid dendritic cell precursors. In line with this, CD35 might be a good option to the identification of CD34+ monocyte precursors. The immunophenotype of this population is depicted in Figure 7.

5. Bone marrow CD34+ B cell precursors
   Even in the absence of an B-cell lineage specific marker, as CD19 or CD79a, CD34+ B cell precursors are clearly identified by the low expression of CD44 and CD45, along with low light scatter properties (Figure 8).

---

[1] According to our experience, CD35 seems to be expressed earlier than CD105 and CD36 on erythroid committed CD34+ precursors, allowing a more accurate quantification of this subset.

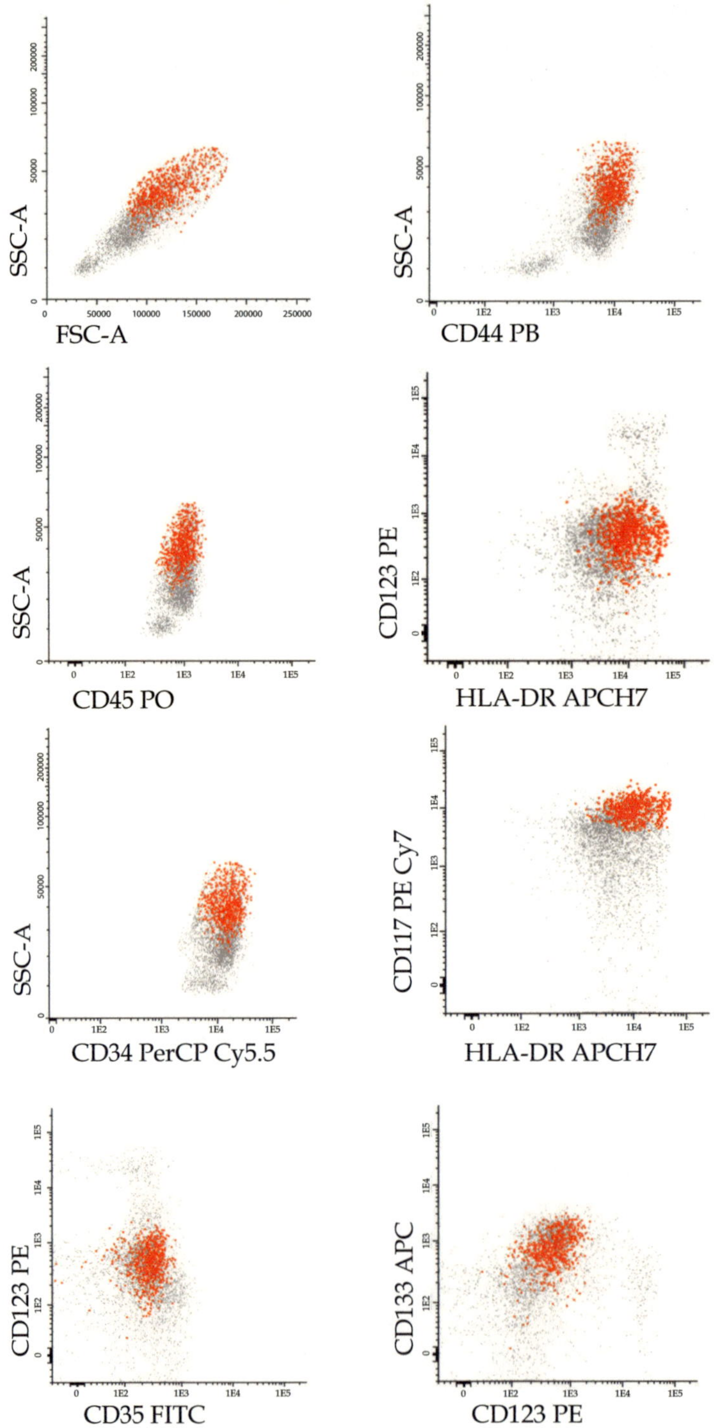

Fig. 6. Neutrophil-committed bone marrow CD34+ precursors (red) immunophenotype. The remaining bone marrow CD34+ cell compartments are presented in grey

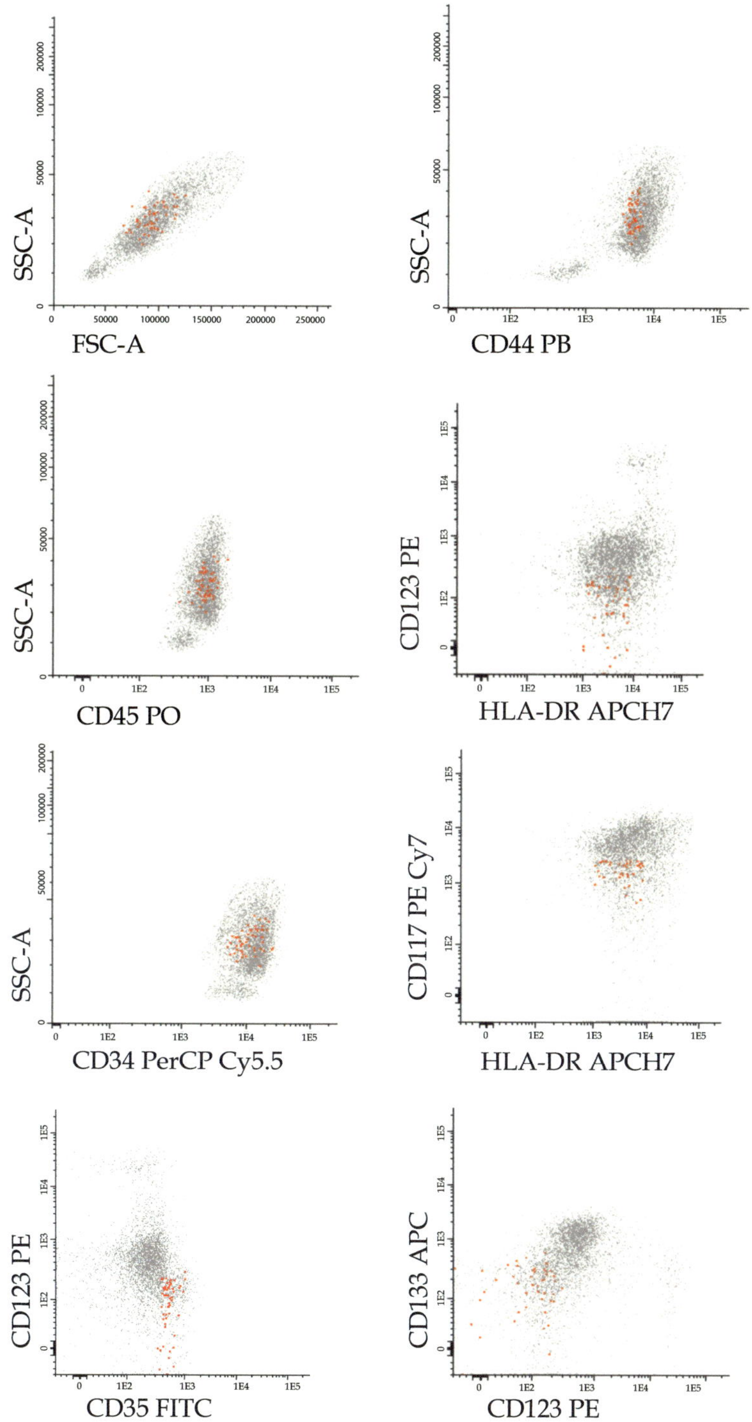

Fig. 7. Monocytic-committed bone marrow CD34+ precursors (red) immunophenotype. The remaining bone marrow CD34+ cell compartments are presented in grey

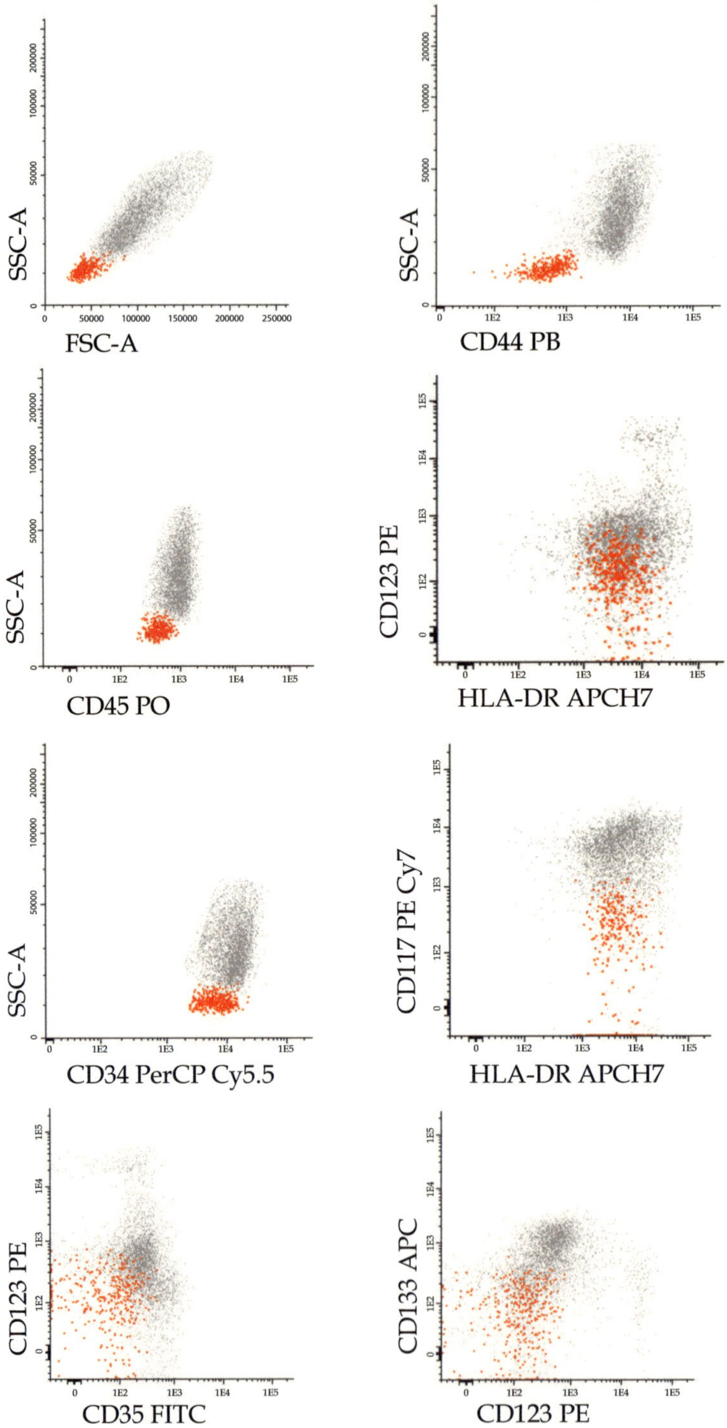

Fig. 8. B-cell-committed bone marrow CD34+ precursors (red) immunophenotype. The remaining bone marrow CD34+ cell compartments are presented in grey

6. Bone marrow CD34+ basophil precursors
   Our protocol allows the identification of basophil precursors using the classical markers and attending to the immunophenotype HLA-DR$^{-/dim}$/CD123$^{int/hi}$. Of note, this CD34+ subset presents the lowest expression of CD44 among all bone marrow myeloid CD34+ cells, being easy to differentiate this precursors from all the other myeloid precursors by using CD44 marker (Figure 9).

7. Bone marrow CD34+ plasmacytoid dendritic cell precursors
   The plasmacytoid dendritic cell precursors are identified using the classical markers, as being HLA-DR^{hi}/CD123$^{hi/int}$. The most immature forms of this precursor express CD133 (CD133^{int}). The immunophenotypic characteristics of this population are represented on Figure 10.

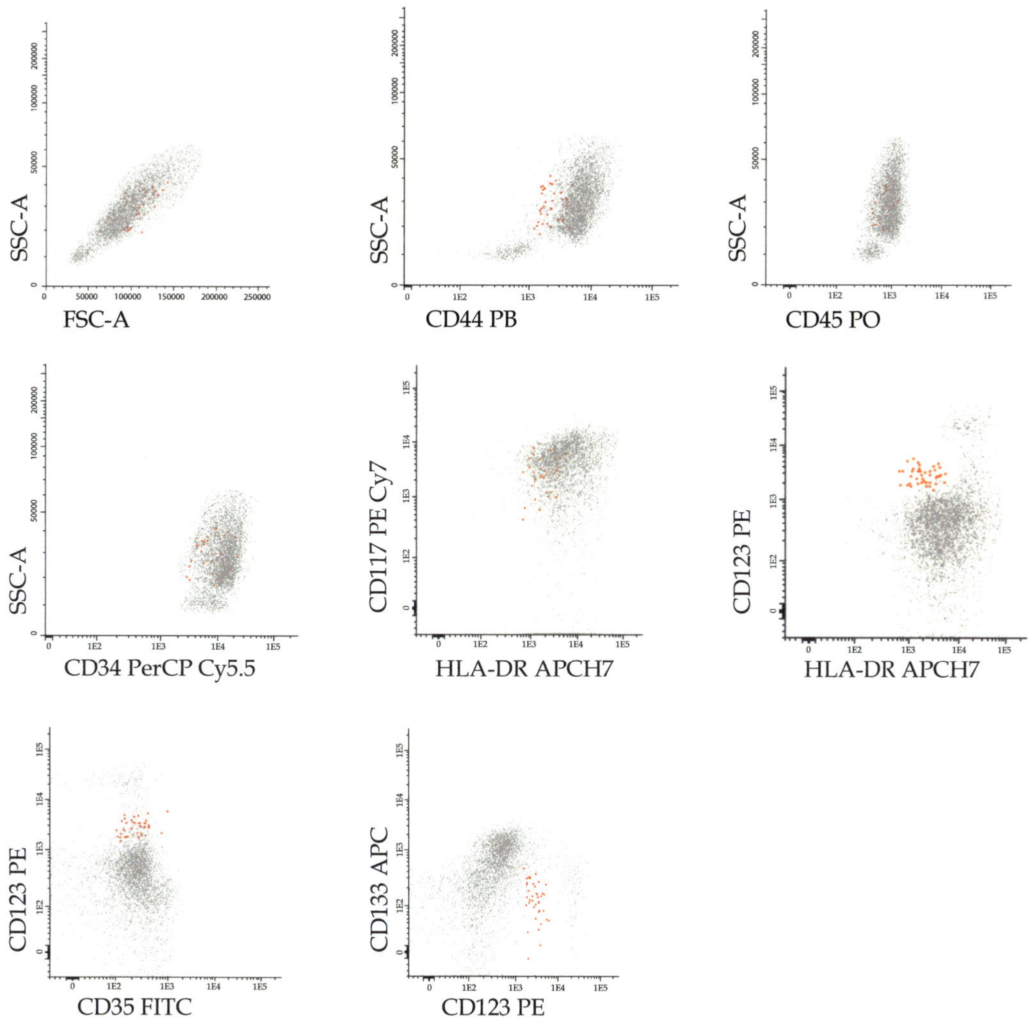

Fig. 9. Basophil-committed bone marrow CD34+ precursors (red) immunophenotype. The remaining bone marrow CD34+ cell compartments are presented in grey

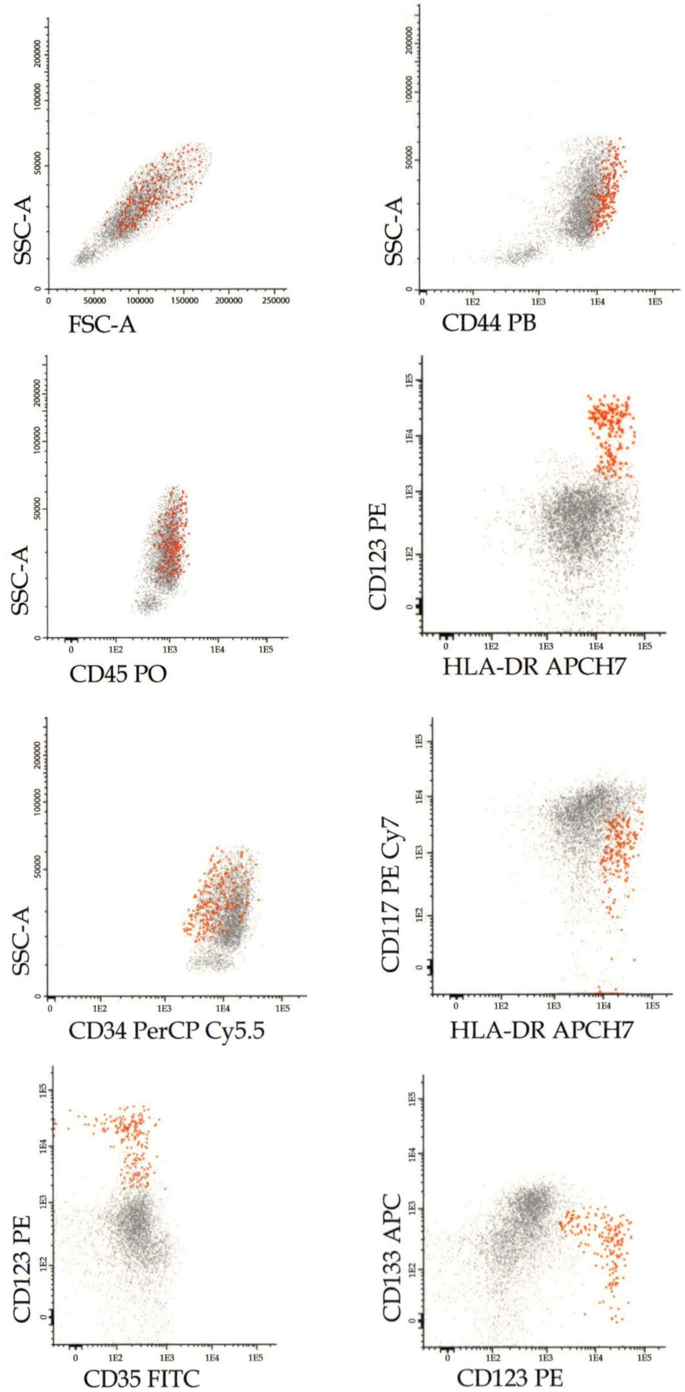

Fig. 10. Plasmacytoid dendritic cell-committed bone marrow CD34+ precursors (red) immunophenotype. The remaining bone marrow CD34+ cell compartments are presented in grey

8. Bone marrow CD34+ mast cell precursors
   The classical markers for the identification of CD34+ mast cell precursors are included in our protocol, and these cells are CD117^{hi}/HLA-DR$^{-/int}$. This subset expresses high levels of CD44. Other immunophenotypic characteristics of this subset are illustrated in Figure 11.

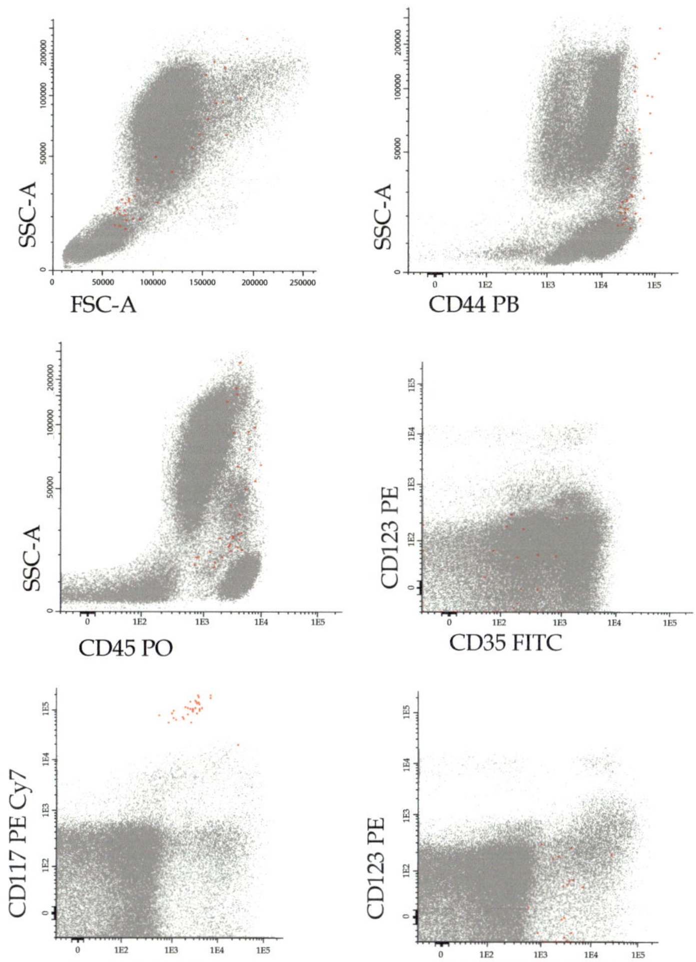

Fig. 11. Mast cell-committed bone marrow CD34+ precursors (red) immunophenotype. The events in grey correspond to remaining whole bone marrow nucleated cells

3.3 The maturation dynamic of bone marrow CD34+ hematopoietic stem cell

The possibility of a multiparameter analysis in a single cell basis conduct to a broader knowledge on the immunophenotypic characteristics of bone marrow CD34+ compartments and how it varies along the differentiation through different hematological cell lineages. Figure 12 depicts the dynamic of the maturation of different bone marrow CD34+ cell compartments.

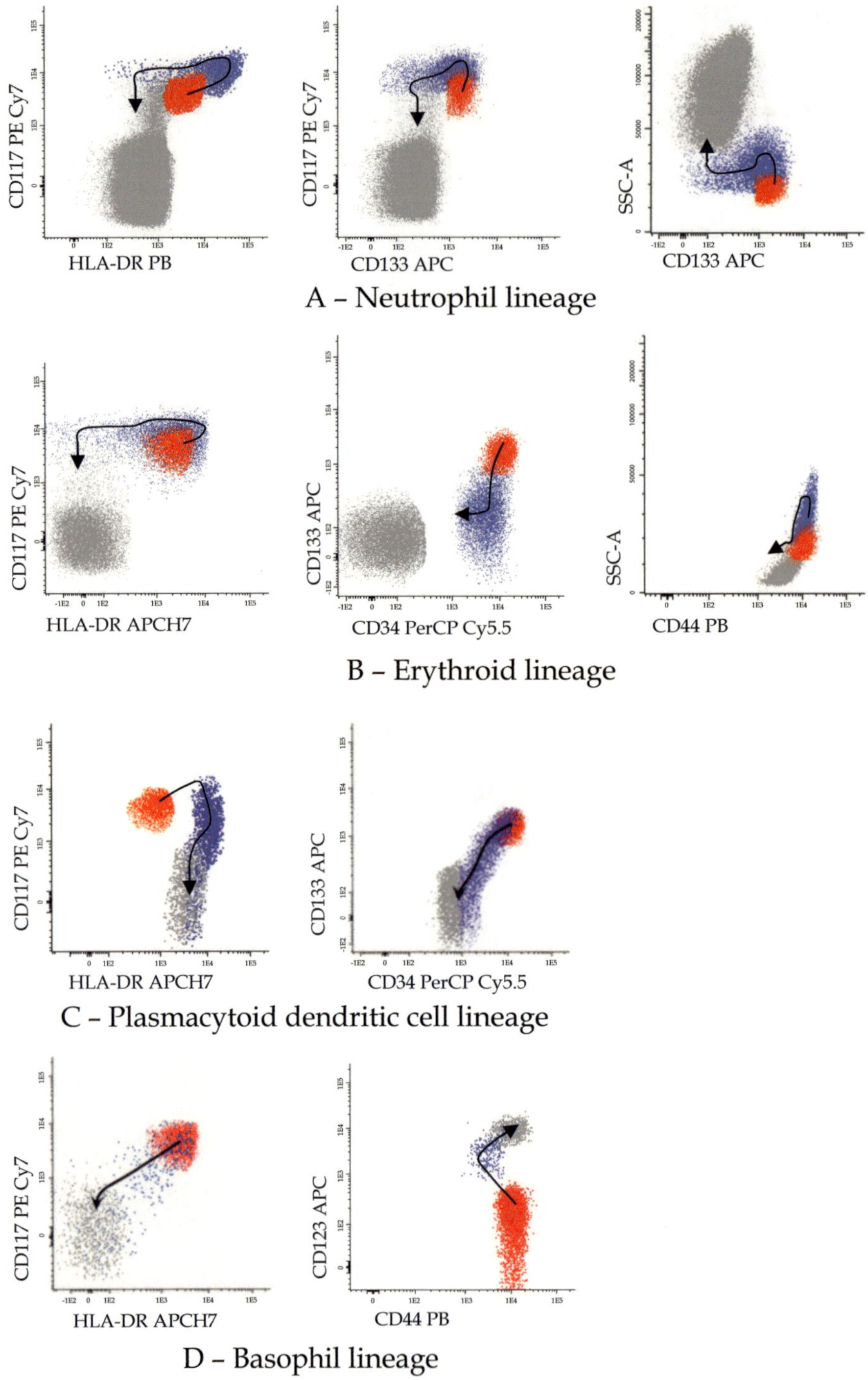

Fig. 12. Maturational dynamic of bone marrow CD34+ HSC. Uncommitted CD34+ cells are presented in red, lineage committed CD34+ cells are presented in blue and the lineage committed CD34- cells correspond to grey events

4. Conclusion

The emergence of high-speed multi-parameter flow cytometers have given an important contribute to unveil the phenotypic characteristics of minor cell populations and/or populations without a known specific cell marker.

Using flow cytometry to characterize bone marrow MSC directly (without in vitro cell culture) represents a great advantage by enabling an analysis closest to the physiologic conditions of the cells, excluding all the phenotypic alterations induced by factors present in the culture medium. Moreover, this direct analysis allows an accurate quantification of these cells in bone marrow. In addition, the strategy used for bone marrow can also be applied in MSC from other tissues, allowing their direct quantification and characterization.

A broader knowledge about the immunophenotypic characteristics of the different compartments of bone marrow HSC could improve their identification, allow a more accurate quantification of those compartments, as well as shed light on the protein expression patterns in the earliest stages of maturation of each hematological cell lineage. Furthermore, a better knowledge of those protein expression patterns might contribute to the development of new strategies to identify aberrant phenotypes in hematological diseases affecting the more immature bone marrow cells compartments, which can be helpful in the classification of acute leukemias, diagnosis of myelodysplastic syndromes and detection of minimal residual disease. A more extensive understanding of the phenotype of CD34+ hematopoietic stem cells in the different maturational stages could also be useful to monitoring and investigate if different mobilization regimens have the capability of mobilizing distinct CD34+ hematopoietic stem cells subpopulations.

Here, we presented a simple, quick and economic approach to identify and quantify the different bone marrow CD34+ HSC compartments.

5. References

Bardin N, Anfosso F, Massé J, Cramer E, Sabatier F, Le Bivic A, Sampol J & Dignat-George F. (2001). Identification of CD146 as a component of the endothelial junction involved in the control of cell-cell cohesion. *Blood*, Vol.98, No.13, (December 2001), pp. 3677-3684, ISSN 0006-4971.

Bühring HJ, Müller CA, Letarte M, Gougos A, Saalmüller A, van Agthoven AJ, Busch FW. (1991). Endoglin is expressed on a subpopulation of immature erythroid cells of normal human bone marrow. *Leukemia*, Vol.5, No.10, (October 1991), pp. 841-847, ISSN 0887-6924.

Caplan A. (2007). Adult mesenchymal stem cells for tissue engineering versus regenerative medicine. *J Cell Phisiol*, Vol.213, No.2, (November 2007), pp. 341-347, ISSN 1097-4652.

Chamberlain G, Fox J, Ashton B & Middleton J. (2007). Concise review: mesenchymal stem cells: their phenotype, differentiation capacity, immunological features, and potential for homing. *Stem Cells*, Vol.25, No.11 (November 2007), pp. 2739-2749, ISSN 1549-4918.

Constantin G, Marconi S, Rossi B, Angiari S, Calderan L, Anghileri E, Gini B, Bach D, Martinello M, Bifari F, Galie M, Turano E, Budui S, Sbarabti A, Krampera M &

Bonetti B. (2009). *Stem Cells,* Vol.27, No.10, (October 2009), pp. 2624-2635, ISSN 1549-4918.

Darlington PJ, Boivin MN, Bar-Or A. (2011). Harnessing the therapeutic potential of mesenchymal stem cells in multiple sclerosis. *Expert Rev Neurother,* Vol.11, no.9, (September 2011), pp. 1295-303, ISSN 1473-7175.

Del Cañizo MC, Fernández ME, López A, Vidriales B, Villarón E, Arroyo JL, Ortuño F, Orfao A & San Miguel JF. (2003). Immunophenotypic analysis of myelodysplastic syndromes. *Haematologica,* Vol.88, No.4, (April 2003), pp. 402-407, ISSN 0390-6078.

Delorme B, Ringe J, Gallay N, Le Vern Y, Kerboeuf D, Jorgensen C, Rosset P, Sensebé L, Layrolle P, Häupl T & Charbord P. (2008).Specific plasma membrane protein phenotype of culture-amplified and native human bone marrow mesenchymal stem cells. *Blood,* Vol.111, No.5, (March 2008), pp. 2631-2635, ISSN 0006-4971.

Ding DC, Shyu WC & Lin S. (2011). Mesenchymal stem cells. *Cell Transplant,* Vol.20, No.1, (2011), pp. 5–14, ISSN 1555-3892.

Ehninger A & Trumpp A. (2011). The bone marrow stem cell niche grows up: mesenchymal stem cells and macrophages move in. *J Exp Med,* Vol.208, No.3, (March 2011), pp. 421-428, ISSN 0022-1007.

Fortunel N, Hatzfeld A, & Hatzfeld J. (2000). Transforming growth factor-b: pleiotropic role in the regulation of hematopoiesis. *Blood,* Vol.96, No.6, (September 2000), pp. 2022-2036, ISSN 0006-4971.

Fox JM, Chamberlain G, Ashton BA & Middleton J. (2007). Recent advances into the understanding of mesenchymal stem cell trafficking. *Br J Haematol,* Vol.137, No.6, (June 2007), pp. 491-502, ISSN 1365-2141.

Goussetis E, Theodosaki M, Paterakis G, Tsecoura C & Graphakos S. (2006). In vitro identification of a cord blood CD133+CD34-Lin+ cell subset that gives rise to myeloid dendritic precursors. *Stem Cells,* Vol.24, No.4, (April 2006), pp. 1137-1140, ISSN 1549-4918.

Gu J, Isaji T, Sato Y, Kariya Y& Fukuda T. (2009).Importance of N-glycosylation on alpha5beta1 integrin for its biological functions. *Biol Pharm Bull,* Vol.32, No.5, (May 2009), pp. 780-785, ISSN 0918-6158.

Halfon S, Abramov N, Grinblat B & Ginis I. (2011). Markers distinguishing mesenchymal stem cells from fibroblasts are downregulated with passaging. *Stem Cell Dev,* Vol.20, No.1, (January 2011), ISSN 1547-3287.

Horwitz EM, Gordon PL, Koo WK, Marx JC, Neel MD, McNall RY, Muul L & Hofmann T. (2002). Isolated allogeneic bone marrow-derived mesenchymal cells engraft and stimulate growth in children with osteogenesis imperfecta: Implications for cell therapy of bone. *Proc Natl Acad Sci USA,* Vol.99, No.13, (June 2002), pp. 8932-8937, ISSN 0027-8424.

Jones E & McGonagle D. (2008).Human bone marrow mesenchymal stem cells in vivo. *Rheumatology (Oxford).* Vol.47, No.2, (February 2008), pp. 126-131, ISSN 1462-0324.

Jurisic G, Iolyeva M, Proulx ST, Halin C & Detmar M. (2010). Thymus cell antigen 1 (Thy1, CD90) is expressed by lymphatic vessels and mediates cell adhesion to lymphatic endothelium. *Exp Cell Res,* Vol.316, No.17, (October 2010) pp. 2982-2992, ISSN 0014-4827.

Kolf CM, Cho E & Tuan RS. (2007). Mesenchymal stromal cells. Biology of adult mesenchymal stem cells: regulation of niche, self-renewal and differentiation. *Arthritis Res Ther,* Vol.9, No.1, (February 2007), pp. 204-214, ISSN 1478-6354.

Martins AA, Paiva A, Morgado JM, Gomes A & Pais ML. (2009). Quantification and immunophenotypic characterization of bone marrow and umbilical cord blood mesenchymal stem cells by multicolor flow cytometry. *Transplant Proc*, Vol.41, No.3, (April 2009), pp. 943-946, ISSN 0041-1345.

Matarraz S, López A, Barrena S, Fernandez C, Jensen E, Flores J, Bárcena P, Rasillo A, Sayagues JM, Sánchez ML, Hernandez-Campo P, Hernandez Rivas JM, Salvador C, Fernandez-Mosteirín N, Giralt M, Perdiguer L & Orfao A. (2008). The immunophenotype of different immature, myeloid and B-cell lineage-committed CD34+ hematopoietic cells allows discrimination between normal/reactive and myelodysplastic syndrome precursors. *Leukemia*, Vol.22, No.6, (June 2008), pp. 1175-1183, ISSN 0887-6924.

Micera A, Lambiase A, Stampachiacchiere B, Bonini S, Bonini S & Levi-Schaffer F. (2007). Nerve growth factor and tissue repair remodeling: trkA(NGFR) and p75(NTR), two receptors one fate. *Cytokine Growth Factor Rev*, Vol.18, No.3-4, (June-August 2007), pp. 245-256, ISSN 1359-6101.

Moody JL, Singbrant S, Karlsson G, Blank U, Aspling M, Flygare J, Bryder D & Karlsson S. (2007). Endoglin is not critical for hematopoietic stem cell engraftment and reconstitution but regulates adult erythroid development. *Stem Cells*, Vol.25, No.11, (November 2007), pp. 2809-2819, ISSN 1549-4918.

Musina RA, Bekchanova ES & Sukhikh GT. (2005). Comparison of mesenchymal stem cells obtained from different human tissues. *Bull Exp Biol Med*, Vol.139, No.4, (April 2005), pp. 504-9, ISSN 0007-4888.

Nimer S. (2008). MDS: a stem cell disorder--but what exactly is wrong with the primitive hematopoietic cells in this disease? *Hematology Am Soc Hematol Educ Program*, (2008), pp. 43-51. ISSN 1520-4391.

Orfao A, Ortuño F, Santiago M, Lopez A & San Miguel J. (2004). Immunophenotyping of Acute Leukemias and Myelodysplastic Syndromes. *Cytometry A*, Vol.58A, No.1, (March 2004), pp. 62-71. ISSN 1552-4930.

Pastore D, Mestice A, Perrone T, Gaudio F, Delia M, Albano F, Russo Rossi A, Carluiccio P, Leo M, Liso V& Specchia G. (2008). Subsets of CD34+ and early engraftment kinetics in allogeneic peripheral SCT for AML. *Bone Marrow Transplant*, Vol.41, No.11, (June 2008), pp. 977-981, ISSN 0268-3369.

Pittenger MF, Mackay AM, Beck SC, Jaiswal RK, Douglas R, Mosca JD, Moorman MA, Simonetti DW, Craig S & Marshak DR. (1999). Multilineage potential of adult human mesenchymal stem cells. *Science*, Vol.284, No.5411, (April 1999), pp. 143-7, ISSN 0036-8075.

Rege TA & Hagood JS. (2006). Thy-1 as a regulator of cell-cell and cell-matrix interactions in axon regeneration, apoptosis, adhesion, migration, cancer, and fibrosis. *FASEB J*, Vol.20, No.8, (June 2006), pp. 1045-54, ISSN: 0892-6638.

Remberger M, Uhlin M, Karlsson H, Omazic B, Svahn BM & Mattsson J. (2011). Treatment with mesenchymal stromal cells does not improve long-term survival in patients with severe acute GVHD. *Transpl Immunol*, 2011 Sep 10 [Epub ahead of print], ISSN 0966-3274.

Rogers ML, Bailey S, Matusica D, Nicholson I, Muyderman H, Pagadala PC, Neet KE, Zola H, Macardle P & Rush RA. ProNGF mediates death of Natural Killer cells through activation of the p75NTR-sortilin complex. *J Neuroimmunol*, Vol.226, No.1-2, (September 2010), pp. 93-103, ISSN: 0165-5728.

Rokhlin OW, Cohen MB, Kubagawa H, Letarte M & Cooper MD. (2005). Differential expression of endoglin on fetal and adult hematopoietic cells in human bone marrow. *J Immunol*, Vol.154, No.9, (May 1995), pp. 4456-4465, ISSN: 0022-1767.

Siatskas C, Payne NL, Short MA & Bernard CC. (2010). A consensus statement addressing mesenchymal stem cell transplantation for multiple sclerosis: it's time! *Stem Cell Rev*, Vol.6, No,4, (December 2010), pp. 500-506, ISSN 1550-8943.

Stagg J. (2007). Immune regulation by mesenchymal stem cells: two sides to the coin. *Tissue Antigens*, Vol.69, No.1, (January 2007), pp. 1-9, ISSN 0001-2815.

Tormin A, Li O, Brune JC, Walsh S, Schütz B, Ehinger M, Ditzel N, Kassem M & Scheding S. (2011). CD146 expression on primary nonhematopoietic bone marrow stem cells is correlated with in situ localization. *Blood*, Vol.117, No.19, (May 2011), pp. 5067-77, ISSN 0006-4971.

Undale AH, Westendorf JJ, Yaszemski MJ & Khosla S. (2009). Mesenchymal stem cells for bone repair and metabolic bone diseases. *Mayo Clin Proc*, Vol.84, No.10, (October 2009), pp. 893-902, ISSN: 0025-6196.

van Lochem EG, van der Velden VH, Wind HK, te Marvelde JG, Westerdaal NA & van Dongen JJ. (2004). Immunophenotypic differentiation patterns of normal hematopoiesis in human bone marrow: reference patterns for age-related changes and disease-induced shifts. *Cytometry B Clin Cytom*, Vol.60, No.1, (July 2004), pp. 1-13, ISSN 1552-4957.

von Bahr L, Sundberg B, Lönnies L, Sander B, Karbach H, Hägglund H, Ljungman P, Gustafsson B, Karlsson H, Le Blanc K & Ringdén O. (2011). Long-Term Complications, Immunologic Effects, and Role of Passage for Outcome in Mesenchymal Stromal Cell Therapy. *Biol Blood Marrow Transplant*, 2011 Aug 4 [Epub ahead of print]. ISSN 1083-8791.

Wang L, Fan J, Thompson LF, Zhang Y, Shin T, Curiel TJ & Zhang B. (2011). CD73 has distinct roles in nonhematopoietic and hematopoietic cells to promote tumor growth in mice. *J Clin Invest*, Vol.121, No.6, (June 2011), pp. 2371-2382, ISSN 0021-9738.

Yin AH, Miraglia S, Zanjani ED, Almeida-Porada G, Ogawa M, Leary AG, Olweus J, Kearney J & Buck DW. (1997). AC133, a novel marker for human hematopoietic stem and progenitor cells. *Blood*, Vol.90, No.12, (December 1997), pp. 5002-5012, ISSN 0006-4971.

Zeng GF, Cai SX, Wu GJ. (2011). Up-regulation of METCAM/MUC18 promotes motility, invasion, and tumorigenesis of human breast cancer cells. *BMC Cancer*, Vol. 11, (March 2011), pp. 113-126, ISSN 1471-2407 .

Zhang B. (2010). CD73: A novel target for cancer immunotherapy. *Cancer Res*, Vol.70, No.16, (August 2010), pp. 6407–6411, ISSN 0008-5472.

24

Ethanol Extract of *Tripterygium wilfordii* Hook. f. Induces G0/G1 Phase Arrest and Apoptosis in Human Leukemia HL-60 Cells Through c-Myc and Mitochondria-Dependent Caspase Signaling Pathways

Chung-Jen Chiang et al.*
Department of Medical Laboratory Science and Biotechnology, China Medical University, Taichung, Taiwan

1. Introduction

Tripterygium wilfordii Hook. f. is a traditional Chinese herb (Murphy, 2006; Qiu et al., 2003). The extract of *Tripterygium wilfordii* Hook. f. has been widely applied to the treatment of immune-related diseases, such as rheumatoid arthritis (RA), nephritis, and systemic lupus erythematosus (SLE) (Chang et al., 1999; Wang et al., 2000). Extracts of *Tripterygium wilfordii* Hook. f. have been shown to inhibit lymphocyte proliferation induced by mitogentic stimulation *in-vitro* (Wu et al., 2003). Triptolide (PG490, one of the most active components in *Tripterygium wilfordii* Hook. f. extract, possesses immunosuppressive, anti-inflammatory and anti-fertility actions *in vivo* and *in vitro* (Zhao et al., 2005; Leuenroth et al., 2005). Many reports have demonstrated that triptolide has anti-proliferate activity against L1210, U937, K562, HL60, and P388 leukemia cells (Lou et al., 2004; Chan et al., 2001; Wei et al., 1991). However, the cellular and molecular mechanisms underlying mediating *Tripterygium wilfordii* Hook. f.-induced differentiation and/or apoptosis in leukemia cells have not been well studied.

Leukemia is a malignant disease characterized by uncontrolled cellular growth and disrupted differentiation of hematopoietic stem cells (Lichtman et al., 2005; O'Hare et al., 2006). Chemotherapy can be effective in certain types of leukemia, but in cases in which it

---

* Jai-Sing Yang[1], Yun-Peng Chao[2], Li-Jen Lin[3] Wen-Wen Huang[4], Jing-Gung Chung[4], Shu-Fen Peng[4], Chi-Cheng Lu[5], Jo-Hua Chiang[5], Shu-Ren Pai[4] and Minoru Tsuzuki[6,7]
[1]*Department of Pharmacology, China Medical University, Taichung, Taiwan*
[2]*Department of Chemical Engineering, Feng Chia University, Taichung, Taiwan*
[3]*School of Chinese Medicine, China Medical University, Taichung, Taiwan*
[4]*Department of Biological Science and Technology, China Medical University, Taichung, Taiwan*
[5]*Department of Life Sciences, National Chung Hsing University, Taichung, Taiwan*
[6]*Nihon Pharmaceutical University, Saitama, Japan*
[7]*Tsuzuki Institute for Traditional Medicine China Medical University, Taichung, Taiwan*

is not effective additional therapeutic strategies are needed. (Faderl et al., 2005; Frankfurt et al., 2006; ter Bals et al., 2005). Several compounds are capable of inducing the differentiation of leukemia cells into mature cells *in vitro*, and differentiation therapy has been shown to be an effective approach for treating leukemia (Altucci et al., 2004; Altucci et al., 2005; Takahashi et al., 2002). Human promyelocytic leukemia HL-60 cells and mouse monocytic leukemia WEHI-3 cells are commonly used to study various properties of leukemia cell proliferation and differentiation *in vitro* (Lin et al., 2006; Abe et al., 1987). Differentiation of HL-60 is induced into granulocytes by dimethyl sulfoxide (DMSO) and all-trans retinoic acid (ATRA), and into monocytic-like cells by phorbol ester (TPA) and 1,25-dihydroxy-vitamin D3 (Tsiftsoglou et al., 2003). In HL-60 cells, differentiation is induce-specific and is characterized by agents to differentiated is a marked increase in the proportion of G0/G1 cells (Yen et al., 2006), and the modulation of cyclin/CDK (Horie et al., 2004; Wang et al., 1996; Barrera et al., 2004; Pizzimenti et al., 1999; Kumakura et al., 1996).

In hematopoietic cells, apoptosis can be coupled to terminal differentiation of myeloid progenitor (Yazdanparast et al., 2005; Samudio et al., 2005). Cells undergoing apoptosis have observable morphology changes expressed as nuclear condensation, DNA fragmentation, and compact packaging of the cellular debris into apoptotic bodies (Fleischer et al., 2006; Bohm et al., 2006). The delivery and performance of apoptotic signals requires a coordinated cascade of caspase activation and action. The initiator caspases include caspase-8 in Fas-induced apoptosis, and caspase-9, the activation of which is triggered by cytochrome *c* release from mitochondria in response to various stimuli. Those caspases can directly activate downstream effectors of caspase-3, -6, and -7, which cleave death substrates, such as poly(ADP-ribose) polymerase (PARP) (Christophe et al., 2006; Lucken et al., 2005; Lockshin et al., 2005).

In this study, we investigated the cytotoxic effects of ethanol extract of *Tripterygium wilfordii* Hook. f. (ETW) on the promotion of cell cycle arrest and apoptosis in HL-60 cells. Our results indicated that ETW effectively induces both G0/G1 phase arrest and apoptosis of HL-60 cells *in vitro*. The mechanisms governing ETW-induced G0/G1 phase arrest included down regulation of cyclin E, Bcl-2 and Bax, and -triggered apoptosis through caspase-9, caspase-8 and caspase-3-dependent pathways.

2. Materials and methods

2.1 Chemicals and reagents

EDTA, Propidium iodide (PI), RNase A, Tris-HCl, Tritox X-100, Tween 20 and Proteinase K were obtained from Sigma Chemical Co. (St.Louis, MO, USA). RPMI-1640 medium, fetal bovine serum (FBS), and L-glutamine, penicillin/streptomycin were obtained from Gibco BRL Co. (Grand Island, NY, USA). The caspase-3, caspase-8 and caspase-9 activity assay kits were bought from R&D Systems, Inc. (Minneapolis, MN, USA)

2.2 Ethanol *Tripterygium wilfordii* Hook. f. (ETW) extraction

Dried and powdered plant materials were subjected to continuous ethanol extraction in a Soxhlet extractor with absolute ethanol for 72 h. The ethanol extract was collected and concentrated by vacuum distillation. The extract was evaporated to dryness and reconstituted in ethanol before experiment.

2.3 Cell culture and viability assay

The human promyelocytic leukemia cell line (HL-60) was obtained from the Culture Collection and Research Center (CCRC, Taiwan, R.O.C.), originally from the American Type Culture Collection (ATCC, USA). Cells were cultured in RPMI-1640 culture medium (Gibco/Life Technologies, Taipei, Taiwan) supplemented with 10% heated-inactive fetal bovine serum (Gibco/Life Technologies), 2 mM L-glutamine, penicillin (100 units/ml), and streptomycin (100 μg/ml) (Gibco/Life Technologies) and incubated at 37°C in humidified 5% CO2 atmosphere.

For viability analysis, 2.5 X 10^5 cells/well were seeded in 24-well culture plates. ETW was added to each well and the plates were incubated at 37°C for 24, 48 and 72 h. Cell viability was estimated by a propidium iodide (PI) incorporation assay and flow cytometry (FACS CaliburTM, Becton Dickinson) analysis (Aouacheria et al., 2002).

2.4 Cell cycle analysis

Cells were incubated with 50, 100 or 200 μg/mL of ETW for 0, 24 or 48 h. After treatment, cells were washed with phosphate-buffered saline (PBS) twice. The cells were re-suspended in hypotonic PI solution (0.1% sodium citrate, 0.1% Triton X-100, and 50 μg/ml propidium iodide), and then cellular DNA content was determined by flow cytometry (Kamikubo et al., 2003).

2.5 Western blotting analysis

Total protein was prepared with protein lysising buffer (PRO-PREP™ protein extraction solution, iNtRON Biotechnology, Seongnam, Gyeonggi-Do, Korea). The concentration of protein was determined by the Bradford method using the Bio-Rad protein assay dye reagent. The lysates containing 40 μg of protein were separated by SDS-PAGE and transferred onto PVDF membrane. Nonspecific binding sites were blocked with 5% non-fat milk in PBST buffer (0.05 % Triton X-100 in PBS) for 1 h. The PVDF membrane was incubated overnight at 4°C with specific primary antibodies against cyclin D1, cyclin E, Bcl-2, and α-tubulin (Santa Cruz Biotechnology, Inc., Santa Cruz, CA, USA). After being washed with PBST buffer, the membrane was incubated with horseradish peroxidase (HRP)-conjugated secondary antibodies (Santa Cruz). Immunoreactive proteins were detected using a Western Blotting Chemiluminescence Reagent Plus kit (NENTM Life Science) and exposed to Chemiluminescence films (Choi et al., 2003).

2.6 Caspase activities assays

Cells were collected in lysis buffer (50 mM Tris-HCl, 1 mM EDTA, 10 mM EGTA, 10 mM digitonin and 2 mM DTT) and placed on ice for 10 min. The lysates were centrifuged at 15,800g at 4°C for 10 min. Cell lysates (50 μg of protein) were incubated with caspase -3, -9, and -8 specific substrates (Ac-DEVD-pNA, Ac-LEHD-pNA, and Ac-IETD-pNA) with reaction buffer in a 96-well plate at 37°C for 1 h. The caspase activity was determined by measuring OD405 of the released pNA (An et al., 2004).

2.7 Statistical analysis

Results are presented as mean ± S.D. Differences between the different treatment groups, which consisted of matched samples, were assessed by the Student's *t*-test. A p value of less than 0.05 was considered to be significant.

3. Results

3.1 Effects of ETW on cell viability in HL-60 and WEHI-3 cells

We treated HL-60 cells with ETW at the concentrations of 0, 50, 100 and 200 µg/ml. The number of viable cells was counted by a PI exclusion method 0, 24 and 48 h later. As shown in Fig. 1, ETW exerted a dose- and time-dependent loss of cell membrane integrity and viability in HL-60 cells.

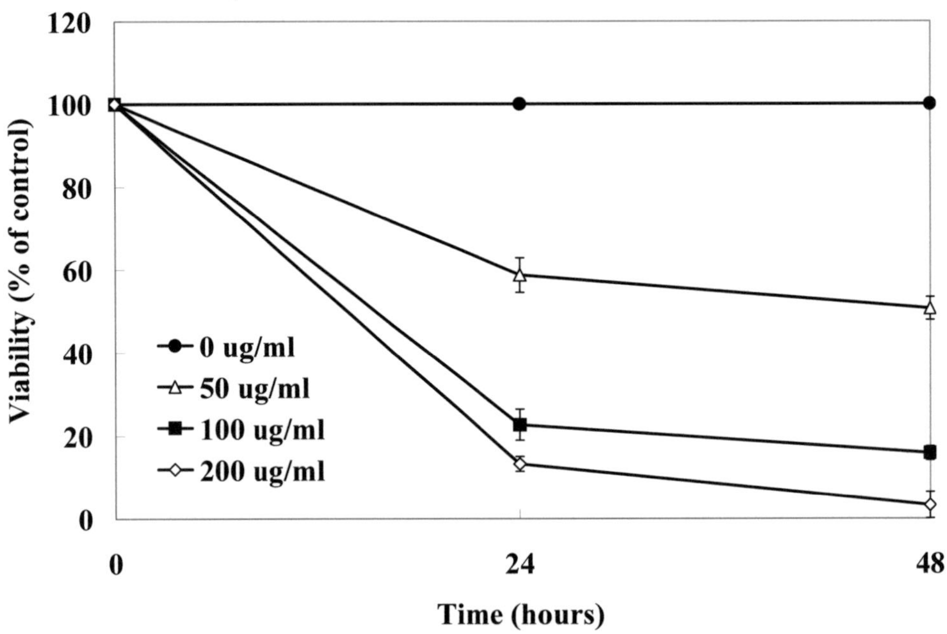

Fig. 1. Effects of cell viability in ETW treated HL-60 cells. Cells were treated with various concentrations of ETW for indicated duration. Viable cells were measured by PI exclusion and immediately analyzed by flow cytometry. The percentage of cell viability was calculated as a ratio between drug-treated cells and control cells. Each value represents mean±S.D. from three independent experiments

3.2 Effects of ETW on cell cycle progression in HL-60 cells

To investigate the mechanisms by which ETW induced cytotoxicity effect in HL-60 cells, we cultured cells for various time periods with 100 µg/ml ETW and analyzed DNA content by flow cytometry. Cell cycle analysis showed that ETW induced a prominent G0/G1 population arrest in HL-60 cells (Fig. 2.). In addition, 100 µg/ml of ETW increased the sub-G0/G1 nuclei population in HL-60 cells in a time-dependent manner (Fig. 2.).

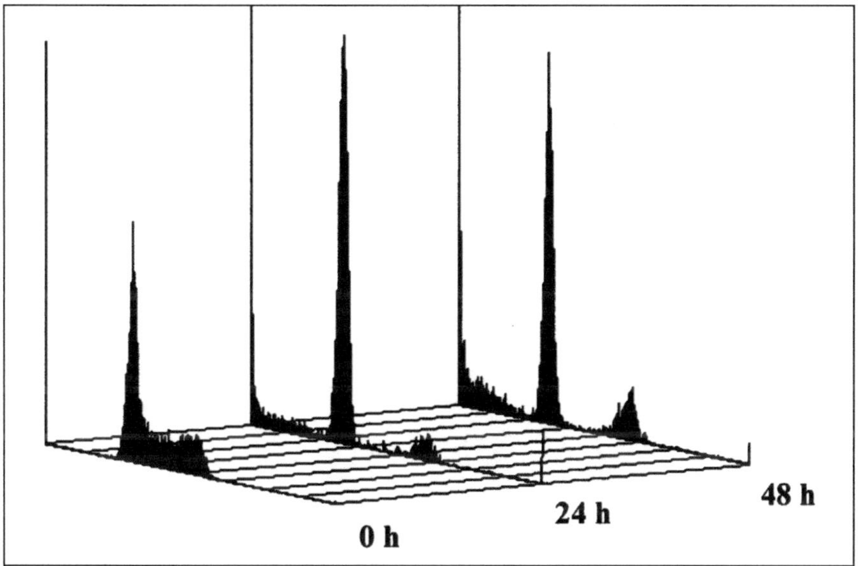

Time	Sub-G1	G0/G1	S	G2/M
0 h	1.19 ± 0.05	52.80 ± 2.64	30.08 ± 1.97	17.12 ± 0.14
24 h	4.58 ± 3.25	77.74 ± 2.59	12.21 ± 2.96	10.05 ± 1.82
48 h	16.68 ± 4.66	81.96 ± 1.35	6.04 ± 1.68	12.00 ± 2.66

Fig. 2. Cell cycle progression on HL-60 cells after treated with ETW. Cells were treated with ETW for the indicated incubation times, then stained for DNA with PI, and analyzed for cell cycle progression or apoptosis by flow cytometry. Cell cycle analysis showed that ETW induced a prominent G0/G1 population arrest and apoptosis in HL-60 cells. Each value represents mean±S.D. from three independent experiments

3.3 Effects of ETW on cyclin D1, cyclin E, Bcl-2 and c-Myc proteins expression in HL-60 cells

To better understand how ETW induces G0/G1 arrest, we investigated the protein expressions of cyclin D1 and cyclin E. After treatment with 100 μg/ml of ETW, there was a marked increase in protein levels of cyclin D1 and a marked decrease in cyclin E (Fig. 3A and 3B.) We also examined the expression levels of Bcl-2 and c-Myc protein. As shown in Fig. 3C and 3D, Bcl-2 and c-Myc protein levels decreased in HL-60 cells relative to controls. Our results suggest that ETW induces G0/G1 arrest and apoptosis in HL-60 cells by regulating cyclin D1, cyclin E, Bcl-2 and c-Myc protein expression.

3.4 ETW induced apoptosis is mediated by the activations of caspase-9, caspase-8 and caspase-3

Activation of caspase plays a key role in the induction of apoptosis. We used a fluorogenic enzymatic assay to detect activated caspase-9, caspase-8 and caspase-3 in ETW-treated HL-60 cells. Both caspase-9 and caspase-3 activities increased 24 h after ETW treatment and caspase-8 activities increased 48 h after ETW treatment (Fig. 4). Our results suggest that ETW-induced apoptosis is mediated through the activation of caspase-9, caspase-3 and then caspase-8.

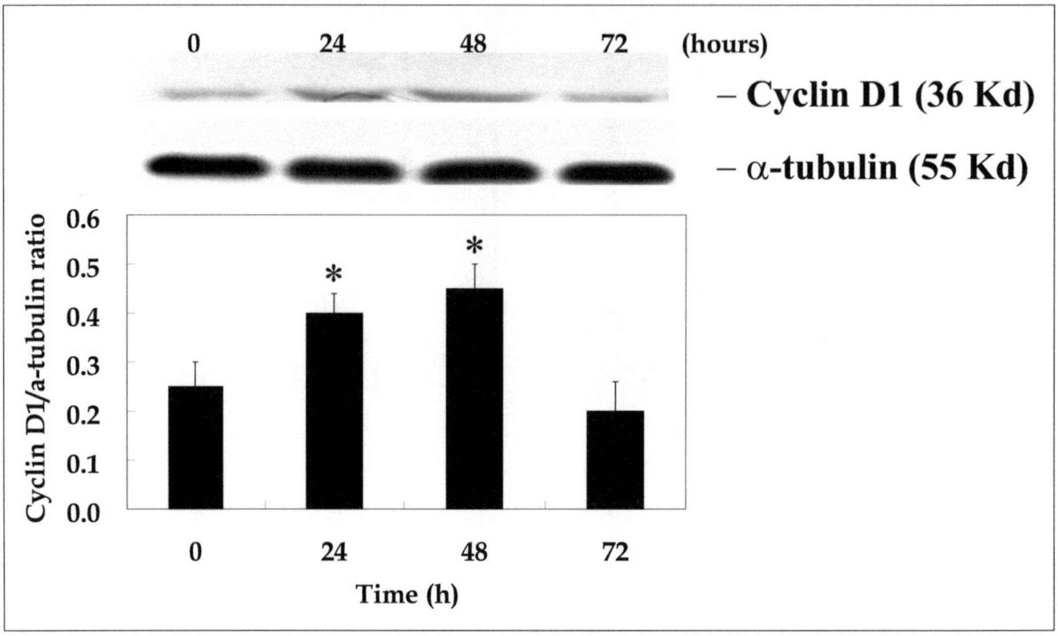
0
24
48
72
(hours)
– Cyclin D1 (36 Kd)
– α-tubulin (55 Kd)
Cyclin D1/a-tubulin ratio
0.6
0.5
0.4
0.3
0.2
0.1
0.0
*
*
0
24
48
72
Time (h)

(a)

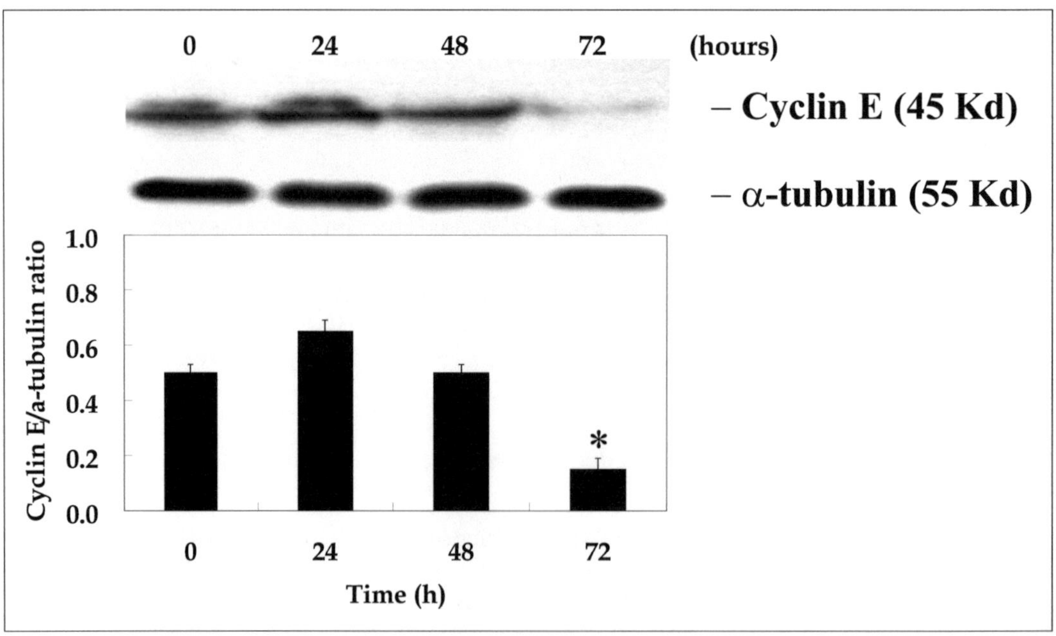
0
24
48
72
(hours)
– Cyclin E (45 Kd)
– α-tubulin (55 Kd)
Cyclin E/a-tubulin ratio
1.0
0.8
0.6
0.4
0.2
0.0
*
0
24
48
72
Time (h)

(b)

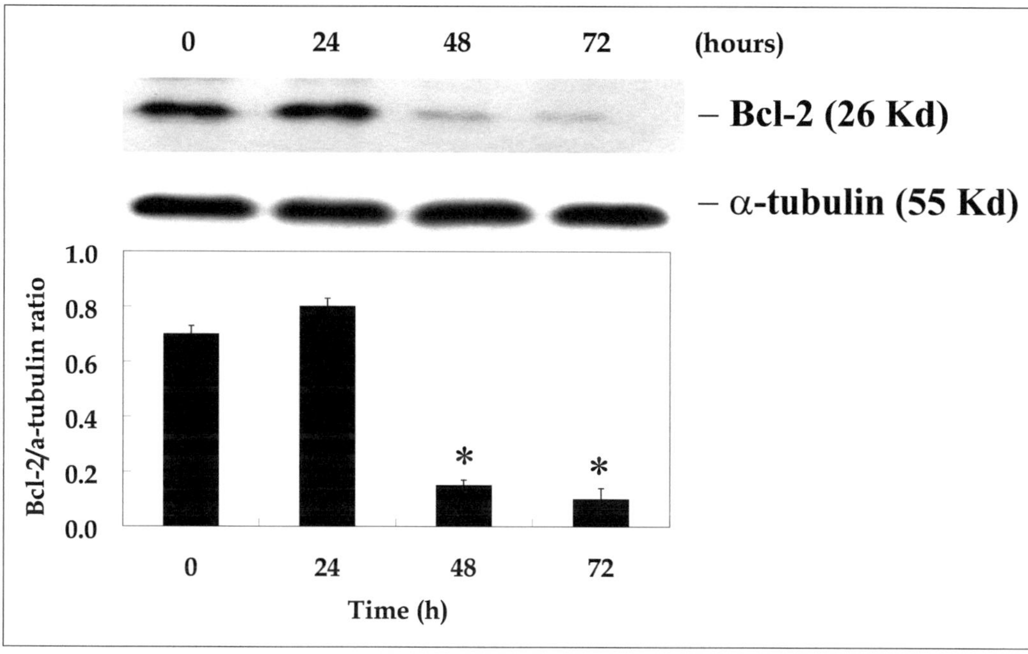

(c)

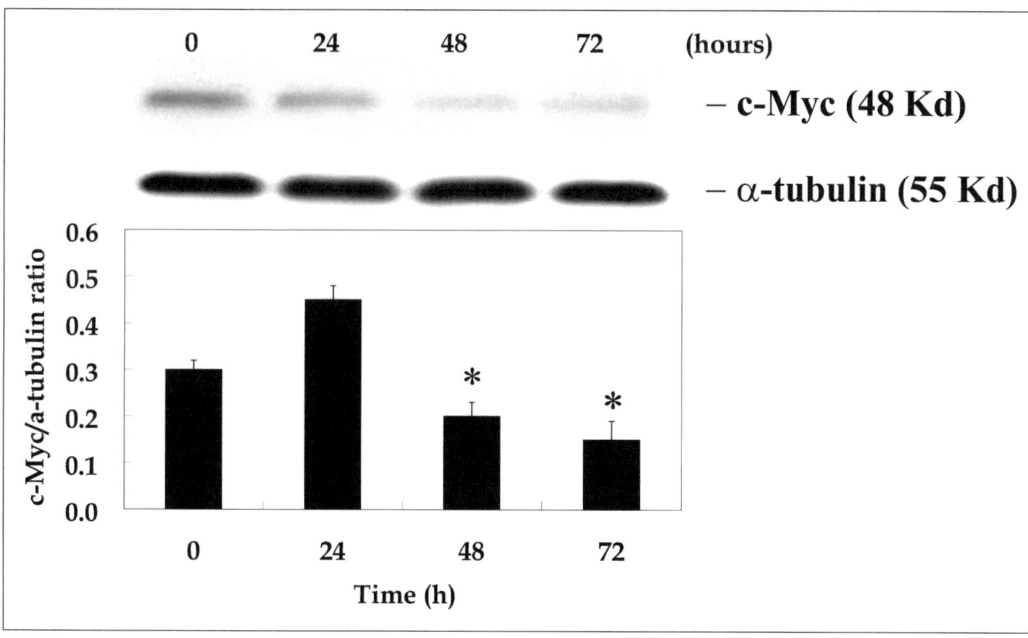

(d)

Fig. 3. Representative Western blotting showing changes on the levels of (A) cyclin D1, (B) cyclin E, (C) Bcl-2 and (D) c-Myc in HL-60 cells after exposure to ETW (100 μg/ml). Cells were treated with ETW for the indicated incubation times then total protein were prepared and determined as described in Materials and Methods

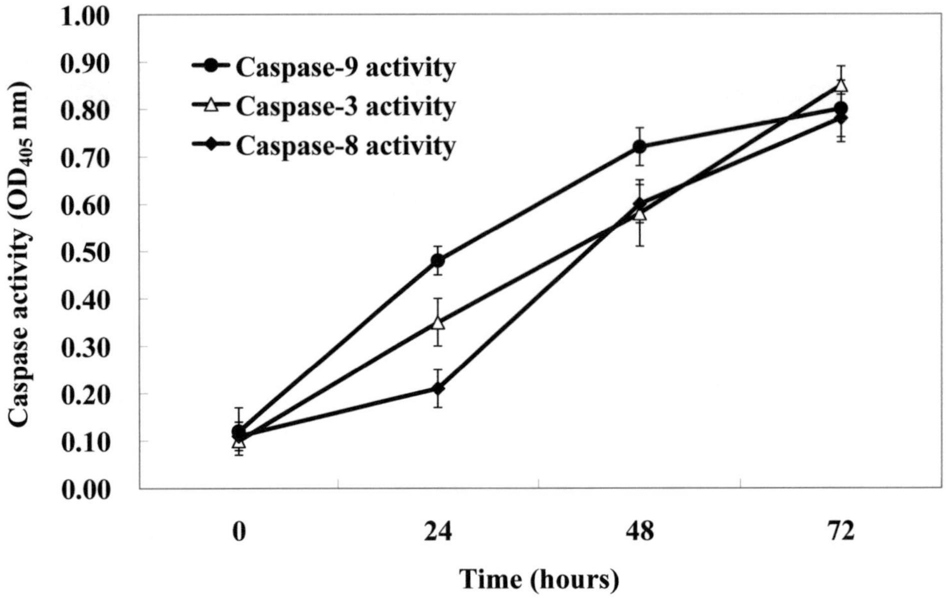

Fig. 4. Effects of ETW induced apoptosis on HL-60 cells by caspases-9, -8 and -3 activities. For caspase activity analysis, aliquots of total cell extracts were incubated with caspases-3, -9 and -8 specific substrates, respectively (Ac-DEVD-pNA, Ac-LEHD-pNA and Ac-IETD-pNA). The release of pNA was measured at 405 nm by a spectrophotometer

4. Discussion

Tripterygium wilfordii Hook. f. (TWHF) is used to treat inflammatory and immune-related diseases. Triptolide, a diterpenoid triepoxide extracted from the TWHF, exerts anti-tumorigenic actions against leukemia cells. In Differentiation -inducing activity study, some triterpene aglycones and Betulinic acid (pentacyclic triterpene) showed differentiation-inducing activity and against human acute promyelocytic leukemia HL-60 cells (Poon, 2004; Umehara et al., 1992). The preclinical laboratory work of identification and testing of potential anti-leukemia agents is designed for three categories: inhibition of cell proliferation, promotion of cell cycle arrest and induction of apoptosis. In the present study, we demonstrated that ETW induces cell cycle arrest and apoptosis in HL-60 cells. Hence, we suggest that ETW is a potent Chinese herb in HL-60 leukemia cells. However, it remains unclear whether ETW effectively induces the elimination of premalignant cells apoptosis *in vivo*.

The effects of ETW on HL-60 cells were associated with a specific disruption of cell cycle events and an induction of G0/G1 arrest. Our results show that ETW led to a loss of cell viability in a dose- and time-dependent manner (Fig. 1). Our study demonstrated that G1 cyclins (cyclin D1 and E) were regulated of HL-60 cells induced by ETW. A recent investigation of leukemia cell differentiation agent-induced differentiation of HL-60 leukemia cells has suggested that TPA to differentiate along the monocyte/macrophage lineage up-regulated of cyclin D1, and all-trans retinoic acid (ATRA) to differentiate along the Granulocyte lineage down-regulated cyclin E expression (Wang et al., 1996; Barrera et al., 2004; Pizzimenti et al., 1999). Thus, it could be suggested that the regulation of cyclin D1 and E as well as CDK2 might anticipate in part the early events in differentiation in ETW-treated HL-60 cells. Our studies found that ETW reduced the level of Bcl-2 and c-Myc in a time-dependent manner. Regulation of the relative levels of Bcl-2 and c-Myc may play an important role in modulating the susceptibility of cells to differentiation (Li et al., 2004; Wu et al., 2002). Previous studies have demonstrated that HL-60 cells exhibited an over-expression of Bcl-2 and c-Myc proto-oncogene and that alteration of cellular oncogenes occur during the differentiation of HL-60 cells (Kumakura et al., 1996). Within myeloid lineage, Bcl-2 is over-expressed in early myeloid precursors but under-expressed or absent in matured myeloid cells and neutrophils (Gazitt et al., 2001; Blagosklonny et al., 1996).

Apoptosis is an evolutionarily conserved process that regulates development and homeostasis, and defects in the mechanisms that regulate cell death are implicated in both tumor genesis and multidrug resistance. Two distinct pathways for apoptosis have been defined, namely the death-receptor pathway and mitochondria pathway (Bohm et al., 2006; Christophe et al., 2006; Lucken et al., 2005; Lockshin et al., 2005). The signal transmitted to the mitochondria pathway causes the release of cytochrome *c* into cytosol. We analyzed apoptosis induction in ETW-treated HL-60 cells by measuring the accumulation of sub-G1 nuclei overtime. We observed the induction of caspase-9 and caspase-8 at 24 h of treatment, and caspase-3 activities at 48 h of treatment before the onset of DNA fragmentation at 72 h treatment by at ETW (Fig. 4). Furthermore, we detected loss of mitochondria membrane potential ($\Delta\Psi m$) in ETW-treated HL-60 cells and release of mitochondrial cytochrome c to cytosol after 18 h of treatment (data not shown). Recent investigation of triptolide-induced apoptosis of U937 cells has suggested that induced caspase-3 activation and down-regulation of the caspase inhibitory protein, XIAP, are involved in this apoptotic process (Choi et al., 2003). Recent reports suggest that DNA damage results in onset of mitochondrial permeability transition, which plays a major role in the apoptotic processes (Choi et al., 2003). A common step in apoptosis involves the loss of mitochondrial membrane potential resulting in increased generation of reactive oxygen species (ROS) from the mitochondrial respiratory chain. Our results suggest that ETW-induced apoptosis is mediated through the loss of mitochondria membrane potential and activation of caspase cascades by activated caspase-9, -8 and caspase-3 in a cytochrome c-dependent manner.

In summary, our results show that ETW induced G0/G1 arrest of HL-60 leukemia cells by regulating the protein expression of cyclin D1, cyclin E, Bcl-2 and c-Myc, and that it induced apoptosis in HL-60 cells by activating caspase-9, caspase-8 and caspase-3. ETW might, therefore, be an alternative cancer therapy in treatment of leukemia patients.

5. References

Abe J., Morikawa M., Miyamoto K., Kaiho S., Fukushima M., Miyaura C., Abe E., Suda T., Nishii Y., 1987. Synthetic analogues of vitamin D3 with an oxygen atom in the side chain skeleton. A trial of the development of vitamin D compounds which exhibit potent differentiation-inducing activity without inducing hypercalcemia. FEBS Letters 226, 58-62.

Altucci L., Rossin A., Hirsch O., Nebbioso A., Vitoux D., Wilhelm E., Guidez F., De Simone M., Schiavone EM., Grimwade D., Zelent A., de The H., Gronemeyer H., 2005. Rexinoid-triggered differentiation and tumor-selective apoptosis of acute myeloid leukemia by protein kinase A-mediated desubordination of retinoid X receptor. Cancer Research 65, 8754-8765.

Altucci L., Wilhelm E., Gronemeyer H., 2004. Leukemia: beneficial actions of retinoids and rexinoids. International Journal of Biochemistry & Cell Biology 36, 178-182.

An WW., Wang MW., Tashiro S., Onodera S., Ikejima T., 2004. Norcantharidin induces human melanoma A375-S2 cell apoptosis through mitochondrial and caspase pathways. Journal of Korean Medical Science 19, 560-566.

Aouacheria A., Neel B., Bouaziz Z., Dominique R., Walchshofer N., Paris J., Fillion H., Gillet G., 2002. Carbazolequinone induction of caspase-dependent cell death in Src-overexpressing cells. Biochemical Pharmacology 64, 1605-1616.

Barrera G., Pizzimenti S., Dianzani MU., 2004. 4-hydroxynonenal and regulation of cell cycle: effects on the pRb/E2F pathway. Free Radical Biology & Medicine 37, 597-606.

Blagosklonny MV., Alvarez M., Fojo A., Neckers LM., 1996. bcl-2 protein downregulation is not required for differentiation of multidrug resistant HL60 leukemia cells. Leukemia Research 20, 101-7.

Bohm I., Traber F., Block W., Schild H., 2006. Molecular imaging of apoptosis and necrosis – basic principles of cell biology and use in oncology. Rofo: Fortschritte auf dem Gebiete der Rontgenstrahlen und der Nuklearmedizin 178, 263-271.

Brown G., Drayson MT., Durham J., Toellner KM., Hughes PJ., Choudhry MA., Taylor DR., Bird R., Michell RH., 2002. HL60 cells halted in G1 or S phase differentiate normally. Experimental Cell Research 281, 28-38.

Chan EW., Cheng SC., Sin FW., Xie Y., 2001. Triptolide induced cytotoxic effects on human promyelocytic leukemia, T cell lymphoma and human hepatocellular carcinoma cell lines. Toxicology Letters. 122, 81-7.

Chang DM., Kuo SY., Lai JH., Chang ML., 1999. Effects of anti-rheumatic herbal medicines on cellular adhesion molecules. Annals of the Rheumatic Diseases 58, 366-371.

Choi YJ., Kim TG., Kim YH., Lee SH., Kwon YK., Suh SI,. Park JW., Kwon TK., 2003. Immunosuppressant PG490 (triptolide) induces apoptosis through the activation of caspase-3 and down-regulation of XIAP in U937 cells. Biochemical Pharmacology 66, 273-80.

Christophe M., Nicolas S., 2006. Mitochondria: a target for neuroprotective interventions in cerebral ischemia-reperfusion. Current Pharmaceutical Design 12, 739-57.

Faderl SJ., Keating MJ., 2005. Treatment of chronic lymphocytic leukemia. Current Hematology Reports 4, 31-38.

Fleischer A., Ghadiri A., Dessauge F., Duhamel M., Rebollo MP., Alvarez-Franco F., Rebollo A., 2006. Modulating apoptosis as a target for effective therapy. Molecular Immunology 43, 1065-1079.

Frankfurt O., Tallman MS., 2006. Strategies for the treatment of acute promyelocytic leukemia. Journal of the National Comprehensive Cancer Network 4, 37-50.

Gazitt Y., Reddy SV., Alcantara O., Yang J., Boldt DH., 2001. A new molecular role for iron in regulation of cell cycling and differentiation of HL-60 human leukemia cells: iron is required for transcription of p21(WAF1/CIP1) in cells induced by phorbol myristate acetate. Journal of Cellular Physiology 187, 124-135.

Hickey EJ., Raje RR., Reid VE., Gross SM., Ray SD., 2001. Diclofenac induced in vivo nephrotoxicity may involve oxidative stress-mediated massive genomic DNA fragmentation and apoptotic cell death. Free Radical Biology & Medicine 31, 139-152.

Ho LJ., Lai JH., 2004. Chinese herbs as immunomodulators and potential disease-modifying antirheumatic drugs in autoimmune disorders. Current Drug Metabolism 5, 181-192,

Horie N., Mori T., Asada H., Ishikawa A., Johnston PG., Takeishi K., 2004. Implication of CDK inhibitors p21 and p27 in the differentiation of HL-60 cells. Biological & Pharmaceutical Bulletin 27, 992-997.

Kamikubo Y., Takaori-Kondo A., Uchiyama T., Hori T., 2003. Inhibition of cell growth by conditional expression of kpm, a human homologue of Drosophila warts/lats tumor suppressor. Journal of Biological Chemistry 278, 17609-17614.

Kumakura S., Ishikura H., Tsumura H., Iwata Y., Endo J., Kobayashi S., 1996. c-Myc and Bcl-2 protein expression during the induction of apoptosis and differentiation in TNF alpha-treated HL-60 cells. Leukemia & Lymphoma 23, 383-394.

Leuenroth SJ., Crews CM., 2005. Studies on calcium dependence reveal multiple modes of action for triptolide. Chemistry & Biology 12, 1259-1268.

Li CY., Zhan YQ., Xu CW., Xu WX., Wang SY., Lv J., Zhou Y., Yue PB., Chen B., Yang XM., 2004. EDAG regulates the proliferation and differentiation of hematopoietic cells and resists cell apoptosis through the activation of nuclear factor-kappa B. Cell Death & Differentiation 11, 1299-1308.

Lichtman MA., Segel GB., 2005. Uncommon phenotypes of acute myelogenous leukemia: basophilic, mast cell, eosinophilic, and myeloid dendritic cell subtypes: a review. Blood Cells Molecules & Diseases 35, 370-383.

Lin CC., Kao ST., Chen GW., Ho HC., Chung JG., 2006. Apoptosis of human leukemia HL-60 cells and murine leukemia WEHI-3 cells induced by berberine through the activation of caspase-3. Anticancer Research 26, 227-242.

Lockshin RA., 2005. Programmed cell death: history and future of a concept. Journal de la Societe de Biologie 199, 169-173.

Lou YJ., Jin J., 2004. Triptolide down-regulates bcr-abl expression and induces apoptosis in chronic myelogenous leukemia cells. Leukemia & Lymphoma 45, 373-376.

Lucken Ardjomande S., Montessuit S., Martinou JC., 2005. Changes in the outer mitochondrial membranes during apoptosis. Journal de la Societe de Biologie 199, 207-210.

Murphy, 2006. Rachel Chinese antirheumatic remedy for the treatment of SLE. Nature Clinical Practice Rheumatology 2, 180-181.

O'Hare T., Corbin AS., Druker BJ., 2006. Targeted CML therapy: controlling drug resistance, seeking cure. Current Opinion in Genetics & Development 16, 92-99.

Peng X., Zhao Y., Liang X., Wu L., Cui S., Guo A., Wang W., 2006. Assessing the quality of RCTs on the effect of beta-elemene, one ingredient of a Chinese herb, against malignant tumors. Contemporary Clinical Trials 27, 70-82.

Pizzimenti S., Barrera G., Dianzani MU., Brusselbach S., 1999. Inhibition of D1, D2, and A-cyclin expression in HL-60 cells by the lipid peroxydation product 4-hydroxynonenal. Free Radical Biology & Medicine 26, 1578-1586.

Poon KH., Zhang J., Wang C., Tse AK., Wan CK., Fong WF., 2004. Betulinic acid enhances 1,25-dihydroxyvitamin D3-induced differentiation in human HL-60 promyelocytic leukemia cells. Anti-Cancer Drugs 15, 619-624.

Qian SZ., 1987. *Tripterygium wilfordii*, a Chinese herb effective in male fertility regulation. Contraception 36, 335-345.

Qiu Daoming, Kao PN., 2003. Immunosuppressive and Anti-Inflammatory Mechanisms of Triptolide, the Principal Active Diterpenoid from the Chinese Medicinal Herb *Tripterygium wilfordii* Hook. f. Drugs in R & D 4, 1-18.

Samudio I., Konopleva M., Safe S., McQueen T., Andreeff M., 2005. Guggulsterones induce apoptosis and differentiation in acute myeloid leukemia: identification of isomer-specific antileukemic activities of the pregnadienedione structure. Molecular Cancer Therapeutics 4, 1982-1992.

Takahashi N., 2002. Induction of cell differentiation and development of new anticancer drugs. Journal of the Pharmaceutical Society of Japan. 122, 547-563.

Ter BE., Kaspers GJ., 2005. Treatment of childhood acute myeloid leukemia. Expert Review of Anticancer Therapy 5, 917-929.

Tsiftsoglou AS., Pappas IS., Vizirianakis IS., 2003. Mechanisms involved in the induced differentiation of leukemia cells. Pharmacology & Therapeutics 100, 257-290.

Umehara K., Takagi R., Kuroyanagi M., Ueno A., Taki T., Chen YJ., 1992. Studies on differentiation-inducing activities of triterpenes. Chemical & Pharmaceutical Bulletin. 40, 401-405.

Veselska R., Zitterbart K., Auer J., Neradil J., 2004. Differentiation of HL-60 myeloid leukemia cells induced by all-trans retinoic acid is enhanced in combination with caffeic acid. International Journal of Molecular Medicine 14, 305-310.

Wang J., Xu R., Jin RL., Chen ZQ., Fidler JM., 2000. Immuno-supperssive activity of the Chinese medicinal plant *Tripterygium wilfordii* Hook.: I. prolongation of rat cardiac and renal allograft survival by the PG27 extract and Immunosuppressive Synergy in Combination Therapy with Cyclosporine. Transplantation 70, 447-455.

Wang QM., Jones JB., Studzinski GP., 1996. Cyclin-dependent kinase inhibitor p27 as a mediator of the G1-S phase block induced by 1,25-dihydroxyvitamin D3 in HL60 cells. Cancer Research 56, 264-267.

Wei YS., Adachi I., 1991. Inhibitory effect of triptolide on colony formation of breast and stomach cancer cell lines. Zhongguo Yao Li Xue Bao/Acta Pharmacologica Sinica 12, 406-410.

Wu LD., Chen YZ., Li NN., Wu Y., 2002. Study on telomerase activity and expression of hTERT, c-myc and bcl-2 during terminal differentiation of HL-60 cells induced by retinoic acid. Zhongguo Shi Yan Xue Ye Xue Za Zhi 10, 395-399.

Wu Y., Wang Y., Zhong C., Li Y., Li X., Sun B., 2003. The suppressive effect of triptolide on experimental autoimmune uveoretinitis by down-regulating Th1-type response. International Immunopharmacology 3, 1457-1465.

Yazdanparast R., Moosavi MA., Mahdavi M., Sanati MH., 2005. 3-Hydrogenkwadaphnin from Dendrostellera lessertii induces differentiation and apoptosis in HL-60 cells. Planta Medica 71, 1112-1117.

Yen A., Varvayanis S., Smith JL., Lamkin TJ., 2006. Retinoic acid induces expression of SLP-76: expression with c-FMS enhances ERK activation and retinoic acid-induced differentiation G0/G1 arrest of HL-60 cells. European Journal of Cell Biology 85, 117-132.

Zhao YF., Zhai WL., Zhang SJ., Chen XP., 2005. Protection effect of triptolide to liver injury in rats with severe acute pancreatitis. Hepatobiliary & Pancreatic Diseases International 4, 604-608.

25

Applications of Quantum Dots in Flow Cytometry

Dimitrios Kirmizis[1], Fani Chatzopoulou[2],
Eleni Gavriilaki[2] and Dimitrios Chatzidimitriou[2]
[1]*Medical School, Aristotle University, Thessaloniki,*
[2]*Laboratory of Microbiology, Aristotle University, Thessaloniki,*
Greece

1. Introduction

Among several applications of flow cytometry is the identification of cell populations, which is a demanding and often daunting task, given the multitude and the often intercalating pattern of protein expression between different cell types. This complexity nescessitated the use of multicolor flow cytometry, a technique that has been given new perspectives with the emergence of Quandum Dot (QD) technology, which permitted overcoming obstacles, such as limited fluorochrome availability or limited sensitivity of combining multiple organic fluorochromes. The first systematic studies of size-dependent optical properties of semiconductor crystals in colloidal solutions were performed at early 1980s (Henglein, 1982; Brus, 1983). Later, Spanhel et al (1987) performed one of the first core–shell syntheses, a major advance in increasing the quantum yield. Major improvements leading to highly fluorescent QDs were made in the mid-1990s (Hines MA & Guyot-Sionnest P, 1996; Dabbousi RO et al, 1997; Peng et al, 1997). Subsequently, CdSe crystals with silane-modified hydrophilic surfaces were introduced for biological applications (Bruchez et al, 1998; Chan, WCW & Nie S, 1998). Even more recent developments include the encapsulation of CdSe/ZnS core–hell nanocrystals into carboxylated polymer, followed by chemical modification of the surface with long-chain polyethylene glycol (PEG) (Quantum Dot Corporation, Hayward, CA).

2. Properties of Quantum Dots

QDs are inorganic fluorochromes manufactured with the use of semiconductor materials (cadmium selenide for QDs emitting light in the 525- to 655-nm range or cadmium telluride for QDs emitting higher wavelength light) that assemble into nanometer-scale crystals (Chan et al, 2002; Bruchez, 2005). The tiny size of the QD nanocrystals gives these materials unique physical properties which seem tailor-made for multicolour flow cytometry compared to typical semiconductors or other fluorochromes. The most important of them is their broad excitation spectra (Bruchez M, 2005). Actually, QDs can be excited over the entire visual wavelength range as well as far into the ultraviolet. Because of their exceptionally large Stokes shifts (up to 400 nm), QDs can potentially be used for the multicolor detection even by a single laser flow cytometer, whereas organic dyes require multiple lasers for excitation in order to be used in multiplexed analysis (Bruchez M, 2005; Perfetto et al, 2004; Chattopadhyay et al, 2006). The light that the flow cytometer detects is the light which the electrons in QDs, after having been excited (excitons) by light absorption, emit as they return back from their conduction to their valence bands. What differentiates QDs from the typical fluorochromes is the so called "quantum confinement" phenomenon (Andersen et al, 2002), i.e. the phenomenon whereby, in contrast with the typical semiconductor materials where the distances between the bands are intimisimal (continuous), the excitons in QDs jump a discrete distance (known as the band gap) between bands, as a result of the very small size of the QD nanocrystal core. The narrow emission spectra of QDs usually overcomes the need for compensation, a standard process used in organic fluorochromes, which subtracts spillover fluorescence by estimating its magnitude as a fraction of the measured fluorescence in the primary detector (Roederer M, 2001) (*see* Fig. 1). In practice, it is reported that most QDs can be used simultaneously with only minimal (<10%) compensation between channels (Roederer et al, 2004). Moreover, when QD reagents are used with common fluorochromes excited by 488, 532, or 633 lasers (e.g., fluoroscein isothiacyanate, phycoerythrin [PE], or allophycocyanin), almost no spillover signal from other fluorochromes in the QD channels is found. Thus, in instruments with two or more lasers, QDs can be multiplexed with other fluorochromes to successfully measure even more colors (Chattopadhyay et al, 2007; 2010). In addition, the signals produced can be extremely bright, such as when an ultraviolet (350 nm) or violet (408 nm) laser is used to excite longer wavelength QDs (like QD605 andQD655), because of their high absorbance and low background levels (Hotz CZ, 2005; Wu et al, 2003). Finally, the emission properties of QDs also offer advantages over organic fluorochromes, albeit to a lesser extent.

Whereas organic fluorochromes of different colors come from a wide variety of source materials, each with distinct (and complex) physical, chemical, and biological properties which may not be compatible with each other or with staining conditions, this becomes less of a concern in QDs since QDs of different colors can be synthesized from the same starting materials (Chan et al, 2002), and thus multiplexed analysis is easier. However, the large surface-to-volume ratio in a nanosized crystal (about 50% of all atoms are on the surface) affects the emission of photons. Photochemical oxidation and surface defects in a crystal with no shell may lead to a broad emission and lower quantum yields. Indeed, early QD nanocrystals did not give stable or bright signals, exhibited poor solubility, and could not be attached to biologic probes (Riegler J & Nann T, 2004). These challenges were overcome by coating the QD nanocrystal with various materials such as inorganic zinc-sulfide, which is in turn coated with organic polymers (Bruchez et al, 1998). These organic polymers increase solubility and provide a platform of functional groups (such as amines, $NH3$) for conjugation to antibodies, streptavidin, and nucleic acids. Because they have similar coatings, QDs of various colors share uniform biophysical properties and a common conjugation procedure. The final QD product is about the size of PE, and can be linked to antibodies using a very similar conjugation chemistry. The shell helps to confine the excitation to the CdSe core and prevent the non-radiative relaxation.

The fluorescent properties of QDs are derived from their nanocrystal cores and not from the overall size of QD, which is actually similar in all QDs as a result of the fact that the cores are coated with various materials as mentioned above. Each QD has its characteristic emission peak, as long as the excitonic energy levels and quantum yields of fluorescence depend on exciton-photon interaction in the crystal and the size of the crystalline core. The primary determinant of the emission spectrum of each particle is its size so that smaller nanocrystals have different quantum confinement properties than bigger ones, as a result of the fact that the distance jumped by the exciton differs (the band gap is larger), and light is emitted at a different wavelength upon return to resting state. Increasing crystal size (from 2-3 to 10-12 nm) results in shift of the emission maximum from 500 to 800 nm. However, although they fluoresce at different wavelengths, they are excited at the same wavelength, allowing detection of multiple QD colors from just one laser. Thus, QDs with the smallest nanocrystal cores (3 nm) emit light in the blue region of the spectrum, whereas QDs with the largest cores (~6 nm) emit far red light (Bruchez et al, 1998). The most commonly used QDs in multicolor flow cytometry emit light at 525 (referred to as QD525), 545, 565, 585, 605, 655, 705, and 800 nm (Perfetto et al, 2004); their nanocrystal cores range in size from 2 to 6 nm (Biju et al, 2008). Other QDs emitting light at intermediate wavelengths (like 625 nm) are also commercially available. Thus, by 'tuning' the size of the nanocrystal core with various procedures (Peng et al, 1998; Smet et al, 1999), the description of which is beyond the scope of this chapter, QDs of different colors can be produced from the same starting material (*see* Fig. 1).

The core-shell nanocrystals have large extinction coefficients and high quantum yields. These parameters describe the capacity of the system to capture and subsequently rerelease light. Although quantum yields of QD conjugates in aqueous buffers (20–50%) are comparable with those of conventional fluorophores, the excitation efficiency of QD conjugates is much higher, making them about two orders of magnitude more efficient at absorbing excitation light than organic dyes and fluorescent proteins. QDs have a fluorescence lifetime of 20–30 ns—about 10 times longer than the background autofluorescence of proteins. Thus, fluorescence from single CdSe crystals has been observed much longer than from other fluorophores, resulting in high turnover rates and a large number of emitted photons (Doose, 2003).

The procedure for conjugation of antibodies to QDs is similar to conjugation of antibodies to PE, with slight variations in the reagents used and ratio of antibodies to fluorescent molecules. Successful conjugation relies on the coupling of malemide groups on the QDs to thiol groups on the antibody. These groups are generated during the initial steps of the procedure, as amine groups on the QDs are activated with a heterobifunctional crosslinker (sulfosuccinimidyl 4-[*N*-maleimidomethyl]cyclohexane-1-carboxylate, sulfo-SMCC) to generate the malemide moieties, and disulfide bonds in the antibody are reduced to thiol groups using dithiothreitol (DTT). Before conjugation, the DTT-reduced antibody is then mixed with two dye-labeled markers, Cyanin-3 (Cy3) and dextran blue, which track the monomeric fraction of antibodies as it passes through purification columns. Activated QDs and reduced antibody are subsequently purified over columns and mixed for conjugation.

A number of laser choices are available to excite QDs. Low wavelength ultraviolet (UV) and violet lasers are typically employed, since they induce maximal fluorescence emission. In theory, QD fluorescence arising from UV excitation is greater than that resulting from violet excitation; however, in practice, UV lasers induce much higher autofluorescence of cells, thereby negating the benefit of higher signal intensity. Still, users who rely on UV-excited probes (like DAPI and Hoechst) should note that QDs are compatible with their systems (Telford WG, 2004). Wheremultiplexed analysis of QDs is important, UV or violet excitation systems can be coupled to as many as eight photomultiplier tubes, allowing simultaneous measurement of QD545, QD565, QD585, QD605, QD655, QD705, QD800, and/or a violet-excitable organic fluorochrome (Chattopadhyay et al, 2010). To detect QD signals, we employ a filter strategy that first selects light sharply with a dichroic mirror, allowing only light above a certain wavelength to pass (long-pass filter). A second filter (known as a band pass filter) is stationed in front of the PMT, in order to collect a broad band of wavelengths for maximal signal. The light reflected by the first long-pass filter is passed to the next detector where it is queried in a similar fashion.

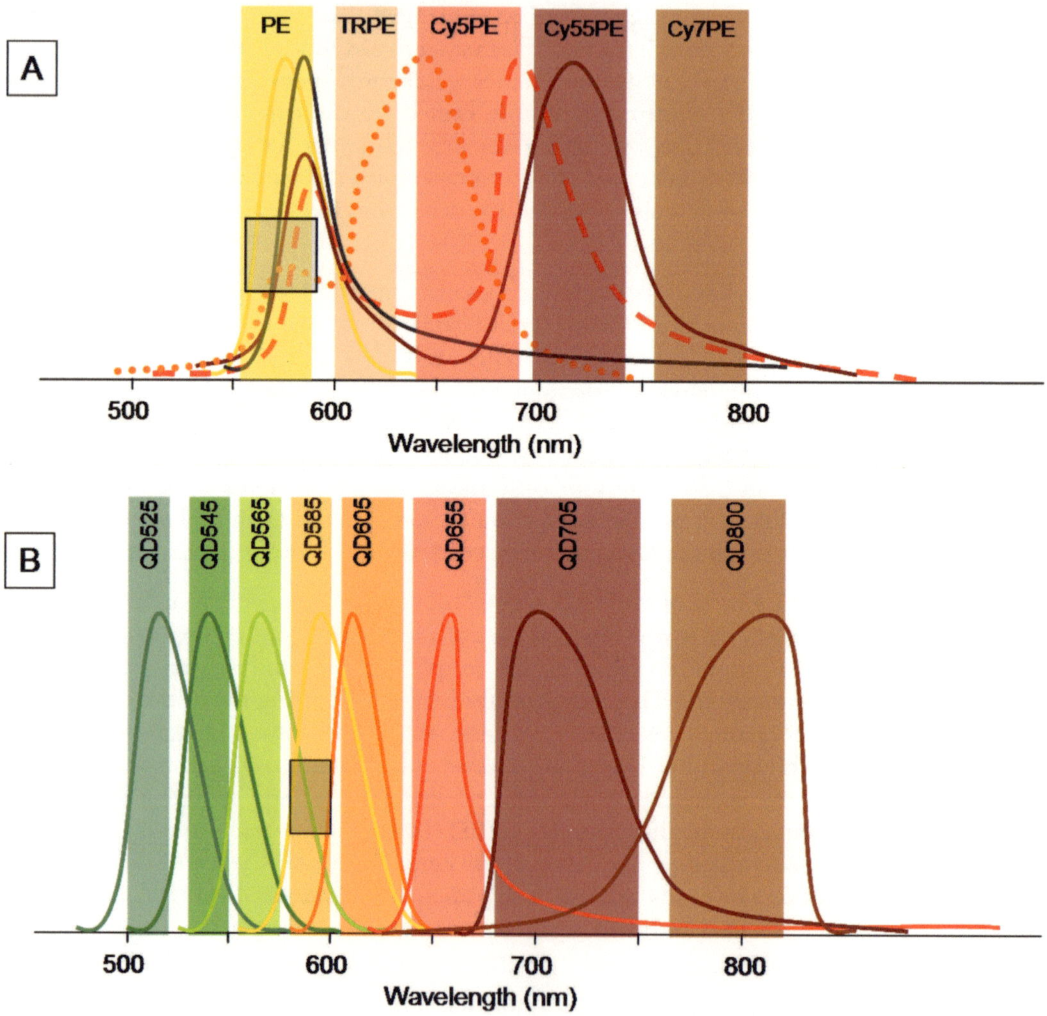

Fig. 1. Emission spectra of fluorochromes. The colored bars represent the wavelength range of filters used for the detection of each fluorochrome. The grey squares note the overlap of neighboring fluorochromes and signify the need for compensation. A significant overlap of phycoerythrin (PE) and PE-based tandems is apparent, which necessitates high compensation values, whereas their long tails of emission can induce significant spreading error (A). In contrast, such an overlap is avoided in QDs, whose emission spectra are narrow and symmetrical, their sensitivity better and the need for compensation less (B)

3. Quantum Dot applications

Multicolor Flow Cytometry: The utility of QDs in multicolor flow cytometry has been documented by several studies. Chattopadhyay et al (2006) in their interesting study analyzed the maturity of various antigenspecific T-cell populations using a 17-color staining panel. This panel consisted of 7 QDs and 10 organic fluorochromes, which were measured simultaneously in the same sample. The QD reagents used were conjugates with conventional antibodies (against CD4, CD45RA, and CD57), as well as peptide MHC Class I (pMHCI) multimers designed to detect those antigen-specific T-cells directed against HIV, EBV, and CMV epitopes. By identifying multiple phenotypically distinct subsets within each antigenspecific T-cell population, the remarkable intricacy of T-cell immunity as well as the power of a multiplexed approach was shown. QDs also allowed the reasearchers to measure many antigen-specific populations simultaneously, an important factor when sample availability is limited.

Markers of interest for use in multicolor flow cytometry are assigned to three categories: primary, secondary, and tertiary (Chattopadhyay et al, 2006, 2010; Perfetto et al, 2004; Mahnke YD & Roederer M, 2007). Primary markers are those that are highly expressed on cells, without intermediate fluorescence (i.e., they exhibit on/off expression). Secondary markers alike are expressed brightly and are well-characterized, but can be expressed at intermediate levels, and therefore resolution of dimly staining populations may be important. Thus, the fluorochromes assigned to secondary markers should be those with the less spreading error. Finally, tertiary markers are particularly dim, poorly characterized, or expressed by only a small proportion of cells. For the latter, bright fluorochromes are necessary. In practice, tertiary markers must be considered first. If these markers are particularly dim, they are assigned to fluorochrome channels that receive very little spreading error. QDs are particularly useful in this regard. However, some QDs are dim (QD 525) (Chattopadhyay et al, 2006), and therefore are not suitable for the measurement of dim cell populations. Among QDs, the brightest choices for tertiary markers are QD655, QD605, and QD585, in order of signal intensity. Secondary markers are ideal candidates for conjugation to QDs, especially for slightly dimmer channels, such as QD545, QD565, or QD800, as long as these are often brightly expressed. Finally, primary markers can be assigned to dim channels or to fluorochrome pairs with significant spectral overlap and spreading error.

Intracellular staining: Although QDs are not always compatible with intracellular staining, there have been recent advances in the ability to stain intracellularly with QDs. One approach, designed to avoid steric issues or intracellular degradation, is to target the QD (with or without conjugated antibody) into a cell using enzymes, such as matrix metalloproteinases (Zhang et al, 2006; Tekle et al, 2008), or nuclear or mitochondrial signal peptides (Hoshino et al, 2004). When coupled to antibodies, QDs bound to delivery molecules might allow organelle directed, specific intracellular staining without fixation/permeabilization.

Tetramer production: In the past, only FITC-, PE-, APC-tetramers were available, which limited panel design because many novel or dimly staining antibodies are only found on these fluorochromes. QDs with SA groups can be used to produce pMHCI multimers (commonly called 'tetramers') (Chattopadhyay et al, 2006), displaying higher valency than PE or APC and, thus, allowing brighter signals and better staining resolution (Chattopadhyay et al, 2008).

Pathogen detection: Efforts to detect whole pathogens have been considerably more successful with the introduction of QDs. When applied to a mixture of pathogenic and harmless *Escherichia coli* strains, QDs conjugated to antibodies against *E. coli* can detect one pathogenic bacterium among 99 harmless ones (Hahn et al, 2008). These detection limits are comparable to current assays that use FITC, but QDs are 10-fold brighter and give more accurate results.

Fluorescence resonance energy transfer (FRET) assays: Another interesting potential application of QDs is for new QD-based FRET assays. In particular, recent studies have reported on efforts to achieve FRET with QDs as the donor or acceptor fluorochrome (Willard DM & VanOrden A, 2003). This might not be so difficult to do, since QDs may be available in a wide variety of colors but share similar biochemistry and, thus, it is easy to find an acceptor dye that emits fluorescence at the desired wavelength. Furthermore, signal from the acceptor and the donor are well discrete and easily recognised, because of their narrow emission spectra. Similarly, donors and acceptors can be chosen such that spectral overlap is minimized; this reduces background emission and increases sensitivity. These advantages are not available in traditional FRET assays using organic fluorochromes.

4. Caveats, safety & toxicity

Although QDs are emerging as useful tools in multicolor flow cytometry, they are not fully characterized and occasionally exhibit peculiar properties. As mentioned above, not all antibodies will successfully conjugate to QDs. In particular, markers for intracellular flow cytometry (e.g., reagents for intracellular cytokine detection) have been problematic to conjugate in our facility, owing in part to the presence of excessive quantities of unconjugated QDs, to limited access to intracellular compartments due to QD size-related steric problems, to uneven dispersion of QDs throughout the intracellular environment, or to high sensitivity of QDs to chemicals used in the fixation and permeabilization process associated with intracellular staining (Riegler J & Nann T, 2004; Jaiswal et al, 2004b; Tekle et al, 2008). Variation within the QDs themselves occasionally might also be considerable, due to difficulties in the control of their production process. Thus, subtle differences in incubation time or injection of precursor solutions can cause differences in size distribution, shape, and surface defects among QDs (Dabbousi et al, 1997). These can potentially impact basic properties like fluorescence. As a rule of thumb, when using QDs in multicolor flow cytometry it might be useful to engage compensation controls using exactly the same reagent as the experimental panel. Another matter of potential concern with QDs is storage method and stability, as long as QDs are prone to form aggregates or precipitate out of solution, albeit the organic coating surrounding QDs has significantly improved solubility (Jaiswal J & Simon S, 2004) and any precipitation does not actually result in loss of activity, nor does it affect staining patterns (since these aggregates stain very brightly in all channels and are easily gated out of analyses). Manufacturers typically recommend storage in glass vials or in specially coated, non-adherent plastic tubes, since in standard microcentrifuge tubes, QDs may bind plastic, precipitate, and lose activity, especially at low volumes.

Two important obstacles to biological applications of commercially available QDs until recently are low quantum yields in aqueous buffers and strong aggregation of conjugates, both determined by the surface chemistry. For the use of QDs as antibody labeled probes, their outer layer must insulate the CdSe/ZnS core structure from the aqueous environment, prevent the nonspecific adsorption of QDs to cells, as well as provide the functional groups necessary for covalent attachment of antibodies. Lately, improvements on both nanocrystal core and shell technologies have enabled production of QD conjugates with exceptional brightness and low nonspecific adsorption (Larson DR et al, 2003). Recently, a new generation of QD nanocrystals was introduced with the application of a novel surface chemistry with the use of polymeric shell modified with long-chain, amino-functionalized PEGs. This new generation of QD nanocrystals has low nonspecific binding to cells and can be directly conjugated to antibodies through the introduced amino groups, using bisfunctional cross-linkers.

Since QDs are a new technology, their safety and toxicity are still a matter of concern. Although preliminary data from literature employing QDs for *in vivo* imaging of mice suggested that QDs are both safe and nontoxic (Voura et al, 2004; Shiohara et al, 2004; Bruchez, 2005; Gao et al, 2007), recent *in vitro* toxicology studies have questioned this assumption (Shiohara et al, 2004; Male et al, 2008). It appears that QDs coated with organic shells are relatively nontoxic for short incubation periods, but their degradation products (in particular Cd and Se), principally as a result of their oxidation and photolysis, may be toxic. Since QD size, charge, and composition of the outer shell are the main factors determinig oxidation and photolysis, toxicity likely differs by QD color and preparation. Regarding their risk on human health, data suggest that this is rather minimal, as long as QDs cannot enter the skin. However, this might not be true upon inhalation or ingestion as well, where there seems to be some potential for toxicity (Oberdorster et al, 2005; Hoet et al, 2004)

5. Conclusion

Although specific applications for QDs are still emerging, the basic technology has matured to the point that it can be relatively easily employed in multicolour flow cytometry. Unfortunately, just as applications for QDs are still nascent, so too is the commercial market for QD reagents. Therefore, to maximize the utility of QDs researchers must turn to in-house conjugations. Once implemented, the powerful potential of QD technology becomes evident. The remarkable spectral properties of QDs allow easy multiplexing, and therefore more information can be acquired from fewer samples. These properties make QDs useful in studying complex biologic systems.

6. References

Andersen KE, Fong C, Pickett W. Quantum confinement in CdSe nanocrystallites. *J Non-Cryst Solids* 2008, 2002:1105–1110.

Bentzen EL, Tomlinson ID, Mason J, Gresch P,Warnement MR, et al. Surface modification to reduce nonspecific binding of quantum dots in live cell assays. *Bioconjug Chem* 2005, 16:1488–1494.

Biju V, Itoh T, Anas A, Sujith A, Ishikawa M. Semiconductor quantum dots and metal nanoparticles: syntheses, optical properties, and biological applications. *Anal Bioanal Chem* 2008, 391:2469–2495.

Brus, L. E. (1983) A simple model for the ionization potential, electron affinity, and aqueous redox potentials of small semiconductor crystallites. *J. Chem. Phys.* 79, 5566–5571.

Bruchez, M., Moronne, M., Gin, P., Weiss, S., and Alivisatos, A. P. (1998) Semiconductor nanocrystals as fluorescent biological labels. *Science* 281, 2013–2016.

Bruchez M. Turning all the lights on: quantum dots in cellular assays. *Curr Opin Chem Biol* 2005, 9:533–537.

Chan, W. C. W. and Nie, S. (1998) Quantum dots bioconjugates for ultrasensitive nonisotopic detection. *Science* 281, 2016–2018.

Chan WC, Maxwell DJ, Gao X, Bailey RE, Han M, et al. Luminescent quantum dots for multiplexed biological detection and imaging. *Curr Opin Biotechnol* 2002, 13:40–46.

Chattopadhyay PK, Price DA,Harper TF, Betts MR, Yu J, et al. Quantum dot semiconductor nanocrystals for immunophenotyping by polychromatic flow cytometry. *Nat Med* 2006, 12:972–977.

Chattopadhyay PK, Perfetto SP, Yu J, et al. Application of Quantum Dots to Multicolor Flow Cytometry. In: Quantum dots : biological applications (editors: Bruchez M, Hotz CZ), 2007, Humana Press Inc., New Jersey

Chattopadhyay PK, Yu J, Roederer M. Application of quantum dots to multicolor flow cytometry. *Methods Mol Biol (Clifton,NJ)* 2007, 374:175–184.

Chattopadhyay PK,Melenhorst JJ, Ladell K, Gostick E, Scheinberg P, et al. Techniques to improve the direct ex vivo detection of low frequency antigen-specific CD8+ T cells with peptide-major histocompatibility complex class I tetramers. *Cytometry A* 2008, 73:1001–1009.

Chattopadhyay PK, Perfetto SP, Yu J, et al. The use of quantum dot nanocrystals in multicolor flow cytometry. *WIREs Nanomed Nanobiotechnol* 2010, 2: 334–348.

Clapp AR, Medintz IL, Mauro JM, Fisher BR, Bawendi MG, et al. Fluorescence resonance energy transfer between quantum dot donors and dye-labeled protein acceptors. *J Am Chem Soc* 2004, 126:301–310.

Dabbousi, R. O., Rodriguez-Viejo, J., Mikulec, F. V., et al. (1997) (CdSe)ZnS coreshell quantum dots: synthesis and characterization of a size series of highly luminescent nanocrystallites. *J. Phys. Chem. B* 101, 9463–9475.

Doose, S. (2003) Single molecule characterization of photophysical and colloidal properties of biocompatible quantum dots. Dissertation, Ruprecht-Karls University, Heidelberg, Germany.

Dwarakanath S, Bruno JG, Shastry A, Phillips T, John AA, et al. Quantum dot-antibody and aptamer conjugates shift fluorescence upon binding bacteria. *Biochem Biophys Res Commun* 2004, 325:739–743.

GaoX, ChanWC, Nie S.Quantum-dot nanocrystals for ultrasensitive biological labeling and multicolor optical encoding. *J Biomed Opt* 2002, 7:532–537.

Gao X, Nie S. Quantum dot-encoded beads. *Methods Mol Biol (Clifton, NJ)* 2005, 303:61–71.

Gao X, Chung LWK, Nie S. Quantum dots for in vivo molecular and cellular imaging. *Methods Mol Biol* 2007, 374:135–145.

Grabolle M, Ziegler J, Merkulov A, Nann T, Resch-Genger U. Stability and fluorescence quantum yield of CdSe-ZnS quantum dots—influence of the thickness of the ZnS shell. *Ann NY Acad Sci* 2008, 1130:235–241.

Hahn MA, Keng PC, Krauss TD. Flow cytometric analysis to detect pathogens in bacterial cell mixtures using semiconductor quantum dots. *Anal Chem* 2008, 80:864–872.

Henglein, A. (1982) Photochemistry of colloidal cadmium sulfide. 2. Effects of adsorbed methyl viologen and of colloidal platinum. *J. Phys. Chem.* 86, 2291–2293.

Hines, M. A. and Guyot-Sionnest, P. (1996) Synthesis and characterization of strongly luminescing ZnS-capped CdSe nanocrystals. *J. Phys. Chem.* 100, 468–471.

Hoet PH, Broske-Hohlfeld I, Salata OV. Nanoparticles— known and unknown health risks. *J Nanobiotechnol* 2004, 2:12–27.

Hoshino A, Fujioka K, Oku T, Nakamura S, Suga M, et al. Quantum dots targeted to the assigned organelle in living cells. *Microbiol Immunol* 2004, 48:985–994.

Hotz CZ. Applications of quantum dots in biology: an overview. *Methods Mol Biol (Clifton, NJ)* 2005, 303:1–17.

Jaiswal JK, Mattoussi H, Mauro JM, Simon SM. Longterm multiple color imaging of live cells using quantum dot bioconjugates. *Nat Biotechnol* 2003, 21:47–51.

Jaiswal J, Simon S. Potentials and pitfalls of fluorescent quantum dots for biological imaging. *Trends Cell Biol* 2004, 14:497–504.

Jaiswal JK, Goldman ER, Mattoussi H, Simon SM. Use of quantum dots for live cell imaging. *Nat Methods* 2004, 1:73.

Larson, D. R., Zipfel,W. R.,Williams, R. M., et al. (2003) Water-soluble quantum dots for multiphoton fluorescence imaging *in vivo*. *Science* 300, 1434–1436.

Medintz IL, Clapp AR, Mattoussi H, Goldman ER, Fisher B, et al. Self-assembled nanoscale biosensors based on quantum dot FRET donors. *Nat Mater* 2003, 2:630–638.

Mahnke YD, Roederer M. Optimizing a multicolor immunophenotyping assay. *Clin Lab Med* 2007, 27:469–485.

Male KB, Lachance B, Hrapovic S, Sunahara G, Luong JH. Assessment of cytotoxicity of quantum dots and gold nanoparticles using cell-based impedance spectroscopy. *Anal Chem* 2008, 80:5487–5493.

Mattoussi H, Mauro JM, Goldman ER, Anderson GP, Sundar VC, et al. Self-assembly of CdSe-ZnS quantum dot bioconjugates using an engineered recombinant protein. *J Am Chem Soc* 2000, 122:12142–12150.

Oberdorster G, Oberdorster E, Oberdorster J. NANOTOXICOLOGY: an emerging discipline evolving from studies of ultrafine particles. *Environ Health Perspect* 2005, 17:823–839.

Peng, X., Schlamp, M. C., Kadavanich, A. V., and Alivisatos, A. P. (1997) Epitaxial growth of highly luminescent CdSe/CdS core/shell nanocrystals with photostability and electronic accessibility. *J. Amer. Chem. Soc.* 119, 7019–7029.

Peng X, Wickham J, Alivisatos AP. Kinetics of II-VI and III-V colloidal semiconductor nanocrystal growth: focusing of size distributions. *J Am Chem Soc* 1998, 120:5343–5349.

Perfetto SP, Chattopadhyay PK, Roederer M. Seventeen-colour flow cytometry: unravelling the immune system. *Nat Rev Immunol* 2004, 4:648–655.

Reiss P, Bleuse J, Pron A. Highly Luminescent CdSe ZnSe core/shell nanocrystals of low size dispersion 781–784. *Nano Lett* 2002, 2:781–784.

Riegler J, Nann T. Application of luminescent nanocrystals as labels for biological molecules. *Anal Bioanal Chem* 2004, 379:913–919.

Roederer M. Spectral compensation for flow cytometry: visualization artifacts, limitations, and caveats. *Cytometry* 2001, 45:194–205.

Roederer, M., Perfetto, S. P., Chattopadhyay, P. K., Harper, T., and Bruchez, M. (2004) Quantum dots for multicolor flow cytometry. Poster, International Society for Analytical Cytology Conference; May 24–28, Montpelier, France.

Shahzi SI,Michael WM, John GB, Burt VB, Carl AB, et al. A review of molecular recognition technologies fordetection of biological threat agents. *Biosens Bioelectron* 2000, 15:549–578.

Shiohara A, Hoshino A, Hanaki K, Suzuki K, Yamamoto K. On the cyto-toxicity caused by quantum dots. *Microbiol Immunol* 2004, 48:669–675.

Smet YD, Deriemaeker L, Parloo E, Finsy R. On the determination of ostwald ripening rates from dynamic light scattering measurements. *Langmuir* 1999, 15:2327–2332.

Spanhel, L., Haase, M.,Weller, H., and Henglein, A. (1987) Photochemistry of colloidal semiconductors. Surface modification and stability of strong luminescing CdS particles. *J. Amer. Chem. Soc.* 109, 5649–5662.

Tekle C, Deurs B, Sandvig K, Iversen T. Cellular trafficking of quantum dot-ligand bioconjugates and their induction of changes in normal routing of unconjugated ligands. *Nano Lett* 2008, 8:1858–1865.

Telford WG. Analysis of UV-excited fluorochromes by flow cytometry using near-ultraviolet laser diodes. *Cytometry A* 2004, 61:9–17.

Voura EB, Jaiswal JK, Mattoussi H, Simon SM. Tracking metastatic tumor cell extravasation with quantum dot nanocrystals and fluorescence emission-scanning microscopy. *Nat Med* 2004, 10:993–998.

Wang HQ, Liu TC, Cao YC, Huang ZL, Wang JH, et al. A flow cytometric assay technology based on quantum dots-encoded beads. *Anal Chim Acta* 2006, 580:18–23.

Willard DM, Carillo LL, Jung J, Van Orden A. CdSe-ZnS quantum dots as resonance energy transfer donors in a model protein-protein binding assay. *Nano Lett* 2001, 1:469–474.

Willard DM, Van Orden A. Quantum dots: resonant energy-transfer sensor. *Nat Mater* 2003, 2:575–576.

Wu X, Liu H, Liu J, Haley KN, Treadway JA, et al. Immunofluorescent labeling of cancer marker Her2 and other cellular targets with semiconductor quantum dots. *Nat Biotechnol* 2003, 21:41–46.

Wu Y, Lopez GP, Sklar LA, Buranda T. Spectroscopic characterization of streptavidin functionalized quantum dots. *Anal Biochem* 2007, 364:193–203.

Wu Y, Campos SK, Lopez GP, Ozbun MA, Sklar LA, et al. The development of quantum dot calibration beads and quantitativemulticolor bioassays in flow cytometry and microscopy. *Anal Biochem* 2007, 364:180–192.

Zhang Y, So MK, Rao J. Protease-modulated cellular uptake of quantum dots. *Nano Lett* 2006, 6:1988–1992.